Thieme

Practical Approach to Glaucoma

Case Based

Ramanjit Sihota, MD, FRCS, FRCOphth
Professor and Head
Glaucoma Research Facility and Clinical Services
Dr Rajendra Prasad Centre for Ophthalmic Sciences
All India Institute of Medical Sciences
New Delhi, India

With the collaboration of
Dewang Angmo
Jyoti Shakrawal
Ajay Sharma
Talvir Sidhu

Thieme
Delhi • Stuttgart • New York • Rio de Janeiro

Publishing Director: Ritu Sharma
Development Editor: Dr Gurvinder Kaur
Director-Editorial Services: Rachna Sinha
Project Manager: Madhumita Dey
Illustrator: Sohaib Alam
Vice President, Sales and Marketing: Arun Kumar Majji
Managing Director & CEO: Ajit Kohli

Thieme Medical and Scientific Publishers Private Limited.
A - 12, Second Floor, Sector - 2, Noida - 201 301,
Uttar Pradesh, India, +911204556600
Email: customerservice@thieme.in
www.thieme.in

Page make-up by RECTO Graphics, India

Printed in India by Nutech Print Services - India

5 4 3 2 1

ISBN: 978-81-948570-1-3
eISBN: 978-81-948570-2-0

Important note: Medicine is an ever-changing science undergoing continual development. Research and clinical experience are continually expanding our knowledge, in particular, our knowledge of proper treatment and drug therapy. Insofar as this book mentions any dosage or application, readers may rest assured that the authors, editors, and publishers have made every effort to ensure that such references are in accordance with **the state of knowledge at the time of production of the book**.

Nevertheless, this does not involve, imply, or express any guarantee or responsibility on the part of the publishers in respect to any dosage instructions and forms of applications stated in the book. **Every user is requested to examine carefully** the manufacturers' leaflets accompanying each drug and to check, if necessary, in consultation with a physician or specialist, whether the dosage schedules mentioned therein or the contraindications stated by the manufacturers differ from the statements made in the present book. Such examination is particularly important with drugs that are either rarely used or have been newly released in the market. Every dosage schedule or every form of application used is entirely at the user's own risk and responsibility. The authors and publishers request every user to report to the publishers any discrepancies or inaccuracies noticed. If errors in this work are found after publication, errata will be posted at www.thieme.com on the product description page.

Some of the product names, patents, and registered designs referred to in this book are in fact registered trademarks or proprietary names even though specific reference to this fact is not always made in the text. Therefore, the appearance of a name without designation as proprietary is not to be construed as a representation by the publisher that it is in the public domain.

Thieme addresses people of all gender identities equally. We encourage our authors to use gender-neutral or gender-equal expressions wherever the context allows.

Contents

Preface vii

Acknowledgments ix

Contributors xi

1. Comprehensive Examination for the Early Diagnosis of Glaucoma 1
2. Glaucomatous Optic Neuropathy and Its Staging 11
3. Gonioscopy 23
4. Perimetry in Glaucoma 39
5. Classifications of Visual Field Loss in Glaucoma 65
6. Optical Coherence Tomography in Glaucoma 75
7. Target Intraocular Pressure in Different Types and Severities of Glaucoma 91
8. Glaucoma Suspect Management—Open Angle 105
9. Glaucoma Suspect Management—Shallow Anterior Chamber with Narrow Angles 111
10. Primary Open-Angle Glaucoma 123
11. Primary Angle-Closure Disease 141
12. Juvenile Open-Angle Glaucoma 161
13. Childhood Glaucomas 173
14. Secondary Glaucomas I: Pseudoexfoliation and Pigment Dispersion 191
15. Secondary Glaucomas II: Pseudophakic, Aphakic, Malignant, and Post-Uveitic Glaucomas 201
16. Traumatic Glaucoma 215
17. Steroid-Induced Glaucoma 227
18. Neovascular Glaucoma 239
19. Medical Therapy in Glaucoma 247
20. Laser Therapy in Glaucoma 259
21. Diagnosing and Managing Progression in Glaucoma 269
22. Trabeculectomy and Its Modifications 295
23. Glaucoma Drainage Devices 319
24. Other Glaucoma Surgeries 327
25. Glaucoma Related to the Lens and Its Surgery 333
26. Low-Vision Aids for Glaucoma Patients 343
27. Lifestyle Modifications for Glaucoma 347

Index 349

Preface

Glaucoma is currently the most common cause of irreversible blindness in India. One out of 20 people over the age of 40 years is likely to be a glaucoma suspect or have glaucoma.

In India, the common problematic areas related to glaucoma are:

- Primary open angle glaucoma (POAG), primary angle closure glaucoma (PACG), and secondary glaucomas are all equally prevalent among patients.
- Primary angle closure suspect (PACS) and primary angle closure (PAC) are more frequent, and if these are diagnosed on time, one can prevent glaucoma.
- Inappropriate lowering of intraocular pressure causing optic nerve damage.

About 30 years ago, we had fewer medications and risky surgeries for treatment of glaucoma, thereby leading to the perpetuation of the Hindi term *kala motia*. Over the years, we have learned about different varieties of glaucomas, increased our understanding of their pathogenesis, reinforcing the need to reduce intraocular pressure, and discovered many more avenues of therapy. As a result, we have a significant reduction in the incidence of blindness due to glaucoma, but still the number of such cases is too high.

In today's age of technology, we have unlimited information available on this topic, but finding the correct and unbiased knowledge is challenging. Also, just having knowledge on the topic is not enough; we need the wisdom to apply it judiciously and in the best interests of our patients.

As per statistics from India, ophthalmologists are likely to encounter equal number of PACG, POAG, and secondary glaucoma cases. The two main reasons of blindness are late diagnosis and wrong diagnosis of the cause of glaucoma, which results in a less targeted approach to treatment. The most common mistakes seen are missing shallow anterior chamber and inadequate lowering of intraocular pressure once a diagnosis of glaucoma is made.

Technology in various forms has entered the glaucoma domain, for example, imaging, better software interpretation, and newer devices. The ones that are evaluated and validated are discussed in this book, and those still under investigation are also mentioned.

This book is aimed to help ophthalmologists understand glaucoma and learn about current best practices. We have tried to avoid undue ambiguities and kept the information simple and practical. All attempts have been made to present the information accurately, and in a simple and logical manner.

There cannot be universal application of a procedure in medicine. However, a trial, as suggested in this book, is a starting point from which further modifications as required over time may be undertaken.

My desire to write this book stems from the fact that so many people lose vision because of glaucoma due to lack of timely and proper treatment. I hope this book helps ophthalmologists to recognize glaucoma suspects and glaucomas, and take appropriate action.

Ramanjit Sihota, MD, FRCS, FRCOphth
Professor and Head
Glaucoma Research Facility and Clinical Services
Dr Rajendra Prasad Centre for Ophthalmic Sciences
All India Institute of Medical Sciences
New Delhi, India

Acknowledgments

I would like to pay tributes to my mentors, Prof. N. N. Sood and Prof. H. C. Agarwal, for their wisdom and forethought, and for teaching meticulous examination and empathetic care of patients.

The privilege of working at Dr Rajendra Prasad Centre for Ophthalmic Sciences, All India Institute of Medical Sciences, New Delhi, India with a host of colleagues, Prof. Tanuj Dada, Prof. Viney Gupta, Dr Shikha Gupta, Dr Dewang Angmo, and all residents, who have worked hard and helped us in glaucoma service is unparalleled. The use of new technology has permitted us to see, learn, record, and review imaging and data over years, all of which are essential for managing glaucoma.

I would also like to thank Mr. Ajay Sharma and Ms. Amisha Gupta who have helped us with imaging systems, perimeters, and data of the patients discussed in the book and made sure that the data is authentic.

This book would not have been as practical without the actual patient data recorded by Dr. Shakrawal, and her comments on the simplified flowcharts. Dr Dewang Angmo has put in a lot of effort for drafting chapters on the topics: lasers, juvenile open angle glaucoma (JOAG), primary open angle glaucoma (POAG), pigment dispersion, pseudoexfoliation syndromes, and drainage devices. Dr Talvir Sidhu helped us collect innumerable photographs and provided her expertise with optical coherence tomography (OCT) and minimally invasive surgery chapter drafts. All these have been put together to provide a coherent narrative of actually practiced glaucoma care. Finally, Dr Shakrawal and Dr Sidhu went through each chapter diligently to ensure presentation and accuracy of information.

Senior residents over the years have helped with documentation of patient problems and their treatment, as well as provided us with many suggestions for better management of Glaucoma. Just to name a few recent ones— Drs Neha Midha, Harathy Selvan, Subodh Lakra, Kishan Azmira, Aswini Behera, Anin Sethi, Monika Yadav, Anand Bukke, and Vaishali Rakheja.

Despite the coronavirus pandemic and its attendant "work from home" policy, I would really like to appreciate and acknowledge the help of the team at Thieme India who continued to push for the completion of the book.

More than anything else, I would like to thank my husband, Dr A. H. Paul, and my children, Nishkaam and Krittika, for their constant encouragement and for being the springboard from which I could launch academic activities such as this.

Ramanjit Sihota, MD, FRCS, FRCOphth
Professor and Head
Glaucoma Research Facility and Clinical Services
Dr Rajendra Prasad Centre for Ophthalmic Sciences
All India Institute of Medical Sciences
New Delhi, India

Contributors

Ajay Sharma, BSc (Ophthalmic Techniques), MSc
Technical officer
Dr Rajendra Prasad Centre for Ophthalmic Sciences
All India Institute of Medical Sciences
New Delhi, India

Dewang Angmo, MD, FRCS, FICO
Assistant Professor
Glaucoma research facility and clinical services
Dr Rajendra Prasad Centre for Ophthalmic Sciences
All India Institute of Medical Sciences
New Delhi, India

Jyoti Shakrawal, MD
Assistant Professor
Department of Ophthalmology
All India Institute of Medical Sciences
Jodhpur, Rajasthan, India

Talvir Sidhu, MD
Assistant Professor
Department of Ophthalmology
Government Medical College
Patiala, Punjab, India

CHAPTER 1

Comprehensive Examination for the Early Diagnosis of Glaucoma

Overview

- Systemic Status of the Patient
- Family History
- Extraocular Examination
- Ocular Examination
  - Visual Status
  - Anterior Segment
  - Anterior Chamber
  - Iris
  - Lens
- Retina
  - Optic Nerve Head Examination
- Tonometry
  - Digital Palpation
- Suggested Readings

Introduction

The diagnosis of a glaucoma or a glaucoma suspect is largely clinical. A *comprehensive examination should be practiced in a regular pattern, for example, estimating visual acuity and field as the patient walks in, and observing the eyelids and any strabismus. On the slit lamp, examining the anterior segment of the left and then right eye with diffuse and then slit beams, followed by examination of the fundus and optic nerve using a 90D lens in the right eye followed by the left should be performed.*

This becomes a reflex over time, which takes less than 5 minutes, and ensures that the ophthalmic review is complete, and no glaucoma suspect or glaucomatous neuropathy is missed (**Flowchart 1.1**).

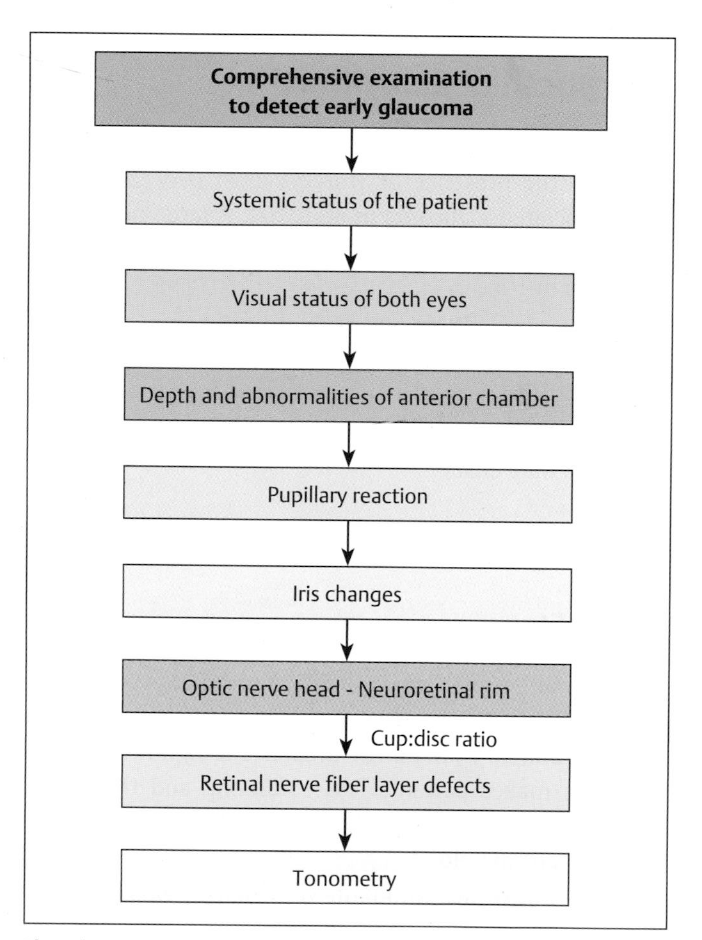

Flowchart 1.1 Systematic examination for the early diagnosis of glaucoma.

Systemic Status of the Patient

A *history of all systemic diseases and medications* is extremely important in any patient having glaucoma, because some of these can raise intraocular pressure (IOP), reduce the ocular perfusion, or can interact with glaucoma medications.

Anticholinergic drugs can precipitate angle closure in predisposed individuals, and are used to treat asthma and chronic obstructive pulmonary disease (ipratropium and tiotropium), Parkinson's disease, incontinence (tolterodine and oxybutynin), and gastric acidity (cimetidine and ranitidine). Other drugs that may also exacerbate glaucoma are: skeletal muscle relaxants (orphenadrine), antidepressants such as selective serotonin reuptake inhibitors and tricyclic antidepressants, antiallergy drugs such as diphenhydramine, medications for nausea (promethazine), antianxiety drugs such as hydroxyzine, and sulfonamide medications such as topiramate and tetracycline.

Steroids are commonly used in most chronic inflammatory diseases including asthma, dermatitis, autoimmune pathologies, arthritis, etc., and are known to cause a raised IOP in patients predisposed to glaucoma and those with glaucoma. This rise is related to the cumulative dose and duration of use of steroids.

Ocular perfusion may be affected in systemic hypotension, or be associated with ischemic heart disease, transient ischemic attack (TIA), stroke, diabetes, etc.

Family History

The primary glaucomas, primary open-angle glaucoma (POAG), primary angle-closure glaucoma (PACG), juvenile open-angle glaucoma (JOAG), and congenital glaucoma, tend to run in families, and a proper history allows an early suspicion or early diagnosis of glaucoma, which can prevent morbidity.

Extraocular Examination

The presence of hemangiomas on the face and eyelid points to the presence of Sturge-Weber (SW) syndrome with associated glaucoma in 40 to70%. A large nevus over the face and eyelid, nevus of Ota, may be associated with glaucoma in 10%.

Exophthalmos can produce a raised IOP in certain cases, and thyroid dysfunction is a risk factor for glaucoma. Proptosis with dilated episcleral veins is generally associated with caroticocavernous fistulas, and a secondary glaucoma may ensue.

Ocular Examination

Visual Status

As a patient enters the examination room, it is possible to approximately assess visual acuity by the ease with which he/she is able to walk in. The presence of significant visual field loss makes patients less confident, and they often have to move their heads to navigate their way with the residual central field.

A history of any problems with *dark adaptation and glare or difficulty in peripheral vision, such as bumping into objects,* should be elicited.

Visual acuity for distance and near should be assessed, and a projection of light in all quadrants elicited in all cases, as central vision may be relatively maintained while peripheral field is lost.

Anterior Segment

Glaucoma is commonly associated with age-related changes in the cornea and lens, which should be recorded, as they can also be involved in different types of glaucoma and contribute to visual prognosis.

Ciliary Congestion

Ciliary congestion is seen in acute angle-closure glaucoma and secondary glaucomas associated with anterior segment inflammation. A red/purplish perilimbal injection indicates inflammation of the iris, ciliary body, cornea, or sclera, and is due to the congestion of deeper, anterior ciliary vessels. This does not blanch with application of vasoconstrictors or direct pressure.

Sclera

Thinning of the sclera with or without ectasia is seen with chronically elevated IOP, forming staphylomata. Staphylomas are classified as anterior if they involve cornea or limbus, intercalary if they are between limbus and ciliary body, ciliary if they are over the ciliary body, and equatorial or posterior whenever the sclera is involved. Pigmentation of the sclera is commonly a nevus, and when there is a greyish blue/brown macular pigmentation of conjunctiva, sclera, and ipsilateral face, it is known as nevus of Ota, or oculodermal melanocytosis. Glaucoma may be seen in approximately 10% of such eyes.

Episcleral hemangiomas, especially at the limbus, are biomarkers for occurrence of glaucoma in SW syndrome.

Cornea

The normal cornea has a smooth, glossy look, and a mild epithelial irregularity may be found with epithelial edema in raised IOP or it may have a ground-glass appearance as seen in congenital glaucoma when stromal and epithelial edema is seen. Inflammations of the cornea, injuries, dystrophies, presence of keratic precipitates, and other pathologies are often associated with glaucoma, and should be looked for. Pigment dispersion on the back of the cornea is seen in angle-closure glaucoma, but a dense Krukenberg spindle is a hallmark of pigmentary glaucoma. Pseudoexfoliative material may also be seen on the corneal endothelium.

In pediatric glaucomas, Haab's striae and iridocorneal adhesions may be seen.

Corneal thickness came into prominence with the Ocular Hypertension Treatment Study, which reported that patients with an IOP of >24 mm Hg but thicker corneas had a significantly lower risk of developing glaucoma, as compared to a normal or thinner cornea. Subsequently many studies have suggested that a thin cornea is an important risk factor for progression of glaucoma, and may be used as a biomarker for structural and physical factors of glaucomatous optic neuropathy. *Ehlers' formula* is commonly referred to, reducing it to a correction factor for applanation tonometry, of an addition or subtraction of 0.7 mm Hg for every 10 µm difference in corneal thickness as compared with normals. Most algorithms presume a linear relationship between central corneal thickness (CCT) and IOP, whereas it appears to be more complex and possibly nonlinear. There is no agreement currently as to the most accurate correction factor till date.

Indian eyes commonly have a corneal thickness of around 520–525 µm. Mean CCT in the Central India Eye and Medical Study was 514+/–33 µm (median, 517 µm; range, 290–696 µm)

Anterior Chamber

Anterior chamber depth is recorded as the distance between the posterior surface of the cornea and anterior surface of the lens, and is normally 2.5 to 3.0 mm deep. It is seen to be physiologically shallow in infancy and in older patients. *In the Central India Eye and Medical Study the mean anterior chamber depth was 3.22 ± 0.34 mm.*

Assessing anterior chamber depth can be easily done using a torch or slit lamp. These are noncontact and subjective assessments, but are easily applied in a busy outpatient clinic.

- *Torch light*: On flashing a beam of light from the temporal limbus, parallel to the surface of the iris, in a normal or deep anterior chamber the beam will pass across, illuminating the entire iris surface and the opposite limbus. In eyes with a shallow anterior chamber, the forward convexity or bowing of the iris obstructs the beam, and a crescentic shadow is observed on the nasal iris and limbus.
- The van Herick test compares the depth of the most peripheral anterior chamber to peripheral corneal thickness. Slit-lamp illumination and viewing arms are placed 60 degrees to each other, with the viewing arm perpendicular to the cornea, at a magnification of 15×. Using a fine slit just inside the temporal limbus, if peripheral anterior chamber depth is equal to or greater than corneal thickness it is grade 4, half corneal thickness is grade 3, quarter thickness of cornea is grade 2, and less than a quarter is Grade 1 (**Table 1.1**). grade 1 anterior chamber depth suggests that angle closure is possible, while in Grade 4, closure is unlikely. Thomas et al found the sensitivity and specificity on the flashlight test were 45.5 and 82.7%, respectively, and for van Herick test they were 61.9 and 89.3% (**Fig. 1.1**).
- A further modification—van Herick Plus—is performed similarly, but at the inferior limbus. A short, thin, vertical slit-lamp beam evaluation straddling the inferior angle is an easy and relatively accurate method for both evaluating peripheral anterior chamber depth and assessing iridocorneal angle (**Fig. 1.2**).

Table 1.1 van Herick system determining the degree of shallowness of the anterior chamber[a]

Grade 4	Angle is wide open	PAC > CT
Grade 3	Angle is narrow	PAC = 1/4–1/2 CT
Grade 2	Angle is dangerously narrow	PAC = 1/4 CT
Grade 1	Angle is dangerously narrow or closed	PAC < CT

[a]Compares peripheral anterior chamber (PAC) depth to corneal thickness (CT).

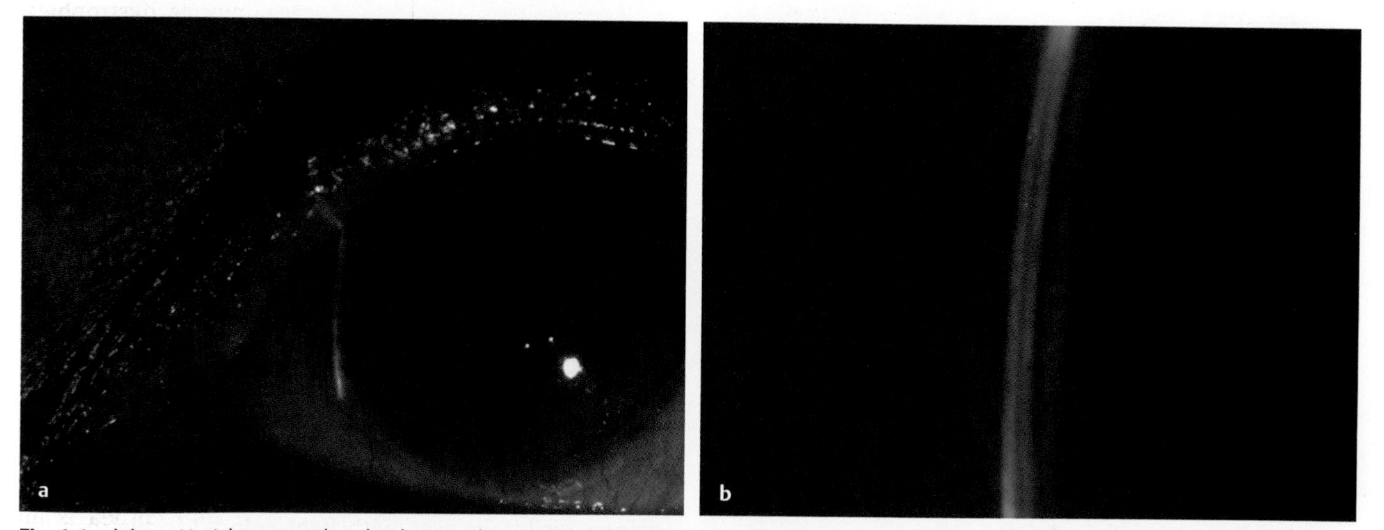

Fig. 1.1 **(a)** van Herick test needs to be done as close to the limbus as possible with the slit-lamp observation and illumination arms at 60 degrees. **(b)** Higher magnification permits a comparison of the thickness of the cornea with the black space of the anterior chamber.

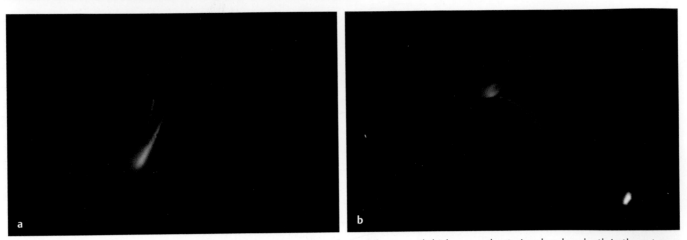

Fig. 1.2 **(a)** A short thin beam of light at 6 o'clock permits a comparison of the corneal thickness and anterior chamber depth in the extreme periphery, as well as an estimation of the iridocorneal angle formed between the most peripheral iris and corneal endothelium. **(b)** Using a short but thin and bright beam, the corneal wedge can be identified, and the proximity and angle formed between the corneal wedge and peripheral iris can be assessed.

- The anterior chamber can be objectively measured by all anterior segment imaging systems such as Pentacam, IOL Master, LenStar, and anterior segment optical coherence tomography, with similar accuracy.

A significantly shallow anterior chamber should cause a suspicion of angle closure, primary or secondary, depending upon other ocular findings present. Although a deep anterior chamber with a concave iris is a hallmark of pigmentary glaucoma, an irregularly deep anterior chamber could be seen with a subluxated lens or angle recession following concussional injury.

Aqueous cells and flare are a feature of uveitis. Flare may also be seen in acute angle-closure and neovascular glaucoma where extravasation of proteins occurs.

Hyphema is commonly seen after trauma, and may presage later traumatic glaucoma. A hypopyon is seen with blebitis or endophthalmitis in glaucoma patients with prior filtration surgery.

Iris

The pupillary reaction is an extremely important biomarker for glaucomatous optic neuropathy. This should be checked using low background illumination and a bright focused light, while asking the patient to look into the distance. A light on one eye will cause constriction of the pupil, which in normal individuals is well maintained. Consensual reaction should always be noted. A swinging flash light highlights unilateral or asymmetrical optic nerve pathology. When the light is shone on the more affected eye both pupils will dilate, and on swinging back to the better eye both pupils will constrict, highlighting a relative afferent pupillary defect.

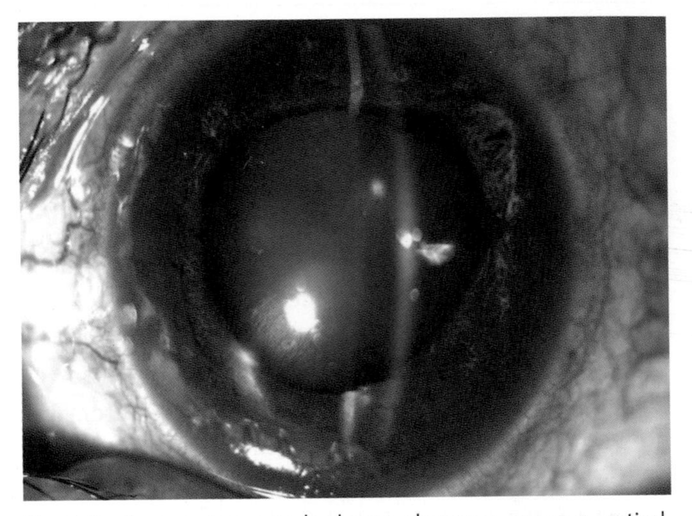

Fig. 1.3 Acute primary angle-closure glaucoma causes a vertical, mid-dilated nonreactive pupil. Sector iris atrophy can be seen at 2 to 4 o'clock.

A vertically mid-dilated, nonresponsive pupil is a hallmark of an acute angle-closure glaucoma (**Fig. 1.3**). A miotic pupil with posterior synechiae is often due to healed uveitis.

The pattern of the iris should be noted, looking specifically for the presence of the pupillary ruff, radial folds, collarette, and peripheral crypts (**Fig. 1.4**). Sectoral loss of pattern occurs after an acute angle-closure glaucoma attack, while a more generalized muddy, featureless iris is associated with uveitis. Neovascularization of the iris starts at the pupillary margin or the angle and then is visible as an irregular network over the surface of the iris, with ectropion uveae. There is a concave iris configuration seen in pigmentary glaucoma with transillumination defects visible in eyes with light-colored irides together

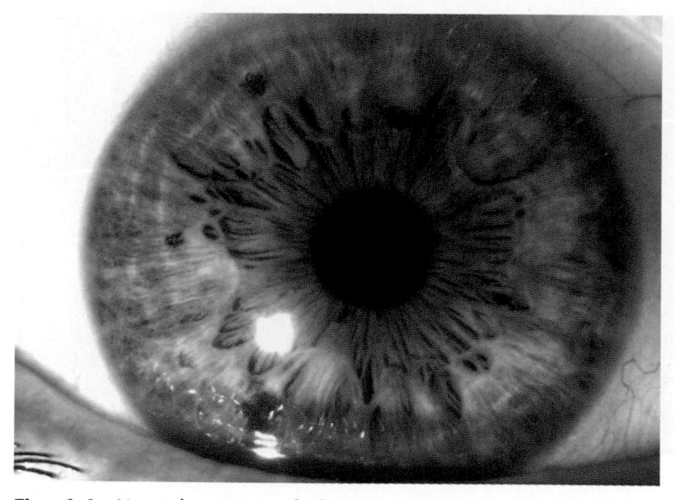

Fig. 1.4 Normal pattern of the iris, pupillary ruff, radial folds, collarette, and peripheral circumferential folds with iris crypts.

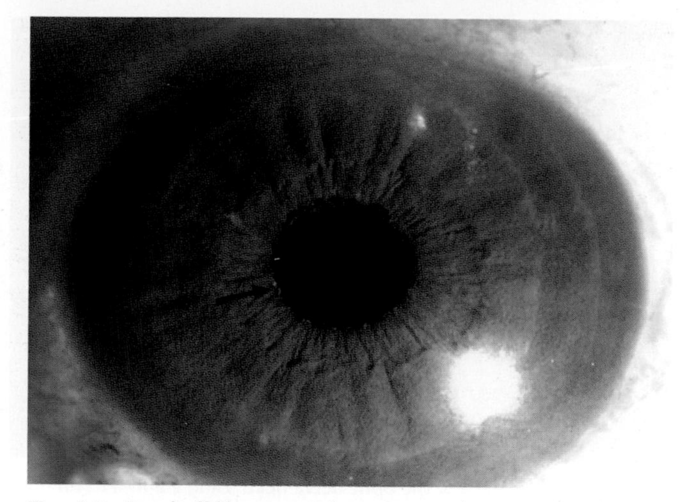

Fig. 1.5 Dandruff-like material at the pupil in pseudoexfoliation syndrome (*black arrow*).

with significant pigment dispersion. Dandruff-like pseudoexfoliative material can be seen at the pupil, with a poorly dilating pupil, due to atrophy or fibrosis of the sphincter muscle (**Fig. 1.5**). Pedunculated nodules and Lisch nodules are seen in neurofibromatosis, while flat nodules are seen in granulomatous uveitis, Koeppe's nodules at the pupil, and Busacca's in the stroma. In Fuch's heterochromic iridocyclitis early iris stromal atrophy is seen, with later heterochromia.

Iridodonesis helps diagnose subluxation of the lens, which in many instances is associated with glaucoma.

Irregularity or loss of the pupillary ruff is commonly seen as a sensitive and specific sign in PACG eyes, but may also be seen after uveitis or in diabetics.

Lens

A small, thick, and mobile lens in microspherophakia can cause intermittent angle closure, while a thicker lens may cause an exaggerated lens vault in some eyes with primary angle-closure disease. An intumescent cataractous lens is seen in phacomorphic glaucoma, while an anteriorly dislocated lens can cause secondary angle closure.

The presence of anterior subcapsular opacities, glaukomflecken, is the result of an acute attack of angle-closure glaucoma.

In pseudoexfoliation syndrome three zones of exfoliative material are seen: an inner central disc which is the size of the pupil, an intermediate clear zone, because of iris moving upon the lens, and most commonly a peripheral area with radial striations.

In pediatric eyes, developmental anomalies are commonly associated with glaucoma, while in oculo-cerebrorenal (Lowe) syndrome, and rubella, cataract and glaucoma are present together.

Retina

Optic Nerve Head Examination

Examine the optic disc in all patients, especially those above 40 years of age, as disc damage generally precedes visual field loss. Assessing the degree of optic nerve damage also helps in guiding treatment goals.

In a busy OPD, the use of a 90-D lens provides a good view of the fundus in an undilated eye of most patients (**Fig. 1.6**).

The optic disc should be documented by inter relationship of two circles, representing the cup edge and outer disc margin, at the time of glaucoma diagnosis, or when a patient is labeled as ocular hypertensive.

- *Normal disc* (**Fig. 1.7**): The ratio of cup diameter-to-disc diameter is normally 0.3 to 0.5:1, and the neuroretinal rim, formed by axons of the ganglion cells, is seen to be of regular thickness 360 degrees, with an orange pink color. The thickness is generally greater at the inferior pole, followed by superior and nasal, while the temporal neuroretinal rim is the thinnest—the *ISNT rule*. Blood vessels emerge from the depth of the cup and the larger superotemporal and inferotemporal arteries and veins course upward before turning temporally. The nasal vessels go directly to the temporal retina. Smaller blood vessels

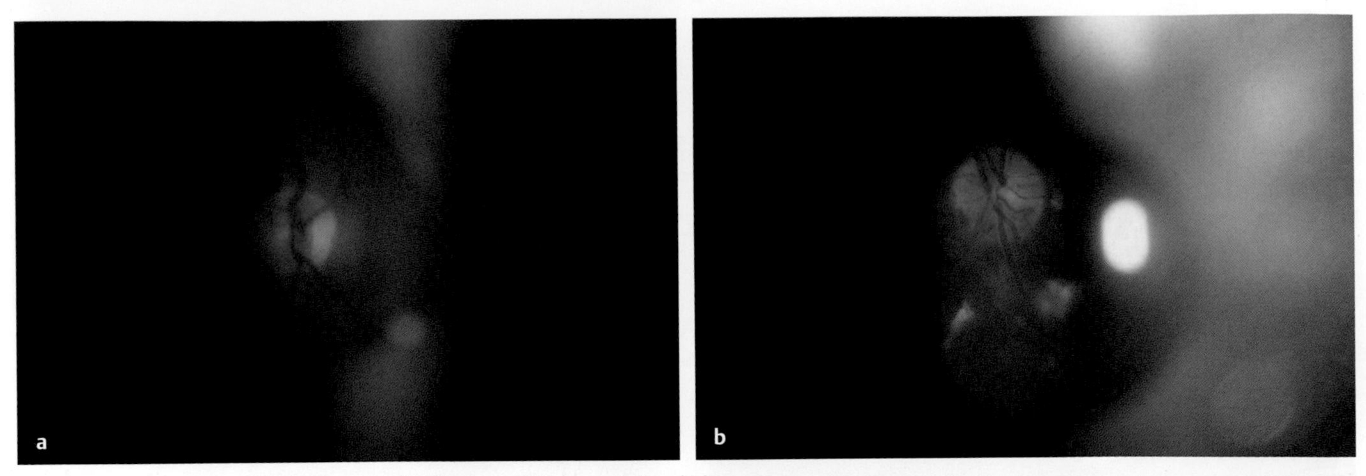

Fig. 1.6 (a, b) View of the optic nerve head using a 90D lens on the slit lamp.

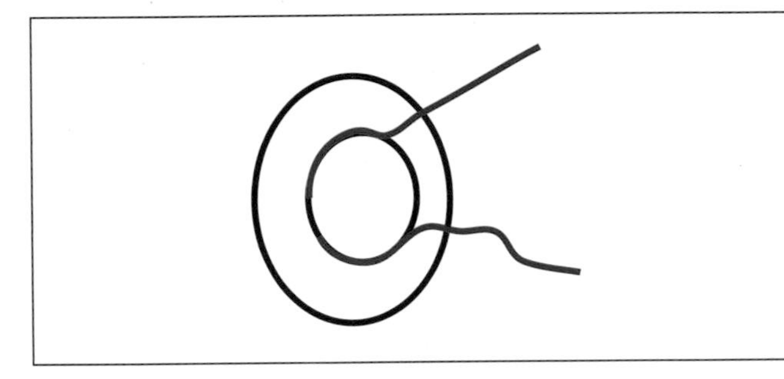

Fig. 1.7 Normal disc and basic diagram.

course along the upper and lower cup margins, and are called circumlinear vessels.

- *Glaucomatous optic neuropathy:*

  Definitive (*hard signs*):

  - Notching, a localized loss or significant thinning of the neuroretinal rim, especially inferotemporal (**Fig. 1.8a**).
  - Optic disc hemorrhage on neuroretinal rim (**Fig. 1.8b**).
  - Retinal nerve fiber layer defects in the area of neuroretinal rim loss, seen best with red free light, and associated perimetry).
  - Localized pallor of the neuroretinal rim associated with thinning.

  Corroboratory signs (*soft signs*):

  - Vertical cup:disc ratio.
  - Beta zone peripapillary atrophy, especially in the region of neuroretinal rim loss.
  - Baring of circumlinear vessels (BCLV) (*black dotted arrow* in **Fig. 1.8a).**
  - Asymmetry in the cup:disc ratio between the two eyes of >0.2.

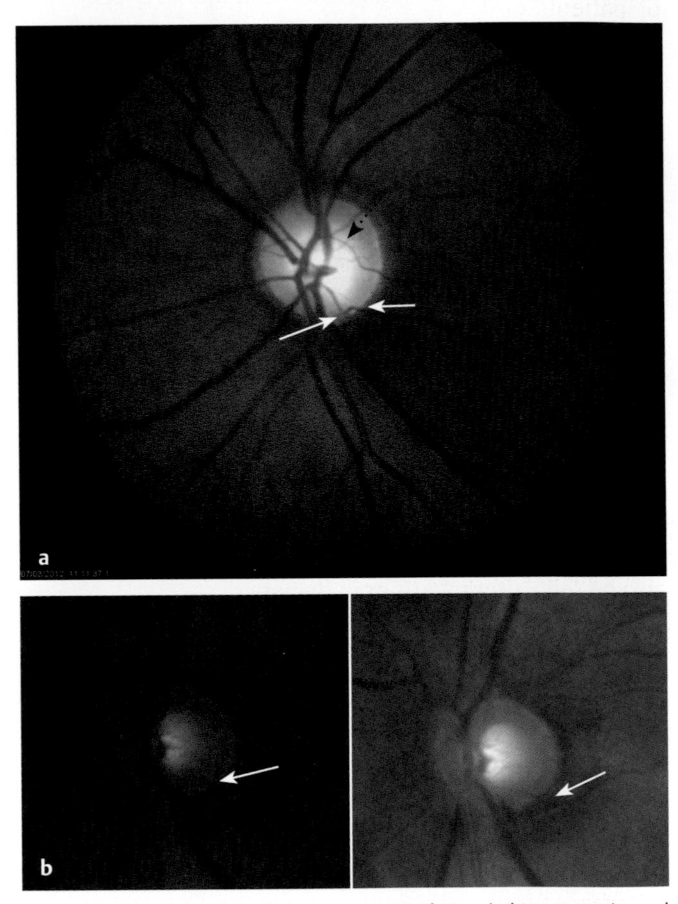

Fig. 1.8 **(a)** Notching of the neuroretinal rim (*white arrows*), and baring of the circumlinear vessel (*dotted arrow*). **(b)** Optic disc hemorrhage (*white arrows*).

  - Thinning or loss of the inferior neuroretinal rim, against ISNT rule.
  - Nasalization of vessels.

A large disc, larger than the small circle of the direct ophthalmoscope, may have a large physiological cup, if the neuroretinal rim is uniform with an orange color.

Tonometry

Tonometry is an indirect measure of IOP, essential in the diagnosis and monitoring of glaucoma therapy.Tonometry measures the IOP more accurately, and should be done in all patients above 40 years of age as part of a screening or cataract work-up. A significant difference >3 mm Hg between the two eyes of a patient alerts one to possible glaucoma.

Tonometers are of many types, with the gold standard being the Goldmann applanation tonometer (**Table 1.2**).

Diurnal phasing or measurements of IOP at different times of the day is important, as both the peak or highest IOP and IOP fluctuations are thought to correlate with the occurrence and progression of glaucoma. Two-thirds of patients in a study, had their highest IOP outside of office hours. Knowing the time at which the IOP is highest allows timing of drug administration, to work maximally at that time.

Tonometry at different times should ideally be done on the same machine. Supine measurement being lower than sitting would mean that a Schiotz tonometer and applanation tonometer should not be used for a diurnal measurement in the same patient.

Specific indications for checking IOP at least as early in the morning as possible and on another visit as late as possible are:

- High-risk glaucoma suspects.
- Normal tension glaucoma.
- To determine compliance/efficacy of drugs in advanced disease.
- Eyes progressing despite achieving "target" IOP.

Digital Palpation

It is a palpation technique alternately using two fingers placed above the superior tarsus, while the patient looks down. Palpation of a few normal eyes provides an assessment of the "feel" or force required to indent an eye having normal IOP. This procedure further provides a means of assessing high IOPs, especially in one eye as compared with the other. An IOP of >30 mm Hg is easily distinguished from normal, and this is a useful tool for assessing IOP in children or patients in whom an accurate applanation tonometry is not possible due to corneal opacification/irregularity, in uncooperative patients, etc.

Applanation Tonometry

It is the most accurate and commonly performed tonometry, applying pressure to flatten an area of the cornea. This is based on *Imbert-Fick principle*, wherein the pressure within a perfectly spherical, dry, flexible, elastic, and infinitely thin sphere is equal to the external force required to flatten a certain area of the sphere. In practice, there are however two other forces because of which the conditions for the Imbert Fick principle are not met: i) corneal rigidity pushing the applanating surface outward and ii) surface tension of the tear film pulling it inwards (**Fig. 1.9**).

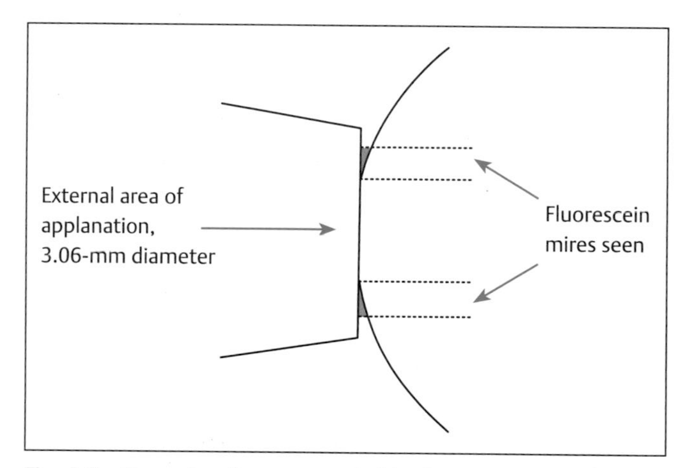

Fig. 1.9 Measuring the pressure inside the eye using applanation tonometry.

Table 1.2 Comparison of different tonometers available

Tonometer	Principle	Advantages	Disadvantages	Differences from applanation
Applanation	Imbert Fick law	Validated by manometry	Large area of contact Influenced by corneal thickness	
iCare	Rebound	Small and very short time of contact Can be used in children and corneal opacification	Influenced by corneal thickness	Reads higher at higher IOP
Dynamic contour tonometer	Transcorneal pressure measured by adjusting to corneal curvature	Least dependent on corneal thickness	Multiple readings take time	Reads higher
Ocular response analyzer	Biomechanical distortion assessed	Measures corneal hysteresis Measures Resistance factor	Expensive	Reads higher

Abbreviation: IOP, intraocular pressure.

The pressure inside the eye would be:

$$P = \frac{F}{\text{Internal corneal area applanated}} + \text{Meniscus surface tension} - \text{corneal rigidity.}$$

Goldmann Applanation Tonometry

To remove the other forces in applanation tonometry, it is seen that when the internal cornea is applanated over an area of 7.35 mm^2, surface tension and corneal rigidity cancel each other. Therefore, the Goldmann applanation prism is designed such that force over an outer area of diameter 3.06 mm applanates an inner corneal area of 7.35 mm^2. The force applied in grams can be directly converted to IOP by multiplying by 10. This displaces only approximately 0.5 µL of fluid, and causes an increase in IOP of only 2.5 to 3%. It is accurate to within ± 0.5 mm Hg for an IOP less than 20 mm Hg.

The following precautions should be taken while measuring IOP with Goldmann applanation tonometry:

- Clean the prism with ethyl alcohol/ sodium hypochlorite before every use, and wait for the cleaned surface to dry.
- Avoid tonometry in infected or injured eyes.
- Scratches/sharp edges and cracks can injure the cornea, while disinfectant can get into the hollow of cracks and cause corneal chemical injury.
- Calibration is required monthly.

Disinfection

For disinfection, 70% isopropyl alcohol as well as 70% ethyl alcohol can be used for rapid germicidal effect against bacteria, fungi, and viruses by denaturating proteins; 10% sodium hypochlorite for 10 minutes is biocidal against HIV, bacteria, bacterial spores, mycoplasma, mycobacterium tuberculosis, and fungi; and 10% hydrogen peroxide deactivates bacteria, fungi, and viruses. The prism should be allowed to dry before use.

Procedure

Inform the patient what you are going to do, and why, so that he/she does not squeeze the eye or hold his/her breath. One to two drops of topical anesthetic work in 15 to 20 seconds, with the effect lasting for 15 minutes. Too many drops can lead to epithelial toxicity.

Align the white line on the prism carrier with the 0- or 180-degree marker of the prism. Set the measuring drum to one (1 g). Place the illumination arm of the slit lamp 60 to 65 degrees temporal to the probe, with a wide open diffuse, bright illumination, using the cobalt blue filter and 16× magnification. The optical system and tonometer are "not aligned" and must be offset by 5 to 10 degrees.

Align the patient's lateral canthus to the black line on the slit-lamp frame, and make sure the patient rests tightly against the head rest. It is best to align the prism to the center of cornea looking from outside the slit lamp, and when the prism touches the cornea, a purple blue limbal glow appears. Then through the observation tube, the opposing semicircular mires are viewed with only one eye, and adjustment made, up or down, to make the semicircles equal above and below. The IOP is read when the inner edges of the mires are just apposed, with visible pulsation (**Fig. 1.10**). If the mires are too wide or pulsations are not seen, pull the slit lamp back slightly. The reading is taken off the measuring drum and multiplied by 10 for mm Hg.

If corneal astigmatism is greater than 3.00 D, measurements are made 43 degrees from the meridian of the lower power. Place the red line on the probe carrier at the 30-degree mark on the probe. The red line and the white line on the probe carrier are separated by 43 degrees.

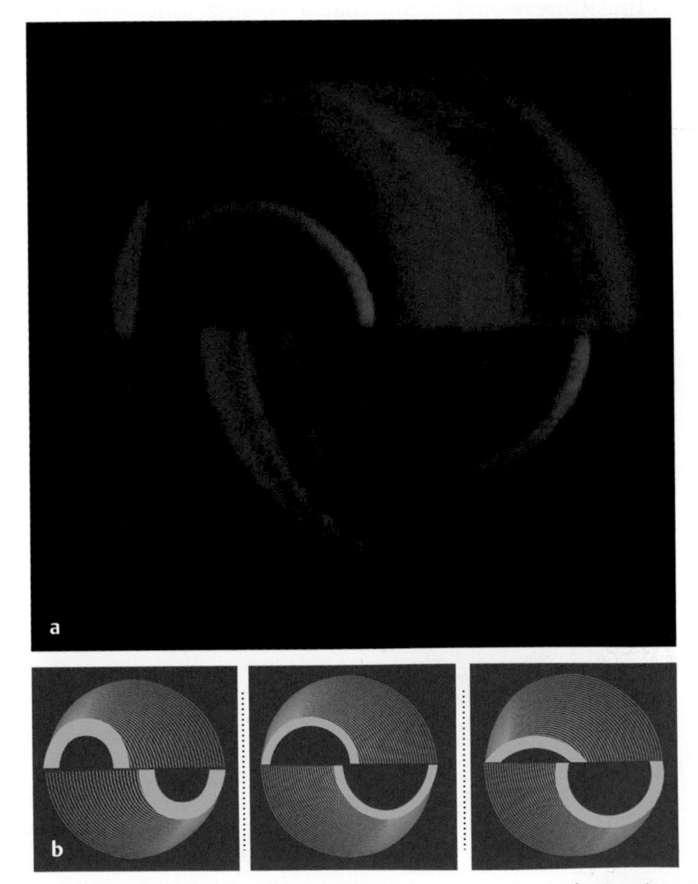

Fig. 1.10 **(a)** End point for measurement is vertically equal mires, just touching internally with oscillations. **(b)** Mires formed should neither be too thick nor too thin, and should be equal above and below.

Sources of Error

- Mires: Too wide or thin, vertical misalignment.
- Corneal variables:
  - Thin corneas, Laser in situ keratomileusis (LASIK), or corneal edema lead to falsely low IOP readings.
  - Thick corneas or corneal scarring may lead to falsely high IOP readings.
  - Astigmatism: 1 mm error for 4D of astigmatism, underestimation with the rule, and overestimation of IOP against the rule.
- Prolonged contact of prism may lower IOP.

Schiotz Indentation Tonometer

This records the depth of indentation by a weighted stylet by means of a lever. The depth and extent of indentation are dependent upon IOP and rigidity of the eye. Weights of 5.5, 7.5, 10, and 15 g can be placed on the stylet to achieve a lever deflection of more than 4, for greatest accuracy. The final reading is then read of a nomogram. Important points while using Schiotz indentation tonometers are:

- *Cleaning of barrel*: Should be done daily to avoid plunger sticking to the barrel.
- *Storage*: In dry, dust-free environment with separable parts separated.
- *Zero error*: Should be checked on artificial cornea in the box.
- Cleaning between cases is best with 3% hydrogen peroxide or 5% sodium hypochlorite.
- Patient should fixate at a target on the ceiling to avoid accommodation.
- Eyelids are separated gently and fingers placed on the superior and inferior orbital rims to avoid pressure on the eye (**Fig. 1.11**).
- Reading should be checked with observer's eye level with weight. Recheck with 7.5 g if reading <3.

Other Tonometers

- *Noncontact tonometers* use a puff of air to applanate the cornea, and this is tracked optically. IOP is estimated either by the force at the time of applanation, or the time taken for applanation. As it is a noncontact procedure, it can be used for screening and in children. A nonaccommodating target is used to decrease the effect of accommodation on IOP.

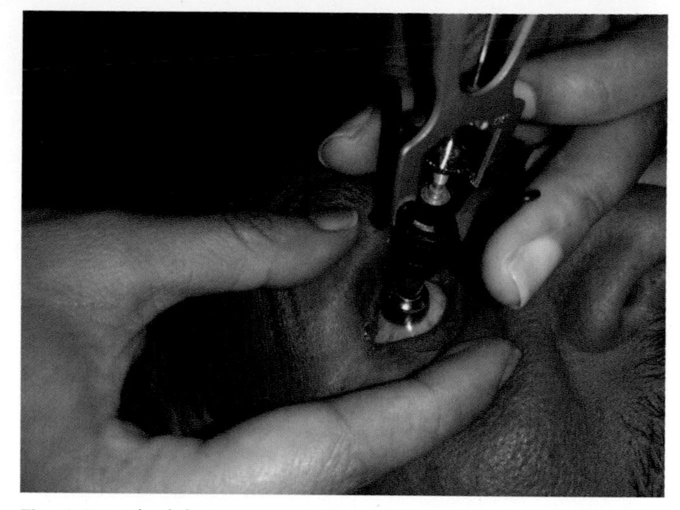

Fig. 1.11 The lids are separated and fingers placed on the superior and inferior orbital rims to prevent pressure on the eye, while checking intraocular pressure.

  The short time required for a reading makes it more sensitive to ocular pulse and even respiratory cycle; therefore, at least three readings should be taken. There is a correlation with Goldmann tonometer up to mid-20s mm Hg, after which variability increases significantly. It also gives variable readings in patients with severe corneal scarring and in uncooperative patients.
- *Tonopen* is based on the Mackay-Marg principle, using both applanation and indentation. It has a small steel probe situated centrally, which indents the cornea till the surrounding surface is applanated. Due to the surrounding applanation, pressure at the plunger suddenly decreases. IOP is measured at the point of applanation. Several measurements are taken and averaged. It correlates well with Goldmann within the normal range, overestimates at lower pressures, and underestimates at higher IOPs. The 1 mm tip makes it useful for irregular corneas, and it can also be used with soft contact lenses in place.
- *Rebound tonometer* is based on the induction rebound principle, with a 1.8-mm plastic ball probe, that strikes the cornea and returns. The speed of its deceleration is converted to IOP. The deceleration is faster if the IOP is high and slower with a lower IOP. The iCare PRO allows measurements to be made in the sitting and lying down positions. It is especially useful in children and for eyes with corneal irregularities. However, there is an additional cost of disposable probes.

- *Dynamic contour/Pascal tonometer (DCT)*: DCT has a probe with a pliable concave surface that adapts to corneal curvature, and a piezoelectric sensor measures transcorneal fluctuations in pressure. There is an average overestimation of IOP of 2 to 3 mm Hg as compared with Goldmann applanation tonometer. It is less affected by corneal thickness but does not give accurate readings if corneal irregularities are present.
- *The ocular response analyzer (ORA)*: ORA uses an air pulse to first applanate the cornea, then to indent it, and finally to return to the applanated surface. The difference in the two pressures at the point of applanation is due to deformability or hysteresis of the cornea. Also measured is the corneal resistance factor which reflects corneal thickness and IOP. A "corrected" IOP is generated.

Conclusion

A comprehensive examination should be practiced in a regular pattern, for example, estimating visual acuity and field as the patient walks in, and observing the eyelids and any strabismus as he/she sits down. On the slit lamp, examining the anterior segment of the left and then right eye with diffuse and then slit beams, followed by examination of the fundus and optic nerve using a 90D lens in the right eye followed by the left should be performed. This becomes a reflex over time, which takes less than 5 minutes, and ensures that the ophthalmic review is complete.

Suggested Readings

Baum J, Chaturvedi N, Netland PA, Dreyer EB. Assessment of intraocular pressure by palpation. Am J Ophthalmol 1995; 119(5):650–651

Ehlers N, Bramsen T, Sperling S. Applanation tonometry and central corneal thickness. Acta Ophthalmol (Copenh) 1975; 53(1):34–43

Herndon LW. Measuring intraocular pressure-adjustments for corneal thickness and new technologies. Curr Opin Ophthalmol 2006;17(2):115–119

Junk AK, Chen PP, Lin SC, et al. Disinfection of tonometers: a report by the American Academy of Ophthalmology. Ophthalmology 2017;124(12):1867–1875

Nangia V, Jonas JB, Sinha A, Matin A, Kulkarni M. Central corneal thickness and its association with ocular and general parameters in Indians: the Central India Eye and Medical Study. Ophthalmology 2010;117(4):705–710

Nelson P, Aspinall P, O'Brien C. Patients' perception of visual impairment in glaucoma: a pilot study. Br J Ophthalmol 1999;83(5):546–552

Ramulu PY, van Landingham SW, Massof RW, Chan ES, Ferrucci L, Friedman DS. Fear of falling and visual field loss from glaucoma. Ophthalmology 2012;119(7):1352–1358

Rödter TH, Knippschild S, Baulig C, Krummenauer F. Meta-analysis of the concordance of Icare® PRO-based rebound and Goldmann applanation tonometry in glaucoma patients. Eur J Ophthalmol 2020;30(2):245–252

Sihota R, Saxena R, Agarwal HC. Entropion uveae: early sphincter atrophy, signposting primary angle closure glaucoma? Eur J Ophthalmol 2004;14(4):290–297

Tan NYQ, Friedman DS, Stalmans I, Ahmed IIK, Sng CCA. Glaucoma screening: where are we and where do we need to go? Curr Opin Ophthalmol 2020;31(2):91–100

Tang J, Liang Y, O'Neill C, Kee F, Jiang J, Congdon N. Cost-effectiveness and cost-utility of population-based glaucoma screening in China: a decision-analytic Markov model. Lancet Glob Health 2019;7(7):e968–e978

CHAPTER 2

Glaucomatous Optic Neuropathy and Its Staging

Overview

- Pathophysiology of Glaucomatous Neuropathy
  - Pressure Dependent or Mechanical Factors
  - Vascular Perfusion Factors
  - Neurodegeneration
  - Cerebral Spinal Fluid Hydrodynamics
  - Genetics
- Examination of the Optic Nerve
  - Normal Optic Nerve Head
  - Glaucomatous Neuropathy
  - Optic Nerve Head Size and Shape
  - Optic Cup
  - Neuroretinal Rim
  - Cup:Disc Ratio
  - Disc Hemorrhages
  - Vascular Signs
  - Peripapillary Atrophy
  - Retinal Nerve Fiber Layer Defects
  - Physiological Cupping
- Staging of Glaucomatous Optic Neuropathy
- Suggested Readings

Introduction

Clinical examination and staging of the optic nerve head in glaucoma is essential in the management of glaucoma, as it is a part of comprehensive examination of all patients seen, and is the *most common reason for suspicion of glaucoma.* Measurable features show significant variation and overlap between normal and glaucomatous eyes, especially in the early stages; therefore, a careful examination of the optic nerve head provides some specific and sensitive features for early diagnosis and staging of glaucoma.

Pathophysiology of Glaucomatous Neuropathy

Glaucomatous neuropathy is a result of various factors as described below.

Pressure Dependent or Mechanical Factors

A significant mechanical effect on the optic nerve head by an intraocular pressure (IOP) that is not commensurate with the structure and function of the optic nerve (ON) could lead to *changes in axoplasmic flow, blood flow, as well as compression and backward bowing of the lamina cribrosa.*

The elevated IOP may also damage *retinal ganglion cell (RGC) axons*, which are *unmyelinated and therefore more vulnerable*, especially at their exit through the lamina cribrosa.

Retrograde and anterograde neuronal transport in glaucomatous eyes can be disturbed or even interrupted by increased IOP.

Vascular Perfusion Factors

Ocular perfusion pressure is the difference between systolic ophthalmic artery pressure and IOP. It can, therefore, be seen that alterations in either, due to abnormal autoregulation, systemic hypotension, microvasculopathies, etc., could result in reduced perfusion to the optic nerve head (**Fig. 2.1**).

Neurodegeneration

RGCs produce neurotrophins, and the antegrade flow to the axons could be hindered at the optic disc in glaucoma. Also, any hindrance to neurotrophin transport from the midbrain tectum/superior colliculus to the RGCs results in the onset of apoptosis. RGCs can also be damaged by glutamate release, which interacts with cell receptors and leads to an increase in intracellular calcium levels. This triggers cell death via apoptosis and leads to further release of glutamate and a vicious cycle occurs.

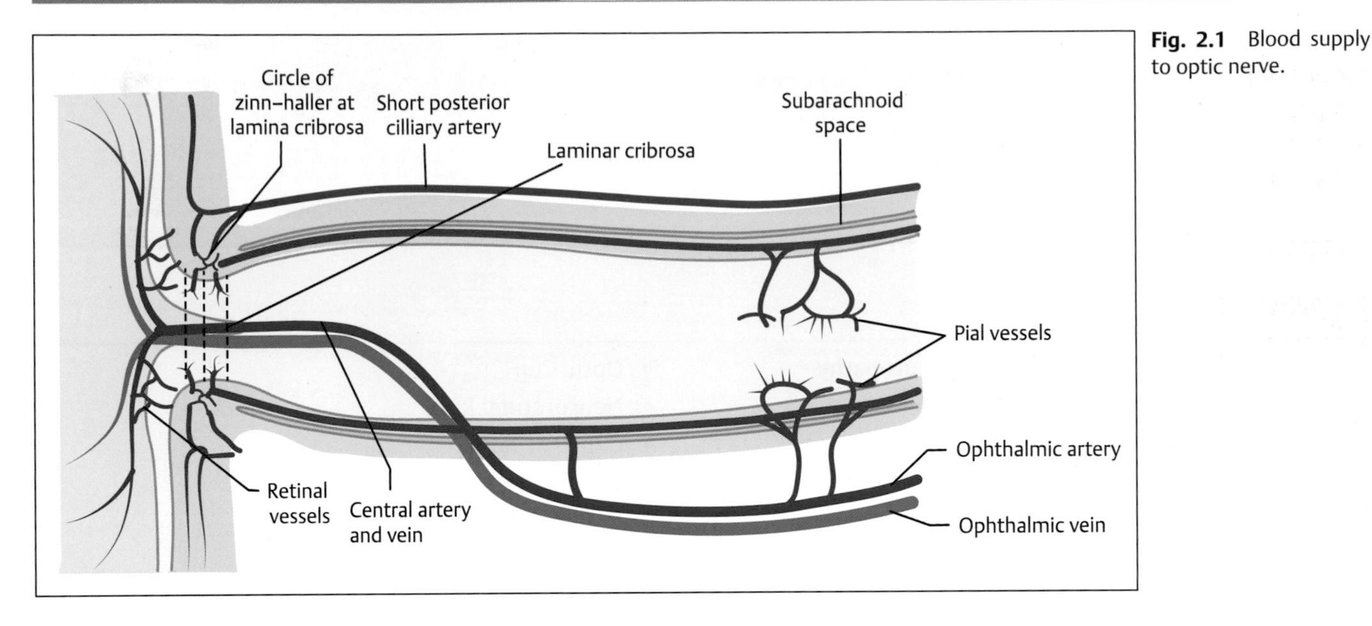

Fig. 2.1 Blood supply to optic nerve.

Cerebral Spinal Fluid Hydrodynamics

A lower intracranial pressure leads to an imbalance in the translaminar pressure, causing backward bowing of the lamina cribrosa. An elevated cerebrospinal fluid pressure could also result in RGC damage, as metabolic toxic substances may accumulate in axons at the lamina cribrosa.

Genetics

Many genes have been reported to contribute to primary open-angle glaucoma (POAG), and many more will probably be found in due time. It is also commonly seen to be more prevalent in families with first-degree relatives having a 9× increased risk.

Examination of the Optic Nerve

Examination of the optic nerve head allows observation of the retinal nerve fiber layer as well as prelaminar and laminar layers of the cup. There are characteristic changes in glaucoma, *usually starting at the inferior neuroretinal rim*. Unfortunately, variations in the size, shape, and morphology of the optic disc in normal individuals overlap with normal variations, and therefore awareness of the many signs—"hard" and "soft" signs suggestive of glaucoma—make evaluation and a final diagnosis of glaucoma more definitive.

Clinical role of optic nerve head examination today is to:

- Differentiate a normal, physiologically large cup from glaucoma.
- Identify and stage glaucomatous neuropathy.
- Identify early damage in at-risk patients.

Direct ophthalmoscopy has been used for examination of the fundus and optic nerve; however, *biomicroscopic examination with high convex lenses provides stereopsis, magnification, and clarity of the optic nerve head and retinal nerve fiber layer*. The lenses commonly used for assessing the optic disc are 78 or 90 diopters (D). Magnification is inversely proportional to the power of the lens and directly proportional to the field of view. Looking at the optic disc alone, one would get a greater magnification with a 78 D as compared with a 90 D; however, 78 D examination requires dilation of the pupil, which is not possible in primary angle-closure disease patients at the first examination, and may not be possible at all visits. The *90D is, therefore, useful for undilated examination of the optic nerve.*

As structural optic nerve head changes are reported to occur earlier than functional visual field (VF) loss in glaucoma, a good optic nerve head examination could identify patients at risk of progression, institute early therapy, and prevent progression.

Normal Optic Nerve Head

In a normal eye the ratio of cup diameter to disc diameter is normally 0.3 to 0.5:1, and the neuroretinal rim formed by axons of the ganglion cells is seen to be of regular thickness 360 degrees, with an orange-pink color. The thickness of the neuroretinal rim is generally greater at the inferior pole, then superior, followed by nasal and temporal, as in the ISNT rule. Blood vessels emerge from the depth of the cup and the larger, superotemporal, and inferotemporal arteries and veins course upward before turning temporally. The nasal vessels go directly to the temporal retina. Smaller blood vessels course along the upper and lower cup margins, and are called circumlinear vessels (**Fig. 2.2**).

Glaucomatous Neuropathy

The following changes are commonly used for screening of glaucoma:

- A vertical cup:disc ratio of >0.7.
- Asymmetry of cup:disc ratio of >0.2 between eyes, in similar-sized discs.

Following are diagnostic signs of glaucoma:

- Definitive:
  - A localized notch or thinning of the neuroretinal rim, especially inferotemporal.
  - Associated retinal nerve fiber layer loss.
  - Disc hemorrhages on neuroretinal rim or in the cup.
  - Localized pallor of the neuroretinal rim.
- Associated signs:
  - ISNT rule not fulfilled.
  - Vascular signs suggestive of an acquired cupping, such as baring of the circumlinear vessels and "overpass" of central vessels.
  - Beta zone parapapillary atrophy.

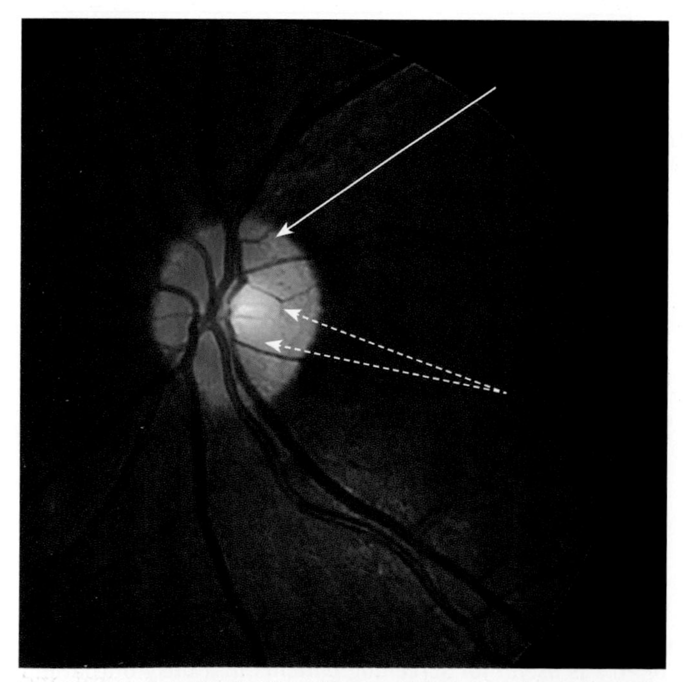

Fig. 2.2 An optic disc that is within normal limits. *Solid arrow* pointing to the disc margin, and the *dotted arrows* to circumlinear vessels on the inner margin of the cup.

Examination should proceed with an initial identification of the outer disc margin, assessment of disc size, followed by noting the inner edge of the cup, the neuroretinal rim width around the disc, vascular changes, presence of disc hemorrhages, retinal nerve fiber layer loss, and any other associated retinal pathology (**Fig. 2.3** and **Flowchart 2.1**).

Optic Nerve Head Size and Shape

The outer margin of the optic nerve head is formed by the edge of the sclera opening, and is identified as the point where the orange color of the neuroretinal rim meets the reflective tissue of the retina. The vertical diameter can be measured using a vertical slit with any high convex lens, applying the appropriate magnification factor, which varies with different manufacturers, and is approximately 0.9 to 1 for a +60 D, 1.1 for +78 D, and 1.3 to 1.6 for a +90 D lens in an emmetrope. Alternatively, the small spot of a direct ophthalmoscope, spanning 5 degrees, can be placed next to the disc, and if the size is the same it could be considered normal, and if smaller or larger, this should be noted. The European glaucoma guidelines have labeled a disc to be small if it is <1.45 mm, medium if 1.45 to 1.9 mm, and large if >1.9 mm. In a small disc, even a small cup may be glaucomatous, and in a large disc, irregularity or pallor of the neuroretinal rim, rather than a large cup, would be suspicious for glaucoma.

The shape of the disc is commonly vertically oval, but may often be round. The neuroretinal rim in vertically oval optic nerve head follows the ISNT rule more closely than those with rounded discs. A tilted disc is seen in myopes, and is often associated with astigmatism. Abnormally shaped discs may be indicators of a congenital anomaly, optic disc dysplasia, pits, or colobomas (**Fig. 2.4a, b**).

Optic Cup

The inner margin of the cup should be identified by observing blood vessels coming from the depth of the cup and along its wall, noting the point of deviation as they turn onto the neuroretinal rim surface, thus identifying the "contour" cup. Often the paler central area of the optic nerve head is mistaken as the cup, the so-called "color" cup, which is extremely likely to be fallacious, especially in elderly individuals having nuclear sclerosis. Another pointer to identifying the cup border are the circumlinear vessels that lie along the superior and inferior edge of the cup in normal individuals. The cup is generally round in healthy eyes, even though the disc is vertically oval. Diffuse loss of the neuroretinal rim is seen as a generalized enlargement of the cup, while focal

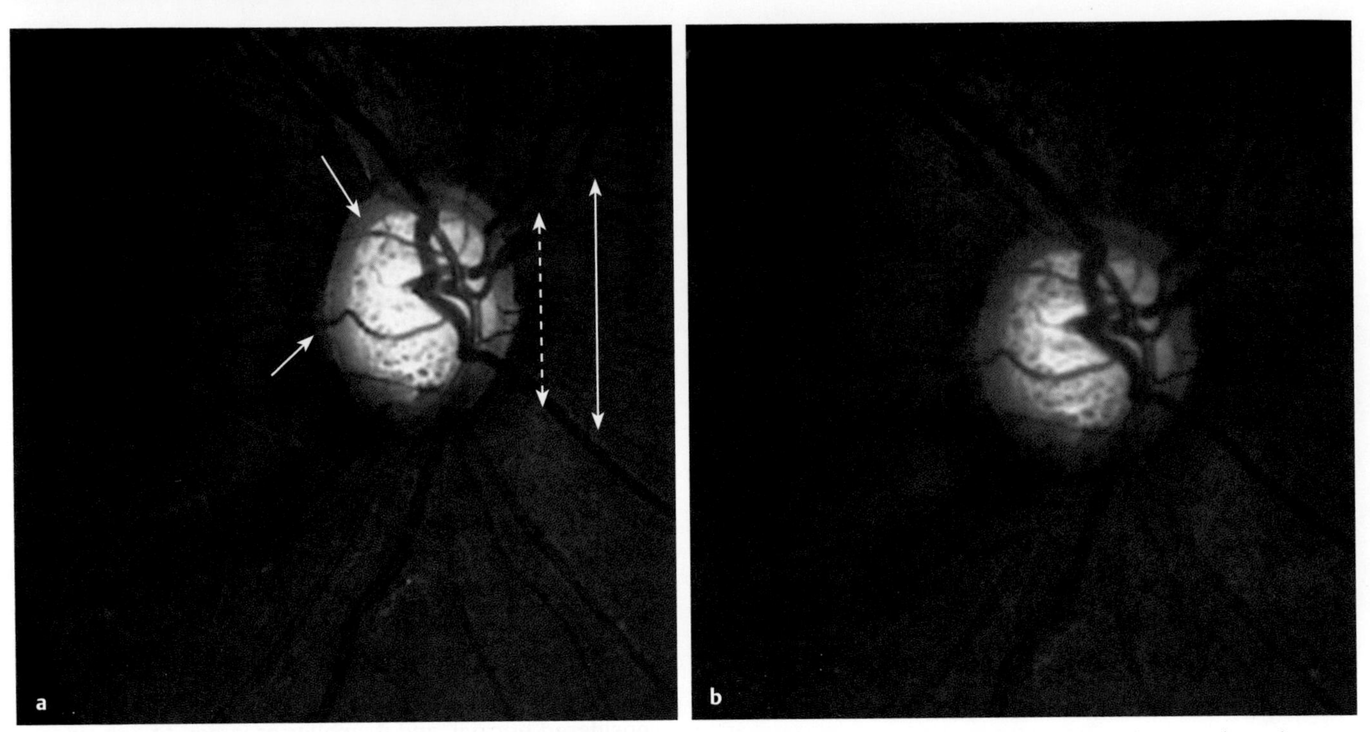

Fig. 2.3 **(a)** Glaucomatous neuropathy. *Vertical white arrow* of vertical disc diameter, and *vertical dashed arrow* marking the vertical cup diameter to give a cup:disc ratio of 0.8:1. *Short white arrows* point to baring of circumlinear vessels which are seen within the cup. *Red arrows* show a wedge-shaped retinal nerve fiber layer loss corresponding to a neuroretinal rim notch from 6 to 7 o'clock. **(b)** The same optic nerve head without markings.

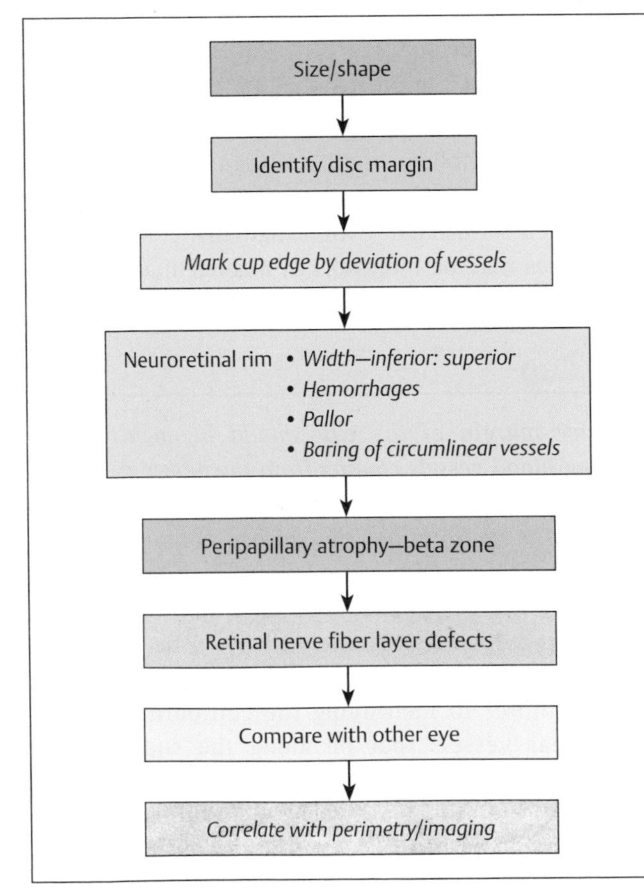

Flowchart 2.1 Structured optic nerve head examination.

damage commonly seen at the inferior and superior poles would cause a vertically oriented cup (**Fig. 2.5a**).

Neuroretinal Rim

The neuroretinal rim containing axons of the ganglion cells is of most importance in glaucoma patients. It is the area between the disc margin and the border of the contour cup (**Fig 2.5a**). In healthy eyes, this is seen to have a pink/orange/yellow color and is regular in width, and follows ISNT rule. As glaucomatous damage commonly starts inferiorly, if the thickness of the inferior rim approaches or becomes less than the superior, the patient should be investigated for glaucoma. *Localized loss of the neuroretinal rim, a notch, is a definitive sign of glaucoma*, and is often seen first inferiorly, and later also superiorly. The temporal neuroretinal rim is often pale in glaucoma, while the nasal is the last to be affected or lost.

Cup:Disc Ratio

Cup:disc ratio has been shown to have poor sensitivity and specificity in the diagnosis of glaucoma, but a *cup:disc ratio of >0.7 is useful for screening patients* in a busy outpatient or community. There is significant interobserver variability in this assessment clinically; however, with measurements on the slit lamp and on imaging devices, the linear cup:disc

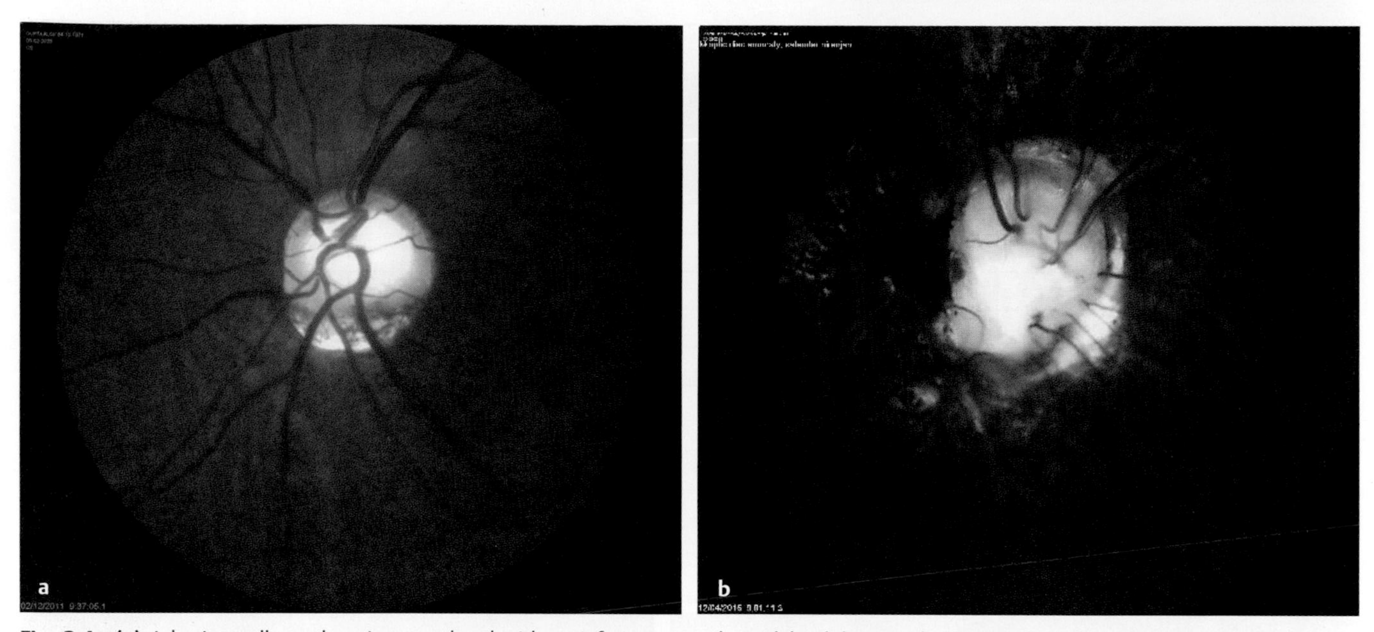

Fig. 2.4 **(a)** A horizontally oval optic nerve head with an inferior retinochoroidal coloboma. Ida Mann type 4. This can be misinterpreted as peripapillary atrophy or show up as a Seidel scotoma on perimetry. **(b)** Coloboma of the optic disc with white glial tissue filling the defect.

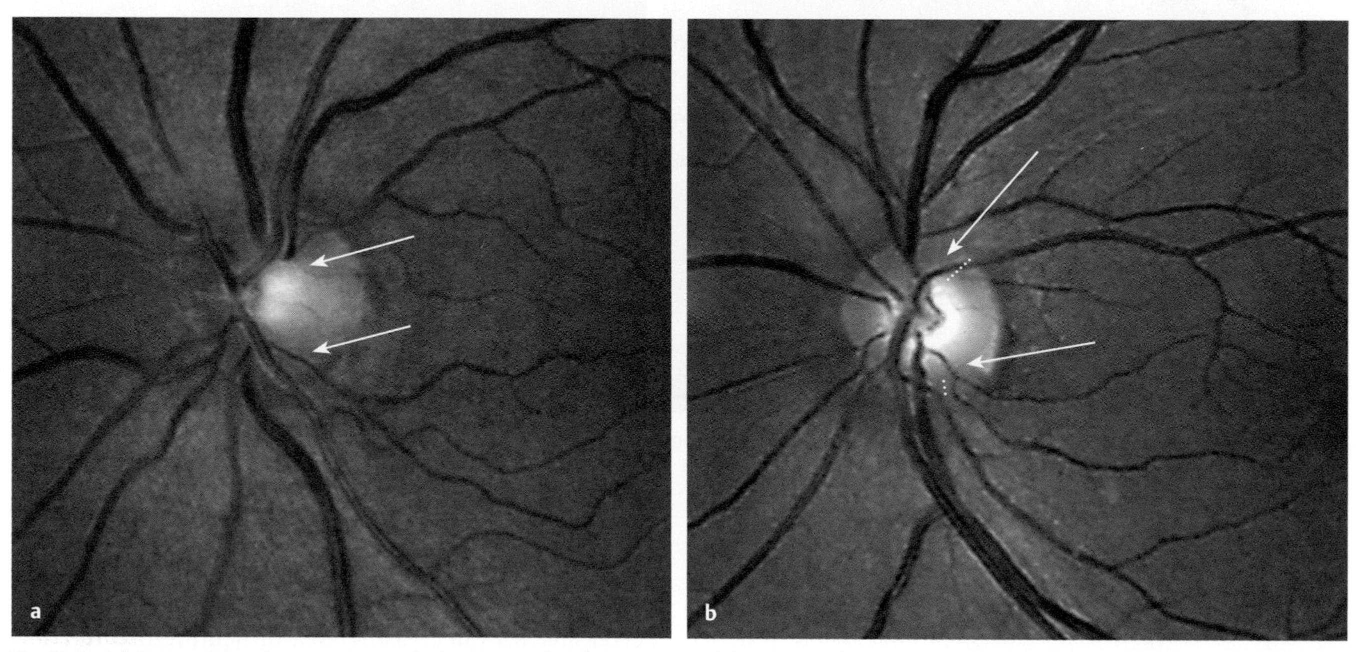

Fig. 2.5 **(a)** Determining the contour cup by looking at the change in vessel direction (*white arrows*) as they reach the surface of the neuroretinal rim. **(b)** Determining the thinnest neuroretinal rim width after identifying the contour (*inferior dotted line*) to determine rim:disc ratio for disc damage likelihood scale (DDLS).

ratio is more reliable. Spaeth et al described the *disc damage likelihood scale* (DDLS), looking at the size of the disc and measuring the width and extent in degrees of the thinnest rim and its meridian, to determine the thinnest cup:disc ratio (**Fig. 2.5b** and **Table 2.1**).

Disc Hemorrhages

The incidence of disc hemorrhages is less than 0.2% in Caucasian populations and can be as high as 3 to 4% in POAG eyes, more so in normal tension glaucoma. These are splinter shaped when present over the neuroretinal rim, but may be more rounded when present within the cup. Such hemorrhages are thought to be *evidence of ischemic damage to the neuroretinal rim, and a predictor of later retinal nerve fiber layer loss, especially when present at the edge of the disc* (**Fig. 2.6**). The presence of posterior vitreous detachment, diabetes, etc., that could cause similar hemorrhages, should be ruled out.

Table 2.1 Disc damage likelihood scale (DDLS)

		The thinnest width of the rim (Rim Disc Ratio)		
	Stage	**Small disc <1.50 mm**	**Average size disc 1.50–2.00 mm**	**Large disc >2.00 mm**
Normal	0a	0.5	0.4 or more	0.3 or more
	0b	0.4 up to 0.5	0.3–0.4	0.2–0.3
At risk	1	0.3 up to 0.4	0.2–0.3	0.1–0.2
	2	0.2 up to 0.3	0.1–0.2	0.05–0.1
Glaucoma damage	3	0.1 up to 0.2	0.01–0.1	0.01–0.05
	4	0.01–0.1	No rim <45 No rim 91–180 degrees	No rim <45 degrees
	5	No rim <45 degrees	No rim 45–90 degrees	No rim 45–90 degrees
Glaucoma disability	6	No rim 45–90 degrees	degrees	No rim 91–180 degrees
	7	No rim >90 degrees	No rim >180 degrees	No rim >180 degrees

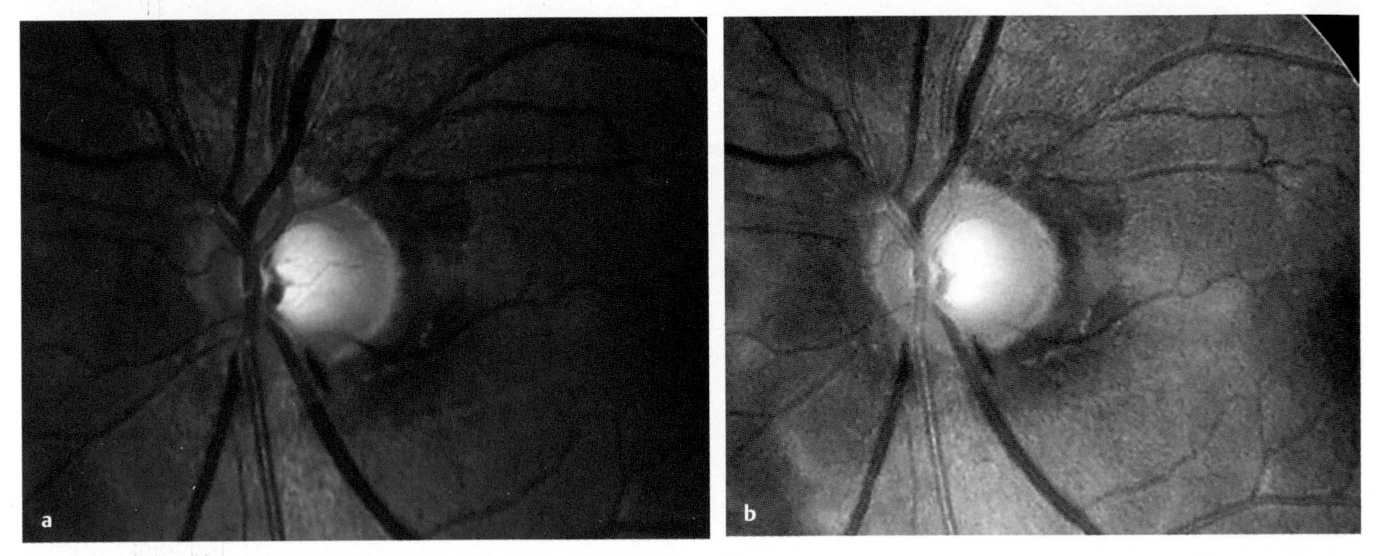

Fig. 2.6 Disc hemorrhage: **(a)** color photograph and **(b)** red-free photograph.

Vascular Signs

Glaucoma causes a progressive enlargement of the cup, due to a loss of axons and their supporting tissues. This also results in changes in vascular arrangement as support tissue to the vessels is lost or pushed peripherally. Circumferential vessels, small branches of the central retinal artery pass along the borders of the cup in healthy individuals, while in patients with glaucoma, they appear to be left within the enlarged cup. This baring of circumlinear vessels is considered to be a sign of acquired loss of the neuroretinal rim, highly sensitive and specific in the diagnosis of glaucoma (*arrows* in **Figs. 2.2** and **2.3**). An "overpass" phenomenon occurs when loss of support makes these vessels appear to float above the cup. As the cup enlarges, the large vessels find support only in the remaining nasal neuroretinal rim, leading to *nasalization of large vessels*, which is a feature but not specific for glaucoma. Retinal arteriolar attenuation is seen to occur in areas of retinal nerve fiber layer loss, with vessel diameter decreasing with decreasing area of neuroretinal rim and retinal nerve fiber layer and presence of VF defects. Vessels emerging from a very deep, bean pot cup pass up wide cup walls, seeming to disappear from view only to reappear and change direction as they reach the neuroretinal rim surface, giving rise to the appearance of *bayonetting*.

Peripapillary Atrophy

In normal and nonmyopic eyes, chorioretinal tissue and retinal pigment epithelium (RPE) are present adjacent to the disc margin. However, in POAG eyes, chorioretinal tissue is thought to undergo ischemic degeneration exposing RPE, with patchy pigmentation. In myopes, a similar appearance can be seen temporally due to the enlargement of the eye leaving the sclera exposed, but this is less pigmented and has a smooth outline. Peripapillary atrophy (PPA) in glaucoma can be divided into two zones: (i) α zone being the more peripheral with mottled pigmentation being commonly seen, sometimes even in normal eyes. (ii) *β zone is juxtapapillary*, correlating with areas of neuroretinal rim loss and VF defects and is irregular, *with large choroidal vessels visible* due to a loss of both the chorioretinal and RPE layers (**Fig. 2.7**).

Retinal Nerve Fiber Layer Defects

Retinal nerve fiber layer in normal eyes has regularly arranged axons, which reflect light uniformly, leading to very fine striations visible on using red-free light. A 20 to 40% loss of these axons is thought to precede VF loss in glaucoma, and an early recognition of this can help in diagnoses and early management. Green light is absorbed by RPE and choroid, while some is reflected back from the retinal nerve fiber layer. Loss of any nerve fiber bundles leads to destructive interference of reflected light, and therefore appears as *dark streaks or wedges around the optic nerve head, seen within two disc diameters from the disc.* Retinal nerve fiber layer defects are first seen inferotemporally or inferiorly associated with neuroretinal rim loss or a prior disc hemorrhage (**Fig. 2.8a, b**). These are generally thicker than the width of a retinal arteriole. In addition, parapapillary blood vessels, which appear indistinct in normal eyes as retinal nerve fiber layer lies over them, become more sharply defined within such areas of retinal nerve fiber layer loss.

Laminar Dot Sign

Laminar pores become visible when there is a loss of RGC axons and supportive tissue over the lamina cribrosa. They may also be seen in some normal eyes, and therefore are not a definitive sign of glaucoma.

Most significant morphological changes identifying glaucoma: Using optic disc photographs, qualitative

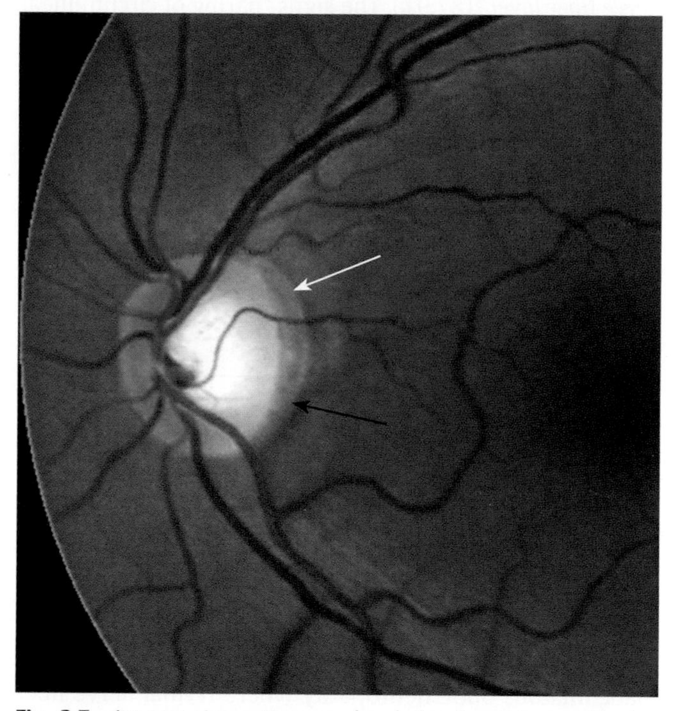

Fig. 2.7 Average size optic nerve head showing extreme thinning and pallor of the neuroretinal rim from 2 to 6 o'clock. There is a corresponding peripapillary atrophy, b zone (*white arrow*), and pigmented a zone (*black arrow*).

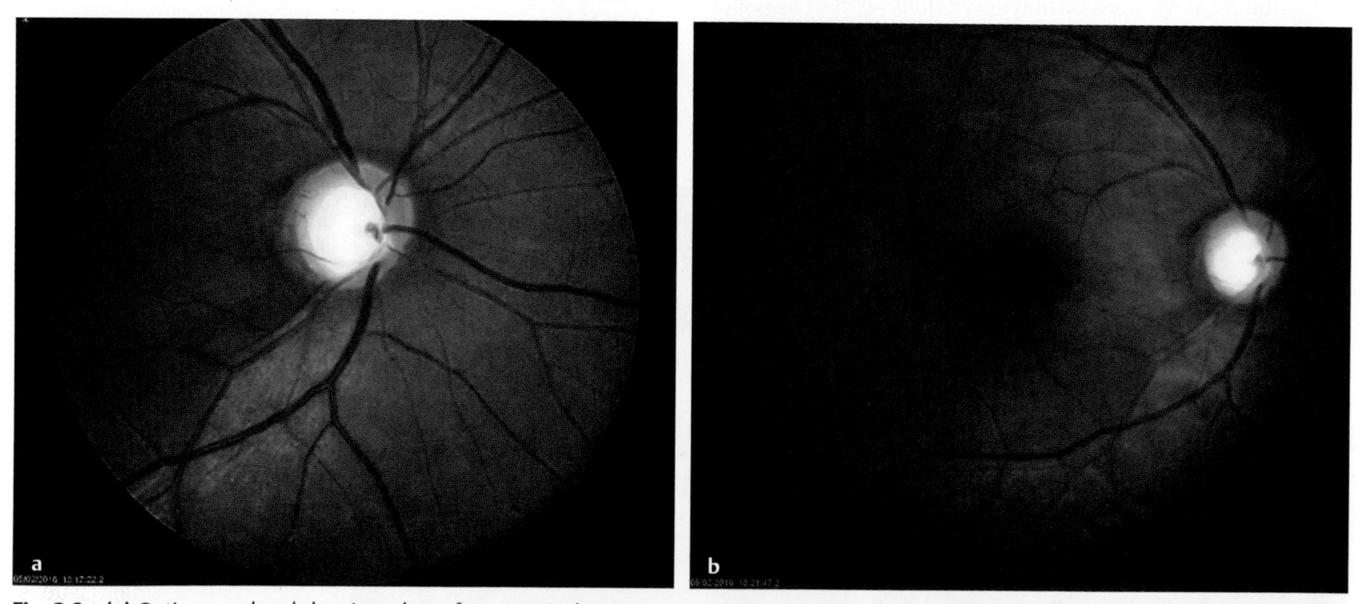

Fig. 2.8 (a) Optic nerve head showing a loss of neuroretinal rim, i.e., a notch from 7 to 8 o'clock, associated with a wedge-shaped retinal nerve fiber layer defect. Peripapillary atrophy, a and a zones, seen. **(b)** On red-free imaging the retinal nerve fiber layer defect is highlighted.

morphologic characteristics of glaucomatous optic neuropathy were determined in 251 nonselected normal eyes and 308 eyes with POAG, and were correlated to perimetric data. The highest degree of accuracy in distinguishing normal from glaucomatous optic discs was found with the characteristics "*localization of narrowest point of neuroretinal rim outside the temporal horizontal optic disc sector*" (85.5%) and "*changes in the parapapillary retinal nerve fiber layer*" (87.9%). The signs "baring of circumlinear vessels," "epipapillary flame-shaped hemorrhages," and "bridging of the vessel trunk" were highly specific for glaucomatous optic nerve damage (94.4–100%), however, less sensitive (5.8–25.3%). "Bayonet-like vessel kinking," "prevalence of cupping nasal to the main vessel trunk," "baring of the lamina cribrosa pores," and "undermining of the cup border" were less useful in qualitative evaluation of the optic disc.

Physiological Cupping

Certain eyes with a normal disc size and most eyes with a large disc size would have a larger than typical cup:disc ratio. In normal size discs, this is due to the Gaussian distribution of optic nerve head parameters. In larger discs, the same number of axons is spread around a greater circumference, leading to a thinner neuroretinal rim and therefore a larger cup. This is called physiological cupping, and is not glaucoma, but needs to be differentiated from glaucomatous optic neuropathy where retinal nerve fiber layer defects, etc., would be present (**Figs. 2.9** and **2.10a, b**).

Such eyes, as stated already, would have a larger optic nerve head, regular but thin neuroretinal rim of normal color, and no associated retinal nerve fiber layer or vascular changes (**Figs. 2.10a, b** and **2.11a, b**). *Both eyes would be similar, with symmetric cupping.*

Staging of Glaucomatous Optic Neuropathy

The extent of glaucomatous optic nerve damage appears to correlate significantly with VF loss and more importantly, also influences progression at a given IOP, and therefore is extremely important in determining Target IOP.

Although reported largely in POAG, this is also applicable to most primary angle-closure glaucoma (PACG) eyes and secondary glaucomas.

Chandler observed that "Eyes with advanced cupping at both ends of the disc worsened, if IOP was not consistently <15 mm Hg ... and require pressures below the average of the population." However, "Eyes with limited cupping,

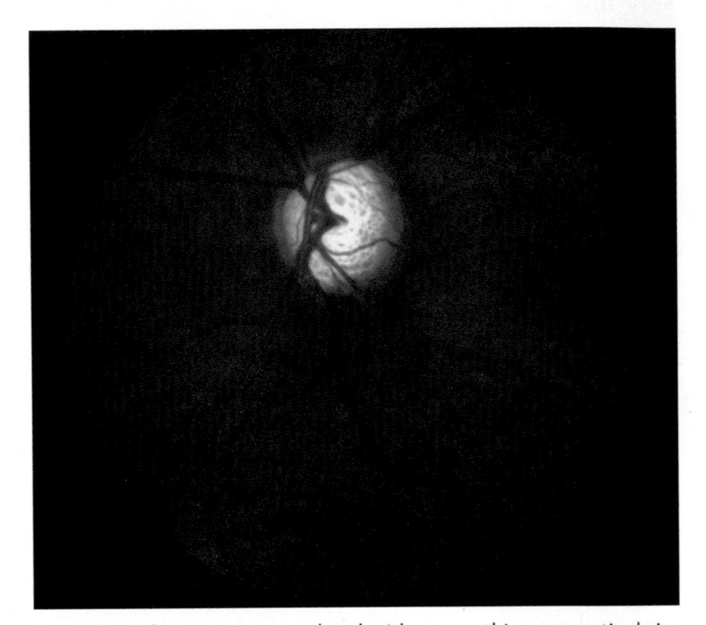

Fig. 2.9 A large optic nerve head with a very thin neuroretinal rim from 2 to 7 o'clock, with corresponding peripapillary atrophy. Extensive retinal nerve fiber layer defects are seen along the same area.

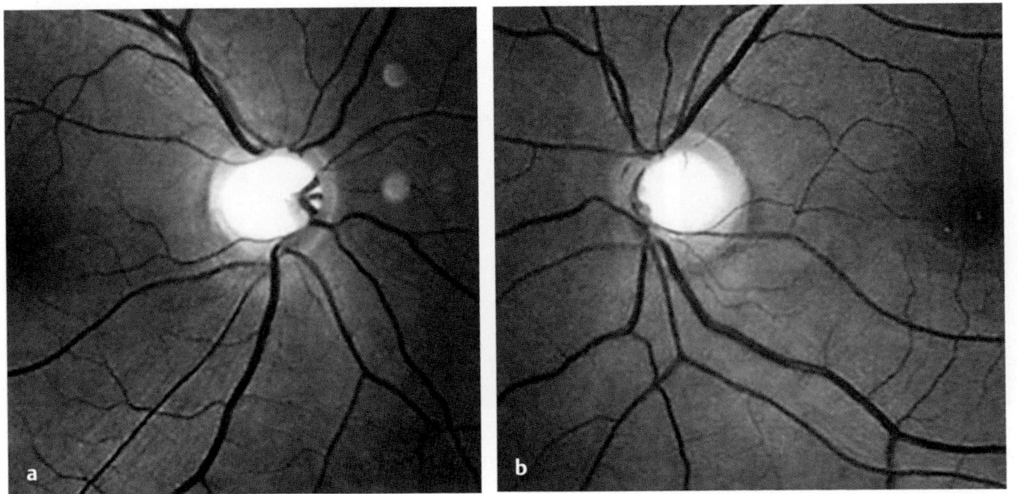

Fig. 2.10 **(a, b)** A physiologically large cup is generally seen to be bilaterally symmetrical and the circumlinear vessels if present will lie along the cup margin.

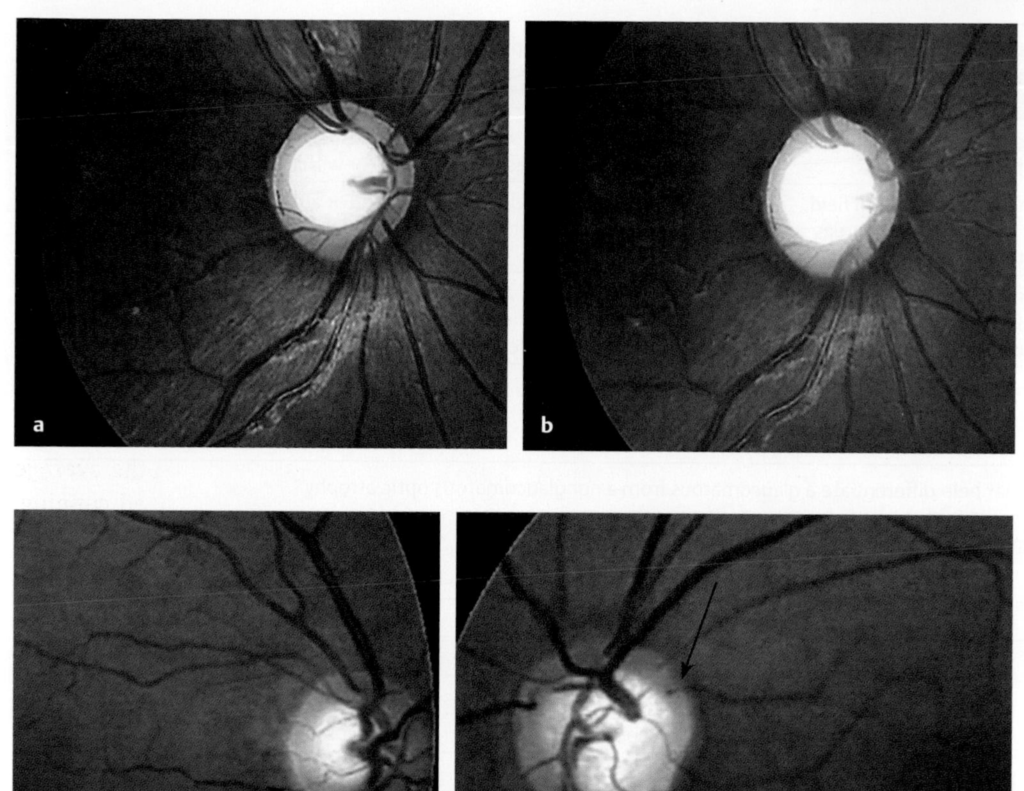

Fig. 2.11 **(a, b)** A physiologically large cup will also follow inferior, superior, nasal, temporal (ISNT) rule, and have no retinal nerve fiber layer defects.

Fig. 2.12 **(a)** Thinning of the inferotemporal neuroretinal rim is most frequently the first sign of mild glaucoma (*black arrow*). **(b)** Localized thinning of the neuroretinal rim seen both superiorly and inferiorly in moderate glaucomatous neuropathy (*black arrows*).

confined to one pole of the disc, appear to withstand tension better, mid to high teens." Finally, "Eyes with a normal disc appear to withstand pressure <30 mm Hg well" for years. Interindividual variability in disc size and shape makes evaluation difficult; however, the extent of thinning of the neuroretinal rim needs to be recorded.

Cup:disc ratio is more commonly employed in clinical practice and recommended as a means of staging glaucomatous damage into: mild with a cup:disc ratio of <0.65, moderate with 0.7 to 0.85, and severe with >0.9. The Ocular Hypertension Treatment Study (OHTS) found baseline cup:disc ratio to be a predictor of further damage in ocular hypertensives. However, in patients with early POAG, the Early Manifest Glaucoma Trial (EMGT) did not find baseline cup:disc ratio to be a significant risk factor for glaucomatous progression. In advanced POAG, the Advanced Glaucoma Intervention Study (AGIS) reported that patients with more severe glaucomatous damage, as measured by larger cup:disc ratio, 0.81 + 0.13, were at the greater risk of progression. Baseline linear cup:disc ratio on Heidelberg retina tomography (HRT) was found to be a significant risk factor for progression at all stages of glaucomatous neuropathy in both POAG and PACG eyes.

Spaeth et al suggested a disc damage likelihood scale (DDLS) based on the radial width of the narrowest neuroretinal rim, and divided optic nerve head changes into 10 stages, with stages 6 to 10 requiring aggressive therapy.

Mild glaucomatous optic neuropathy with a cup:disc ratio of <0.65 may show a thinned inferior neuroretinal rim or notch (**Fig. 2.12a**).

Moderate glaucomatous optic neuropathy has been reported if there is a localized loss of both inferior and superior neuroretinal rim, an inferior neuroretinal rim notch, or retinal nerve fiber layer defect in both superior and inferior arcuate area with a cup:disc ratio of 0.7 to 0.85 (**Fig. 2.12b**).

Severe glaucomatous optic neuropathy should have a cup:disc ratio of >0.9, extensive neuroretinal rim thinning, and pallor, possibly with b zone parapapillary atrophy (**Fig. 2.13** and **Table 2.2**).

Table 2.2 Differentiating features between mild, moderate, and severe glaucomatous optic neuropathy

	Mild	Moderate	Severe
AAO	Optic disc cupping but no visual field loss	Glaucomatous neuropathy with visual field loss not within 5 degrees of fixation	Visual field loss in both hemispheres or within 5 degrees of fixation
Canadian guidelines	CDR <0.65 or mild visual field defect not within 10 degrees of fixation	CDR 0.7 to 0.85 or visual field defect not within 10 degrees of fixation or both	CDR >0.9 or visual field defect within 10 degrees of fixation or both
International Classification of Diseases–10	Optic nerve abnormalities consistent with glaucoma + normal fields	Optic nerve abnormalities consistent with glaucoma + one hemifield abnormality, not within 5 degrees	Optic nerve abnormalities consistent with glaucoma + both hemifield abnormality or within 5 degrees

Abbreviations: AAO, American Academy of Ophthalmology; CDR, cup:disc ratio.

Table 2.3 Some clinical features that help differentiate a glaucomatous from a nonglaucomatous optic atrophy

	Glaucomatous optic neuropathy	Nonglaucomatous optic neuropathy
History	Gradual progressive loss of vision	Sudden loss of vision
Age	Older	<50 years
Visual acuity	Affected late	Low at the start
Pupil reflexes	Sluggish bilaterally	Ipsilateral RAPD
Neuroretinal rim	Neuroretinal rim left has a good color	Significant pallor >> cup
Regional loss of neuroretinal rim	Present	Never complete rim loss
Peripapillary atrophy	Corresponds to neuroretinal rim loss	Absent
Visual field defects	Respect the horizontal midline	Respect the vertical midline or maybe centrocecal scotoma
Correlating cupping with visual field loss	Good correlation	Visual field loss much more than cupping

Abbreviation: RAPD, relative afferent pupillary defect.

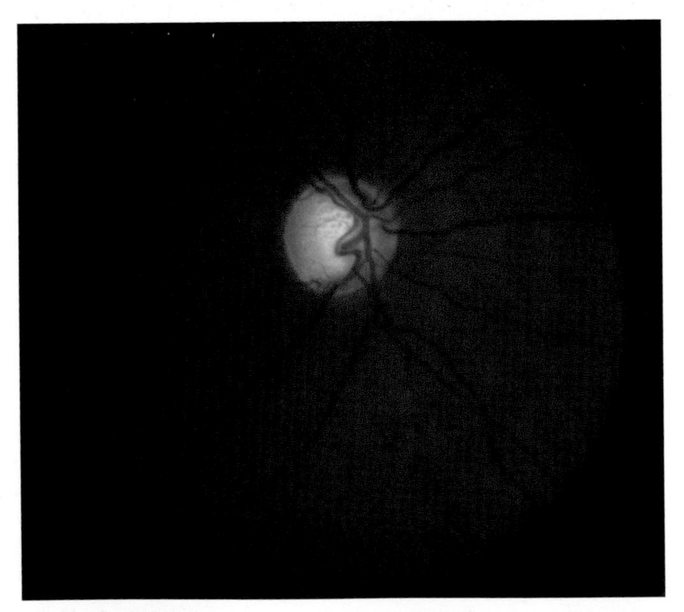

Fig. 2.13 Extensive neuroretinal rim loss/thinning and pallor is seen in severe glaucomas.

Nonglaucomatous cupping seen in central nervous system (CNS) and other diseases may be difficult to differentiate from glaucomatous optic neuropathy (**Table 2.3**). Cupping seen in an eye with a sudden, significant fall in visual acuity, generalized optic nerve pallor in excess of cupping, normal IOP, and the presence of vertically aligned VF defects in a young patient should suggest nonglaucomatous cupping. Evaluation for anterior ischemic optic neuropathy, optic nerve or sellar tumor or hemorrhage, trauma, and certain inherited optic neuropathies is mandatory in such eyes (**Fig. 2.14a, b**).

There is significant inter- and intraobserver variability in the evaluation of cup:disc ratio even among glaucoma specialists. Therefore, more specific signs of neuroretinal rim notching, retinal nerve fiber layer loss, and disc hemorrhages improve the specificity of diagnosing glaucomatous optic neuropathy clinically. The advent of imaging in glaucoma helps in the diagnosis of glaucoma, but can only be used in conjunction with clinical examination.

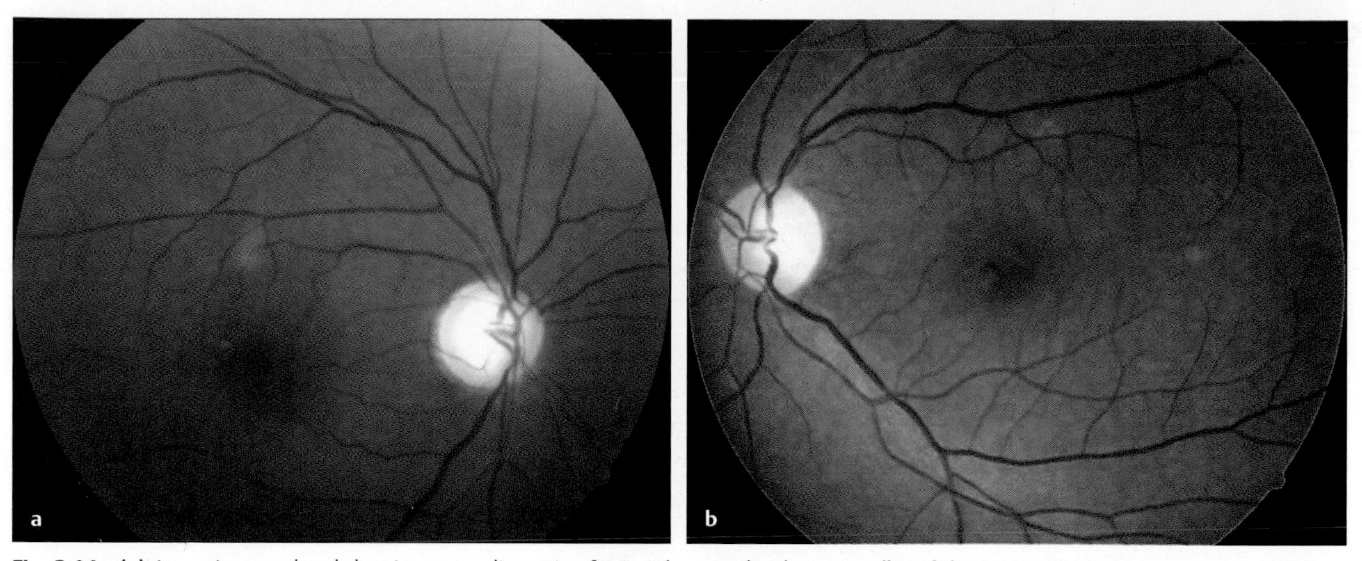

Fig. 2.14 **(a)** An optic nerve head showing a cup:disc ratio of 0.7 with generalized severe pallor of the neuroretinal rim due to a large pituitary adenoma. **(b)** An optic nerve head with a vertical cup:disc ratio of 0.6 but pallor of the temporal half of the optic disc due to a pituitary adenoma.

Suggested Readings

Bengtsson B, Leske MC, Yang Z, Heijl A; EMGT Group. Disc hemorrhages and treatment in the early manifest glaucoma trial. Ophthalmology 2008;115(11):2044–2048

Broadway DC, Nicolela MT, Drance SM. Optic disk appearances in primary open-angle glaucoma. Surv Ophthalmol 1999; 43(Suppl 1):S223–S243

Brusini P, Johnson CA. Staging functional damage in glaucoma: review of different classification methods. Surv Ophthalmol 2007;52(2):156–179

Budenz DL, Anderson DR, Feuer WJ, et al; Ocular Hypertension Treatment Study Group. Detection and prognostic significance of optic disc hemorrhages during the Ocular Hypertension Treatment Study. Ophthalmology 2006;113(12):2137–2143

Chandler PA. Progress in the treatment of glaucoma in my lifetime. Surv Ophthalmol 1977;21:412–28

Fingeret M, Medeiros FA, Susanna R Jr, Weinreb RN. Five rules to evaluate the optic disc and retinal nerve fiber layer for glaucoma. Optometry 2005;76(11):661–668

Foster PJ, Buhrmann R, Quigley HA, Johnson GJ. The definition and classification of glaucoma in prevalence surveys. Br J Ophthalmol 2002;86(2):238–242

Greenfield DS, Siatkowski RM, Glaser JS, Schatz NJ, Parrish RK II. The cupped disc. Who needs neuroimaging? Ophthalmology 1998;105(10):1866–1874

Hitchings RA, Spaeth GL. The optic disc in glaucoma. I: Classification. Br J Ophthalmol 1976;60(11):778–785

Jasty U, Harris A, Siesky B, et al. Optic disc haemorrhage and primary open-angle glaucoma: a clinical review. Br J Ophthalmol 2020;104(11):1488–1491

Jonas JB, Gusek GC, Naumann GO. Optic disc morphometry in chronic primary open-angle glaucoma. I. Morphometric intrapapillary characteristics. Graefes Arch Clin Exp Ophthalmol 1988;226(6):522–530

Jonas JB, Gusek GC, Naumann GO. Optic disc morphometry in chronic primary open-angle glaucoma. II. Correlation of the intrapapillary morphometric data to visual field indices. Graefes Arch Clin Exp Ophthalmol 1988;226(6):531–538

Jonas JB, Budde WM. Diagnosis and pathogenesis of glaucomatous optic neuropathy: morphological aspects. Prog Retin Eye Res 2000;19(1):1–40

Malik R, Swanson WH, Garway-Heath DF. 'Structure-function relationship' in glaucoma: past thinking and current concepts. Clin Exp Ophthalmol 2012;40(4):369–380

Martínez-De-La-Casa JM, Saenz-Francés F, Fernandez-Vidal AM, et al. Agreement between slit lamp examination and optical coherence tomography in estimating cup-disc ratios. Eur J Ophthalmol 2008;18(3):423–428

Quigley HA, Dunkelberger GR, Green WR. Retinal ganglion cell atrophy correlated with automated perimetry in human eyes with glaucoma. Am J Ophthalmol 1989;107(5):453–464

Spaeth GL, Lopes JF, Junk AK, Grigorian AP, Henderer J. Systems for staging the amount of optic nerve damage in glaucoma: a critical review and new material. Surv Ophthalmol 2006;51(4):293–315

Tezel G, Kolker AE, Kass MA, Wax MB, Gordon M, Siegmund KD. Parapapillary chorioretinal atrophy in patients with ocular hypertension. I. An evaluation as a predictive factor for the development of glaucomatous damage. Arch Ophthalmol 1997;115(12):1503–1508

Tezel G, Kolker AE, Wax MB, Kass MA, Gordon M, Siegmund KD. Parapapillary chorioretinal atrophy in patients with ocular hypertension. II. An evaluation of progressive changes. Arch Ophthalmol 1997;115(12):1509–1514

Tielsch JM, Katz J, Quigley HA, Miller NR, Sommer A. Intraobserver and interobserver agreement in measurement of optic disc characteristics. Ophthalmology 1988;95(3): 350–356

Uhm KB, Lee DY, Lee JS, Hong C. Sensitivity and specificity of qualitative signs to detect glaucomatous optic nerve damage. J Korean Ophthalmol Soc 1998;39:153–162

CHAPTER 3

Gonioscopy

Overview

- Gonioscopes
  - Direct Gonioscopes
  - Indirect Gonioscopes
- Importance of Doing Gonioscopy
- Anterior Chamber Angle Structures
- Grading Systems for Gonioscopy
- Techniques to Visualize Angle Structures in a Narrow Angle
  - Manipulative Gonioscopy
  - Indentation Gonioscopy
- Commonly Encountered Gonioscopic Patterns
  - Open Angle
  - Narrow Angles
- Recording Gonioscopy
- Cases
- Suggested Readings

Introduction

The major risk factor or cause for glaucomatous optic neuropathy is a raised intraocular pressure (IOP), and this is due to changes in aqueous outflow pathways. Normally the most important means of aqueous outflow is through the conventional or trabecular pathway, the intracameral surface of which is easily visible on gonioscopy. Any abnormality seen on the surface would reflect changes within the trabecular meshwork, which could decrease the spaces available for draining aqueous (**Fig. 3.1a, b**).

Direct visualization of the iridocorneal angle is not possible, as light emanating from here exceeds the critical angle of 46 degrees at the cornea–air interface, and is totally internally reflected. Trantas first used the term *gonioscopy* in 1907 while observing the angle with a direct ophthalmoscope after applying pressure over the limbus

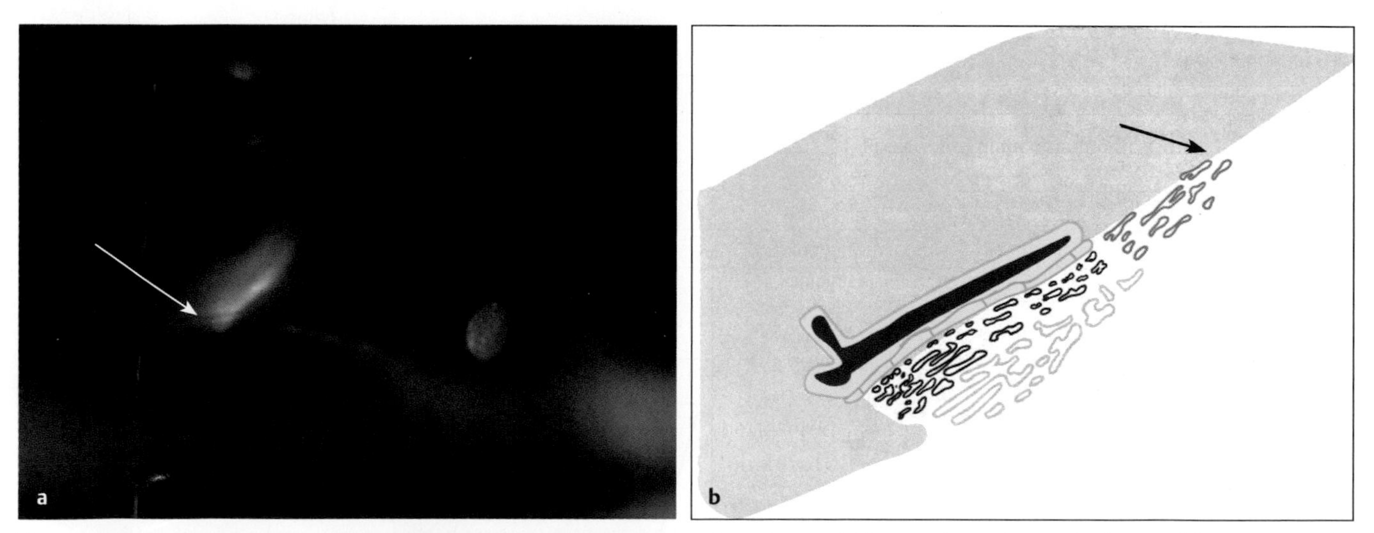

Fig. 3.1 (a) Gonioscopy with a 2-mm height, narrow and bright slit away from the pupil. The anterior and posterior layers of the cornea can be seen meeting at the Schwalbe's line forming the corneal wedge (*white arrow*). **(b)** Diagrammatic representation of the corneal wedge (*black arrow*), the landmark for the Schwalbe's line, the anterior boundary of the trabecular meshwork, which lies within the sclera sulcus. The *light brown* anterior trabecular meshwork is considered to be nonfunctional, while the posterior trabecular meshwork is divided into the uveal (*gray*), corneoscleral (*purple*), and the juxtacanalicular (*pink*). The canal of Schlemm and collector channels lie within the scleral spur (*black arrow*).

in an eye with keratoglobus. Koeppe used a thick, convex contact lens with an operating microscope or a slit lamp for direct gonioscopy, and Goldmann in 1936 developed a contact lens with an angled mirror for an indirect evaluation of the angle (**Table 3.1**).

Gonioscopes

There are two types of gonioscopes, namely, direct and indirect gonioscopes (**Fig. 3.2**).

Direct Gonioscopes

Direct gonioscopes have a thick convex contact lens whose refractive index is the same as that of the cornea, thereby nullifying the effect of the anterior corneal surface and allowing light rays from the angle to pass through the contact lens–air interface.

Direct gonioscopes give a panoramic view of the angle, with little distortion. Both eyes can be visualized and compared simultaneously. However, the disadvantages are that it requires a supine patient and an operating microscope or handheld slit lamp.

Direct surgical gonioscopes, namely, Hoskins-Barkan, Swan Jacob, Richardson Schaffer, and Thorpe, have been used for goniotomy in congenital glaucoma. With the popularization of new angle surgeries such as iStent, Trabectome, etc., knowledge of direct gonioscopy is now essential.

Indirect Gonioscopes

These can be used on a slit lamp, with bright illumination, magnification, and stereopsis permitting localization of each angle structure. However, the image is inverted and of the opposite angle.

Gonioscopes can be *sterilized with 1:10 household bleach (sodium hypochlorite) for 5 minutes, or 3% hydrogen peroxide*, while operating gonioscopes need ethylene oxide sterilization.

Importance of Doing Gonioscopy

Gonioscopy is the technique used to visualize the irido-corneal or anterior chamber angle, which is the intracameral surface of the trabecular meshwork. Angle configuration is

Table 3.1 Comparison between Goldmann and four-mirror gonioscopes

Specifications of lens criteria	Goldmann one- or two-mirror gonioscope	Four-mirror gonioscopes
Diameter of corneal contact	12 mm	9 mm
Overall diameter	15 mm	9 mm
Size of rim	1.5 mm	None
Mirror angulation	62 degrees	64 degrees
Mirror height	17 mm	12 mm
Distance from central cornea	3 mm	5 mm
Radius of curvature	7.4 mm	7.85 mm
Coupling fluid	Required	Not required
Dynamic gonioscopy	Manipulation	Indentation

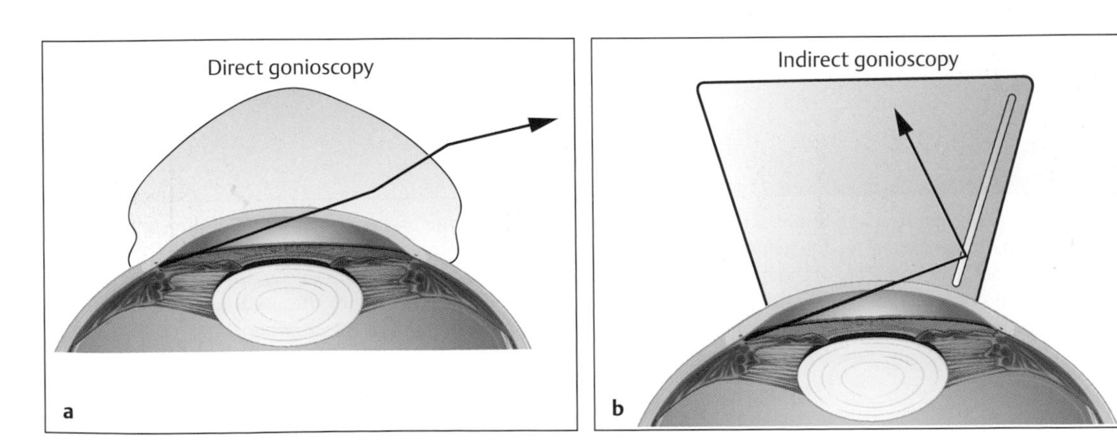

Fig. 3.2 Types of gonioscopes. **(a)** Direct and **(b)** indirect gonioscopes.

dependent on pupil size, lens thickness, and ciliary tone. Gonioscopy is extremely helpful in assessing this area and provides information about:

- Anatomy—narrow or open angle.
- Developmental abnormalities.
- Acquired pathologies of the trabecular outflow pathways—recession, neovascularization, etc.
- Changes over time or with age.

It also helps in management:

- Determines the reason for IOP rise in any glaucoma.
- Identifies the possibility of angle-closure glaucoma.
- Identifies structures for laser trabeculoplasty, laser gonioplasty, goniotomy, and synechiolysis and newer angle surgeries can be performed.

Anterior Chamber Angle Structures

The iridocorneal angle is bordered by the Schwalbe's line superiorly, and then the intracameral surface of the trabecular meshwork, scleral spur, anterior face of the ciliary body seen as a gray band, and the most peripheral iris can be seen inferiorly (**Fig. 3.3**).

It is ideal to start gonioscopy with a short, thin, bright slit at low magnification to judge the iridocorneal angle, so that pupillary constriction is avoided, as that would open up a narrow angle. Then identify the anterior landmark after increasing magnification—Schwalbe's line is almost always identifiable by the corneal wedge. If in primary position only the Schwalbe's line or anterior trabecular meshwork is visible due to a convex iris; *manipulation*, moving the lens toward the angle being viewed or asking the patient to look toward the mirror, may help see other structures. Alternately, *indentation* of the central cornea is possible with a gonioscope having a diameter less than the cornea, so that aqueous is displaced to the periphery, pushing the iris posteriorly, and opening the angle (**Flowchart 3.1**).

Schwalbe's line marks the end of the Descemet's membrane, and is the transition between transparent corneal tissue and the sclera. It is seen as a prominent white band, and can be identified easily by the *"corneal wedge,"* the point where lines of reflected light from anterior and posterior surfaces of the cornea meet (**Figs. 3.4** and **3.5a, b**). Also, at this point, the three-dimensional appearance of light on the gonioscopic view of the cornea is replaced by the two-dimensional appearance of trabecular meshwork.

The *trabecular meshwork* has a grayish translucency, and can be divided into an anterior nonpigmented trabecular meshwork and posterior pigmented surface. The latter is thought to be the area of aqueous outflow. The size of spaces between trabecular beams decreases from the anterior chamber toward Schlemm's canal, and aqueous has a tortuous path to traverse, permitting the progressive sieving of any large to small particulate matter that may be present (**Fig. 3.6**).

The *scleral spur* is seen as a white line immediately posterior to the trabecular meshwork in open angles. Neovascular vessels are seen as irregularly branching vessels that cross the scleral spur.

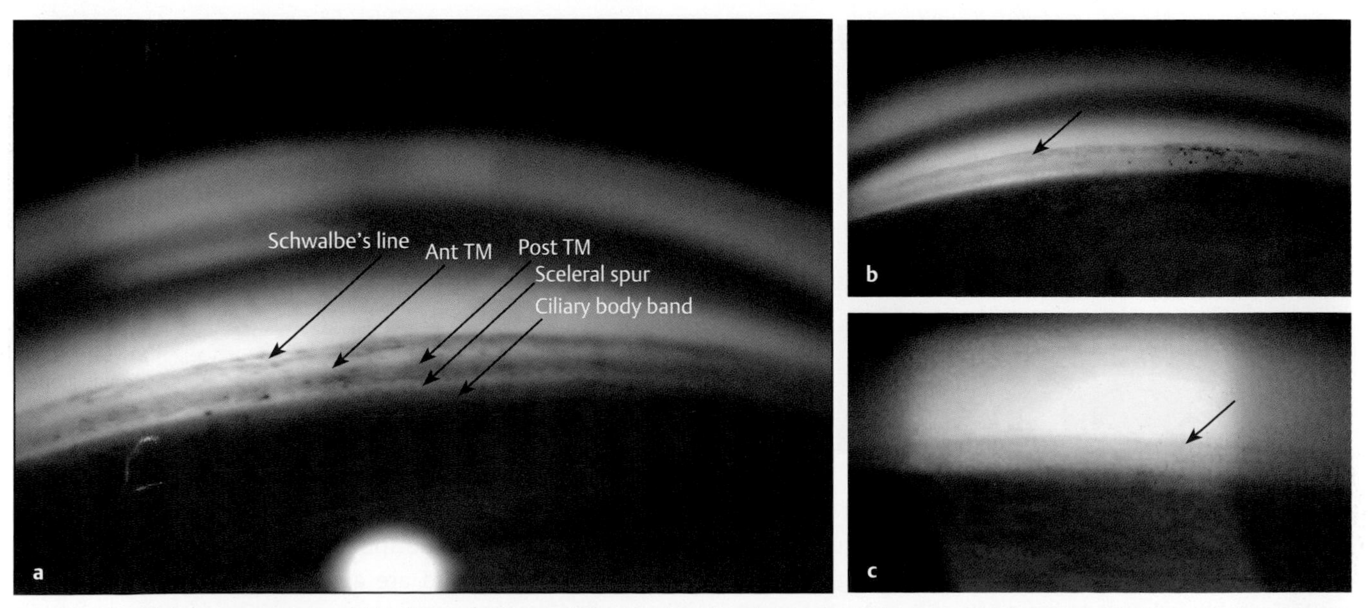

Fig. 3.3 **(a, b)** An open angle in which all the structures of the anterior chamber angle can be seen. The presence of pigment in the posterior trabecular meshwork and anterior to Schwalbe's line has highlighted the different structures. **(c)** Normal eyes do not show such pigment. Elderly Indians may have mild pigmentation seen in the posterior trabecular meshwork. TM, trabecular meshwork. (*Black arrows* in **(b, c)** denote Schwalbe's line.)

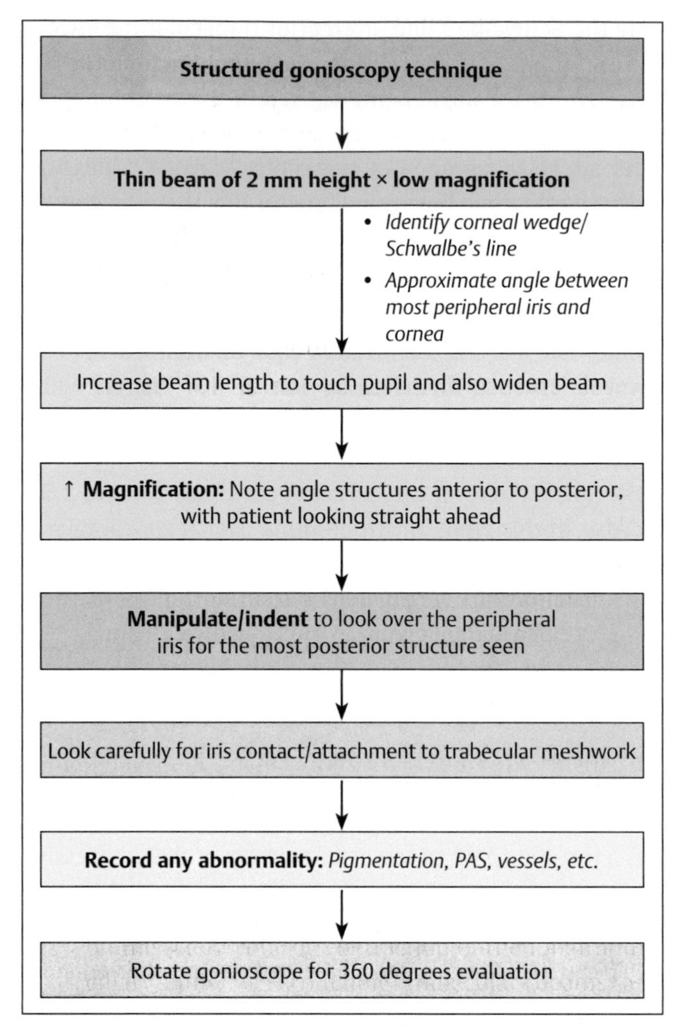

Flowchart 3.1 Algorithm explaining the technique of structured gonioscopy. PAS, peripheral anterior synechiae.

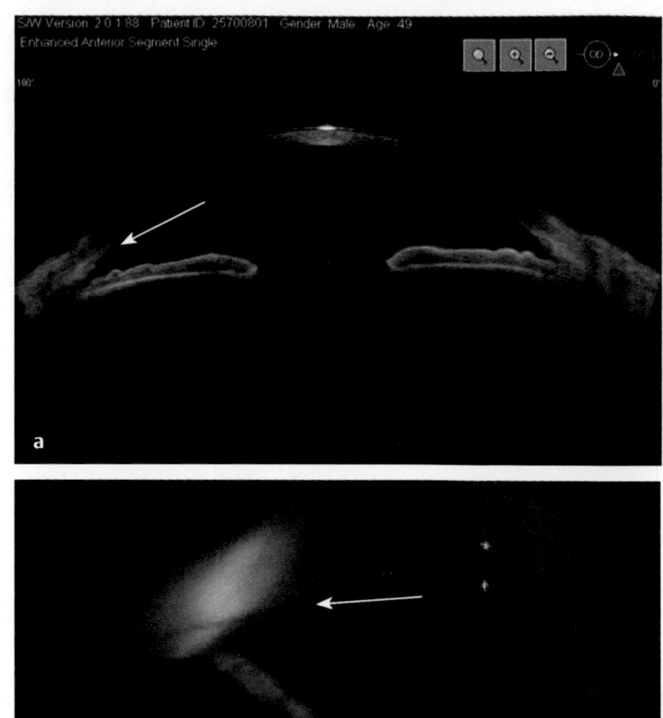

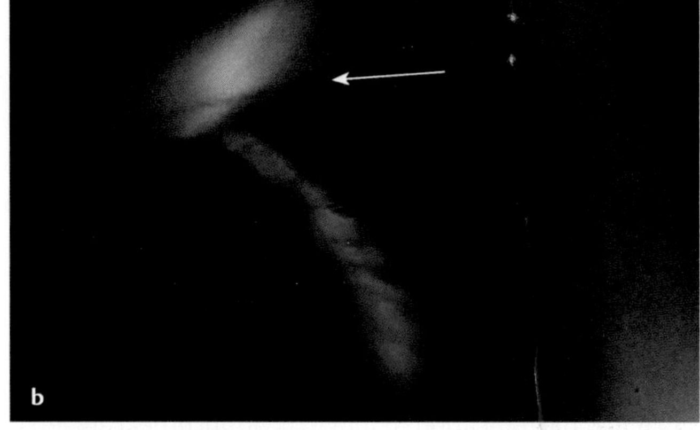

Fig. 3.4 **(a)** Corneal wedge of light (*white arrow*) as landmark for Schwalbe's line, the beginning of the anterior chamber angle. **(b)** Anterior segment optical coherence tomography (AS-optical coherence tomography) shows the corneal wedge, and its distance from the iris with *white arrow* at Schwalbe's line.

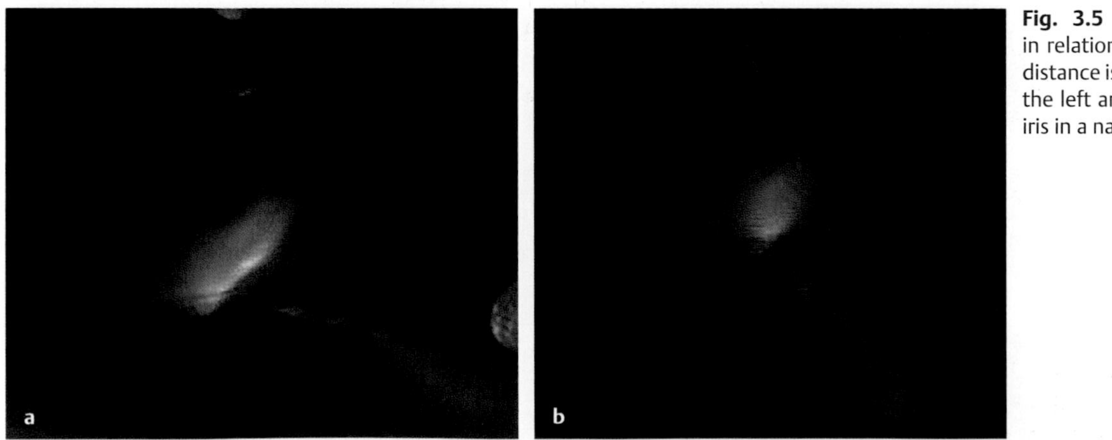

Fig. 3.5 **(a, b)** Corneal wedge in relation to the iris. A significant distance is seen in an open angle to the left and close proximity to the iris in a narrow angle to the right.

The gray *ciliary body band* is the anterior face of the ciliary body, from which the iris originates. Visualization of this signifies an open angle, and traumatic angle recession leads to an irregular widening of the ciliary body band.

The *root of the iris* can be seen originating from the ciliary body band. Sometimes fine iris processes extend anteriorly to the trabecular meshwork, following the contour of the angle. In contrast, peripheral anterior synechiae (PAS) bridge the angle and are almost always associated with surrounding pigmentation.

The view of the angle structures is influenced by the curvature of the iris and any synechiae that are present.

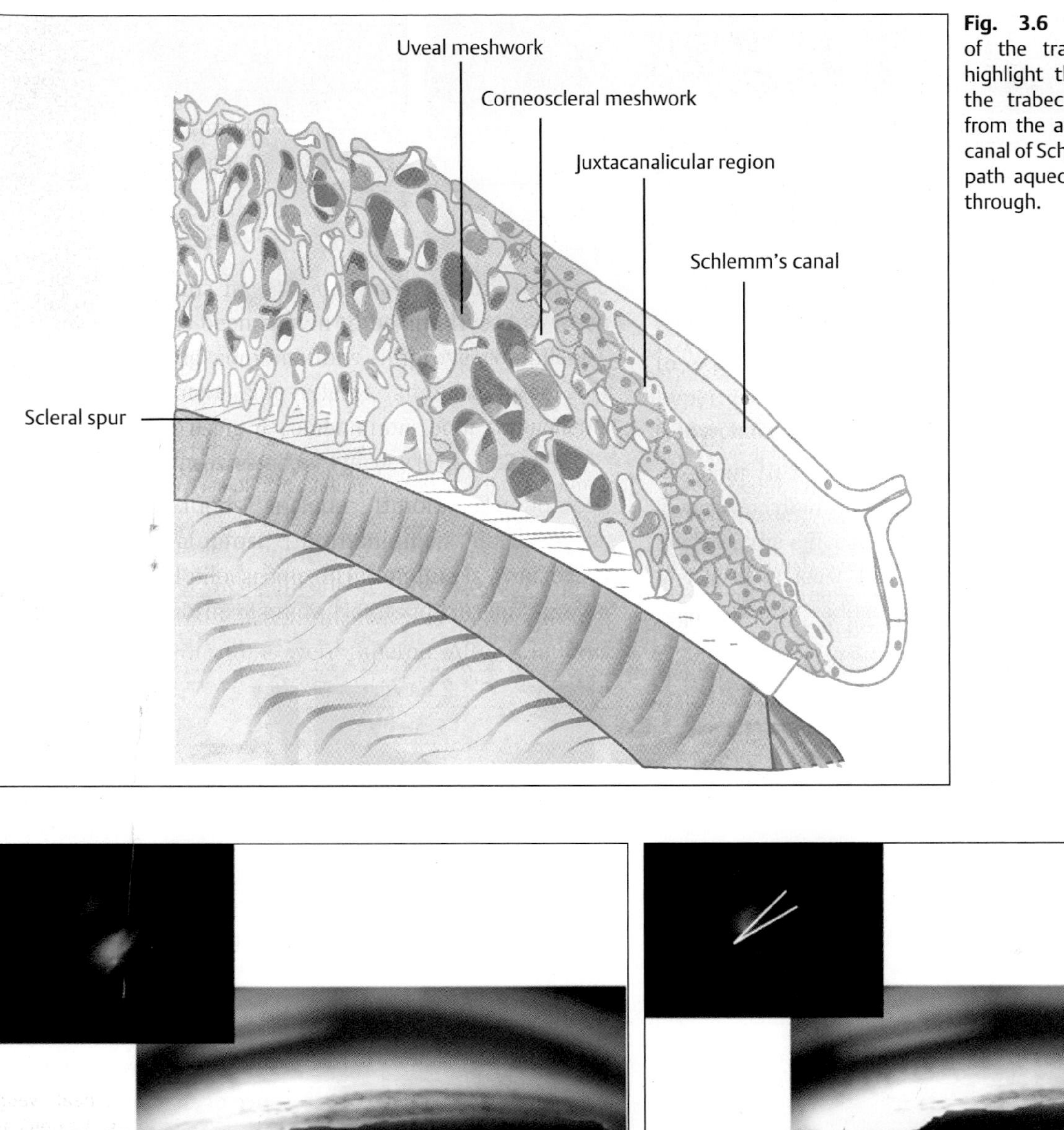

Fig. 3.6 A transverse section of the trabecular meshwork to highlight the decrease in size of the trabecular meshwork spaces from the anterior chamber to the canal of Schlemm, and the tortuous path aqueous has to take to pass through.

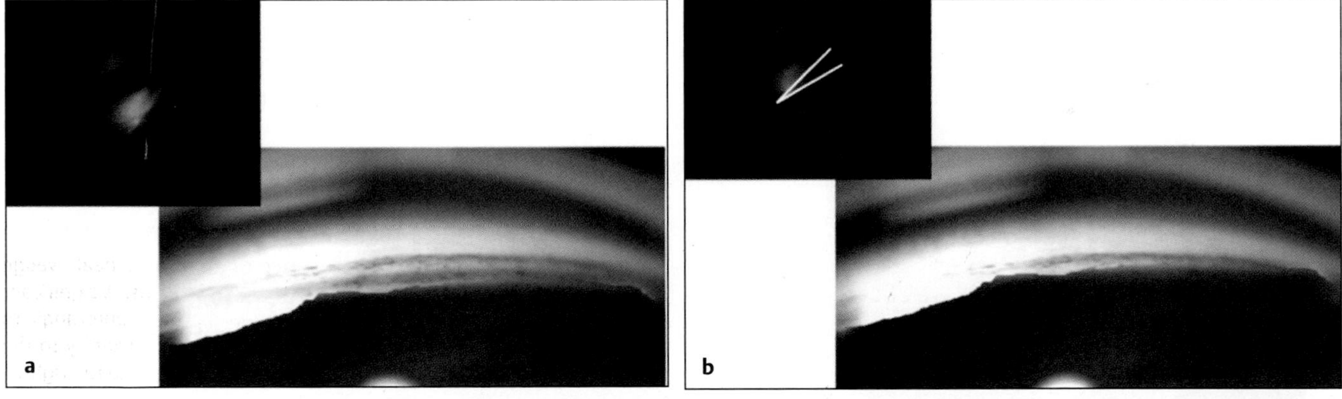

Fig. 3.7 (a) A narrow angle viewed in primary position does not allow visualization of the ciliary body band and scleral spur as seen in an open angle (**Fig. 3.4**). Also, a part of the posterior trabecular meshwork is obscured by a possible synechiae. **(b)** A very steep iris with a very narrow angle obscures the posterior trabecular meshwork all around, also obscuring the anterior trabecular meshwork around the circumference.

With a patient looking straight ahead and the gonioscope placed centrally, a wide open angle shows all structures, while a steeper iris and a narrow angle will obscure the more posterior structures. If >180 degrees of the posterior trabecular meshwork is not visualized in primary gaze, i.e., a steep iris obscures the view, an occludable angle is diagnosed (**Fig. 3.7a, b**).

Grading Systems for Gonioscopy

Grading of gonioscopy is done to determine features such as angle recess, or iridotrabecular angle, and iris configuration that help determine the type of glaucoma in the patient being seen. The iridotrabecular angle is estimated clinically from the angle formed by an edge of the slit-lamp beam, between the most peripheral cornea and a tangent to the iris (**Fig. 3.8**).

There are many grading systems for gonioscopy, with the simplest being *Shaffer's* grading that relies on the anterior chamber *angle, estimated by a tangent drawn on the surface of the midperipheral iris to a tangent on the trabecular meshwork* (**Fig. 3.9** and **Table 3.2**). *Spaeth's* classification looks at other features to corroborate the angle measured,

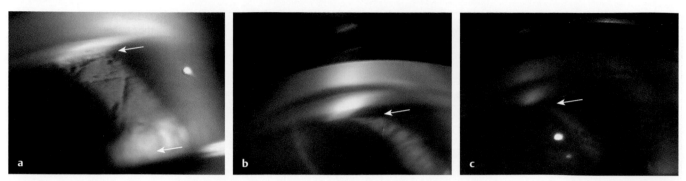

Fig. 3.8 Estimating the iridocorneal angle by following one edge of the light beam (*white arrow*): **(a)** 40 degrees, **(b)** 20 degrees, and **(c)** less than 10 degrees.

Table 3.2 Shaffer's system for grading angle widths

Grade number	Angle width	Description	Structures visible	Risk of closure
4	45–35°	Wide open	SL to CB	Impossible
3	35–20°	Wide open	SL to SS	Impossible
2	20°	Narrow	SL to TM	Possible
1	≤10°	Extremely narrow	SL only	Probable
Slit	Slit	Narrowed to slit	SL maybe	Probable
0	0°	Closed	SL maybe	Closed

Abbreviations: CB, ciliary body; SL, Schwalbe's line; SS, scleral spur; TM, trabecular meshwork.

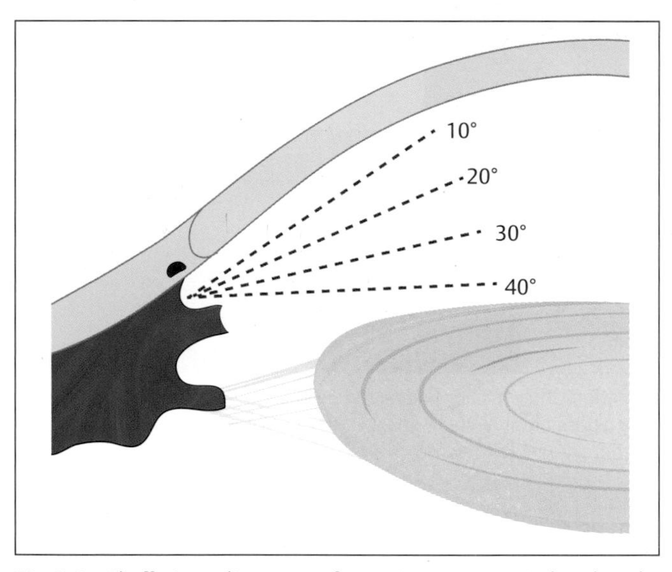

Fig. 3.9 Shaffer's grading system for gonioscopy using iridotrabecular angle. Less than 20 degrees being more likely to develop angle closure.

noting iris configuration and other abnormalities on the trabecular meshwork (**Figs. 3.10** and **3.11** and **Table 3.3**).

These were formulated for populations with largely open angles. In India there is a large percentage of population with a narrow angle and *evidence and extent of iridotrabecular contact must be added.*

Techniques to Visualize Angle Structures in a Narrow Angle

For populations as in India where about a third of the population may have narrow angles, it is necessary to be able to visualize the trabecular meshwork for any abnormalities, even in the presence of a steep convexity of the iris. In such a situation there are two techniques that help: manipulation of the gonioscope and indentation with a four-mirror gonioscope (**Fig. 3.12**).

Manipulative Gonioscopy

On finding a narrow angle in primary position, i.e., iris obscuring the trabecular meshwork, the mirror can be slid toward the angle being visualized, or the patient can be asked to look in the direction of the mirror. This permits the observer to look over the "hill" of the iris into the angle.

Another way to help visualize structures in a narrow angle is to use the length of the light beam. The examination is started using a fine, bright, and short light beam at the angle to avoid the pupil. This allows an estimation of the angle width and the anterior-most structure is visualized. The light beam is then lengthened to reach the pupil, when the pupil constricts, flattening the iris and allowing a view of angle structures (**Fig. 3.13**).

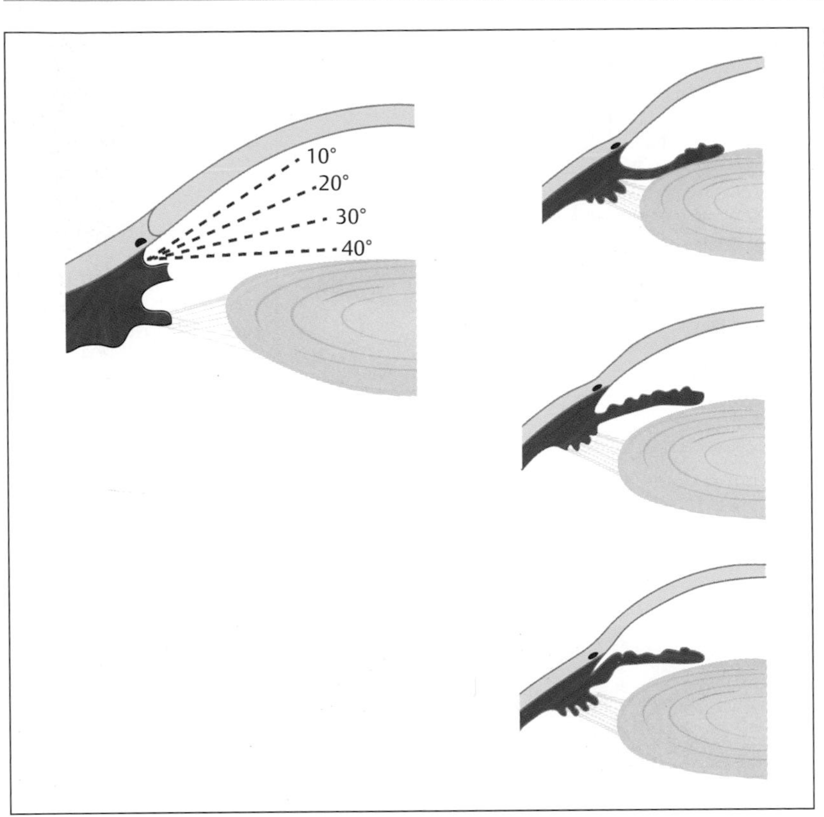

Fig. 3.10 Spaeth's classification system for gonioscopy. Iridotrabecular angle with iris configuration—concave, steep, and plateau.

Table 3.3 Spaeth's gonioscopic grading system

Angular approach	Peripheral iris		Pigmentation of posterior trabecular meshwork	Iris insertion
0 to 50 degrees	**r** regular	**f** flat	**0** no pigment	**A** Anterior to Schwalbe's line
	s steep	**b** bowed anteriorly	**1+** minimal	**B** Between Schwalbe's line and scleral spur
		p plateau iris	**2+** mild	**C** Scleral spur visible
	q queer	**c** concave	**3+** moderate	**D** Deep with ciliary body visible
			4+ intense	**E** Extremely deep with >1 mm of ciliary body visible

Note: Add presence and extent of peripheral anterior synechiae in India.

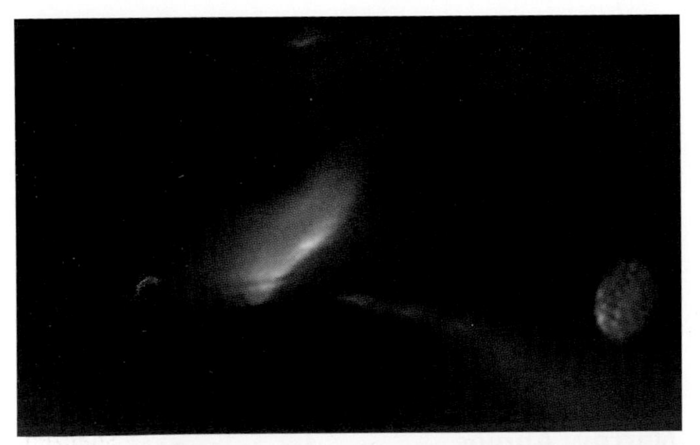

Fig. 3.11 Spaeth's system in an eye: angular width of 30 degrees, and iris configuration, slightly steep. The level of iris insertion, synechiae, pigmentation, or other abnormality can be identified only after manipulation.

Indentation Gonioscopy

A four-mirror gonioscope such as Posner, Sussman, or Zeiss has a diameter less than that of the cornea. Therefore, when the cornea is indented by these, central aqueous is displaced into the periphery, pushing the iris backward and allowing visualization of the trabecular meshwork over a flattened iris. The lens should be applied carefully and lightly, just till air in the tear film disappears. Central indentation requires some expertise to stabilize the view and keep just enough pressure on the cornea so that folds do not appear. This is a dynamic procedure by which *iridocorneal apposition, just contact*, can be differentiated from *iridocorneal adhesions, PAS* (**Fig. 3.14**).

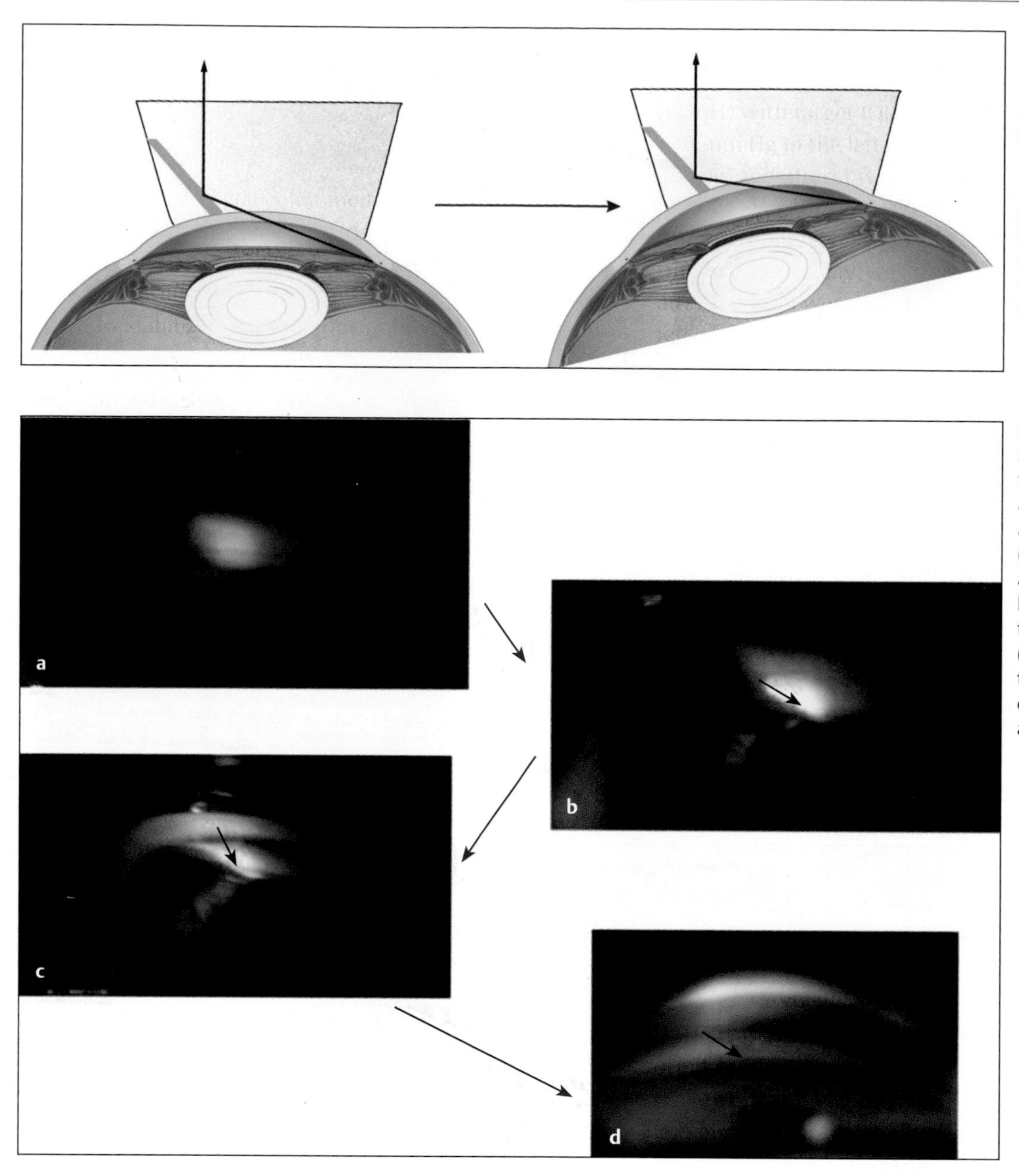

Fig. 3.12 Manipulative gonioscopy. A steep iris obscures visualization of trabecular meshwork in a narrow angle. Moving the indirect gonioscope toward the angle being observed or asking the patient to look toward the mirror allows the observer to look over the iris, into the angle recess in most cases.

Fig. 3.13 **(a)** Using a short, 2-mm slit away from the pupil to estimate angular width and view anterior-most structure. **(b)** Increasing the length and then width of the beam to reach the pupil, thereby flattening the iris. **(c, d)** Widening the beam to view up to 120 degrees of the angle. (*Black arrows* are at Schwalbe's line.)

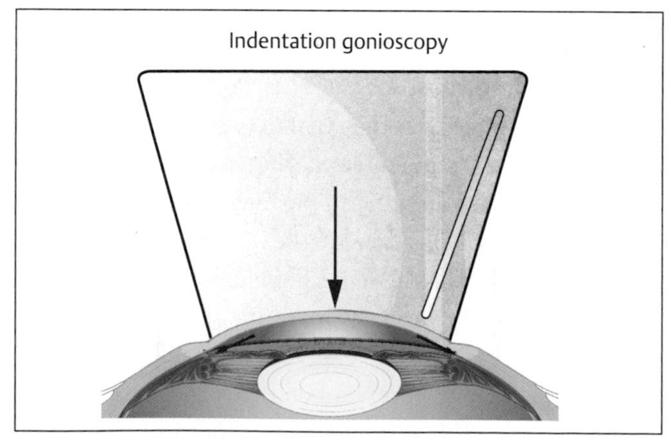

Fig. 3.14 Dynamic gonioscopy. A gonioscope with a diameter less than the cornea can be used to push central aqueous peripherally, and thereby iris posteriorly, exposing angle structures.

Commonly Encountered Gonioscopic Patterns

Open Angle

An *anterior chamber angle of >20 degrees* allows visualization of the trabecular meshwork surface and angle closure is unlikely to occur. Anomalies such as iris processes and abnormalities such as pigmentation, debris, and recession may be seen and documented (**Figs. 3.15–3.21**).

Narrow Angles

In India *narrow angles, <20 degrees*, are very common, as is the prevalence of primary angle-closure glaucoma (PACG).

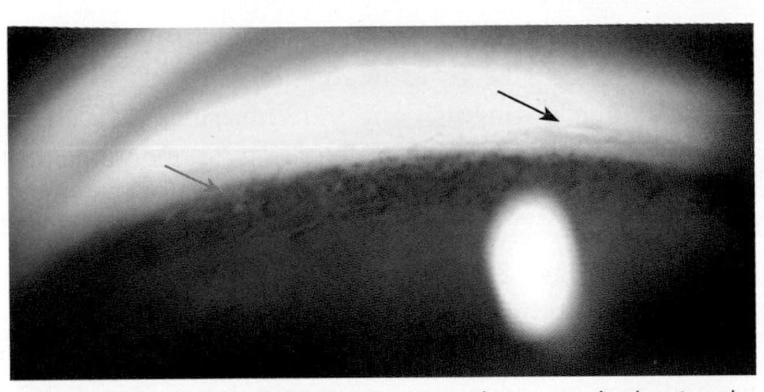

Fig. 3.15 Gonioscopic picture of a normal open angle showing the Schwalbe's line above and the gray brown ciliary body band inferiorly. *Blue arrow* is at the ciliary body band and the *black arrow* at Schwalbe's line.

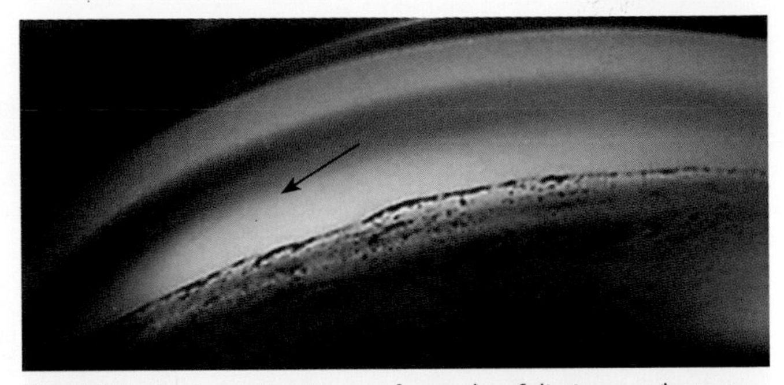

Fig. 3.16 Gonioscopic picture of pseudoexfoliation syndrome: an open angle showing a line of pigment anterior to Schwalbe's line (*black arrow*), Sampaolesi's line, and a moderately pigmented, stippled trabecular meshwork with the *gray brown* ciliary body band inferiorly.

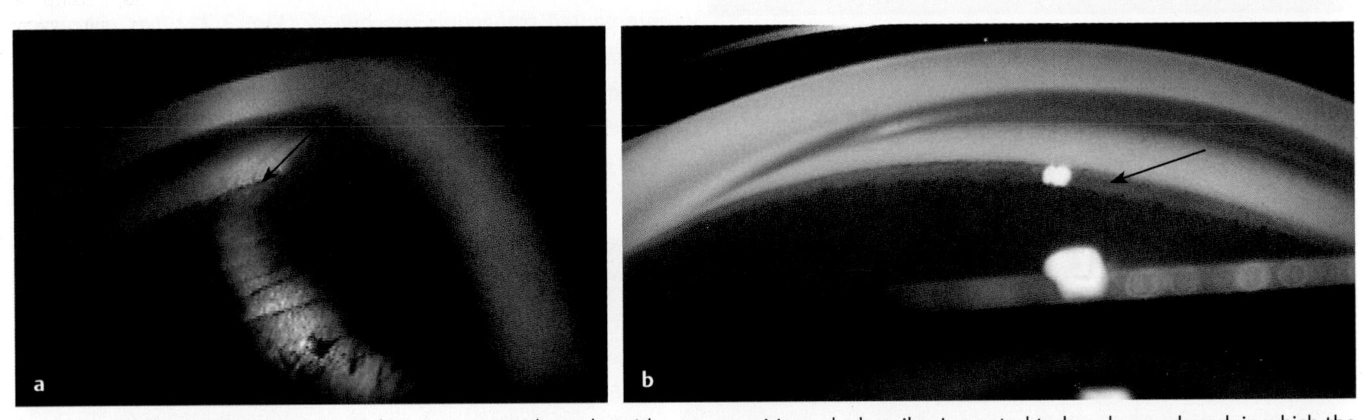

Fig. 3.17 **(a)** Pigment dispersion syndrome: a very wide angle, with a concave iris, and a heavily pigmented trabecular meshwork in which the individual structures cannot be identified (*black arrow*). **(b)** Moderate pigmentation of an open angle. Schwalbe's line is highlighted with the *black arrow*.

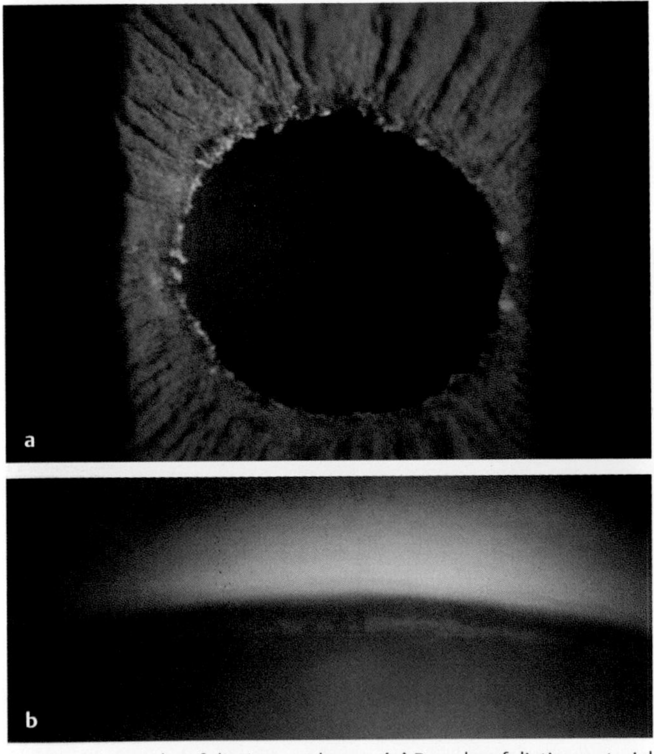

Fig. 3.18 Pseudoexfoliation syndrome: **(a)** Pseudoexfoliative material at the pupil. **(b)** An open angle showing a highly pigmented, trabecular meshwork and scleral spur inferiorly.

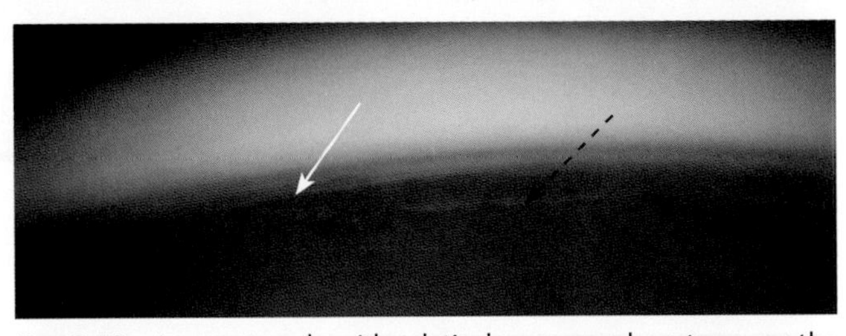

Fig. 3.19 An open angle with relatively preserved anatomy on the extreme left, and pigmentation anterior to Schwalbe's line and on the trabecular meshwork. The gray ciliary body band can be seen to increase in width gradually from the left to the right (*white arrow*) with white sclera; a cyclodialysis (*dashed arrow*) is also visible posterior to it.

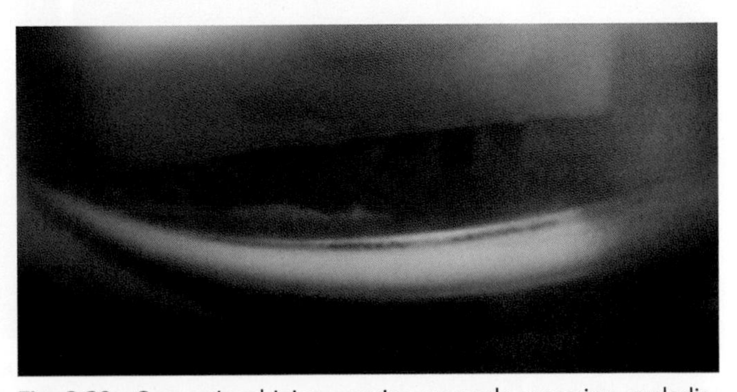

Fig. 3.20 Concussional injury causing an angle recession, cyclodialysis, and iridodialysis.

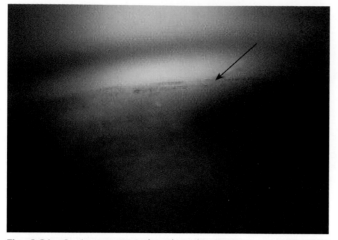

Fig. 3.21 Gonioscopy in iridocyclitis showing a translucency and moderate scattered trabecular pigmentation (*black arrow*), with a snow ball-like deposit seen.

It is therefore necessary for all ophthalmologists treating glaucoma to be able to estimate the iridocorneal angle (**Fig. 3.7**), and distinguish any *iridotrabecular apposition,* which can be relieved by indentation or manipulation (**Figs. 3.13** and **3.14**), from *PAS*, which are structural adhesions between the peripheral iris and trabecular meshwork (**Figs. 3.22** and **3.23**), or Schwalbe's line (**Fig. 3.24**). In chronic PACG, the iridotrabecular adhesions cover the entire trabecular meshwork, and cannot be pushed back by indentation or manipulation (**Fig. 3.25**). PAS also need to be differentiated from iris processes. *PAS appear as tented elevations of the peripheral iris, which are seen to bridge the angle recess and attach to a pigmented trabecular meshwork (***Fig. 3.22***). Iris processes, on the other hand, follow the contour of the angle wall and have no trabecular meshwork pigmentation*, as they are developmental anomalies seen frequently in congenital and juvenile open-angle glaucomas (**Fig. 3.26**).

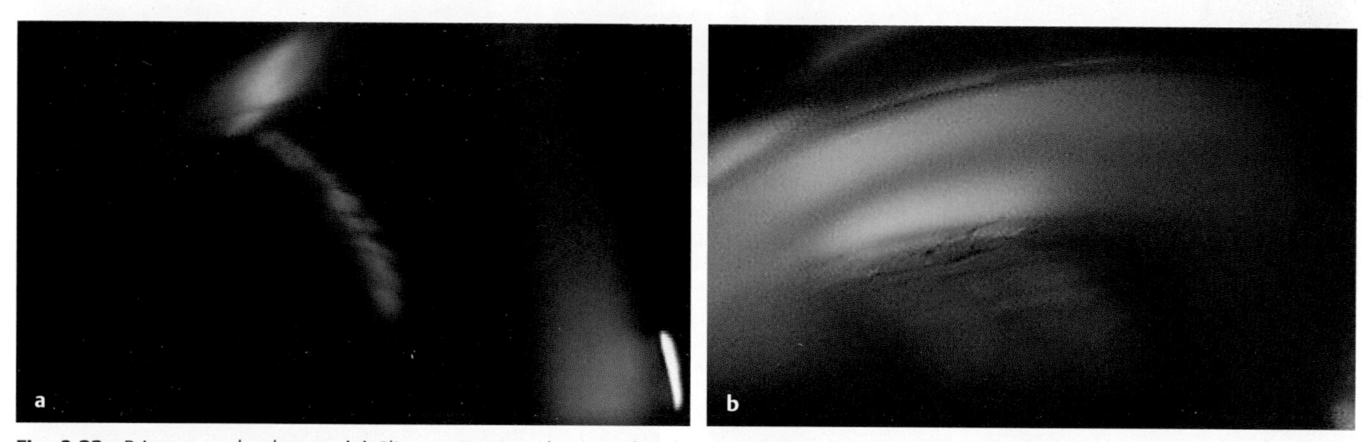

Fig. 3.22 Primary angle closure. **(a)** Slit examination showing the close proximity of the corneal wedge to the iris, and an angle width of approximately 15 degrees. **(b)** Blotchy pigment in the angle and a few filiform synechiae of past iridotrabecular contact are seen.

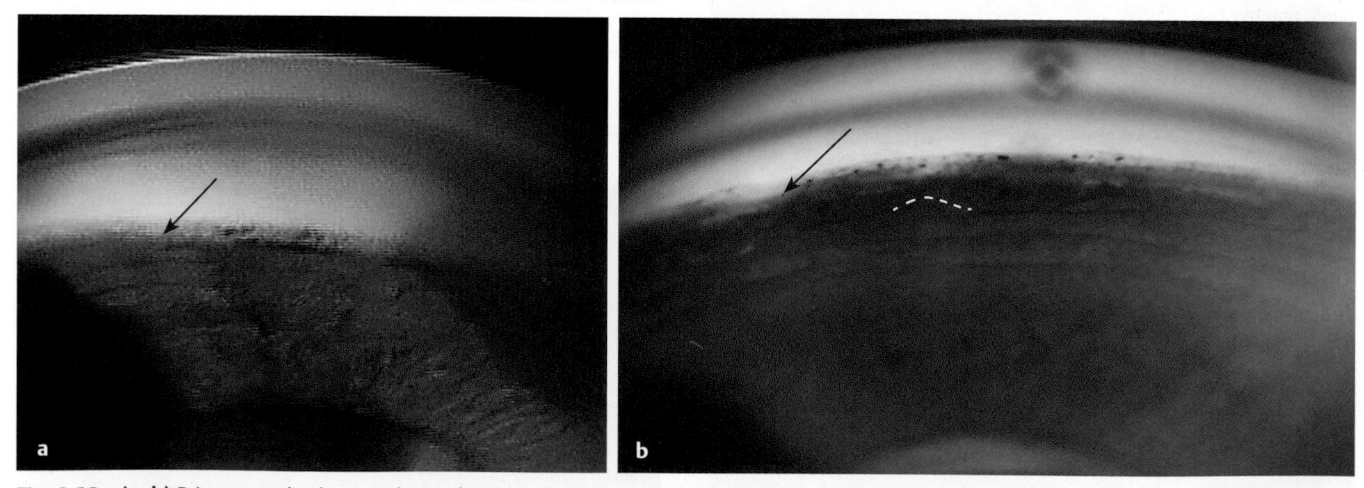

Fig. 3.23 **(a, b)** Primary angle closure. The angle width is approximately 20 degrees as seen by the edge of the beam, with blotchy pigment and some synechiae to the trabecular meshwork, goniosynechiae, tenting the iris up (*white dashed line*), but not extending to Schwalbe's line (*black arrows*).

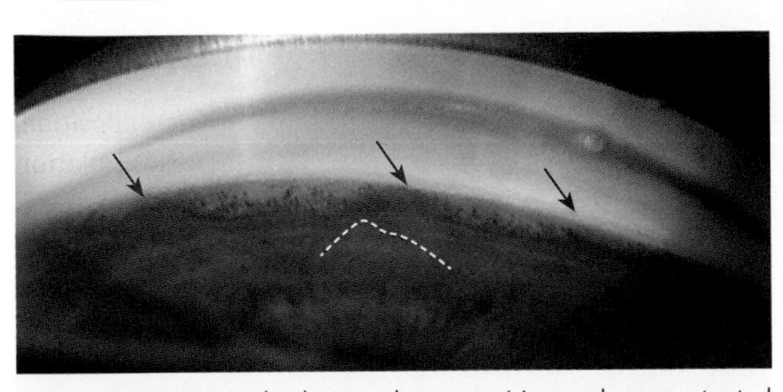

Fig. 3.24 Acute angle-closure glaucoma. Iris can be seen tented up (*white line*) and stuck to the trabecular meshwork, iridotrabecular or goniosynechiae (*black arrow*), and to Schwalbe's line, iridocorneal synechiae (*red arrows*).

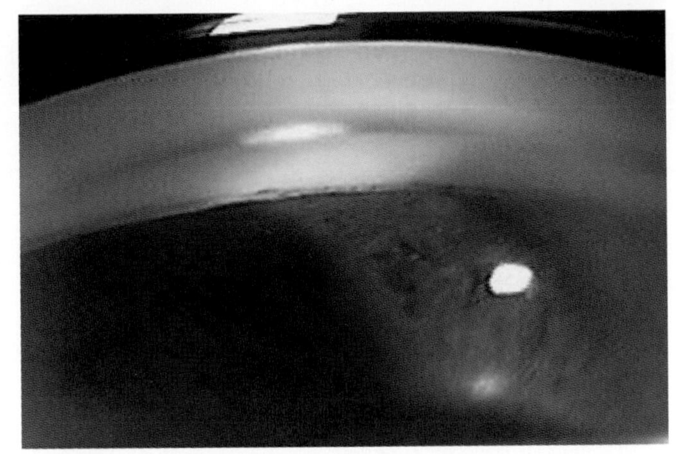

Fig. 3.25 Closed angle in primary angle-closure glaucoma (PACG). No dipping of the light beam between the steep iris and cornea was visible in this eye, signifying apposition or adhesion up to Schwalbe's line. On manipulation/indentation, the iris could not be separated due to extensive peripheral anterior synechiae (PAS). The mild pigmentation on the cornea could be mistaken for speckled pigmentation of the trabecular meshwork, and is known as a "false" angle.

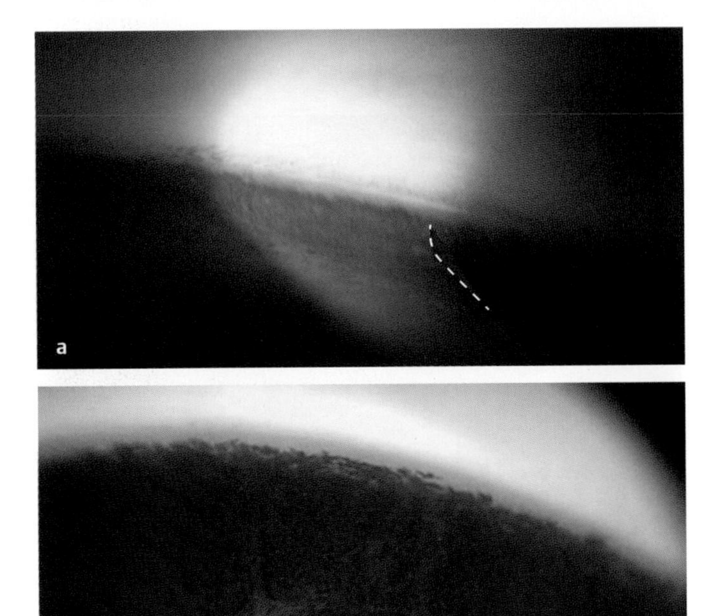

Fig. 3.26 (a) Primary congenital glaucoma. Iris can be seen to be wrapped around the angle recess along the wall (*white dashed line*), reaching almost up to Schwalbe's line. **(b)** Primary congenital glaucoma. Iris processes can be seen on the trabecular meshwork.

Fig. 3.27 Plateau iris. An eye with a narrow angle width, approximately 15 degrees, being indented to show a double hump pattern. The peripheral hump is caused by ciliary processes pushing up the iris, and the central is due to the lens.

A *plateau iris configuration* is seen with a flat iris, having a shallow anterior chamber peripherally but relatively normal centrally. This is caused by the upward push of peripheral iris by anteriorly rotated ciliary processes, approximating the iris to trabecular meshwork. Indentation in such eyes leads to a double hump appearance—peripheral hump due to ciliary process pushing upwards and central hump due to the lens (**Fig. 3.27**).

Secondary Glaucomas and Miscellaneous Angle Abnormalities

A rise in IOP is caused by obstruction to outflow of aqueous, and gonioscopy allows a broad differentiation between angle-closure and open-angle secondary pathologies. Further detailed evaluation *provides clues as to the possible cause*, against which appropriate therapy can be initiated, such as pseudoexfoliative material, inflammatory cells, traumatic damage, etc. (**Figs. 3.28–3.33**).

Recording Gonioscopy

A record of the gonioscopic picture seen is important, for justifying a diagnosis and its further treatment, and to be able to detect changes over time. Many diagrams have been suggested. One possible gonioscopy diagram has been suggested by Shaffer (**Fig. 3.34**).

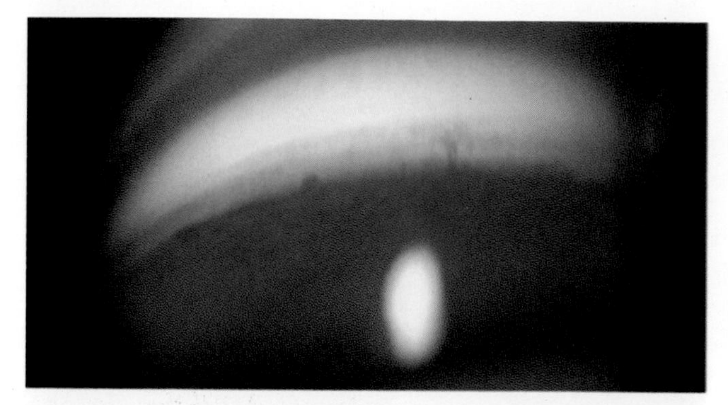

Fig. 3.28 Secondary open and angle closure. Gonioscopy illustrating neovascularization of the angle (NVA), crossing the scleral spur and trabecular meshwork. Early signs of iridotrabecular synechiae can be seen as well.

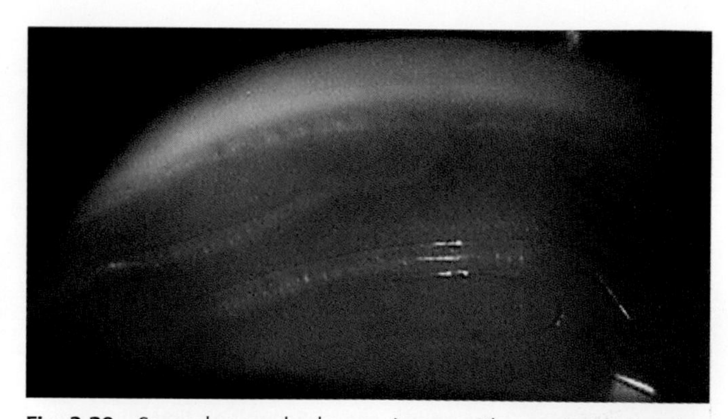

Fig. 3.29 Secondary angle closure. An eye with an anterior chamber intraocular lens (IOL) shows a highly pigmented trabecular meshwork and iridocorneal adhesions caused by the malposition of the haptic.

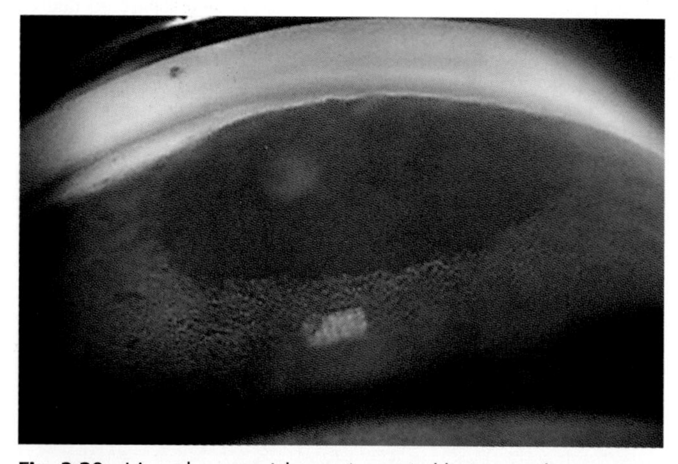

Fig. 3.30 Iris melanoma. A large pigmented lesion can be seen over the iris, which is extending into the angle up to the cornea.

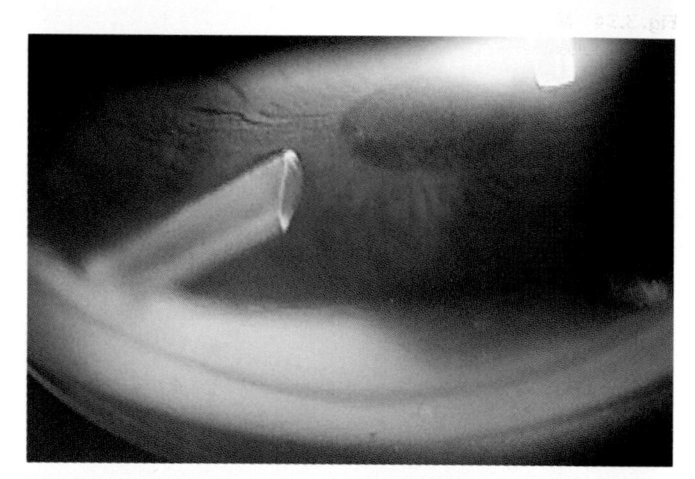

Fig. 3.31 Gonioscopy showing the placement of the tube of a glaucoma drainage device. This is rubbing on the iris, away from the cornea, and the opening is clear. There is evidence of pigment dispersal and healed iritis.

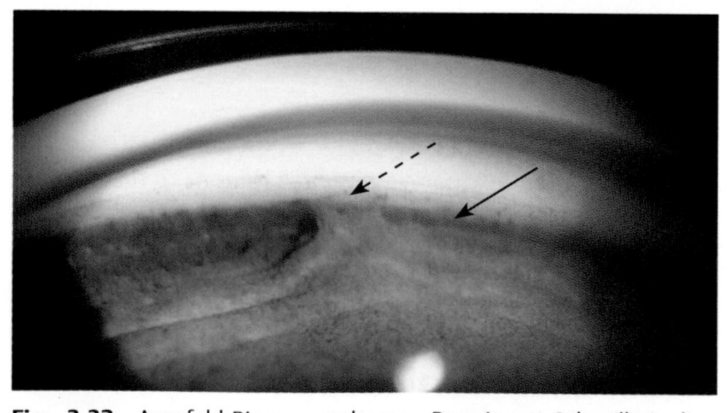

Fig. 3.32 Axenfeld-Rieger syndrome. Prominent Schwalbe's line (*black arrow*), with a midperipheral iridocorneal adhesion present (*dashed arrow*). Such developmental adhesions can be distinguished from acquired angle closure by the lack of pigment dispersal.

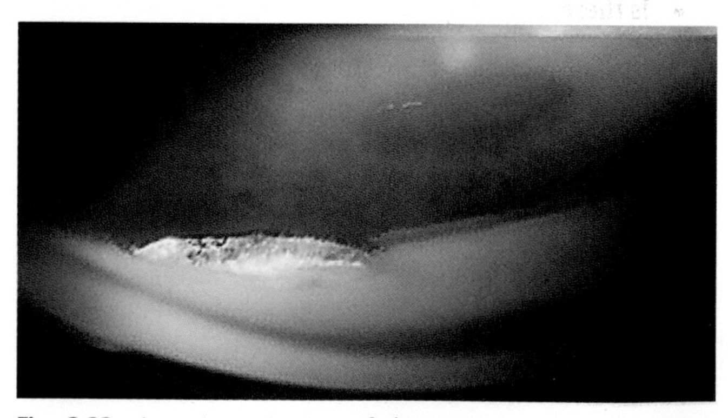

Fig. 3.33 A gonioscopic view of the internal ostium of a trabeculectomy showing an open ostium with no obstruction by iris, etc.

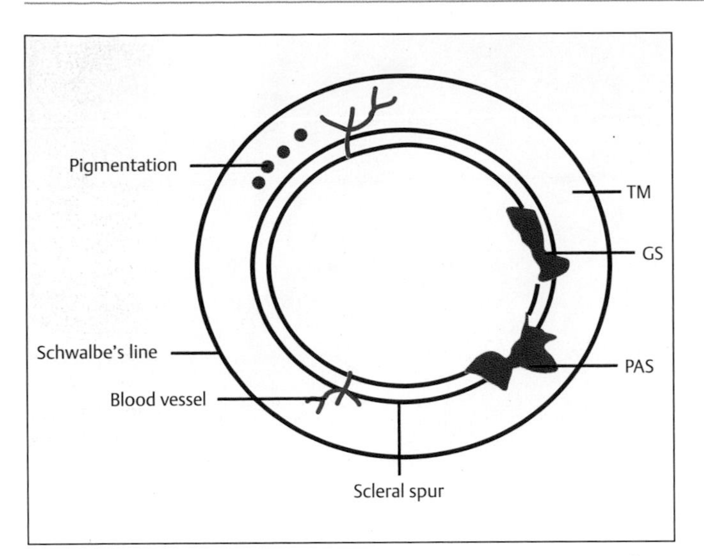

Fig. 3.34 Modified Shaffer gonioscopic diagram. GS, goniosynechiae; PAS, peripheral anterior synechiae; TM, trabecular meshwork.

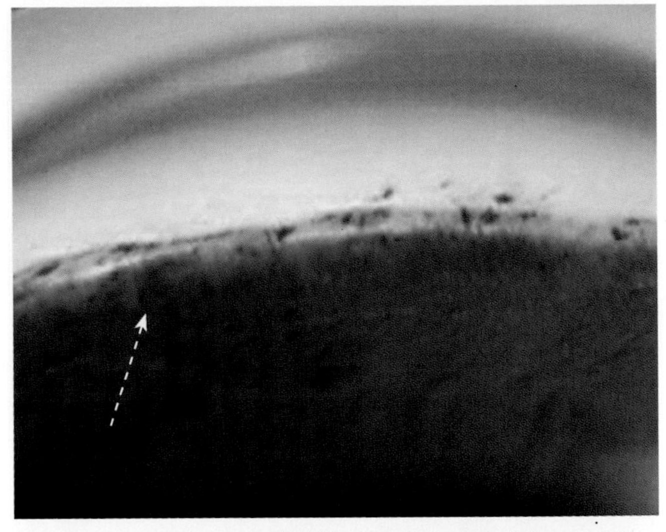

Case 1-1 The angle was occludable, and after manipulation, by asking the patient to look toward the mirror being observed, blotchy pigment is seen on the trabecular meshwork and anterior to Schwalbe's line. Few intermittent synechiae can be seen (*dashed arrow*), with a generalized increase in pigmentation of the posterior trabecular meshwork.

Cases

Case 1

A 60-year-old male diagnosed to have chronic glaucoma 10 years ago had a nasal step in both eyes. He was on regular treatment and follow-up, with IOPs recorded from 14 to 16 mm Hg. He was using an increasing number of medications over time, but continued to show visual field progression.

Points to consider

- Is the patient compliant?
- Has target IOP been achieved?
- Is the diagnosis correct?
- Is there tolerance to medications?
- Are there ongoing gonioscopic changes?

Diagnosis and Management

On doing a gonioscopy, an angle recess of 15 degrees with PAS of >180 degrees was seen (**Case 1-1**). An iridotomy done at first diagnosis could have prevented progression of PAS in a narrow angle, and the progressive increase in IOP, medications, and visual field defects over time.

Case 2

A 62-year-old man presented after noticing a diminution of vision in his left eye. The anterior chambers were deep and optic nerve head examination showed an almost total cupping in the left eye with a thin and pale neuroretinal rim, and 0.5:1 cup in the right with normal rim color. IOPs were 12 and 32 mm Hg.

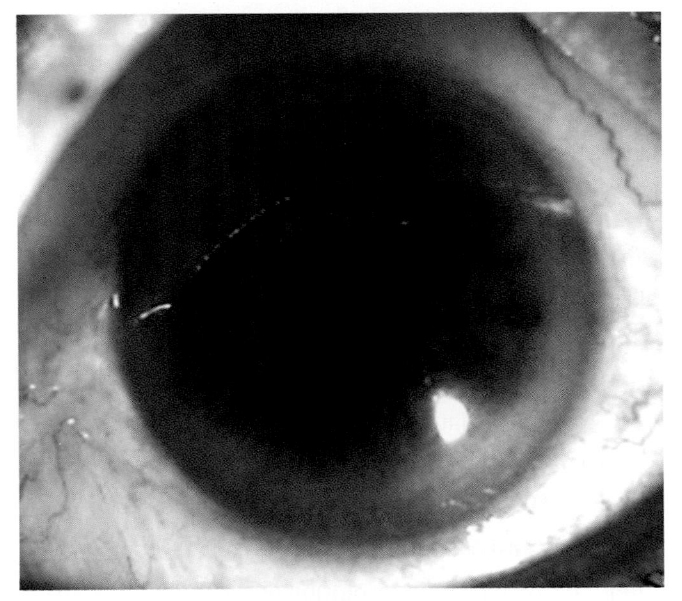

Case 2-1 Irregularity and mild dilation of the pupil is seen from 2 to 7 o'clock.

Point to consider

- Primary open-angle glaucoma (POAG) does not present with such asymmetry, so secondary glaucomas should be kept in mind.

Diagnosis and Management

Minimal irregularity of the pupil was seen in the left eye, and gonioscopy revealed an angle recession of 240 degrees in the left eye. Therefore a diagnosis of left traumatic glaucoma was made (**Cases 2-1** and **2-2**).

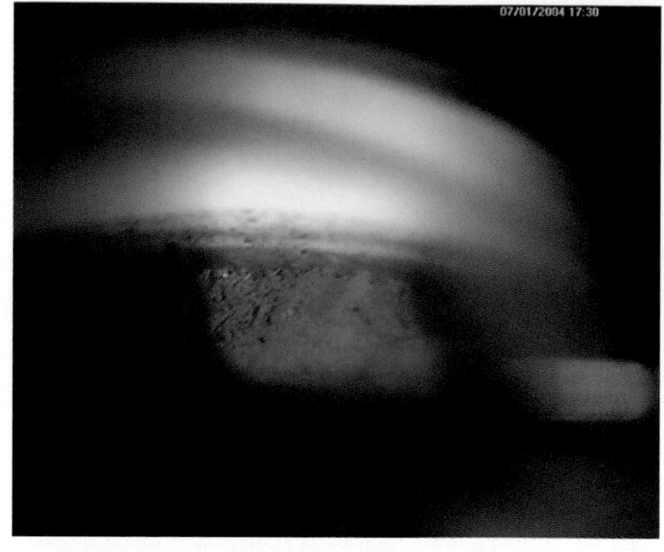

Case 2-2 Inferior angle showing a relatively intact angle to the left of the photograph, with a gradual widening of the ciliary body band toward the right, an angle recession.

Case 3

A 25-year-old male presented with pain and diminution of vision in the left eye. He had no significant past history. On examination there was ciliary congestion inferiorly, corneal edema, and an IOP of 42 mm Hg, with a visual acuity of 6/60. After maximal medical therapy of bimatoprost, timolol, brimonidine, Diamox 250 mg Q8 hourly, and syrup glycerol 1 oz Q8 hourly, the cornea cleared the next day and a gonioscopy could be done.

Points to consider

- Unilateral glaucoma in a young male.
- Juvenile open-angle glaucoma (JOAG) or a secondary glaucoma could be considered.

Diagnosis and Management

After control of IOP and resolution of corneal edema, an iris hole was visible at 6 o'clock. Gonioscopy showed PAS from 4 to 7 o'clock, and pigmentation anterior to Schwalbe's line. A glass foreign body could be seen in the angle, suggesting a diagnosis of traumatic foreign body with chronic uveitis and secondary glaucoma (**Case 3-1**).

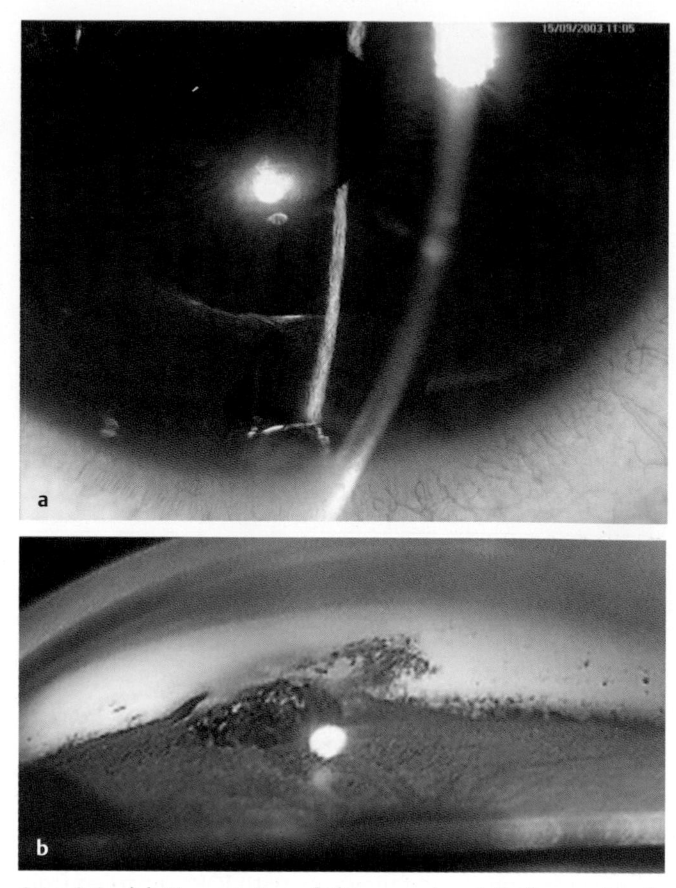

Case 3-1 **(a)** Pigmentation of the corneal endothelium, refractile object, and an iris hole at 6 o'clock. **(b)** Gonioscopy showing endothelial pigmentation, glass foreign body, and peripheral anterior synechiae on either side of an iris defect.

Case 4

A 54-year-old lady presented for a routine evaluation and gave a family history of glaucoma. On examination a peripherally shallow anterior chamber was seen to be present, with a cup:disc ratio of 0.7:1 and 0.6:1 in right and left eye and IOPs of 18 and 20 mm Hg, respectively. Gonioscopy showed a recess of 15 degrees and blotchy pigment on the trabecular meshwork.

Points to consider

- Possibility of primary angle-closure disease (PACD), wherein a smaller size of optic nerve head may be present, and in which even a cup:disc ratio of 0.5/0.6 is significant.
- neuroretinal rim irregularity or pallor should be looked for.

Diagnosis and Management

The patient was reexamined and an inferotemporal notch in the right eye with neuroretinal rim pallor was recorded. A corresponding narrow retinal nerve fiber layer defect was seen (**Case 4-1**). A superior nasal step field defect was present in the right eye.

The patient was diagnosed to have PACG with mild glaucomatous neuropathy, and an iridotomy was done, followed by diurnal phasing 2 weeks later. IOP was 14 to 24 mm Hg. She was advised a prostaglandin analog at bedtime in both eyes, 6 monthly review, and imaging.

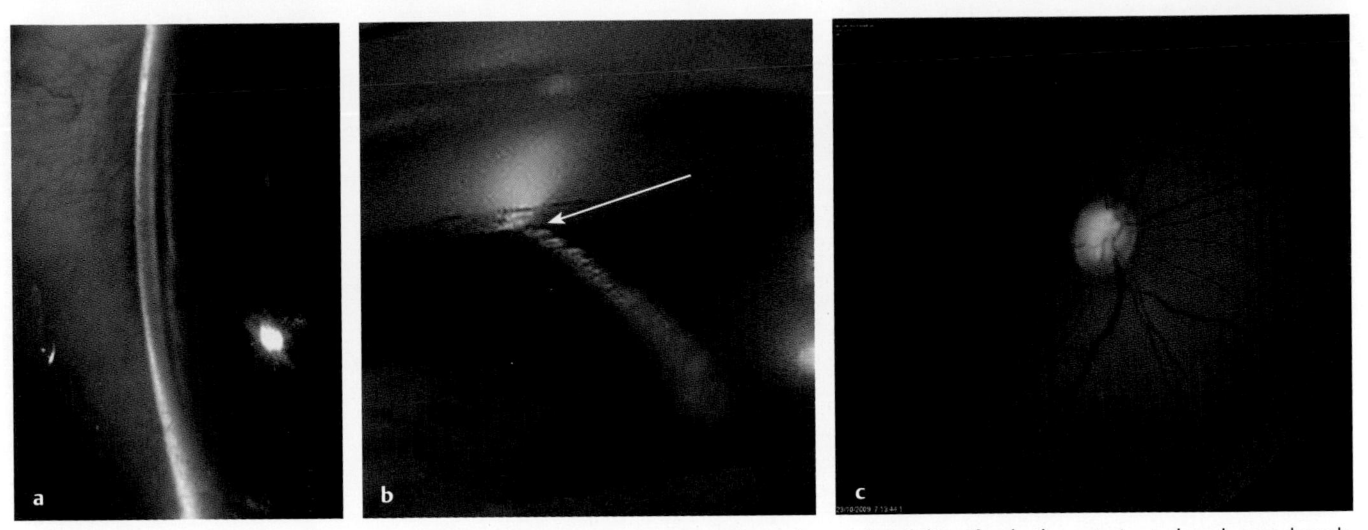

Case 4-1 **(a)** van Herick grade 2. **(b)** Gonioscopy showing a convex iris configuration, and visibility of only the anterior trabecular meshwork. Scattered, blotchy pigmentation of the trabecular meshwork and also anterior to Schwalbe's line (*white arrow*) is seen. **(c)** Small optic nerve head with a notch at 7 o'clock seen on careful noting of the contour cup. There is a narrow retinal nerve fiber layer defect corresponding to this neuroretinal rim loss.

Suggested Readings

Atlas of gonioscopy. www.gonioscopy.org

Alward W. Color atlas of gonioscopy. Barcelona: Mosby-Wolfe; 1994

Alward WL. A history of gonioscopy. Optom Vis Sci. 2011 Jan;88(1):29–35

Foster PJ, Devereux JG, Alsbirk PH, et al. Detection of gonioscopically occludable angles and primary angle closure glaucoma by estimation of limbal chamber depth in Asians: modified grading scheme. Br J Ophthalmol 2000;84(2):186–192

Shaffer RN. Primary glaucomas: gonioscopy, ophthalmoscopy and perimetry. Trans Am Acad Ophthalmol Otolaryngol 1960; 64:112–127

Smith SD, Singh K, Lin SC, et al. Evaluation of the anterior chamber angle in glaucoma: a report by the American Acade-my of Ophthalmology. Ophthalmology. 2013;120(10):1985–1997

Spaeth GL. Gonioscopy: uses old and new. The inheritance of occludable angles. Ophthalmology 1978;85(3):222–232

van Herick W, Shaffer RN, Schwartz A. Estimation of width of angle of anterior chamber. Incidence and significance of the narrow angle. Am J Ophthalmol 1969;68(4):626–629

Wojciechowski R, Congdon N, Anninger W, Teo Broman A. Age, gender, biometry, refractive error, and the anterior chamber angle among Alaskan Eskimos. Ophthalmology 2003;110(2): 365–375

CHAPTER 4

Perimetry in Glaucoma

Overview

- Kinetic Perimetry
- Static Perimetry
  - Reading a Single Field
  - Printouts of Different Perimeters
  - Diagnosing a Glaucomatous Scotoma on Standard Automated Perimetry
  - Patterns of Visual Field Loss Seen in Glaucoma
  - Perimetric Artifacts
  - Nonglaucomatous Causes of an Arcuate Scotoma
- Illustrating the Reading of a Single Visual Field
- Cases
- Suggested Readings

Introduction

The *visual field is defined as the area perceived simultaneously by a fixating eye*. Perimetry records the sum of all directions from which the eye may perceive visual stimulation at a defined moment in time and documents perception of this stimulation.

Using perimetry one can evaluate and quantify the visual field using targets of various sizes, illumination, and colors. *Perimetry depends upon responses provided by the patient, and is therefore a subjective test, with many variables*. The first fields recorded need to be interpreted with caution, as they appear to improve as the patient "learns" to respond more accurately to stimuli. Perimetry has advanced over the years to become more standardized, with as few variables as possible, as in automated static perimetry.

The ability to detect a spot of light against a uniformly illuminated background is called differential light sensitivity at a given point of the retina. It is highest at the macula and gradually decreases toward the periphery, with recordings across the retina forming a "hill of vision." It varies with the size and illumination of the spot and background, and is documented in numeroalphabetical notations or decibels (dB) (**Fig. 4.1a, b**). Perimetry is commonly done with a white target, but when recorded with a blue on yellow target it is about 10 degrees less and with a red on green target 20 degrees constricted as compared to a white target. These are necessary for patients having neuritis, toxic neuropathy, or chloroquine retinopathy.

Two techniques are commonly used:

- Kinetic: A target is slowly moved in front of the eye to map out the extended area where it is seen.
- Static: This is more standardized and graded, with stimuli of different luminance projected at the same position to *ascertain differential light sensitivity*, at points of the retina, with additional information of depth and area of the field.

Kinetic Perimetry

This is a simple and adaptable method of evaluating the visual field, in the hands of a trained operator. The patient has to be carefully explained the procedure as he/she may not understand what is required of him/her, or may find it difficult to respond.

Kinetic perimetry was initially described using a Bjerrum screen, and was further standardized by Goldmann using a half sphere with standard background illumination of 31.5 apostilbs, and a movable arm with a light of variable illumination and size.

The patient has one eye occluded, and is asked to keep his or her chin on the chin rest throughout the test. He or she is asked to fix on the central white dot/light with the eye under observation, and press a buzzer when the target is *clearly seen, not just a blur*. The target is moved from the periphery along a meridian until the patient responds (**Fig. 4.2**). A reverse movement from seeing to nonseeing can be used to more clearly delineate the edge of the visual field. Such points are recorded across all meridians, and represent points of a given retinal sensitivity. A line drawn through all these points is an isopter, designated by the size and illumination of the target used, e.g., I4e. *The largest and brightest target will have the largest isopter and the dimmest the smallest one.* Patients with good vision should have their field assessed with I4e target, while those with poor vision, up to 6/60, can have V4e utilized

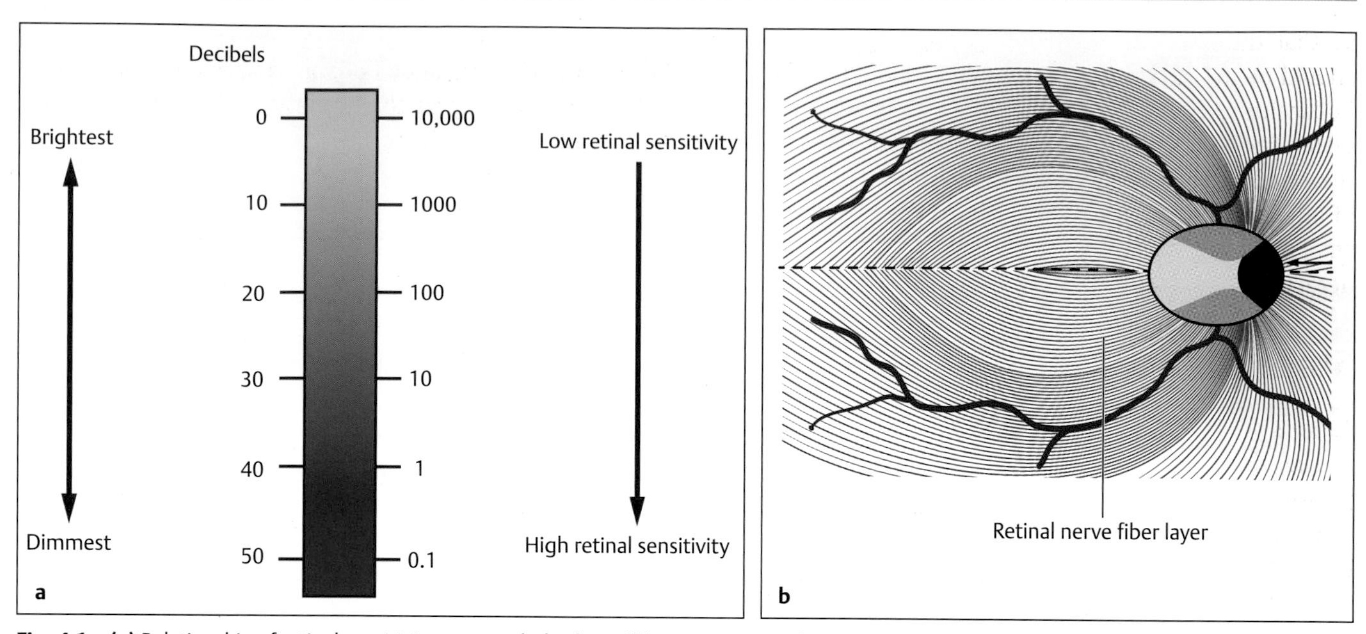

Fig. 4.1 **(a)** Relationship of retinal sensitivity to recorded values. **(b)** Arrangement of nerve fiber layers in the optic nerve and retina.

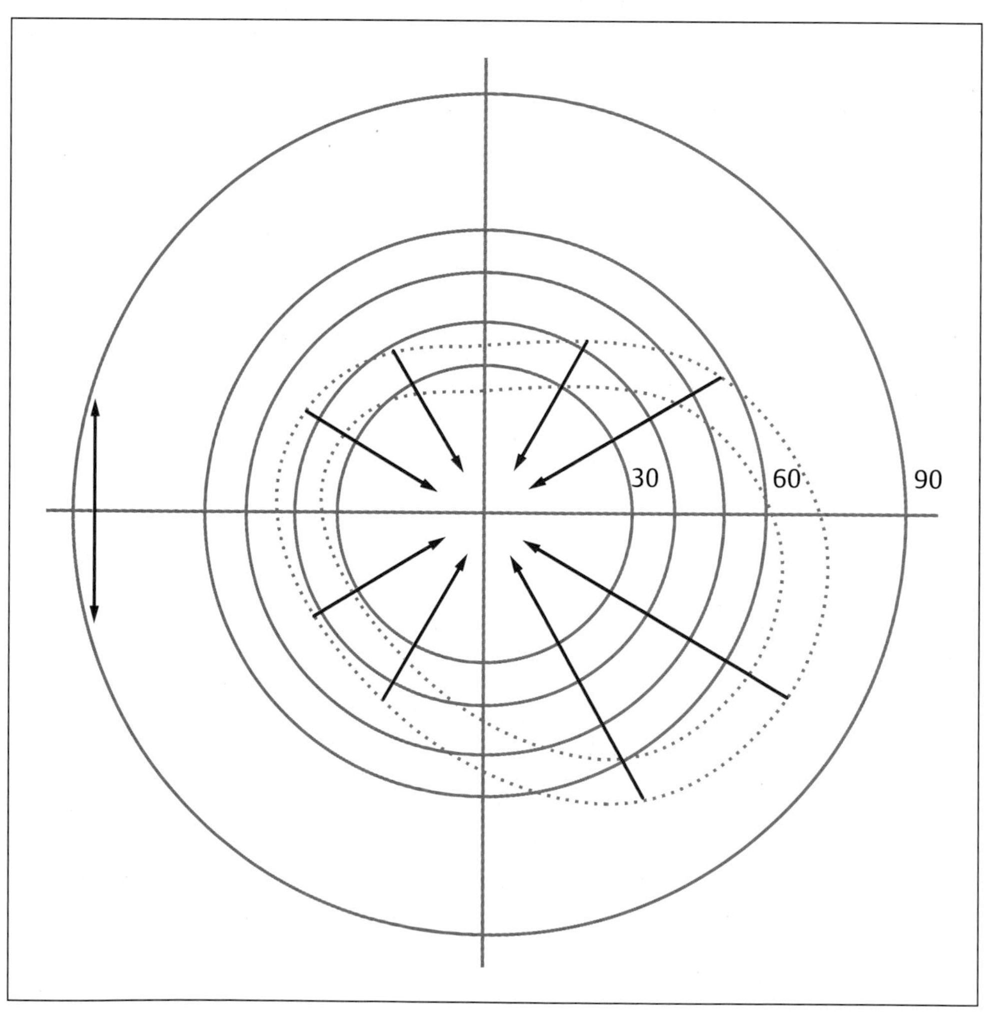

Fig. 4.2 Directions of movement of a target in kinetic perimetry for glaucoma, periphery to the center and across the nasal raphe.

so that the field can still be recorded. The white target should be moved up to fixation in all meridians to detect nonseeing areas within the field as well. These are again tested from seeing to nonseeing and the reverse to map out the scotomas. Absolute scotomas are detected by targets of all sizes, but relative scotomas are detected only with smaller and dimmer targets. Kinetic perimetry may fail to detect relative scotomas.

Static Perimetry

Targets of different luminance can be projected anywhere in the visual field in a random fashion, obviating false-positive responses, such as in kinetic perimetry where the sameor adjacent meridian is tested and the patient soon becomes aware of this. Randomization used in automated perimeters has made perimetry less dependent on trained technicians, and is more accurate and reproducible.

Automated perimeters allow a constant monitoring of fixation, retest abnormal points automatically, and can be customized to look at specific areas of the field of interest. *The most commonly used standard automated perimeter (SAP) uses a white-on-white stimulus.*

A number of strategies are possible, the most common being the following:

- *Suprathreshold for screening*: Targets of supranormal luminance, which would be visible to normal people, but would not be seen in areas having moderate to severe loss of sensitivity are presented. Points are recorded by the machine as "seen" or "not seen." This would not be able to detect mild loss of function.
- *Threshold strategy*: At each point, targets of increasing and decreasing luminance are randomly projected till just visible, to ascertain the differential light sensitivity at each locus. A *"staircase" strategy* increases light intensity in larger steps of 4 dB, and then fine tunes the sensitivity measurement by decreasing intensity in smaller steps of 2 dB. *Sensitivity measurements indicating that the patient has seen the stimulus 50% of the time are recorded.*

The algorithms test 50 to 100 spots, in grids that are 3 to 6 degrees apart, on or straddling the vertical and horizontal meridians.

- *Swedish interactive threshold algorithm* (SITA): On Humphrey field analyzer (HFA), it uses Bayesian statistics and predetermined normal and glaucomatous thresholds for each locus and interpoint correlations, so that the time for bracketing at each point is reduced. It dynamically monitors patient's responses and compares them with adjacent areas. SITA automatically postprocesses information to provide a likelihood of abnormality. Use of listening windows rather than repeat catch trials also helps decrease test duration.
- *Tendency oriented perimetry* (TOP): TOP, which is available on Octopus style perimeters, similarly estimates thresholds using information of adjacent loci and bracketing, to reduce duration of testing.

The patient is seated at a half sphere or screen with appropriate lens correction for near, on a chin rest, with one eye occluded. He or she is asked to fixate at a central light. In case of macular pathology, the patient can be asked to fixate at the center of a diamond of lights (**Fig. 4.3**). The patient is demonstrated a few targets in the field and is counseled to maintain constant central fixation. On perception of a light stimulus randomly presented at any point, a buzzer has to be pressed, to record sensitivity, and the next target can then be projected. The test can be paused in case the patient is fatigued.

The program starts with *4 seed locations in each quadrant, 13 degrees from fixation*, and then progresses randomly around the field. If the patient gets fatigued or inattentive, a clover leaf pattern is seen on the pattern deviation plot and grayscale (**Fig. 4.4**). The testing can be done for various extended areas of the visual field and with a larger or smaller number of stimuli and can also be customized (**Table 4.1**).

Fixation is monitored by different means in perimeters. In the Heijl-Krakau method, the stimulus is projected on the blind spot randomly. If the patient responds, it is because the eye has been moved, and this is recorded as a fixation loss. Gaze tracking monitors eye movements by monitoring the corneal reflection, and records even small movements over the test duration, providing a measure of the quality of fixation. The Octopus perimeter uses a video monitor display and an automatic eye tracking system. However, these do not quantify or identify the direction of fixation losses.

Once the test is complete, the sensitivity of the individual is compared to age-matched controls and a printout generated.

Reading a Single Field

Fig. 4.5 represents an example of Humphrey type perimeter single-field printout. **Flowchart 4.1** illustrates the algorithm for reading a single field.

Patient Parameters

First check that an *appropriate refractive correction for near* has been given and the patient has a *vision of at least 6/18.*

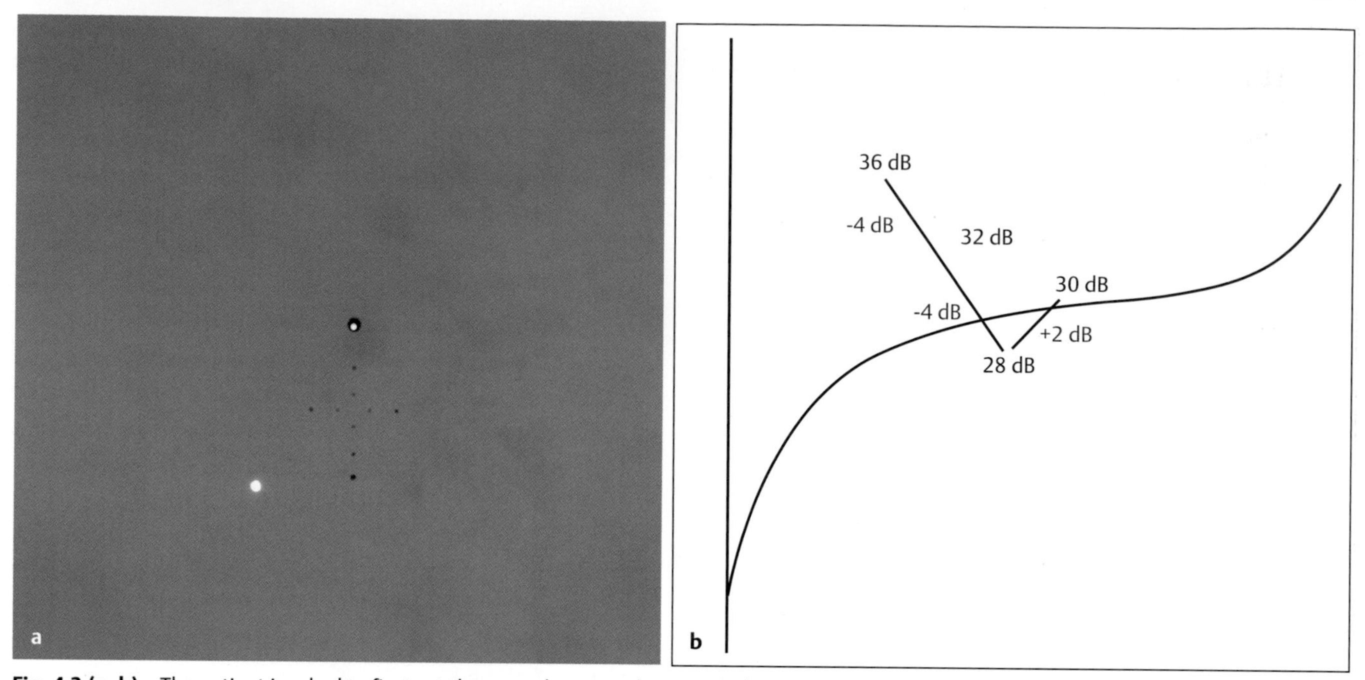

Fig. 4.3 (a, b) The patient is asked to fixate at the central spot, and respond when a stimulus is visible elsewhere.

Check that the date of birth is accurate as results are compared to age-matched normals. Pupils should be recorded as between 2 and 4 mm.

Test Parameters

The correct strategy should be chosen—30-2 or 24-2 for mild-to-moderate glaucoma and an additional 10-2 *is advised for all patients now to identify early involvement of the central field. In severe glaucoma with only a central island remaining, 24-2 and 30-2 test only 12 loci in the central 10 degrees, therefore a 10-2 program is used, and a macular threshold protocol may provide additional testing of 16 points in the central 5 degrees for very advanced glaucomas.*

Background illumination should be periodically calibrated. *Foveal threshold evaluation* provides a correlation with visual acuity, and a pointer to possible involvement of the central field.

Table 4.1 Testing strategies on Humphrey field analyzer

Threshold test	Extent of visual field tested	Number of loci tested
10-2	10 degrees	68-point grid
24-2	24 degrees	54-point grid
30-2	30 degrees	76-point grid
60-2	30–60 degrees	60-point grid
Full field 120	120 degrees	120 points

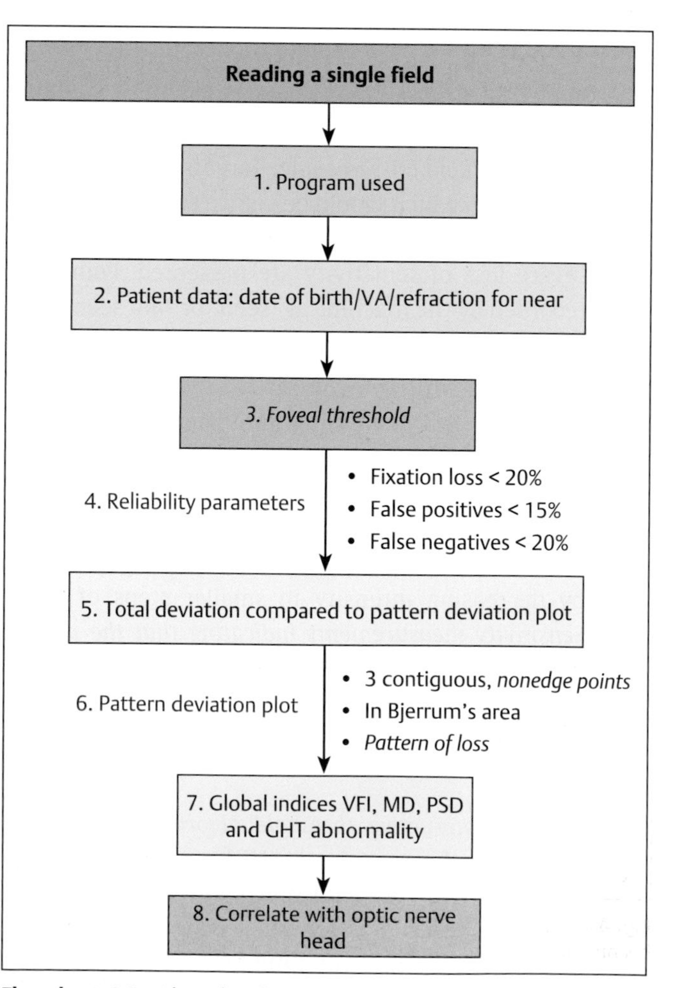

Flowchart 4.1 Algorithm for reading a single field. GHT, glaucoma hemifield test; MD, mean deviation; PSD, pattern standard deviation; VA, visual acuity; VFI, visual field index.

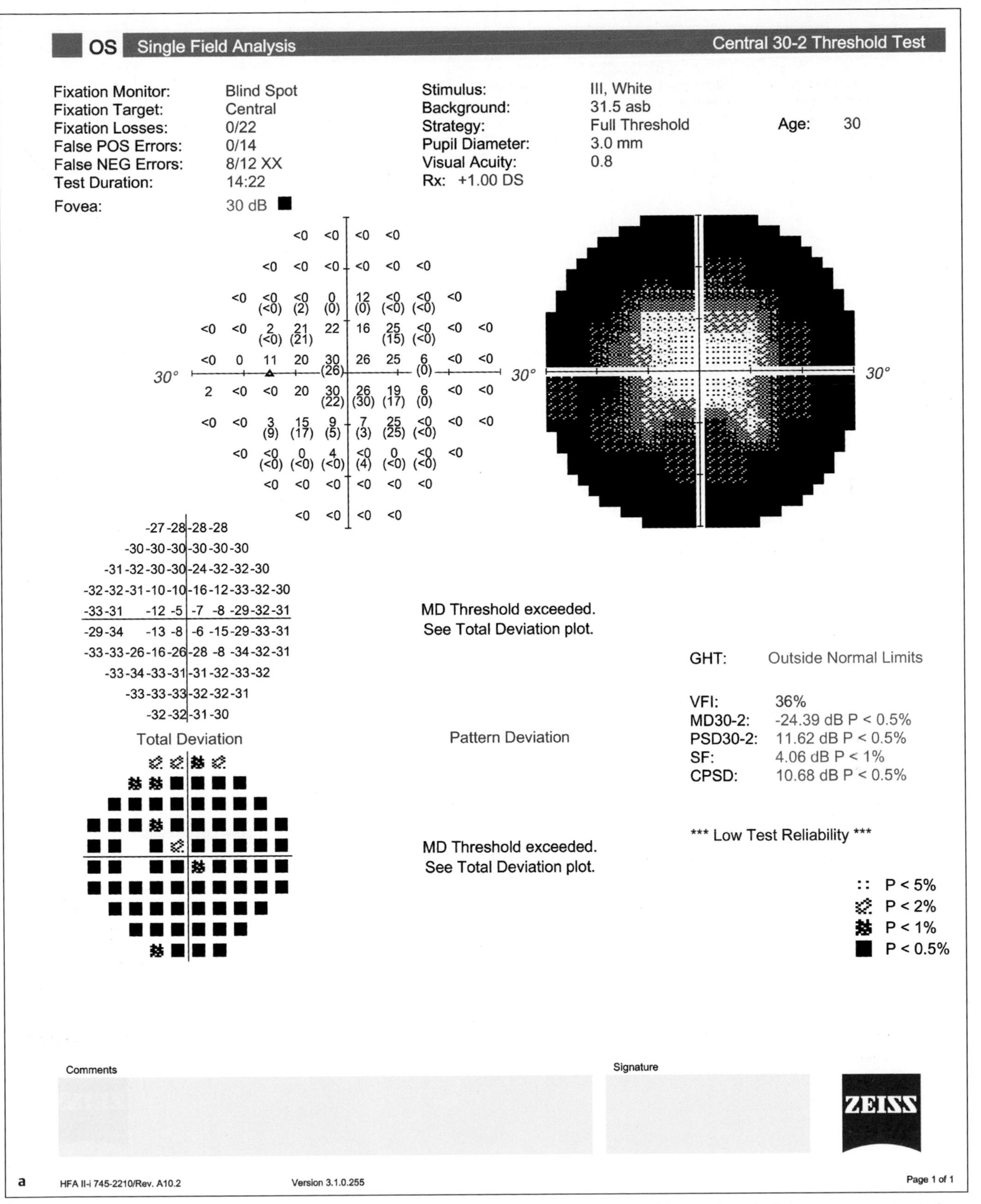

Fig. 4.4 (a) The initial 4 seed locations in the middle of three quadrants are grossly within normal limits, after which the patient appears to have become inattentive, leading to a clover leaf pattern on the pattern deviation plot and grayscale. *(Continued)*

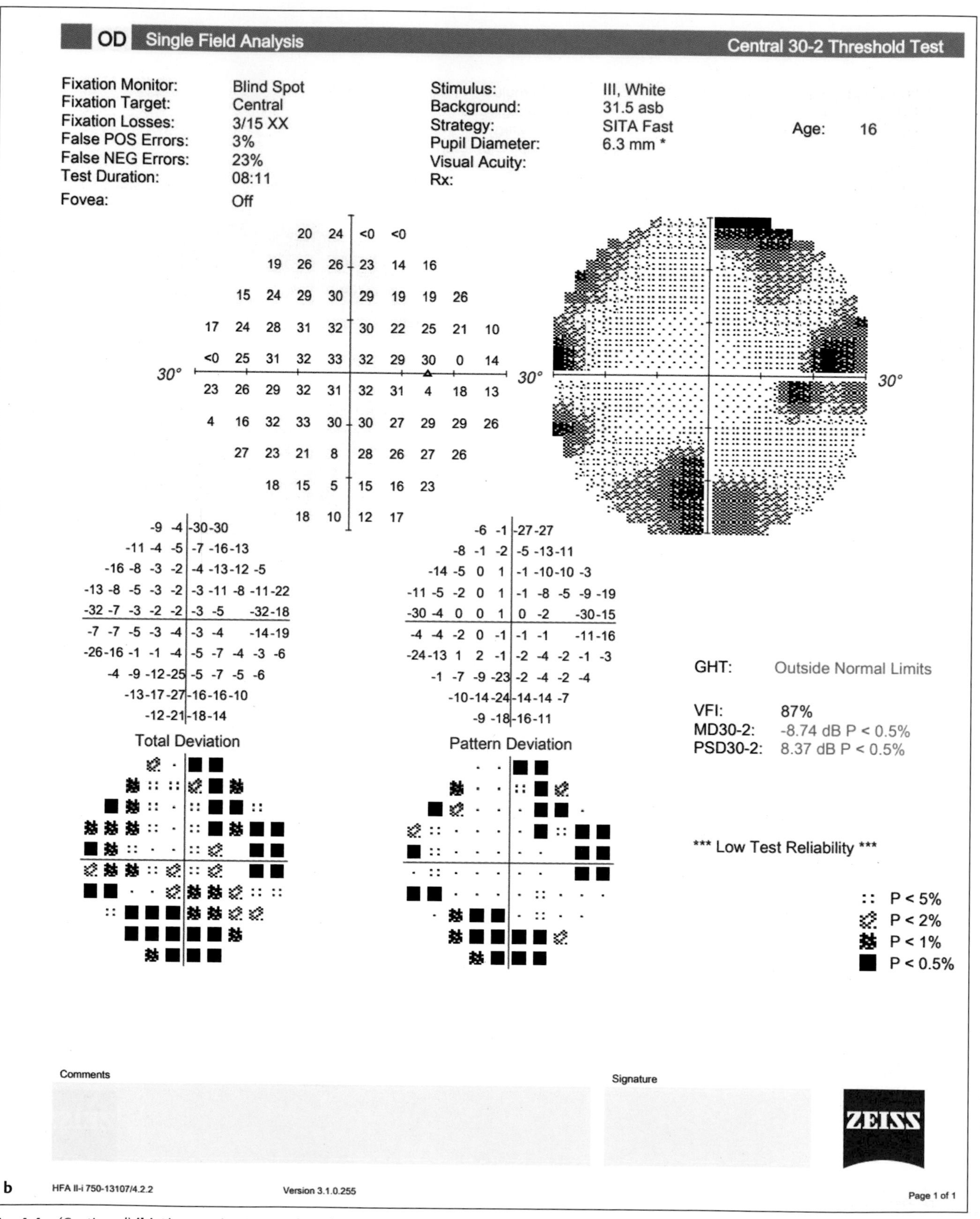

Fig. 4.4 *(Continued)* **(b)** Abnormal points are largely peripheral, and should not be considered in a 30-2 printout. There are high fixation losses and false negative responses, making this an unreliable field.

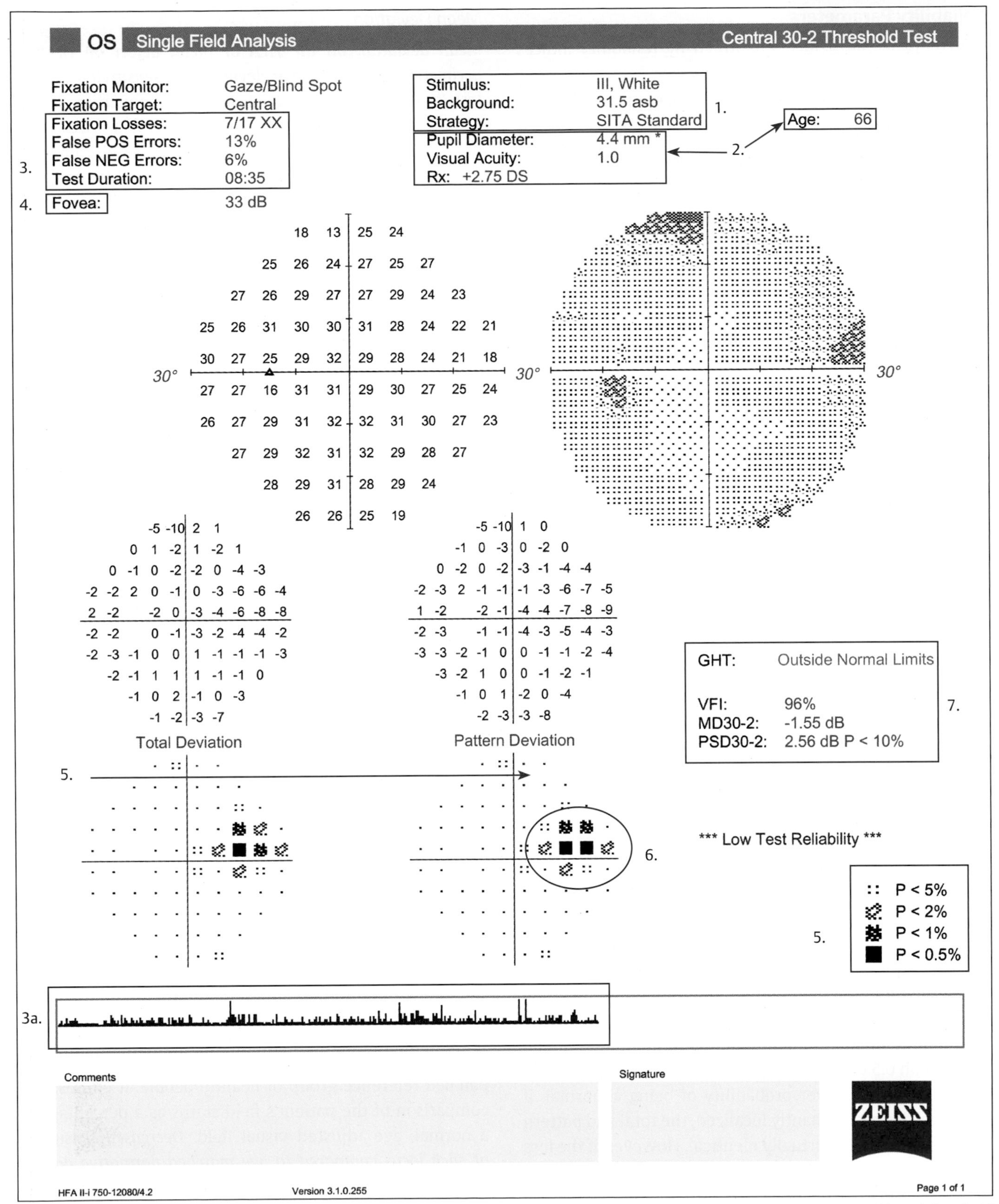

Fig. 4.5 A representative Humphrey field analyzer (HFA) single-field printout. Reliability criteria are met, and the visual acuity and foveal threshold correspond. A cluster of 5 nonedge, contiguous points with one having a probability of being seen in < 1% of age matched normals.

Reliability Parameters

Reliability of the field is quantified by reliability indices generated:

- Fixation losses of >20% render the field unreliable.
- False-positives: Patient responses in the absence of projected stimuli of >15% are marked with an xx as unreliable.
- False-negatives: If a patient records seeing the stimulus at a location initially, but fails to respond a second time to a brighter stimulus shown at the same location, by over 20%, this is considered an unreliable field. However, in advanced glaucoma this is more common and even >30% may still be considered for evaluation.

The test duration, if longer than average, may alert one to the possibility of inattentiveness or fatigue, and hence a less reliable field.

Total Deviation

Total deviation is the difference of a patient's retinal sensitivity at each location tested, compared to an age-matched normative database. The box plot presents one of a group of symbols, indicating whether the sensitivity is within age-adjusted normal limits or has a *probability of being seen in less than 5, 2, 1, or 0.5% of age-matched normal individuals*. This provides an immediate graphical representation of the locations that are abnormal and the degree to which they vary from normal.

Pattern Deviation

Pattern deviation shows retinal sensitivity levels, after the "average" or "overall" sensitivity loss has been subtracted, thereby revealing localized deviations compared to normal age-matched individuals. Pattern deviation plot values are calculated by subtracting the value of the 85th percentile of highest sensitivity deviation from all the values in the total deviation plot. This is achieved by subtracting all values on the total deviation by the 7th highest value, thereby adjusting the whole field. *The pattern of true visual field loss is best seen here by shape and location.* On the probability plot, solid black squares indicate a probability of being seen in less than 0.5% of the normal population, with less dense squares having a lower probability of being abnormal. If the deficit is predominantly localized, the total and pattern deviation plots look virtually identical. However, if the loss is widespread as in the presence of a cataract, abnormalities may be present on the total deviation plot, but the pattern deviation plot could be virtually normal.

Global Indices

Evaluation of perimetric damage is further aided by global indices provided on the printout.

Mean Deviation

Mean deviation on the HFA or mean defect on Octopus perimeters is the average deviation of sensitivity at each test location from age-adjusted normal population values. It indicates the degree of generalized or widespread loss present in the visual field, and is therefore less likely to pick up early, localized loss, and *is only good for assessing moderate-to-severe field loss, −6 to −12 dB.* Normal eyes have an mean deviation value of 0 to −2 dB.

Pattern Standard Deviation (PSD)

PSD on the HFA or loss variance (LV) on the Octopus system is a calculation of the average deviation of individual visual field sensitivity values from the normal slope of the visual field, after correcting for any overall sensitivity differences. It is the sum of the differences between absolute values recorded at each locus and the average sensitivity at each point, calculated by age-matched normal values + mean deviation. PSD is a measure of localized visual field loss or scotomas. A high value indicates an irregular field of vision, while a low value could signify either a smooth hill of vision, or severe visual field loss. *It is only useful in detecting early to moderate loss.*

Glaucoma Hemifield Test (GHT)

GHT compares sensitivity of five clusters of points above and below the horizontal midline which resemble the nerve fiber bundle pattern to identify any asymmetry, a common finding in glaucoma. The GHT summary could read:

- Outside normal limits (ONL): Lower sensitivity than seen in <1% of population.
- Borderline: Lower sensitivity than seen in <3% of population.
- Within normal limits (WNL): No significant difference.
- Abnormally high sensitivity: Higher sensitivity than seen in <0.5% of population.

Visual Field Index (VFI)

VFI provides a means of evaluating visual field loss as a percentage, relative to the sensitivity of an age patched reference group of healthy people. It expresses a comparison of the patient's field status as a percentage of a normal, age-adjusted visual field. *Decreased sensitivity at each locus compared to age-matched normative data is expressed as percentiles. There is greater weightage toward the central field, and the mean of all loci is expressed as a percentage.* Values range from 100% in an age-adjusted normal eye to *0% in one perimetrically blind.* VFI is less influenced by generalized loss seen with a cataract, and can be tracked over time as a measure of progression.

The index is calculated by considering the pattern deviation for defects up to −20 dB and the total deviation for more advanced visual field loss.

Grayscale: It has to be understood that this is an extrapolation of results, so that a general idea of a depression and its location can be seen. On the grayscale, areas of high sensitivity are denoted by a lighter color, and areas of low sensitivity by a darker color. *It cannot be used for diagnosis or assessment of the depth of visual field loss. The clinician should glance at it, but evaluate a field from total and pattern deviation records.*

Gaze monitor: At the bottom of the printout is a graphical representation of corneal movements, that is, loss of fixation or a movement of the head of even 1 to 2 degrees, as an upstroke and loss of pupil visibility, such as by blinking, as a downstroke.

Perimetry should always be correlated with the clinical picture, that is, the optic nerve head findings of the patient (**Fig. 4.6** and **Table 4.2**).

Printouts of Different Perimeters

These can be similarly read. Octopus type perimeter printouts (**Fig. 4.7**) provide the same data under slightly different terminology, with an additional Bebie or cumulative defect curve.

Octopus terminology and matching Humphrey equivalents:

- Catch trials: Reliability indices.
- Comparisons: Total deviation.
- Corrected comparisons: Pattern deviation.
- Mean defect: mean deviation.
- Mean sensitivity: Mean value of all data.
- Loss variance: PSD.
- Reliability factor provides an analysis from 1 to 15%.
- Bebie curve is a cumulative defect curve that ranks any deviation from normal values, providing an indicator of generalized depression of the field or extent of localized loss.

Diagnosing a Glaucomatous Scotoma on Standard Automated Perimetry

On evaluating a visual field, the first step is to determine whether there is a scotoma, and the second is to ascertain the possible causes of the field defect.

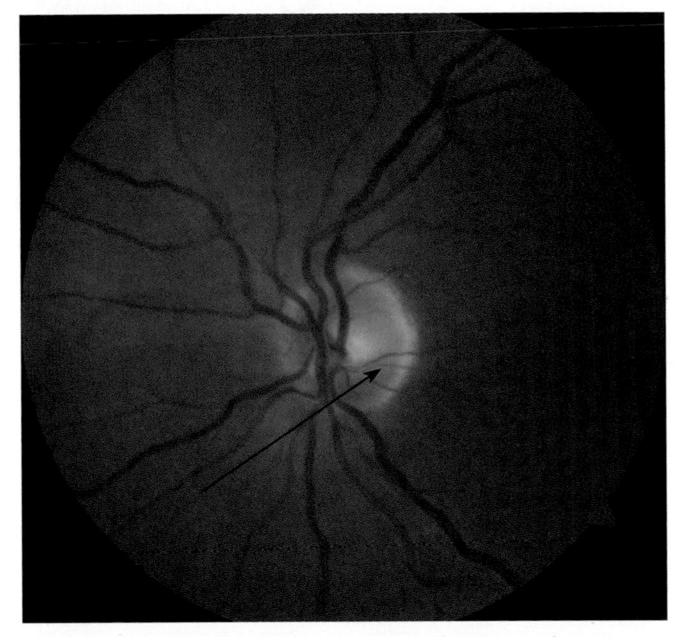

Fig. 4.6 Thinning of the inferior neuroretinal rim more than superior (*black arrow*), correlating with the superior nasal step in the field in **Fig. 4.5**.

Table 4.2 Commonly used perimeters

	Humphrey perimeter	Octopus perimeter
Background illumination	31.5 apostilbs (10 cd/m²)	31.4 apostilbs (10 cd/m²)
Luminance for 0 dB	10,000 apostilbs	4,000 apostilbs
Stimulus exposure time	200 ms	100 ms
Spacing of test locations	Equal spacing at 6-degree separation and off-set from vertical and horizontal meridian	Spacing is 2.8 degrees centrally and greater spacing toward the periphery
Strategy	SITA standard: 4-2 bracket process SITA fast: 3-1 bracket process	G-dynamic: 10-2 bracket process G-tendency-oriented perimetry: Interpolation process
Global indices recorded	Mean deviation Pattern standard deviation Fixation losses False-positives False-negatives	Mean sensitivity Mean deviation Standard loss variance Catch trials—positive/negative

Abbreviation: SITA, Swedish interactive threshold algorithm.

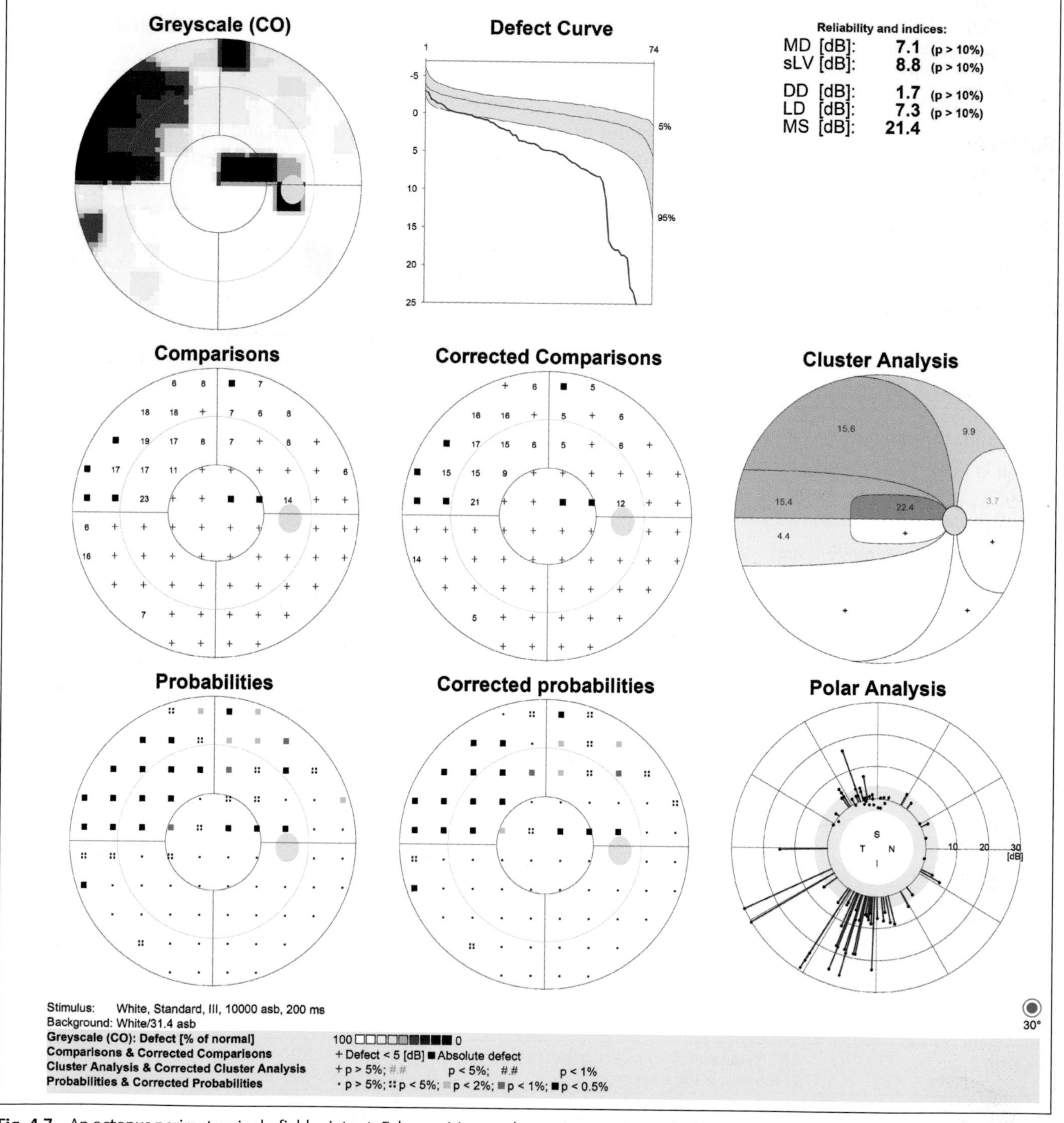

Fig. 4.7 An octopus perimeter single-field printout. False positives and negatives are 0%, with abnormal loci stretching from the blind spot to the superior nasal area. A superior arcuate scotoma is present, with a defect curve showing a largely localised loss. Polar analysis shows the expected loss of neuroretinal rim to be at both poles, inferior more than superior.

Anderson's criteria for the diagnosis of a scotoma is the presence of any of the three below, but the specificity increases if all are present and are reproducible on at least two consecutive fields:

- GHT should be marked as abnormal.
- Three contiguous, nonedge points on the pattern deviation plot within Bjerrum area have a probability of <5% of being seen in a normal population, one of which should have a probability of <1%.
- PSD should have a probability of <5%.

Patterns of Visual Field Loss Seen in Glaucoma

Visual field loss in glaucoma is due to loss of ganglion cells and their axons, which have a specific arrangement in the retina and the optic nerve. Loss of the axons is seen as thinning/notching of the neuroretinal rim, commonly inferotemporal and then superotemporal. *This results in a loss of function in Bjerrum area, that is, 5 to 20 degrees from fixation.* Loss of superficial axonal fibers causes a more central loss—paracentral scotomas—and extension of loss to deeper axons is probably related to formation of a nasal step. More extensive loss of the neuroretinal rim causes an expanding scotoma, arcuate or biarcuate with breakthrough to the periphery, finally leaving only central and temporal islands of vision (**Fig. 4.8**).

Relative paracentral scotomas: These are areas where smaller or dimmer targets are not visualized by the patient but larger or brighter targets are noticed, above or below fixation in Bjerrum area.

Nasal step: The appearance of a cluster of abnormal loci having a horizontal shelf in the nasal visual field is caused by an asymmetric nerve fiber loss at the two poles of the optic nerve.

Seidel scotoma is one that appears to start at a pole of the blind spot arching over the macula, without reaching the horizontal meridian nasally.

Arcuate scotomas also appear to start at the superior or inferior poles of the blind spot and arch over the macular area, widening as they curve down or up, to end at the horizontal meridian nasally.

Double arcuate or ring scotoma: Arcuate scotomas may occur in both hemispheres to form a ring-shaped loss in the midperipheral visual field.

End-stage or near-total field defect: Two arcuate scotomas expand to involve the entire peripheral visual field with only a central and residual temporal island of vision.

At least two consecutive, corroborative fields plotted on different occasions are required before a diagnosis of any glaucomatous loss can be made, as there is often a significant improvement in the field when plotted a second time, as patients become more familiar with the machine and test process, that is, the *learning effect. Clustering of perimetry, that is, performing field examinations frequently, initially permits the recognition of a learning effect, while determining reproducible defects, and also the rate of change in a given individual.* All results need to be considered together with clinical examination.

Artifacts on automated perimetry commonly appear as defects in the extreme periphery of a field, or a moth-eaten appearance of a field defect, or appear as diffuse abnormalities in the visual field (**Fig. 4.2**). *Glaucomatous defects are almost always dense and occur within Bjerrum area in defined patterns.*

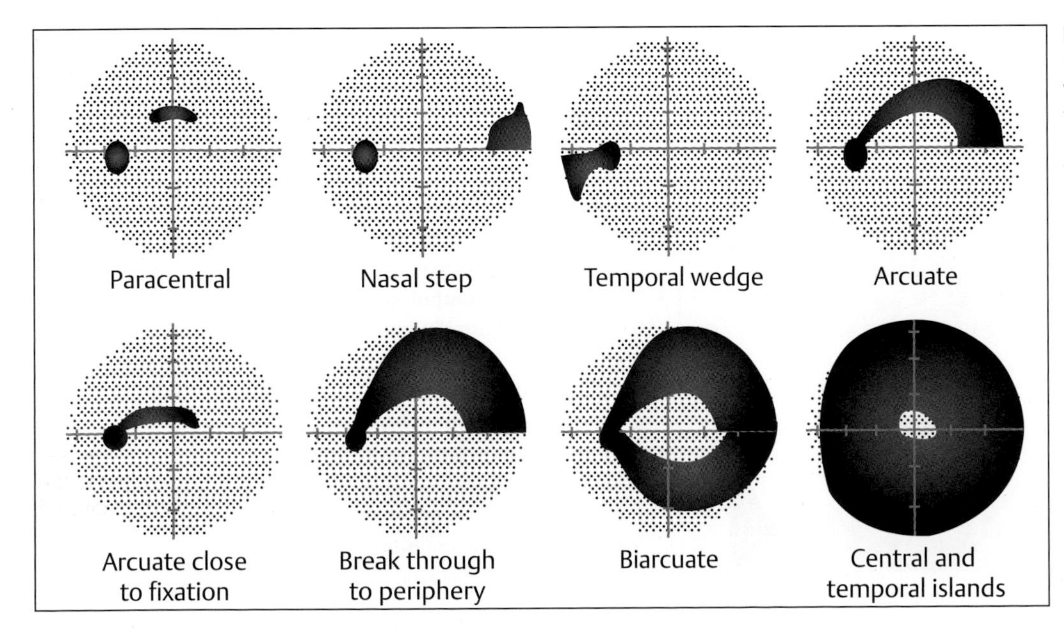

Fig. 4.8 Progression of glaucomatous visual field loss, starting with Bjerrum area in the superior field and progressing to the other hemisphere and peripherally, is frequently seen.

Perimetric Artifacts

Perimetric artifacts are often due to procedural problems or patient-related factors.

Procedural problems could be:

- Incorrect name.
- Incorrect date of birth.
- Patient's head not placed against the bar.
- Use of a lens that is not full field.
- Inappropriate refractive correction for near.
- Pupil not 2 to 4 mm.

Patient-related factors are as follows:

- Inattention over time leading to a "clover leaf" pattern.
- False-positives leading to supranormal thresholds being recorded as a "white-out" field or swiss-cheese pattern.
- Media opacification.
- Irregular refractive surfaces as in keratoconus and posterior staphylomas.

Other ocular or systemic pathology could also appear glaucomatous, such as:

- Medullated nerve fibers (**Fig. 4.9**).
- Chorioretinal scars.
- Diabetic retinopathy.

Nonglaucomatous Causes of an Arcuate Scotoma

An arcuate scotoma is considered to be definitive for glaucoma in the presence of corroborating changes on the optic nerve head and retinal nerve fiber layer. However, other ocular lesions and some along the optic pathway can also result in an arcuate scotoma (**Box 4.1**). These should be kept in mind if a discordance is seen between the field defect and optic nerve head picture.

Illustrating the Reading of a Single Visual Field

A 63-year-old underwent an HFA, 30-2 SITA standard test (**Fig. 4.10**). Visual acuity was 6/6, a near correction was used, and the pupil was 3 mm. Reliability indices showed 10% fixation losses. But the false-positives and false-negatives were nil. The Foveal threshold of 32 dB corresponds with visual acuity. Total deviation values and plot show a significant loss of sensitivity in the superior and inferior nasal area and superior paracentral loss. This is mirrored in the pattern deviation numbers and plot; therefore, there appears to be no significant media opacification, such as a cataract, etc.

Looking at the pattern deviation plot, in the superonasal area, there are three contiguous loci having a probability of being seen in the age-matched normal population of <5% with one likely to be seen in <1% of the age-matched normal population. This substantiates the presence of a scotoma. On identifying Bjerrum area, this scotoma falls within it, and GHT is "outside normal limits," making it likely to be glaucomatous. The pattern of the defect appears to be a definite superior nasal step, and some paracentral loss. The VFI is 91% and the mean deviation, PSD and corrected pattern standard deviation (CPSD), and short-term fluctuation (SF) are all significantly abnormal. These should correlate with the appearance of the optic nerve head in this patient, and will need to be confirmed on the next perimetry. Similarly read, **Figs. 4.11–4.13** show

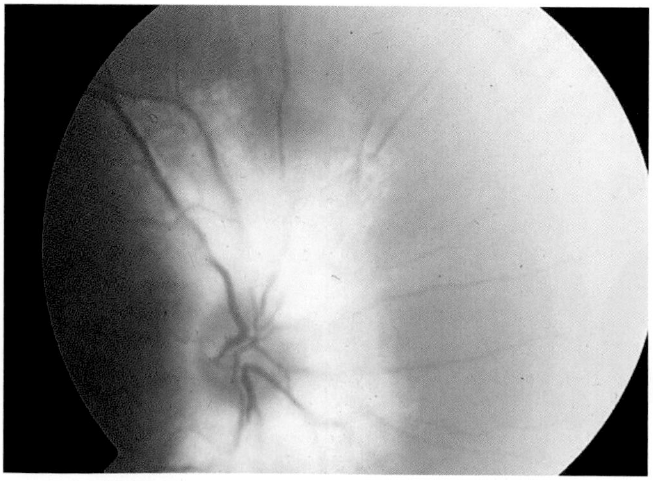

Fig. 4.9 Medullated nerve fibers that would cause an abnormal field.

Box 4.1 Nonglaucomatous causes of an arcuate scotoma

- **Retinal pathology**
  - Retinal branch vein occlusion
  - Retinal coloboma
  - Juxtapapillary choroiditis
- **Optic nerve head pathology**
  - Anterior and posterior ischemic optic neuropathy
  - Optic disc pit
  - Optic disc drusen
  - optic nerve head dysplasia
- **Central nervous system pathology**
  - Pituitary tumors
  - Meningioma—optic nerve, dorsum sella
  - Internal carotid aneurysms
  - Opticochiasmatic arachnoiditis

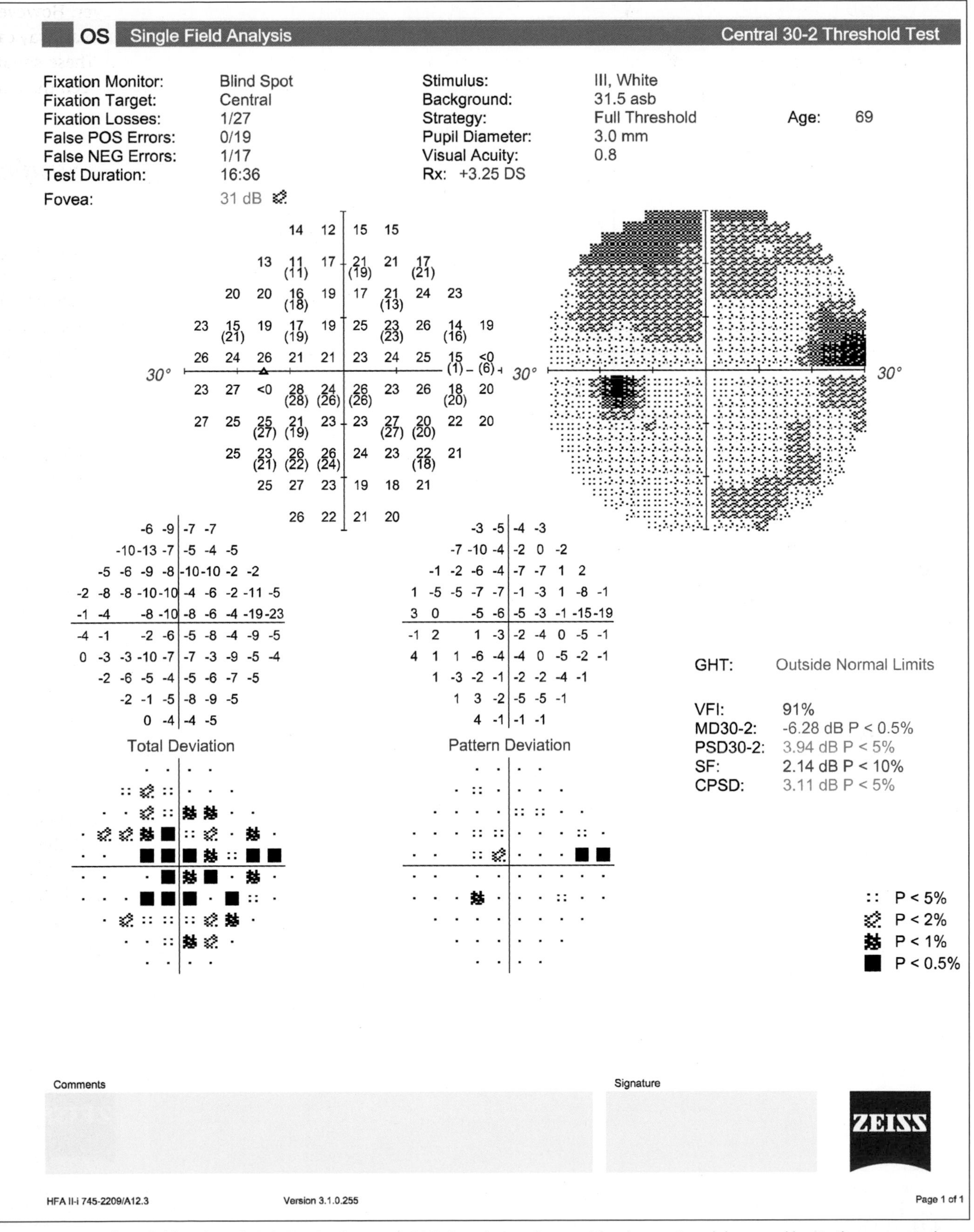

Fig. 4.10 Humphrey field analyzer (HFA). Fixation losses are 10%. Superior nasal step, with other scattered depressed loci in the paracentral area are seen. This needs to be reproduced in the next field done.

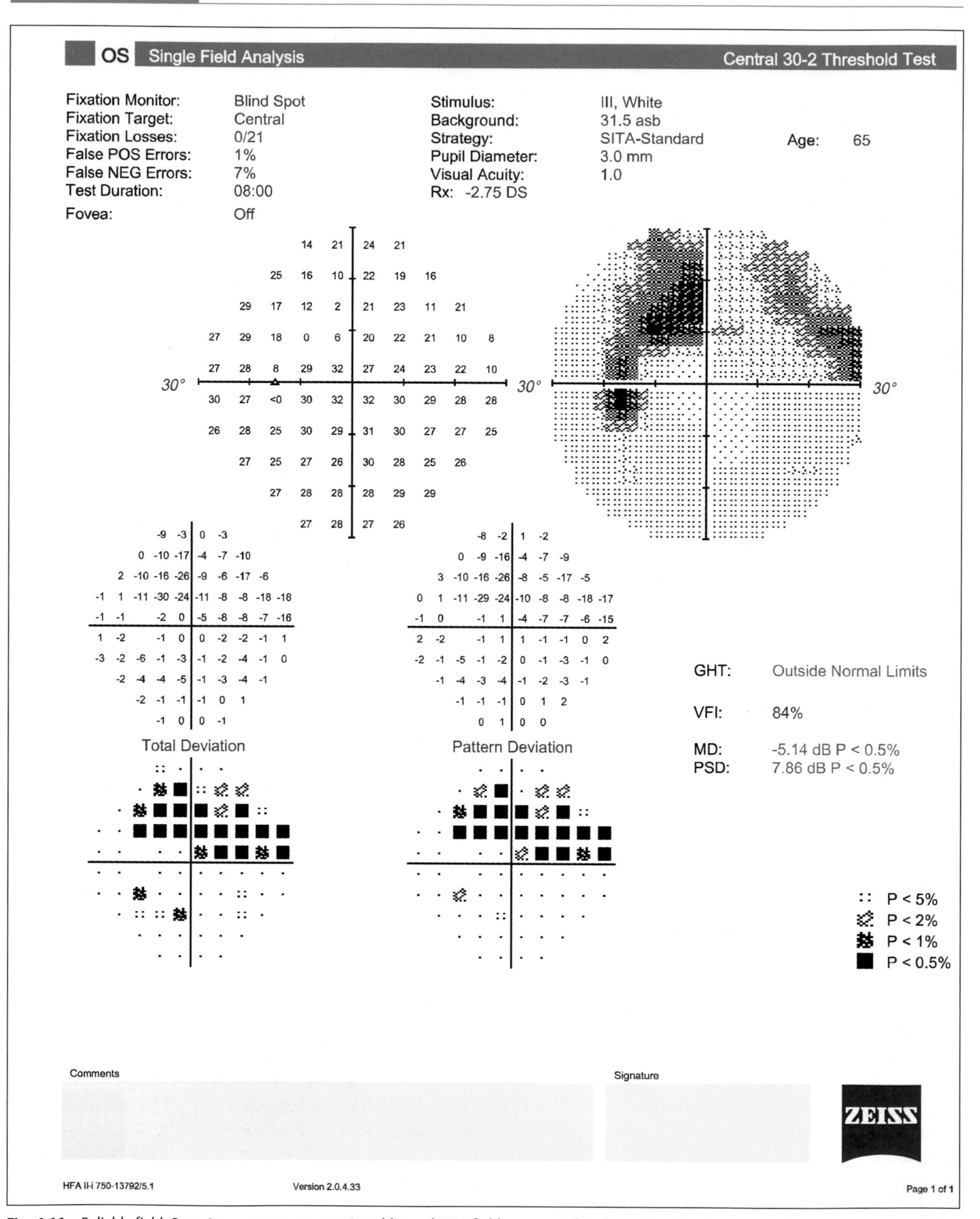

Fig. 4.11 Reliable field. Superior arcuate scotoma. An additional 10-2 field may provide information about any central loss.

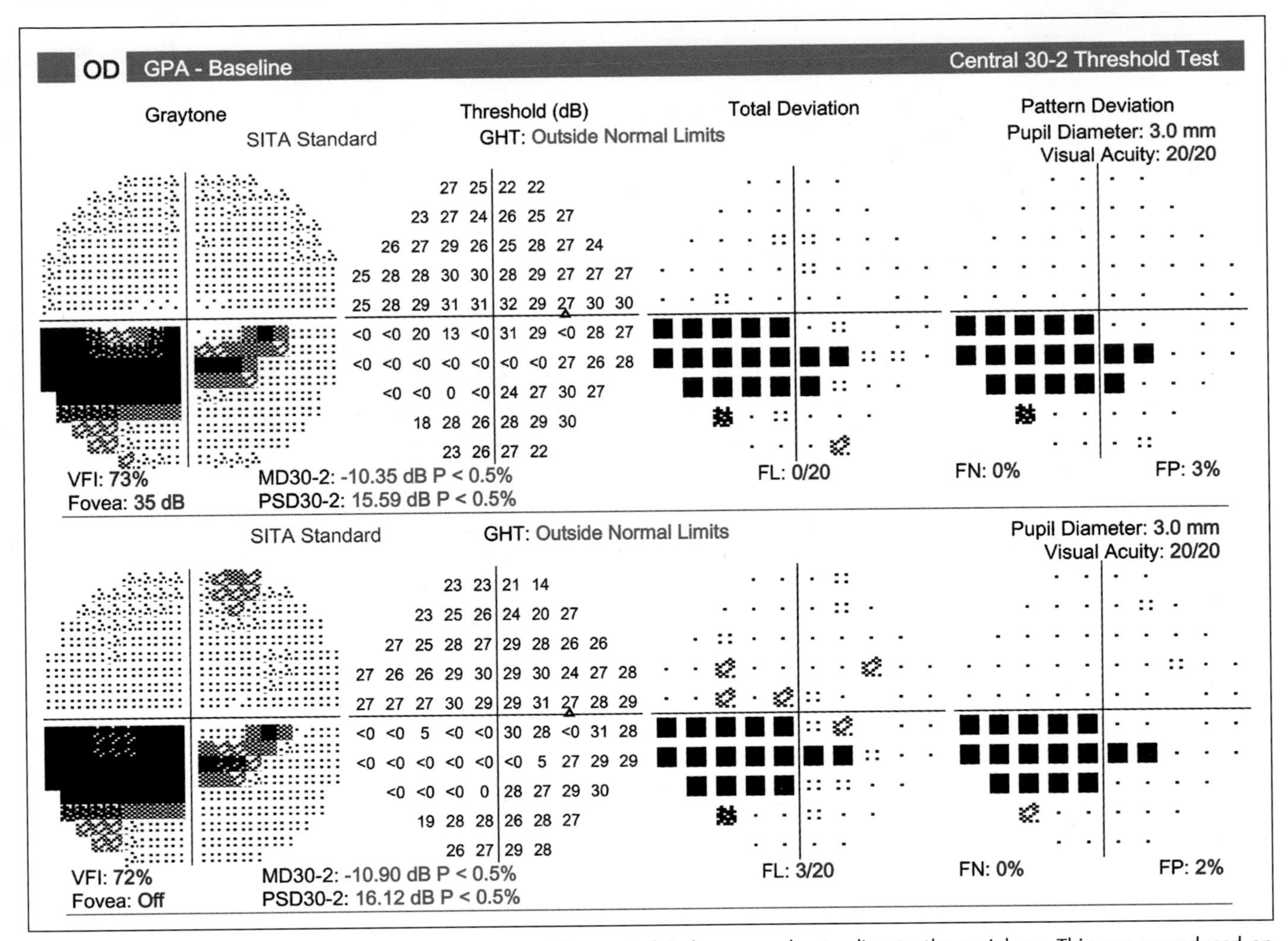

Fig. 4.12 Reliable field. Inferior arcuate scotoma encroaching central 5 degrees and extending to the periphery. This was reproduced on consecutive fields and should also have a 10-2 field done.

reliable and reproducible fields. **Fig. 4.14** shows the better appreciation of central 10 degree filed loss with a 10-2 or central 5 degrees with a macula program.

Newer perimetric techniques for glaucoma include microperimetry or fundus-tracked perimetry for the central field, perimeters that provide a standard automated field and optical coherence tomography confocal images at the same time to correlate changes, and a free iPad app, e.g., Melbourne Rapid Fields test, which uses a moving fixation target in order to increase the field area to test up to 30 degrees of field. Many inexpensive, lightweight, mobile virtual reality goggles, and software are also being evaluated.

Diagnosing progression on perimetry is very important, and will be discussed in the chapter on Progression.

Perimetry records a subjective response of the patient and could be influenced by fatigue, stress, and attentiveness of the patient. The search for an objective measure of visual function continues. Optical coherence tomography, multifocal visual-evoked potentials (VEPs), multifocal pupillographic objective perimetry, and a brain–computer interface using Goggle for objective assessment of the field are currently being evaluated. The advent of artificial intelligence and automated algorithms will dramatically change perimetry in the near future.

Currently, standard automated perimetry remains the gold standard for assessing and quantifying visual field loss, but it is commonly complemented by detection of optical coherence tomography changes. Some perimeters now provide a combined printout for glaucoma, including optical coherence tomography and fundus photography, separately and as an overlay.

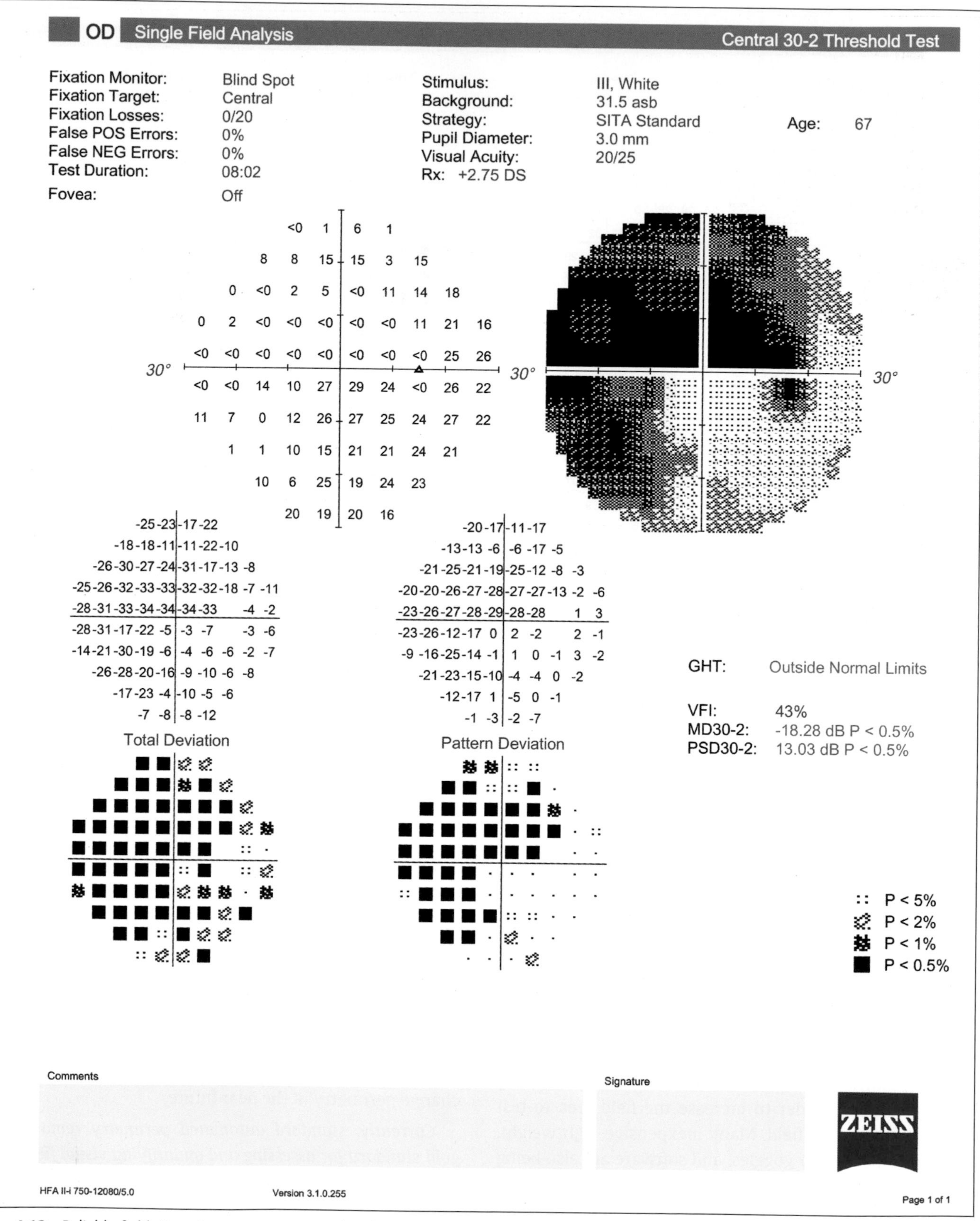

Fig. 4.13 Reliable field. Superior arcuate scotoma breaking into the periphery, with involvement of the central 5 degrees and a large inferior nasal step.

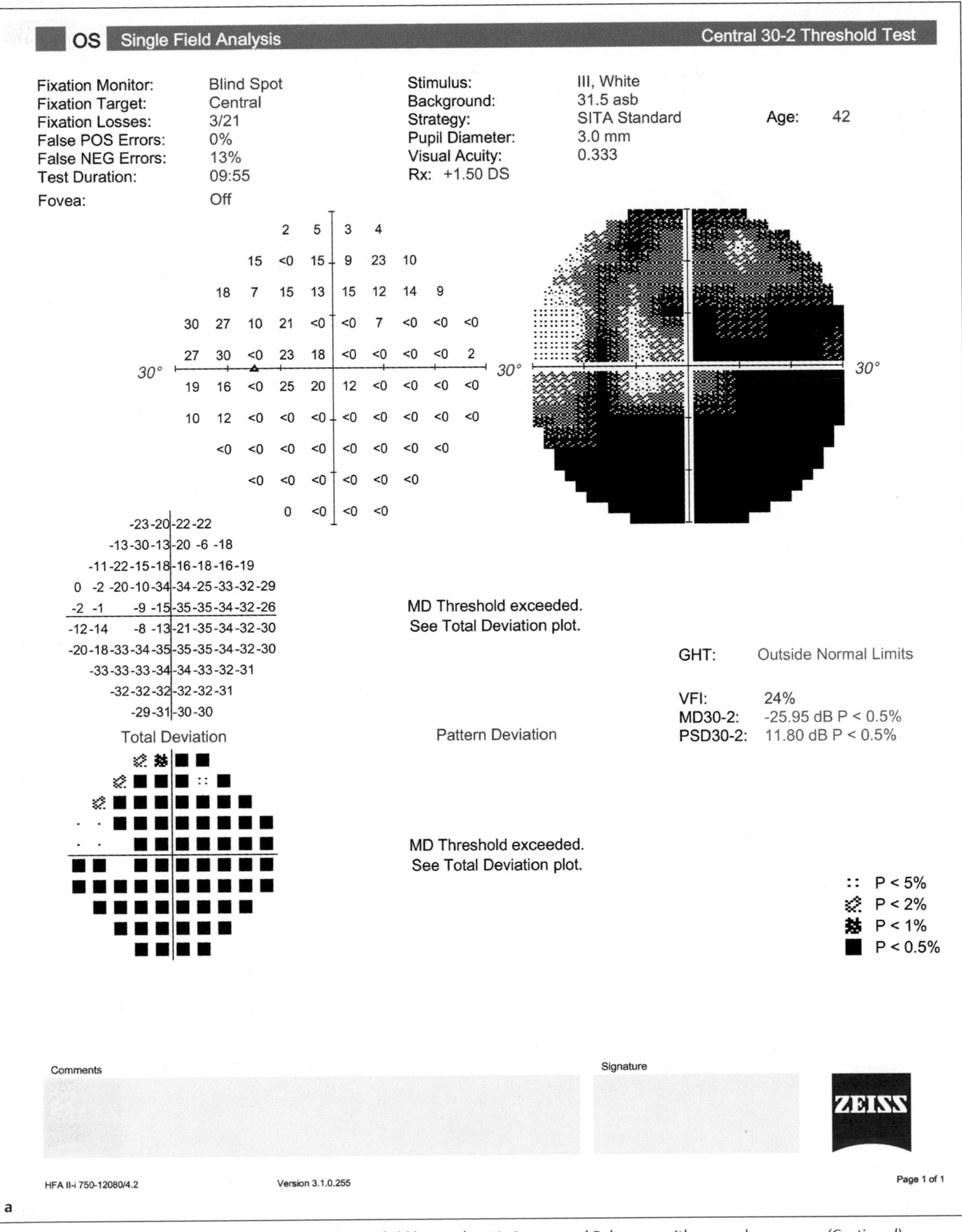

Fig. 4.14 (a–c) Better appreciation of central 10 degree field loss with a 10–2 or central 5 degrees with a macula program. *(Continued)*

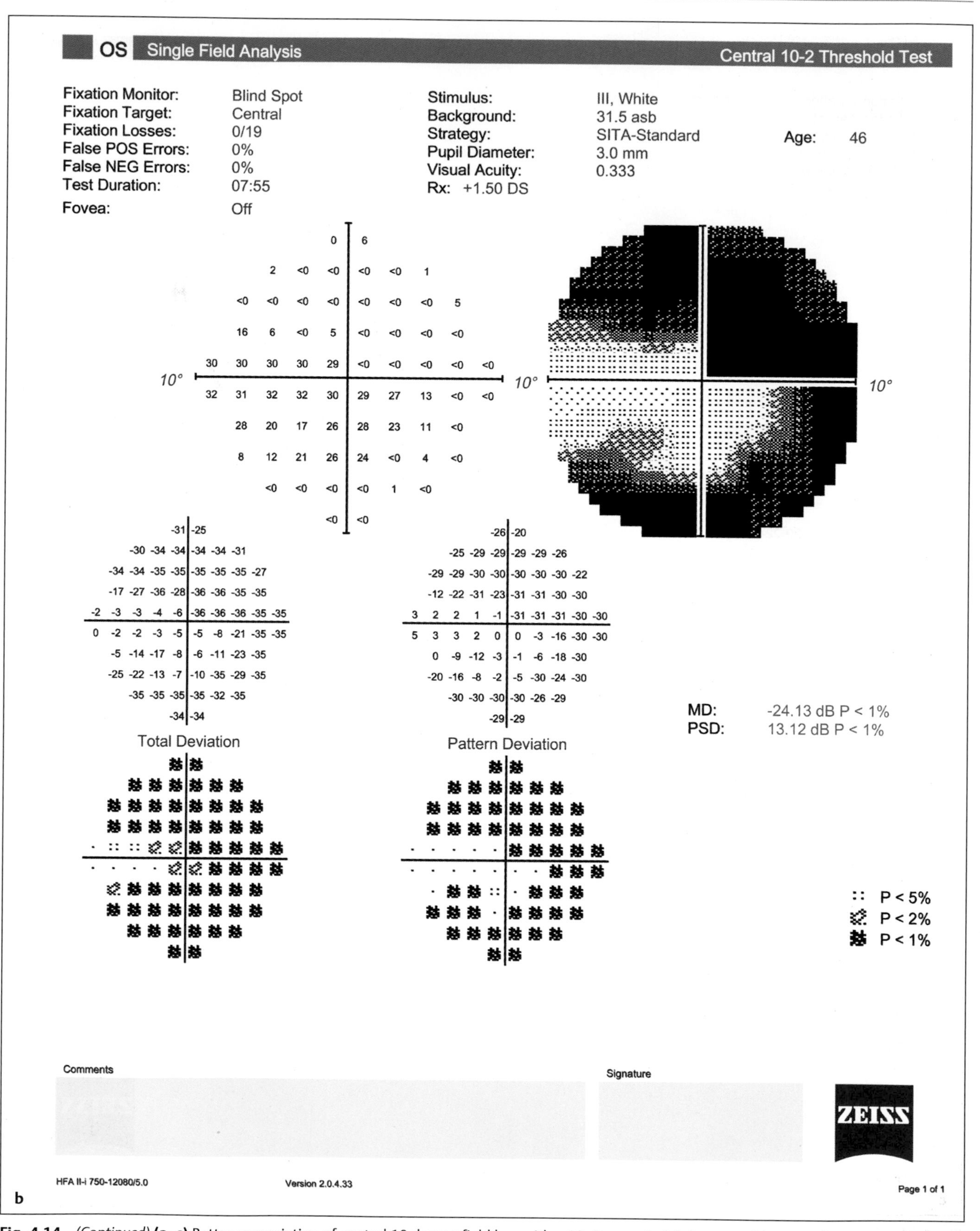

Fig. 4.14 *(Continued)* **(a–c)** Better appreciation of central 10 degree field loss with a 10–2 or central 5 degrees with a macula program.

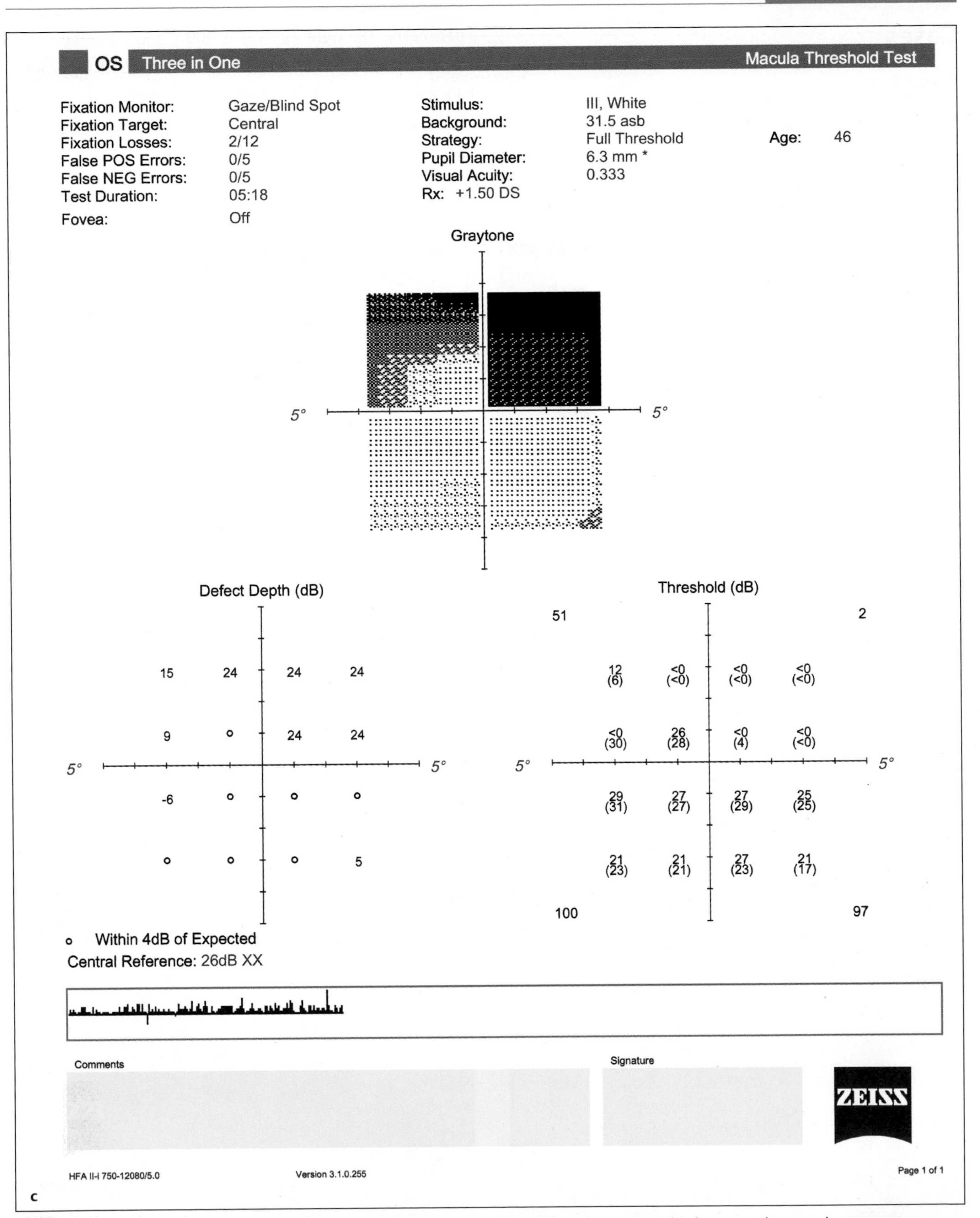

OS Three in One
Macula Threshold Test
Fixation Monitor: Gaze/Blind Spot
Fixation Target: Central
Fixation Losses: 2/12
False POS Errors: 0/5
False NEG Errors: 0/5
Test Duration: 05:18
Fovea: Off
Stimulus: III, White
Background: 31.5 asb
Strategy: Full Threshold
Pupil Diameter: 6.3 mm *
Visual Acuity: 0.333
Rx: +1.50 DS
Age: 46
Graytone
5°
5°
Defect Depth (dB)
15 24 24 24
9 o 24 24
-6 o o o
o o o 5
Threshold (dB)
51
2
12 (6) <0 (<0) <0 (<0) <0 (<0)
<0 (30) 26 (28) <0 (4) <0 (<0)
29 (31) 27 (27) 27 (29) 25 (25)
21 (23) 21 (21) 27 (23) 21 (17)
100
97
o Within 4dB of Expected
Central Reference: 26dB XX
Comments
Signature
ZEISS
HFA II-i 750-12080/5.0
Version 3.1.0.255
Page 1 of 1
c

Fig. 4.14 *(Continued)* **(a–c)** Better appreciation of central 10 degree field loss with a 10–2 or central 5 degrees with a macula program.

Cases

Case 1

A 62-year-old patient with a suspicion of primary open-angle glaucoma (POAG) due to a cup:disc ratio of 0.6 and 0.7, and intraocular pressure (IOP) of 24/26 mm Hg, underwent perimetry. The right eye VFI is 100%, and mean deviation and PSD are within normal limits. There are no loci having a significant loss of sensitivity. This corresponds with the optic nerve head picture of thinning of the neuroretinal rim inferiorly but no focal or generalized loss (**Cases 1-1** and **1-2**).

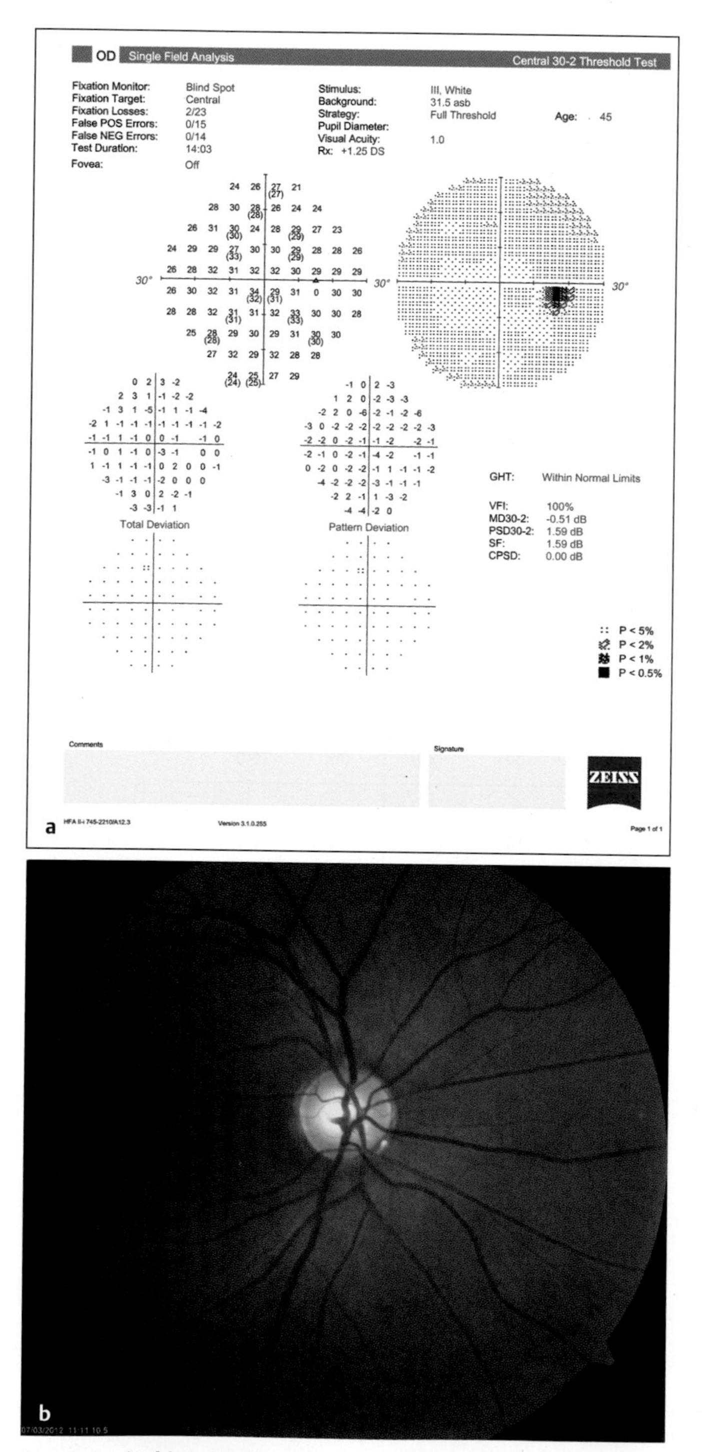

Case 1-1 (a, b) Perimetry within normal limits corresponding to the optic nerve head picture of thinning of the neuroretinal rim without neuroretinal rim loss at any point.

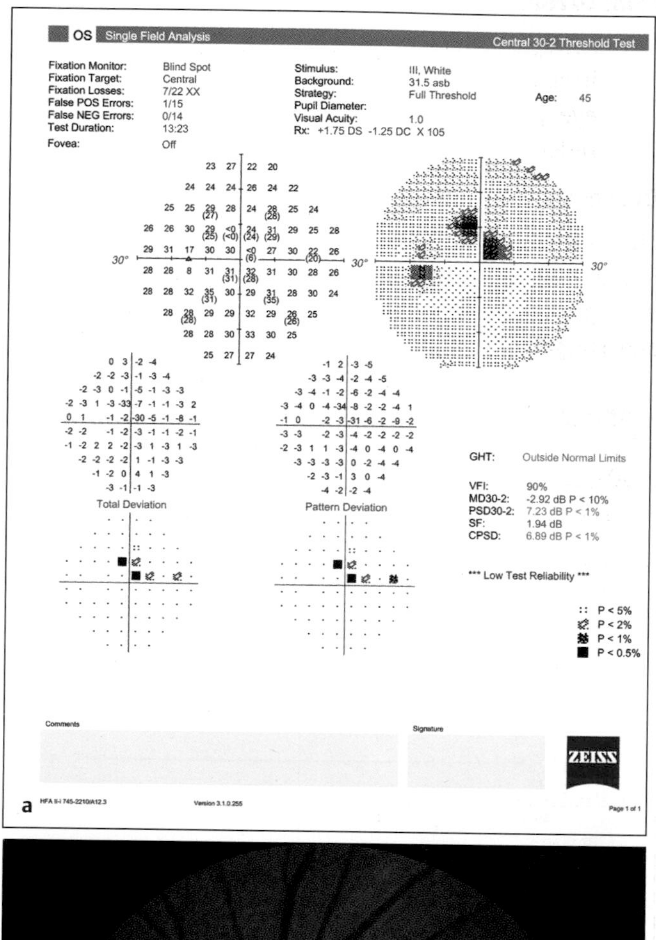

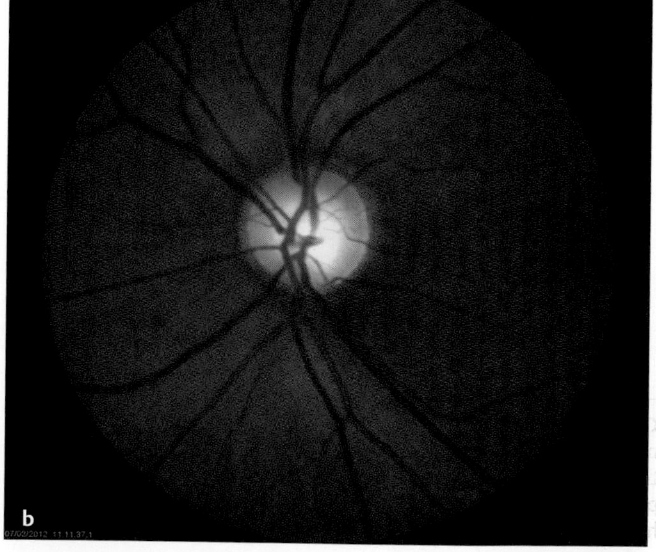

Case 1-2 (a, b) Left eye of the same patient. Humphrey field analyzer (HFA) shows a superior arcuate scotoma, and the optic nerve head photograph reveals a corresponding loss of neuroretinal rim from 4 to 6 o'clock.

The other eye of the same patient has a significant Seidel or early arcuate scotoma on pattern deviation plot, VFI of 92%, mean deviation of −2.43, and PSD of 5.76. Even though it corresponds with the focal loss of neuroretinal rim between 5 and 6 o'clock positions, fixation losses are high. The field is therefore unreliable, and would need to be repeated to reach a final diagnosis.

Point to consider

- Always look at both ONHs, as an asymmetry of >0.2 in cup:disc ratio or a loss of neuroretinal rim in either eye is probably glaucomatous, and this would be reflected on perimetry.

Diagnosis and Management

The patient underwent a gonioscopy and the angle was found to be wide open with a normal trabecular meshwork. A diagnosis of POAG with mild visual field loss was made and a target IOP range of 15 to 17 mm Hg was decided upon.

Case 2

A 50-year-old lady with a cup:disc ratio of 0.6 in the right eye and 0.5 in the left underwent a perimetry on HFA. Her fields showed a severe loss on total deviation plot and a possible inferior nasal step on pattern deviation plot in the left eye (**Case 2-1**).

Point to consider

- As the left optic nerve head was grossly normal and did not correlate with the field, this was probably an artifact or "learning effect."

Diagnosis and Management

Perimetry was repeated twice and the last total and pattern deviation plots did not show any defect.

Case 3

A 59-year-old lady presenting with a gradual painless diminution of vision was found to have a normal anterior segment, cup:disc ratio of 0.7:1 in both eyes with inferior neuroretinal rim thinning, and an open angle. Diurnal phasing IOPs ranged from 14 to 22 mm Hg, and perimetry showed severely depressed points scattered and in the periphery of the 30-2 field of the left eye (**Case 3-1**).

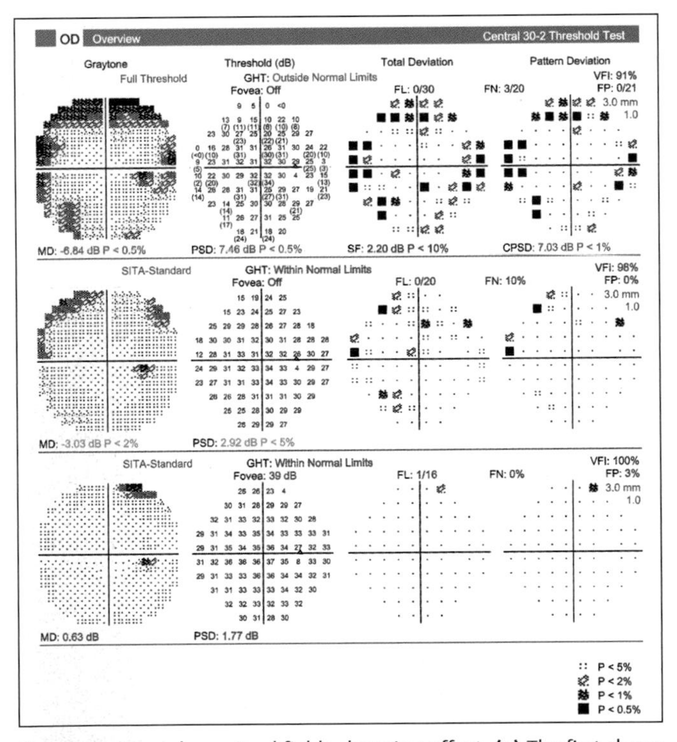

Case 2-1 Humphrey visual fields—learning effect. **(a)** The first shows many points of decreased sensitivity on total deviation plot and few on the pattern deviation plot. **(b)** The second field had fewer depressed points on both total and pattern deviation plots, while the third field had no non edge depressed loci.

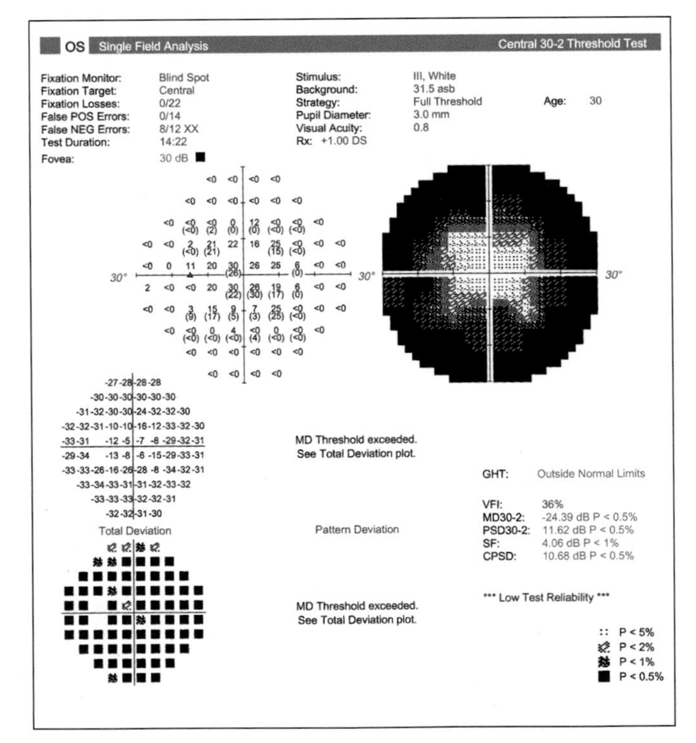

Case 3-1 Partial clover leaf pattern on perimetry, suggesting inattention after the first cardinal points were recorded and an unreliable field.

Points to consider

- Perimetric defects having scattered defects suggest inattention after the first four cardinal points were recorded.
- It was thought to be an unreliable field, and needs repitition.

Diagnosis and Management

A repeat perimetry revealed a "moth-eaten" appearance of peripheral defects not within Bjerrum area. A third perimetry in 1 to 2 months was advised, as all of the clinical parameters were within normal limits.

Case 4

A 70-year-old lady is being followed up for her POAG over the last 5 years. Her fields show an apparent progression, despite IOPs of 10 to 12 mm Hg (**Case 4-1**).

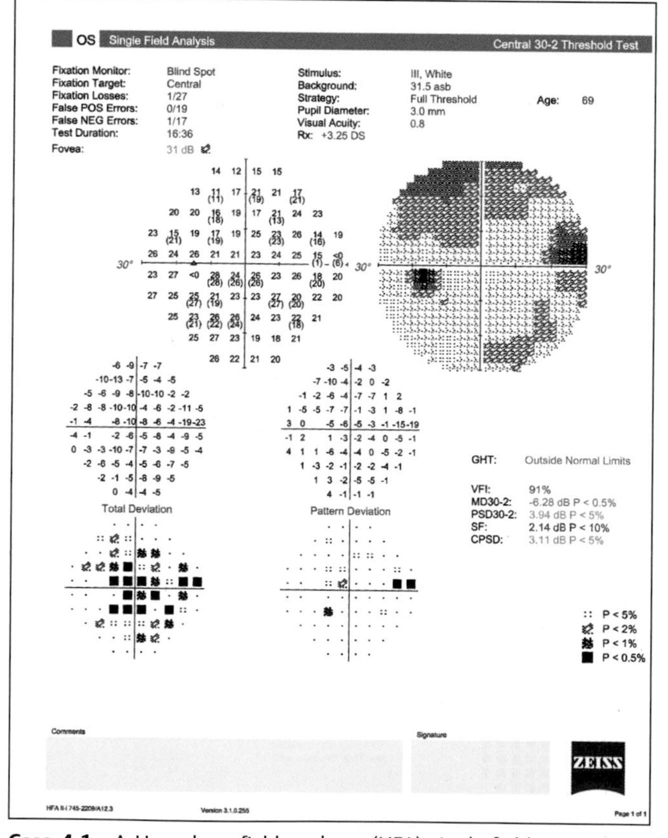

Case 4-1 A Humphrey field analyzer (HFA) single-field report total deviation plot showing a diffuse, moth-eaten appearance of depressed points, while the pattern deviation highlights a superior nasal step only. Diffuse loss due to a posterior subcapsular cataract was responsible for the discrepancy.

Point to consider

- The last field shows a total deviation plot depressed in significantly more loci than pattern deviation plot. This could mean that media opacification, probably a cataract, was causing the increased generalized depression of fields, and mistakenly diagnosed as progression.

Diagnosis and Management

On examination a posterior subcapsular cataract was seen. A repeat perimetry after cataract surgery showed an improvement in central points.

Case 5

A 12-year-old boy with a family history of glaucoma underwent perimetry. His fields showed scattered loci of significant abnormality in both total deviation plots (**Case 5-1**).

Point to consider

- There is no normative data for children in the Humphrey machine.

Diagnosis and Management

There were large areas of "white-out" in the fields, and the significant loci are highlighting difference between normal to supranormal responses. A kinetic perimetry was done, and was normal.

Case 6

A 70-year-old male underwent cataract surgery, and was then diagnosed to have advanced glaucoma on perimetry. It showed a superior hemispheric loss with inferior nasal step in the right eye and an inferior arcuate scotoma with a superior paracentral defect in the left (**Case 6-1**). His children were concerned about his safety while driving.

Point to consider

- There are severe defects in each eye which could affect visibility within the field of vision. However, uniocular fields overlap, and the binocular status could be almost normal.

Diagnosis and Management

An Esterman binocular field was done and showed some defects, but only in the periphery, suggesting that the patient could be a safe driver for now.

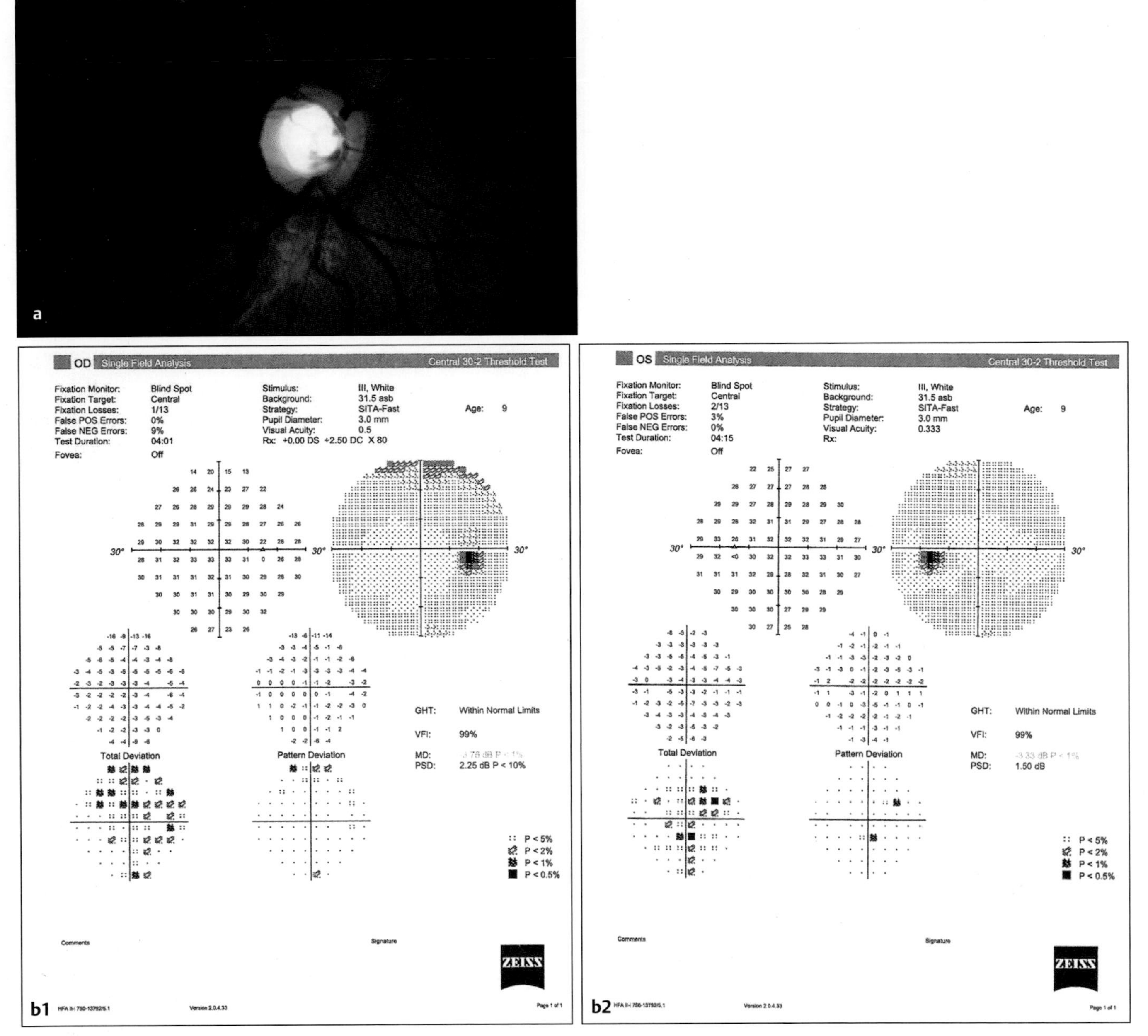

Case 5-1 (a) Fundus photo of the right eye showing a cup:disc ratio of 0.6 with a regular, normal colored neuroretinal rim. **(b)** Humphrey field analyzer (HFA) field showing scattered defects on total deviation plot but none on pattern deviation. The grayscale shows a central area of more widely spaced dots—"white-out" areas signifying supranormal sensitivity, with the patient pressing the buzzer even when stimulus was not seen, a "trigger happy" patient. There is no normative data for a 12-year-old.

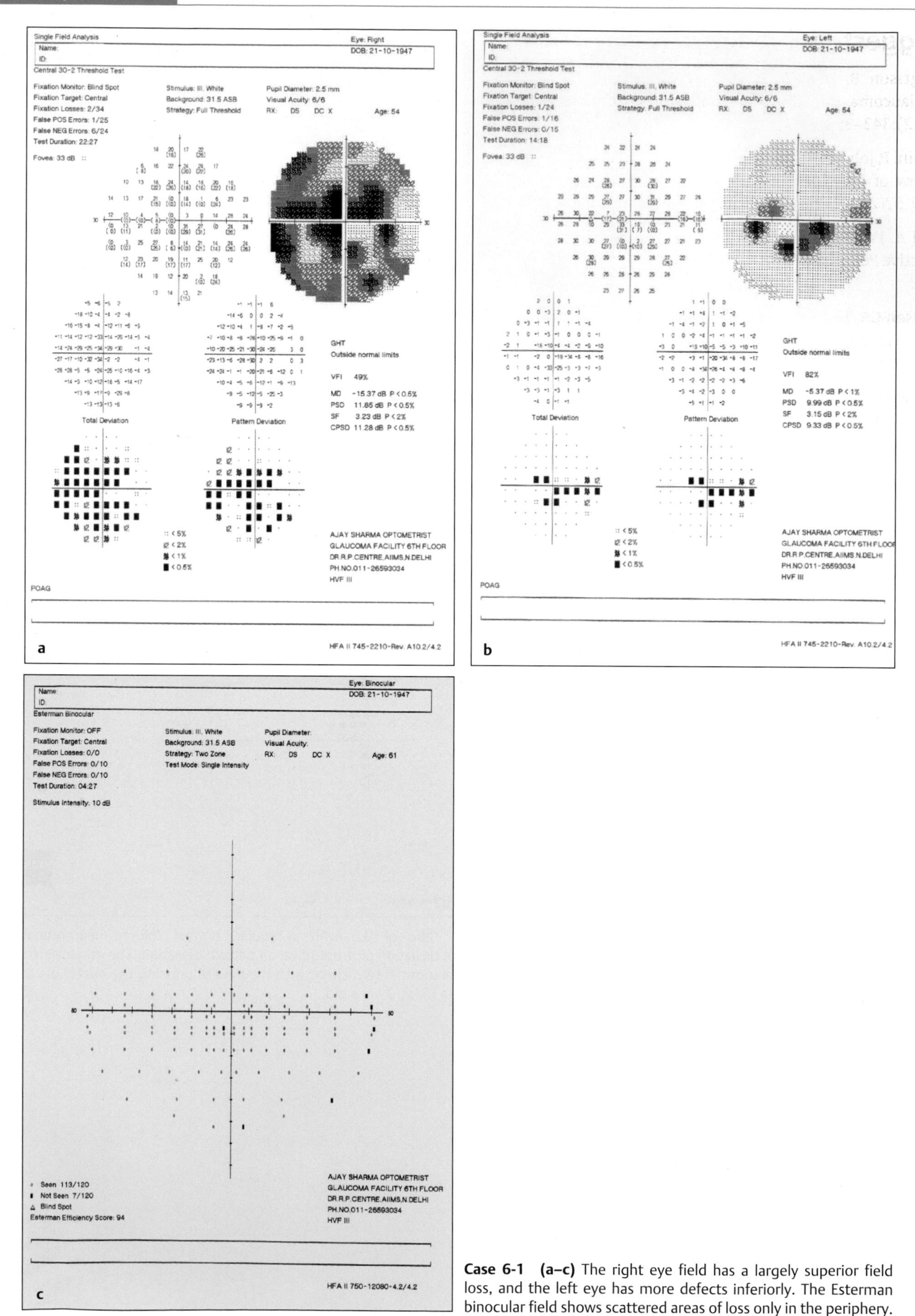

Case 6-1 (a–c) The right eye field has a largely superior field loss, and the left eye has more defects inferiorly. The Esterman binocular field shows scattered areas of loss only in the periphery.

Suggested Readings

Bengtsson B, Heijl A. A visual field index for calculation of glaucoma rate of progression. Am J Ophthalmol 2008; 145(2):343–353

Brusini P, Johnson CA. Staging functional damage in glaucoma: review of different classification methods. Surv Ophthalmol 2007;52(2):156–179

Heijl A, Patella VM, Bengtsson B. The Field Analyzer Primer: Effective Perimetry. 4th ed. Dublin, CA: Carl Zeiss Meditec, Inc; 2012

Johnson CA, Thapa S, George Kong YX, Robin AL. Performance of an iPad application to detect moderate and advanced visual field loss in Nepal. Am J Ophthalmol 2017;182: 147–154

Johnson CA, Wall M, Thompson HS. A history of perimetry and visual field testing. Optom Vis Sci 2011;88(1):E8–E15

Mills RP, Budenz DL, Lee PP, et al. Categorizing the stage of glaucoma from pre-diagnosis to end-stage disease. Am J Ophthalmol 2006;141(1):24–30

Phu J, Khuu SK, Yapp M, Assaad N, Hennessy MP, Kalloniatis M. The value of visual field testing in the era of advanced imaging: clinical and psychophysical perspectives. Clin Exp Optom 2017;100(4):313–332

Susanna R Jr, Vessani RM. Staging glaucoma patient: why and how? Open Ophthalmol J 2009;3:59–64

The AGIS Investigators. The advanced glaucoma intervention study, 6: effect of cataract on visual field and visual acuity. Arch Ophthalmol 2000;118(12):1639–1652

Thomas R, George R. Interpreting automated perimetry. Indian J Ophthalmol 2001;49(2):125–140

CHAPTER 5 Classifications of Visual Field Loss in Glaucoma

Overview

- Anderson's Criteria for Diagnosing a Scotoma
- Aulhorn and Karmeyer Classification
- Simple Classification Based on Optic Nerve Head and Extent of Visual Field Loss
- Classifications Based on Mean Deviation and Extent of Visual Field Loss
- Other Classifications Using Staging
- Illustration of Staging Perimetric Loss by Different Classifications
- Cases
- Suggested Readings

Introduction

Glaucoma is a chronic progressive optic neuropathy and an assessment of visual function is imperative for definitive diagnosis, as well as early diagnosis of progression. In both these situations the degree of loss determines "target" intraocular pressure (IOP) and the therapy required to achieve it.

Classifying visual field loss is important because they:

- Provides a basis of identifying definitive glaucomatous defects.
- Helps determine target IOP and therefore management.
- Determines the efficacy of therapy over time.
- Enables comparisons with patients in literature.

The following are helpful in determining the visual field damage in glaucoma:

- Anderson's criteria for diagnosing a scotoma.
- Aulhorm and Karmeyer classification.
- Classifications based on optic nerve head and extent of visual field loss.
- Classifications based on global indices and extent of visual field loss:
  - Hodapp, Parrish, and Anderson (HPA) classification.
  - Mills classification.
  - Glaucoma staging system.
  - Enhanced glaucoma severity staging.
- Classifications by number and depth of loss on total deviation—Advanced Glaucoma Intervention Study (AGIS) and Collaborative Initial Glaucoma Treatment Study (CIGTS).
- Illustration of staging perimetric loss by different classifications.

Anderson's Criteria for Diagnosing a Scotoma

The criteria for the presence of a glaucomatous scotoma are any one of the three below, but the specificity increases if all are present and reproducible on at least two consecutive fields:

- Glaucoma hemifield test (GHT) should be marked as abnormal.
- Three contiguous, nonedge points on the pattern deviation plot within Bjerrum area have a probability of <5% of being seen in a normal population, one point should have a probability of <1%.
- Corrected pattern standard deviation (PSD) should have a probability of <5%, confirmed on two consecutive tests.

The ideal classification or staging would be simple and easy to interpret, while allowing subtle changes to be definitively identified over time. It should be evidence based and validated. There are many suggested classifications of the severity of glaucomatous damage—HPA classification, glaucoma severity staging system, enhanced glaucoma severity staging system, etc. They are based on the extent of damage and proximity to fixation, using global indices and number/percentage of significantly depressed loci, with multiple and varied staging. They need time and effort to analyze and stage a patient's perimetric loss, and are largely used for research purposes at present and are difficult to apply clinically, by most ophthalmologists.

Aulhorn and Karmeyer Classification

The earliest classification was by *Aulhorn and Karmeyer* for *kinetic perimetry*, to classify glaucomatous damage into the following five stages (**Fig. 5.1**):

- Relative defects in Bjerrum area.
- Absolute defects that do not reach the blind spot.
- Absolute scotomas that merge with blind spot: Arcuate or Seidel.
- Ring-shaped loss with central island left.
- Only temporal island left.

On automated perimetry, the corresponding gray scale would be as depicted in **Fig. 5.2**.

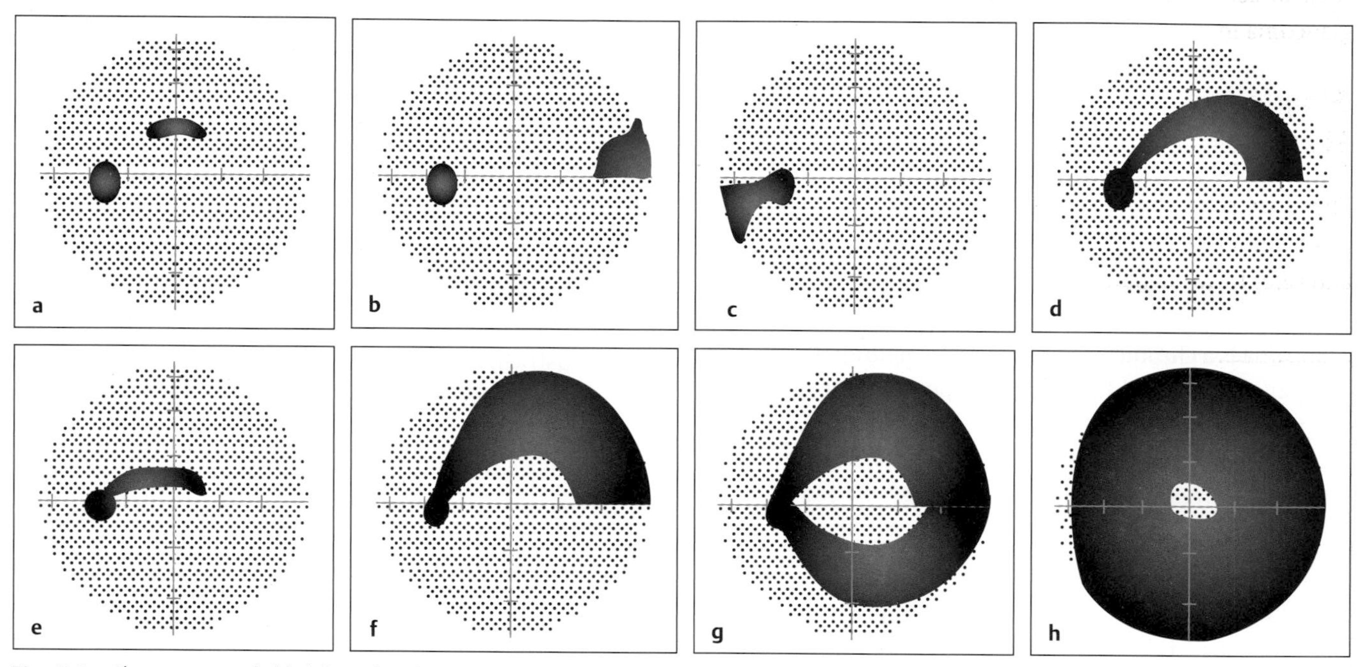

Fig. 5.1 Glaucomatous field defect classification of Aulhorm and Karmeyer for kinetic perimetry transposed to its possible appearance on automated perimetry. **(a)** Paracentral. **(b)** Nasal step. **(c)** Temporal wedge. **(d)** Arcuate. **(e)** Arcuate close to fixation. **(f)** Break through to periphery. **(g)** Biarcuate. **(h)** Central and temporal islands.

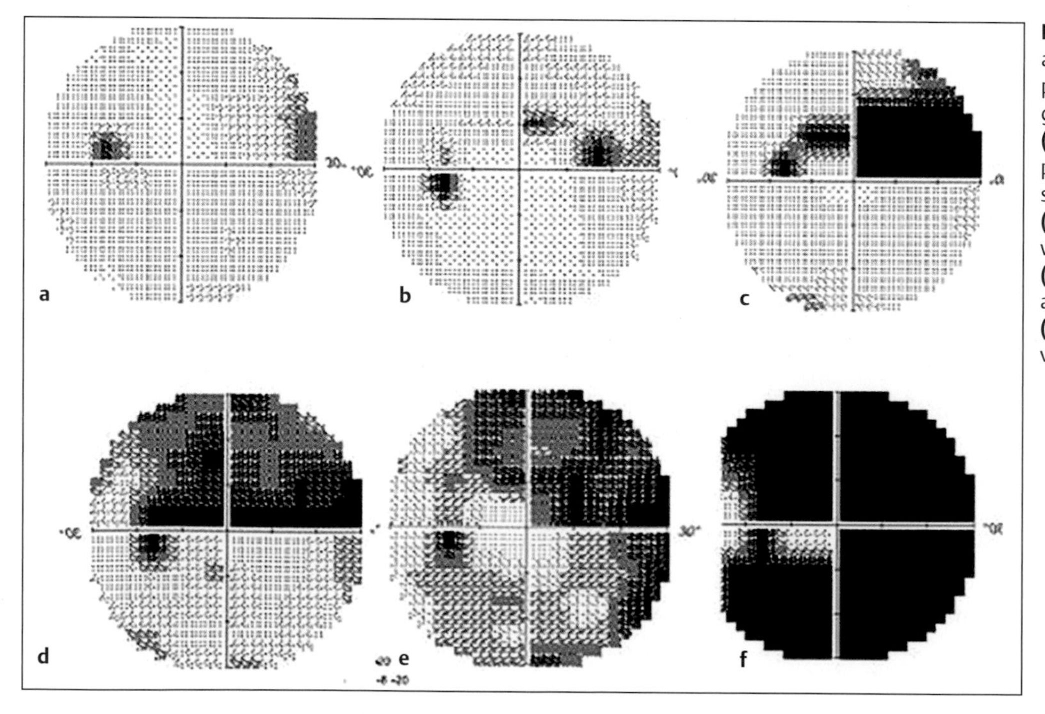

Fig. 5.2 Gray scale printouts of automated perimetry showing progressive visual field loss in glaucoma, as commonly seen. **(a)** Superior nasal step. **(b)** Superior paracentral scotoma and a nasal step. **(c)** Superior arcuate scotoma. **(d)** Superior arcuate scotoma with peripheral breakthrough. **(e)** Additional inferior nasal step and possible arcuate scotoma. **(f)** Central and temporal islands of vision remaining.

There are many glaucoma staging systems; however, it is not known whether any of them actually represents equal steps of damage. Further validation needs to be done so that appropriate management algorithms can be developed. All perimeters with normative data provide global indices and contain a plot highlighting localized loss in the visual field that is definitive of glaucoma, similar to the pattern deviation plot on Humphrey field analyzer (HFA). Therefore, all perimetric printouts can be similarly read to ascertain the pattern of loss and the severity of glaucoma in each eye (**Fig. 5.3**).

Simple Classification Based on Optic Nerve Head and Extent of Visual Field Loss

These are simplified to be easily determined clinically, so as to initiate therapy and enter into databases (**Table 5.1** and refer to **Table 2.2**).

Classifications Based on Mean Deviation and Extent of Visual Field Loss

On automated perimetry, ***Hodapp, Parrish, and Anderson,*** HPA, proposed a classification based on the extent of significant depression of loci. This was based on mean deviation, mean deviation, the percentage of significantly defective points on the pattern deviation plot, and their proximity to fixation. It is easy to apply clinically, but does not allow the diagnosis of small changes in a few loci over time. There is also no information about the location or depth of the defect (**Table 5.2**).

Mills Classification

Mills et al subdivided visual field loss into five stages allowing for an earlier diagnosis of change from one stage to another (**Table 5.3**). Being more time consuming it has not generally been used clinically, and suffers from some of the same problems as the HPA classification.

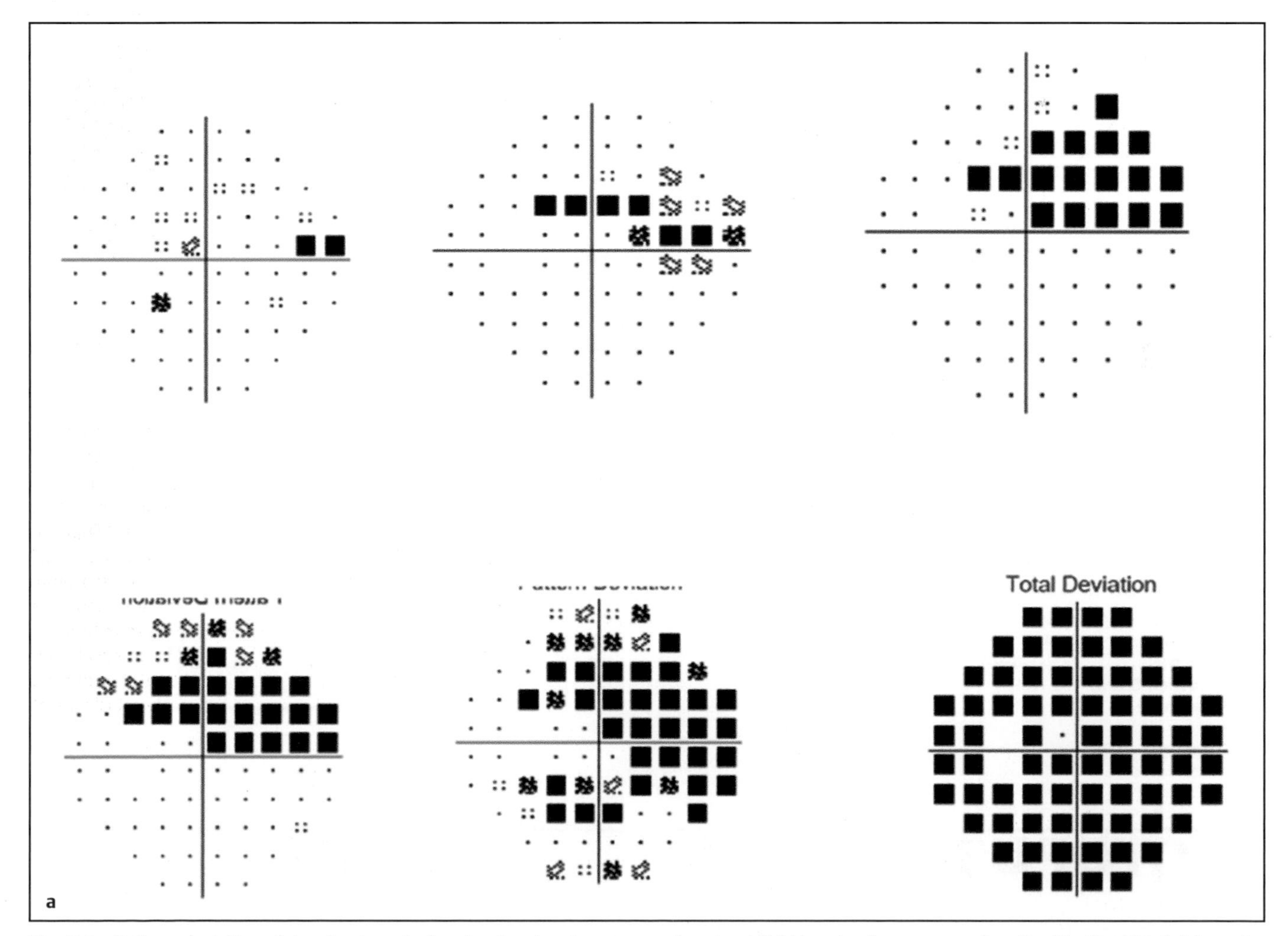

Fig. 5.3 Pattern deviation plots of automated perimetry showing progressive visual field loss in glaucoma, as described in **Fig. 5.2. (a)** Superior nasal step. *(Continued)*

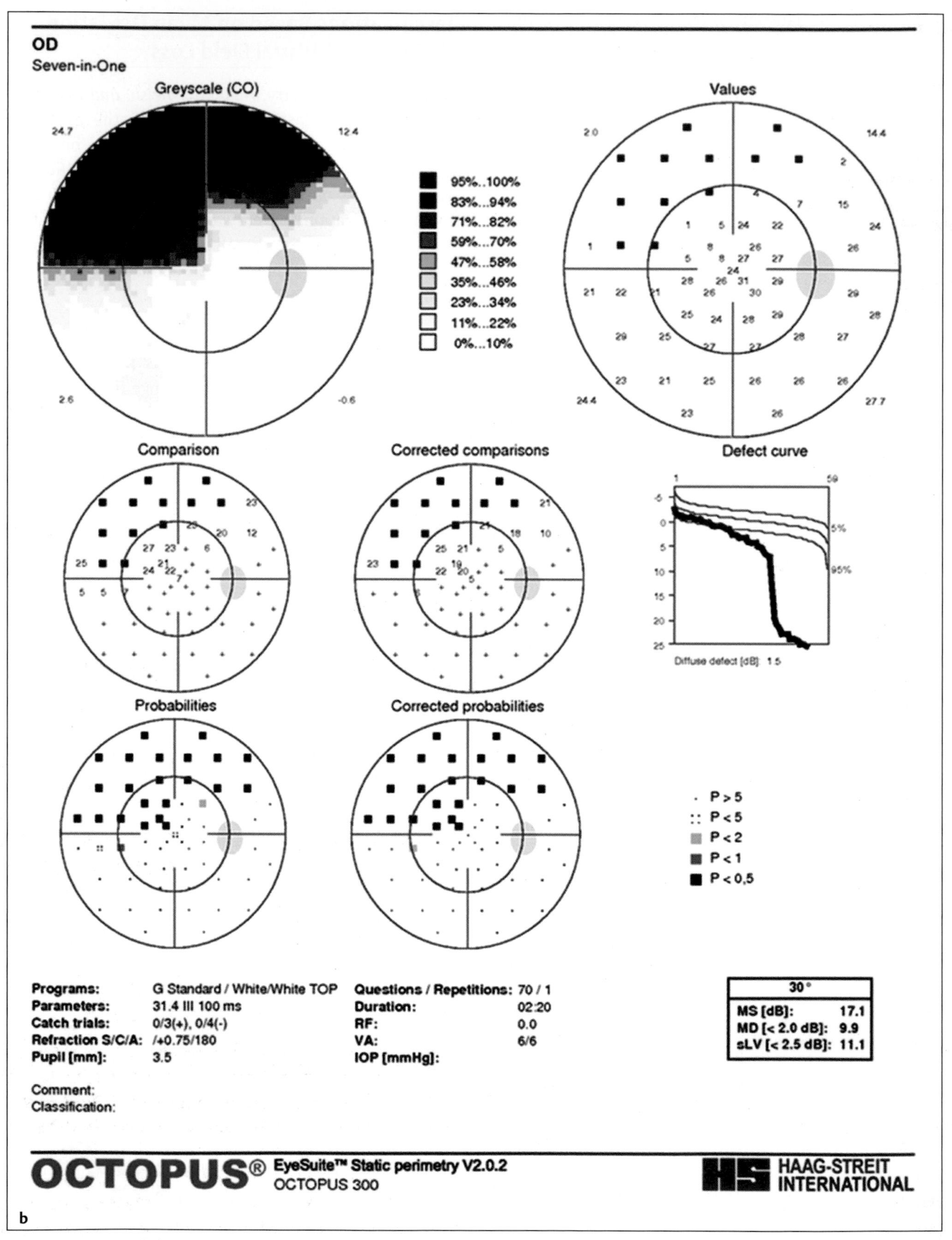

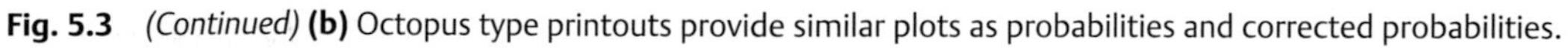

b

Fig. 5.3 *(Continued)* **(b)** Octopus type printouts provide similar plots as probabilities and corrected probabilities.

Table 5.1 Simple classification to use in the clinical setting

	Mild glaucoma	Moderate glaucoma	Severe glaucoma
Perimetric loss	One hemifield nasal step/paracentral scotoma	One hemifield arcuate scotoma not within 10 degrees of fixation	Both hemifields affected or defect within 10 degrees of fixation
Optic nerve head cup:disc ratio	<0.65	0.7 to 0.85	≥0.9

Note: Modification of American Academy of Ophthalmology and Canadian guidelines.

Table 5.2 Hodapp, Parrish, and Anderson classification based on Humphrey visual fields

	Mean deviation	Points depressed, $p < 5\%$	Points depressed $p < 1\%$	Central five-degree points
Early	More than −6 dB	18 (<25%)	<10	All points >15 dB
Moderate	More than −12 dB	<37 (<50%)	<20	One hemifield at <15 dB No point at 0 dB
Severe	Less than −12 dB	>37 (50%)	>20	Both hemifields at <15 dB At least 1 point at 0 dB

Table 5.3 Glaucoma staging system based on Humphrey visual fields (Mills et al)

Stage	Humphrey MD score		Probability plot/ pattern deviation		dB Plot (Stages 2–4) or CPSD/PSD (Stage 1)		dB Plot (Stages 2–4) or hemifield test (Stage 1)
Stage 0—Ocular hypertension/ earliest glaucoma	>0.00	AND		OR	Does not meet any criteria for Stage 1	OR	
Stage 1—Early glaucoma	−0.01 to −5.00 (p<0.05)		Points below 5%: >3 contiguous and >1 of the points below 1%		CPSD/PSD significant at p < 0.05		Glaucoma hemifield test "outside normal limits"
Stage 2—Moderate glaucoma	−5.01 to −12.00		Points below 5%: 19–36 and Points below 1%: 12–18		Point(s) within the central 5 degrees with sensitivity of <15 dB: >1 and point(s) within the central 5 degrees with sensitivity of <0 dB: None (0)		Point(s) with sensitivity <15 dB within 5 degrees of fixation: only 1 hemifield (1 or 2)
Stage 3—Advanced glaucoma	−12.01 to −20.00		Points below 5%: 37–55 and Points below 1%: 19–36		Point(s) within the central 5 degrees with sensitivity of <0 dB: 1 only		Point(s) with sensitivity <15 dB within 5 degrees of fixation: both hemifields, at least 1 in each
Stage 4—Severe glaucoma	−20.01 or worse		Points below 5%: 56–74 and Points below 1%: 37–74		Point(s) within the central 5 degrees with sensitivity of <0 dB: 2–4		Point(s) with sensitivity <15 dB within 5 degrees of fixation: both hemifields, 2 in each (All)
Stage 5—End-stage glaucoma/blind	No HVF in "worst eye"		HVF not possible attributable to central scotoma in "worst eye" or "worst eye" acuity of 20/200 or worse attributable to glaucoma. "Best eye" may fall into any of above stages				

Abbreviations: CPSD/PSD, corrected pattern standard deviation/pattern standard deviation; dB, decibel; HVF, Humphrey visual field; MD, mean deviation.

Glaucoma Staging System and Enhanced Glaucoma Severity

It is a modification of the HPA classification, with many additions. It is based on visual field global indices, mean deviation and PSD, GHT, number and location of depressed points on the pattern deviation plot, and visual acuity. It is, therefore, able to detect focal and generalized field loss. It is divided into six stages—0: no defect, 1: mild, 3: moderate, 4: severe, 5: end stage—but does not provide information about the pattern or location of defects. Some of the additional parameters used to stage the glaucoma were not found to be useful, restricting its use currently. The enhanced glaucoma severity staging can also be used with Octopus fields using mean defect and loss variance. A chart is required for interpretation.

Other Classifications Using Staging

The AGIS divided glaucomatous visual field loss by a score of 20, based on the number and depth of adjacent loci on the total deviation plot, with 0 denoting no depression, while a score of 20 had two depressed points in the nasal and nine each in the superior and inferior hemifields. Adjacent points reaching a defined depression of sensitivity were noted to produce a score. Stage 1 is a score of 0, Stage 2 is mild loss of 1 to 5, Stage 3 is moderate loss of 6 to 11, Stage 4 is severe loss of 12 to 17, and Stage 5 is end stage of 18 to 20. This is again time consuming, and not suitable for use clinically.

The CIGTS also used total deviation readings on a 24 -2 printout, and based change on a minimum loss of sensitivity at a locus and two adjacent defective points. The score of all points was then divided by 10.4 to get a scale of damage. Being based on the total deviation plot these may be affected by media opacification.

Illustration of Staging Perimetric Loss by Different Classifications

All classifications look at the extent of visual field loss, but by different criteria and in different steps, which make comparisons or interchangeable use difficult (**Figs. 5.4** and **5.5**).

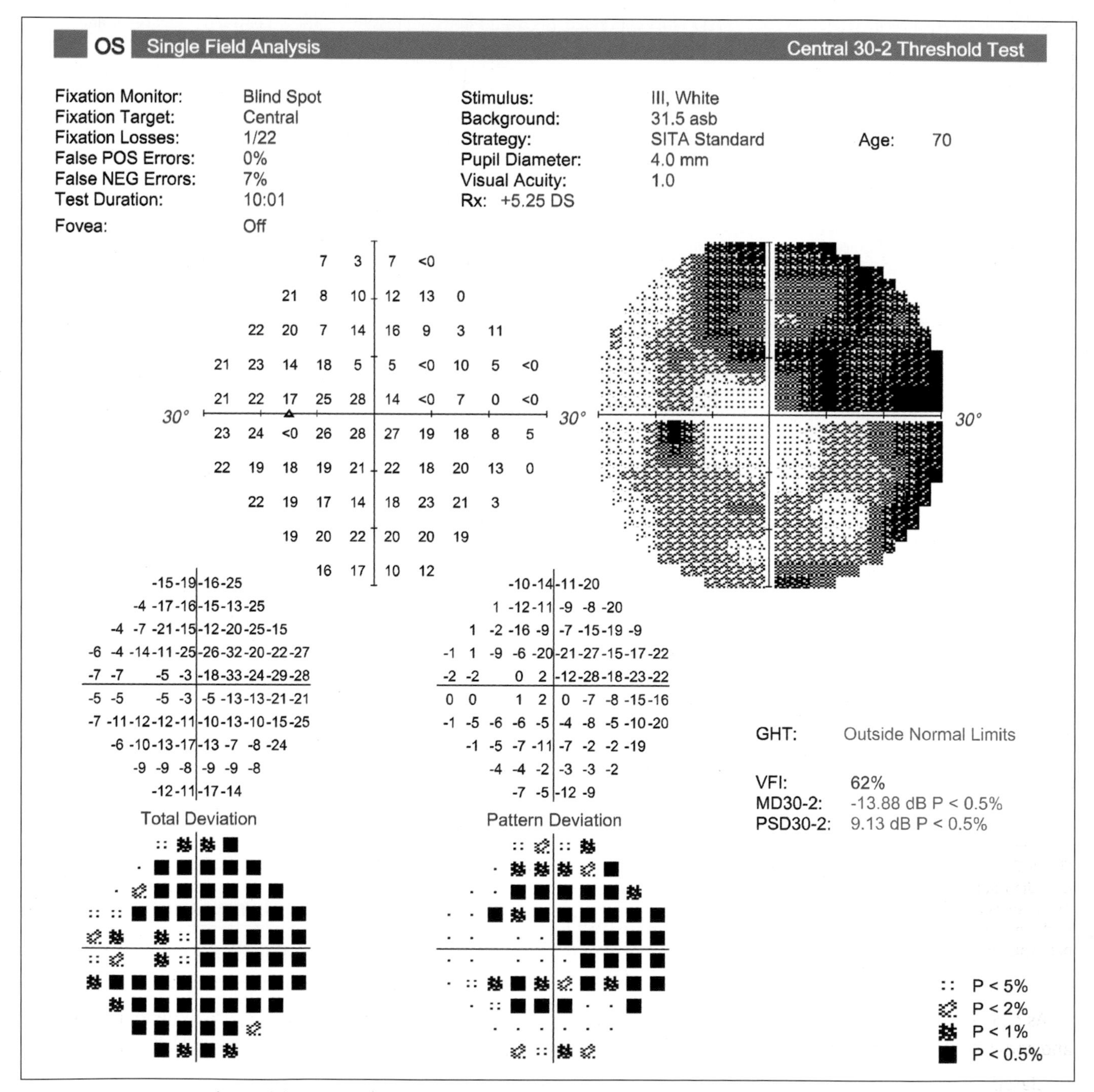

Fig. 5.4 On comparing the guidelines, American Academy of Ophthalmology (AAO), International Classification of Diseases (ICD) 10, and Canadian guidelines classified as severe—as both hemispheres are involved. Hodapp, Parrish, and Anderson classification classified as severe—mean deviation 13, >37 loci values likely to be seen in <5% of the normal population, >20 loci values likely to be seen in <1% of the normal population, central 5 degrees show values of <15 dB in both hemispheres with one point at 0 dB. Mills classification classified as moderate—11 loci <1%, no loci with values <0 dB, one hemisphere involved.

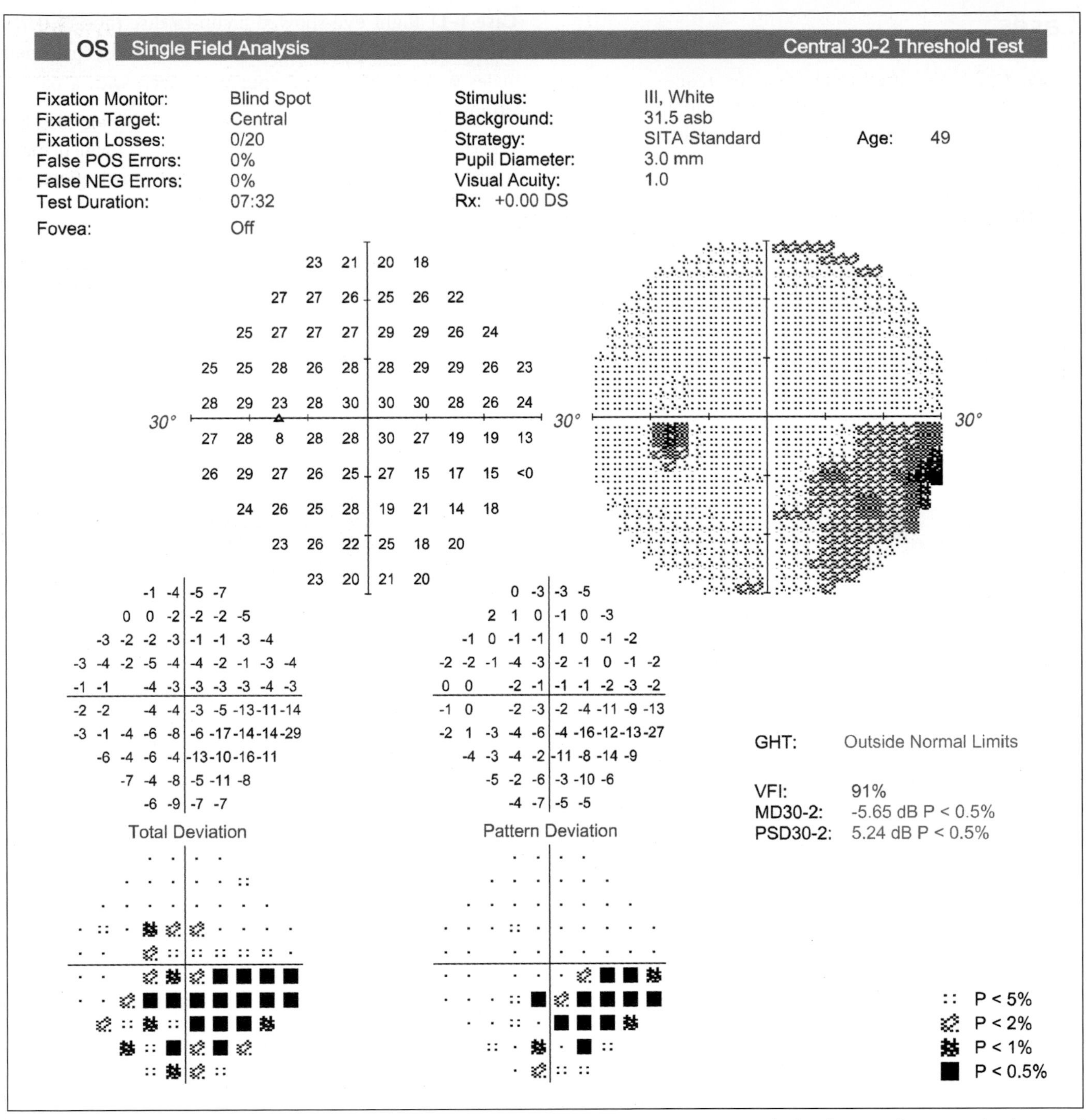

Fig. 5.5 On comparing the guidelines, American Academy of Ophthalmology (AAO), International Classification of Diseases (ICD) 10, and Canadian guidelines classified as moderate—as one hemisphere is involved and the central 5/10 degrees are uninvolved. Hodapp, Parrish, and Anderson classification classified as early or moderate (may be one or both stages)—mean deviation −5.65 dB, 14 loci values likely to be seen in <5% of the normal population. However, central points are <15 dB. Mills classification classified as early or moderate—mean deviation −5.65 dB, one hemisphere, 14 loci <5%, all central loci with values <15 dB.

As can be seen, the classifications do not always concur, and some fields fall between two stages.

Classification of the severity of visual field loss in glaucoma is important, as it is one of the *most important criteria determining the functional extent of damage to the optic nerve head.* This then provides a basis for reaching an estimate of the IOP that may stabilize and maintain optic nerve head function for the patients' lifetime. *As perimetry is a subjective test and perimetric loss is different in all individuals, it is important to understand the basis of such classifications, and not base it on just one parameter, for example, mean deviation.*

Cases

Case 1

A 19-year-old male, diagnosed as juvenile open-angle glaucoma (JOAG) with baseline IOP of 42 mm Hg in right eye and 44 mm Hg in left eye, underwent a trabeculectomy in both eyes 10 years ago and IOPs were well controlled till a year earlier without medications. He complained of gradual and painless diminution of vision in right eye, with a best corrected visual acuity of 6/12 in right eye and 6/6 in left eye, and IOPs of 34 mm Hg and 22 mm Hg in right eye and left eye, respectively.

On examination, anterior chamber of van Herick grade 3 was present with sluggish pupillary reaction in right eye. Mildly elevated but vascular blebs were seen in both eyes (**Case 1-1**). Right eye showed a cup-to-disc ratio of 0.9:1 and left eye cup:disc ratio of 0.7:1. On gonioscopy, open angles with visible scleral spur were seen with a patent ostium.

Perimetry right eye 10–2 showed involvement of both hemispheres, and left eye had a relatively normal field.

Points to consider

- Failing blebs due to subconjunctival fibrosis are present, which lead to inappropriately high IOPs.
- Target IOPs should be lower as patient is young with severe glaucomatous neuropathy, and is expected to live for at least 60 years.
- As perimetry has high fixation losses, it needs to be repeated.

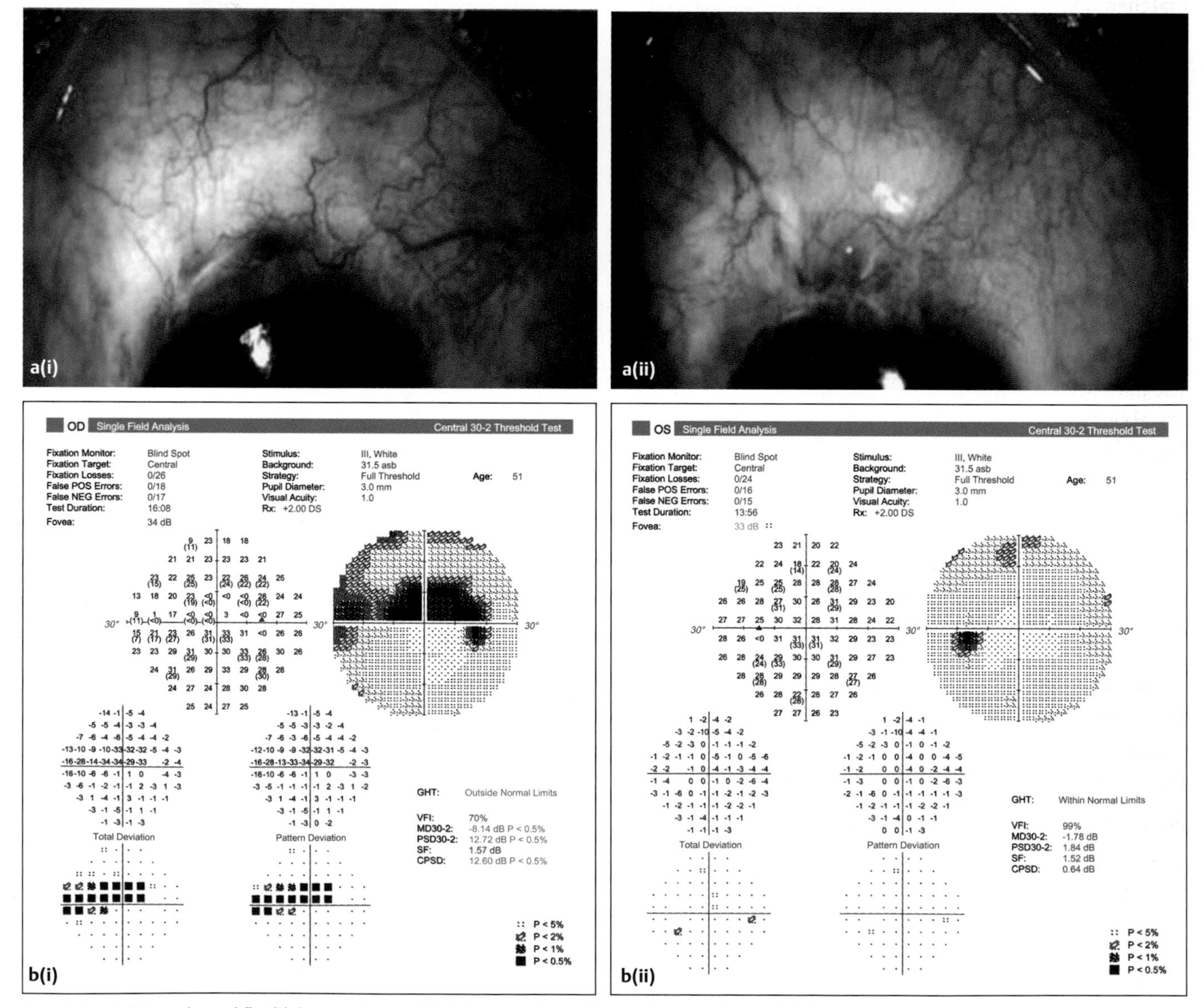

Case 1-1 **(a)** Vascularized flat bleb on right eye. **(b)** Left eye with mildly vascular but elevated bleb.

Diagnosis and Management

Both eyes were started on a prostaglandin (PG) analog, with additional β-blocker in right eye. IOP remained at 24/14 mm Hg. In right eye, 360-degree selective laser trabeculoplasty (SLT) was then done. After 6 months, peak diurnal IOPs were 14 mm Hg in both eyes and perimetry was stable.

Case 2

A 65-year-old male was diagnosed as a glaucoma suspect on routine evaluation. Both eyes anterior chamber was shallow and van Herick grade 2, iris atrophy was present, and cup:disc ratio was 0.7 in the right eye and 0.5 in the left. Highest IOPs were 28 and 22 mm Hg.

The right eye HFA showed seven contiguous loci in the superonasal field, likely to be seen in <5% of the age-matched population, with three points likely to be seen in <1% of the normal population (**Case 2-1**).

Points to consider

- The abnormal points are in the nasal extent of Bjerrum area and respect the horizontal midline; therefore, glaucoma is likely.
- Anderson's criteria are fulfilled (more than 3 contiguous points/likely to be seen in <5% of age-matched population and one point <1%/GHT outside normal limits).

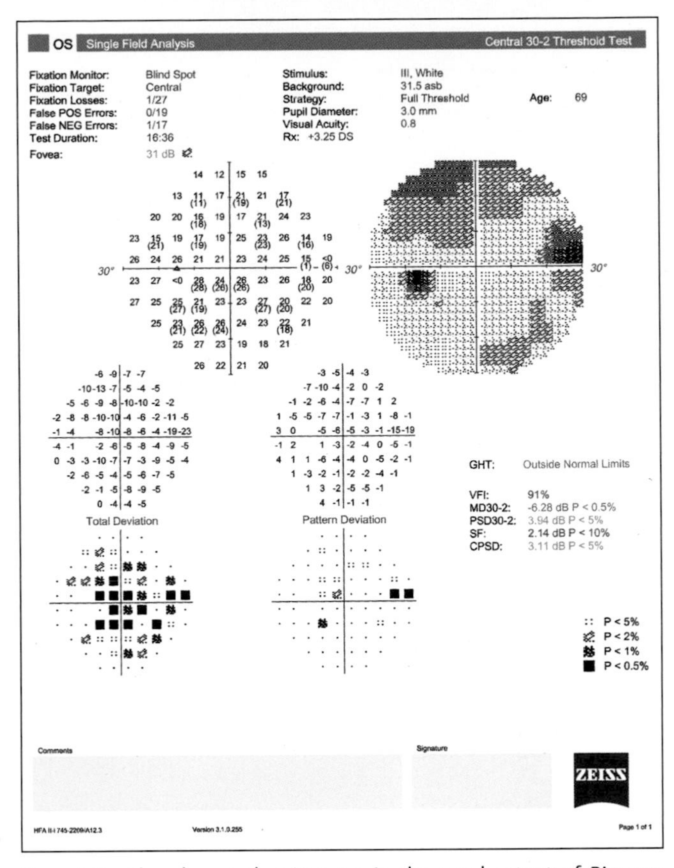

Case 2-1 The abnormal points are in the nasal extent of Bjerrum area and respect the horizontal midline; therefore, glaucoma is likely. Anderson's criteria are fulfilled (more than 3 contiguous points/likely to be seen in <5% of age-matched population and one point <1%/ glaucoma Hemifield test [GHT] outside normal limits).

Diagnosis and Management

The patient has mild glaucoma by HPA criteria, <25% of loci are abnormal, no central points are significantly affected. Target IOP should be 15 to 18 mm Hg initially.

Case 3

A 65-year-old male with dysthyroid ophthalmopathy was recorded to have an applanation tonometry of 24/26 mm Hg 8 years ago, with normal fields, for which he was on intermittent glaucoma medication with one drug. He presented with a superior arcuate scotoma in the left eye. On examination, there was a deep anterior chamber, cup:disc ratio of 0.5 and 0.7 with a thin neuroretinal rim inferiorly, and an IOP of 26/30 mm Hg.

Points to consider

- Anderson's criteria for a visual field defect are fulfilled (more than 3 contiguous points/likely to be seen in <5% of age-matched population and one point <1%/GHT outside normal limits).
- The field defect is in Bjerrum area and respects the horizontal midline (**Case 3-1**).

Diagnosis and Management

The patient has a moderate glaucoma by HPA criteria: <50% of loci are abnormal, no central points are affected significantly, and a superior arcuate defect is found. Target IOP was initially set at 12 to 15 mm Hg, for which a PG analog hs and a β-blocker bd were prescribed.

Case 4

A 68-year-old male was referred with uncontrolled IOP, 22/20 mm Hg, on four glaucoma medications. On examination, he was a myope with deep ACs, and a cup:disc ratio of 0.9 in both eyes. His perimetry was done.

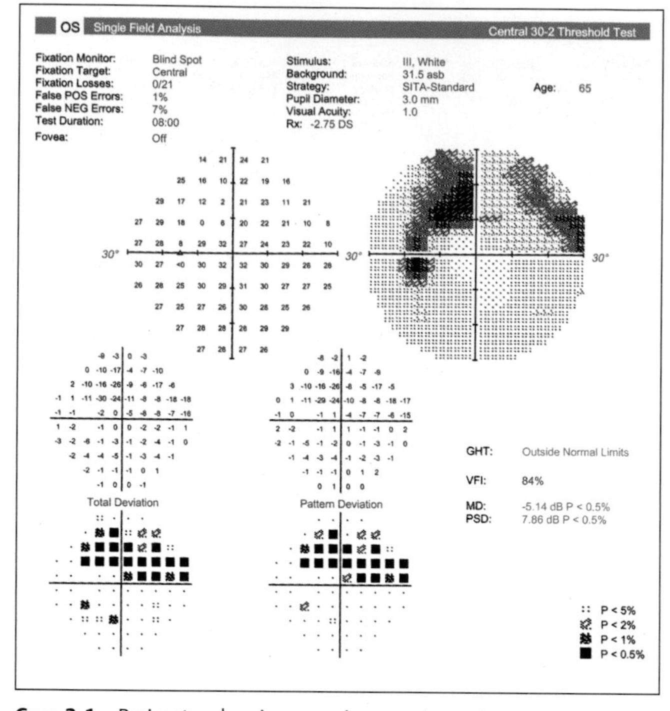

Case 3-1 Perimetry showing superior arcuate scotoma.

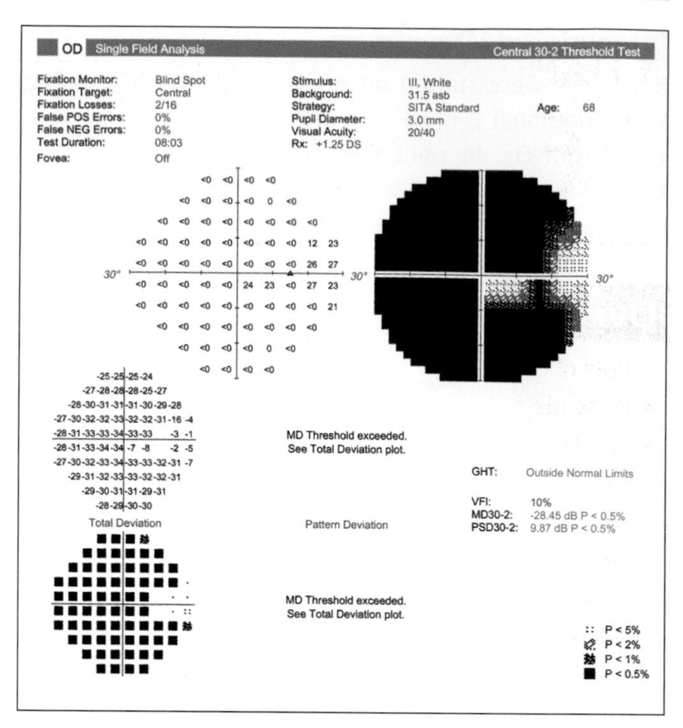

Case 4-1 Perimetry showing a central and temporal island of vision remaining; severe by all classifications.

Points to consider

- Anderson's criteria are fulfilled and the pattern deviation plot shows that >50% of loci are abnormal and central 10 degrees are affected significantly.
- This is a severe glaucoma by HPA criteria (**Case 4-1**).
- Such patients need a low IOP, 10 to 12 mm Hg, which was achieved by a trabeculectomy in both eyes. His fields are stable 15 years later.

Suggested Readings

Advanced Glaucoma Intervention Study. 2. Visual field test scoring and reliability. Ophthalmology 1994;101(8): 1445–1455

Bengtsson B, Heijl A. A visual field index for calculation of glaucoma rate of progression. Am J Ophthalmol 2008;145(2): 343–353

Brusini P. Clinical use of a new method for visual field damage classification in glaucoma. Eur J Ophthalmol 1996;6(4): 402–407

Brusini P, Filacorda S. Enhanced Glaucoma Staging System (GSS 2) for classifying functional damage in glaucoma. J Glaucoma 2006;15(1):40–46

Hirasawa K, Shoji N, Morita T, Shimizu K. A modified glaucoma staging system based on visual field index. Graefes Arch Clin Exp Ophthalmol 2013;251(12):2747–2752

Hodapp E, Parrish RK II, Anderson DR. Clinical decisions in glaucoma. St Louis: CV Mosby Co; 1993: 52–61

Lau LI, Liu CJ, Chou JC, Hsu WM, Liu JH. Patterns of visual field defects in chronic angle-closure glaucoma with different disease severity. Ophthalmology 2003; 110(10):1890–1894

Mills RP, Budenz DL, Lee PP, et al. Categorizing the stage of glaucoma from pre-diagnosis to end-stage disease. Am J Ophthalmol 2006;141(1):24–30

Ng M, Sample PA, Pascual JP, et al. Comparison of visual field severity classification systems for glaucoma. J Glaucoma 2012;21(8):551–561

Öhnell H, Bengtsson B, Heijl A. Making a correct diagnosis of glaucoma: data from the EMGT. J Glaucoma 2019;28(10): 859–864

Quigley HA, Tielsch JM, Katz J, Sommer A. Rate of progression in open-angle glaucoma estimated from cross-sectional prevalence of visual field damage. Am J Ophthalmol 1996; 122(3):355–363

Susanna R Jr, Vessani RM. Staging glaucoma patient: why and how? Open Ophthalmol J 2009;3:59–64

CHAPTER 6

Optical Coherence Tomography in Glaucoma

Overview

- Role of Optical Coherence Tomography in Glaucoma
- Principle
- Spectral Domain Optical Coherence Tomography
- Swept Source Optical Coherence Tomography
- Normative Data for Glaucoma in Optical Coherence Tomography
- Parameters Relevant to the Detection of Glaucomatous Abnormalities
    - Retinal Nerve Fiber Layer Analysis
    - Macular Ganglion Cell Complex
    - Optic Nerve Head Analysis
- How to Read a Retinal Nerve Fiber Layer Optical Coherence Tomography Report
- How to Read a Macula Report
- Optic Nerve Head Analysis
- Factors Leading to Misinterpretation in Optical Coherence Tomography
- Diagnosing Progression
- Cases
- Suggested Readings

Introduction

Progressive loss of retinal ganglion cells (RGCs) and their axons is characteristic of any glaucoma. RGCs synapse with bipolar and amacrine cells in the inner plexiform layer, and their axons form the retinal nerve fiber layer. RGC axons converge toward the scleral canal and form the neuroretinal rim of the optic nerve. Optical coherence tomography can image all these anatomical structures in high resolution, allowing imaging of each retinal layer and optic nerve head, to be used for objective evaluation of glaucomatous neuropathy.

Role of Optical Coherence Tomography in Glaucoma

Optical coherence tomography is a noncontact, noninvasive method of examining the optic nerve head and retina, and providing ultra-high spatial resolution, cross-sectional, and three-dimensional images.

The importance of optical coherence tomography in glaucoma is manifold, and lies especially in:

- Early diagnosis by detecting objective, progressive change in parameters.
- Diagnosis of progression to guide and reassess therapy over time.
- Providing prognostic parameters for counseling.

The fallacies of optical coherence tomography, however, have to be kept in mind, and some are:

- High false positives reported.
- Frequent artifacts seen.
- Parameters influenced by optic nerve head size.
- Age-related changes vary in individuals.
- Other retinal and neurological disease changes overlap with those of glaucoma.
- Inability to compare data from different machines.

Principle

It is based on the principle of interferometry, as in Michelson interferometer, wherein interference between reflected light and a reference beam is used to reconstruct depth and identify tissue discontinuities. The interferometer splits incoming light into two, one to the tissue and the other to a reference beam of known length. Light returning from both paths is again combined at the interferometer output. The superimposed waves can add or cancel each other, and the different intensity of combined light is interpreted through an electrical signal and photodetector, as a difference in the length of the optical path of both beams. Differences in the reflecting properties and echo delay of ocular tissues permit the delineation of different layers of the anterior segment, retina, and optic nerve.

Optical coherence tomography uses light in the near-infrared spectrum to permit a penetration in tissue of 2 to 400 µm. A scanning beam acquires many two-dimensional cross-sectional images, which are then put together to form a three-dimensional image of the tissue. In *time domain optical coherence tomography*, the reference length is modulated for each scan using broadband light source with a point detector. *Spectral domain optical coherence tomography* uses an interference spectrum to compute A-scans. *Swept source optical coherence tomography* utilizes an optical light source to sweep scan a narrow width. Each wavelength of the interferometric signal is detected sequentially. This picks up details of the entire depth at one go, from which an A-scan is computed by Fourier transformation, allowing for greater speed of imaging and an increase in signal to noise ratio.

Spectral Domain Optical Coherence Tomography

Spectral domain optical coherence tomography uses Fourier domain transformation and is also called spatially encoded frequency domain optical coherence tomography. A broad beam light source is used with a fixed reference mirror and the images are formed by a spectrometer and a linear charge-coupled devices (CCD) using Fourier transformation (**Fig. 6.1**). This increases the image acquisition speed by 200 times that of time domain optical coherence tomography, thus also reducing the artifacts caused by eye movements. The axial resolution of this system approaches 5 to 7 µm.

Swept Source Optical Coherence Tomography

Swept source optical coherence tomography uses a narrow bandwidth of light rather than broad wavelength used in time domain or spectral domain. The narrow wavelength light is changed in frequency by the swept source laser over time, leading to changed echo delay times. Since the light changes over time, a spectrometer is not used, instead a high-speed detector picks up the change in interference signal and further uses Fourier domain to analyze the signal (**Fig. 6.2**). Axial resolution with this is 5 to 7 µm at 1,050 nm wavelength.

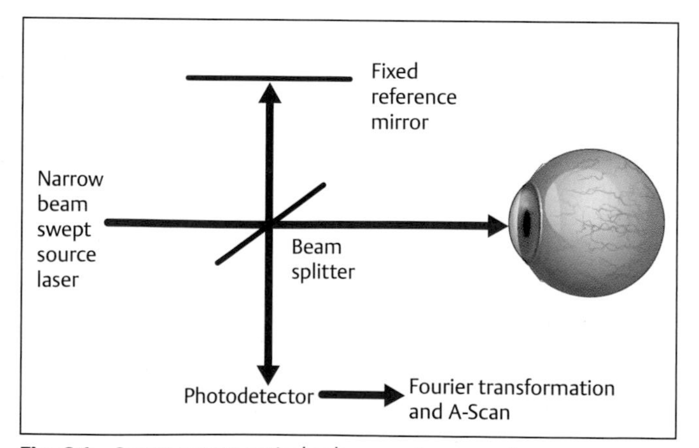

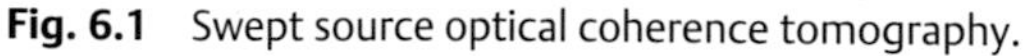

Fig. 6.1 Swept source optical coherence tomography.

Normative Data for Glaucoma in Optical Coherence Tomography

Normative data is generated by evaluation of normal individuals of different ages, and is different in different optical coherence tomography machines. The normative age-matched data differs due to differences in the machines themselves, as well as the fact that different individuals are scanned in each. Most of the data is of Caucasians, with the Cirrus, Optovue, and some other machines incorporating data of other ethnicities as well. *As the normative data used by machines is different, it follows that they cannot be used interchangeably.* For example, average thickness of the retinal nerve fiber layer is 84 to 94 µm +/− 13.68 on Cirrus, 89 to 97.3 µm +/− 9.6 to 15.87 µm on Spectralis, and 107.9 µm +/− 10 µm on Optove (**Table 6.1**).

Further, each machine has different scan protocols, analysis methodology, and printouts, so that evaluation of each report has to be done carefully. Each update leads to more features, such as real-time eye tracking system that couples confocal scanning laser ophthalmoscope (CSLO) and spectral domain optical coherence tomography scanners in the Spectralis machine, and differences in marking of the outer retinal boundary, outer retinal pigment epithelium (RPE) or Bruch's membrane.

It is seen that all of them project any significant differences from normative data in color, coded as yellow for likelihood of being seen in 1 to 5% and red for likelihood of being seen in less than 1% of an age-matched normal cohort.

Parameters Relevant to the Detection of Glaucomatous Abnormalities

Retinal nerve fiber layer thinning and ganglion cell and neuroretinal rim loss are considered to be the most useful for diagnosis of glaucoma, as well as for an early detection of progression. Optical coherence tomography permits an objective and quantitative determination of these parameters and changes can be analyzed both quantitatively and qualitatively.

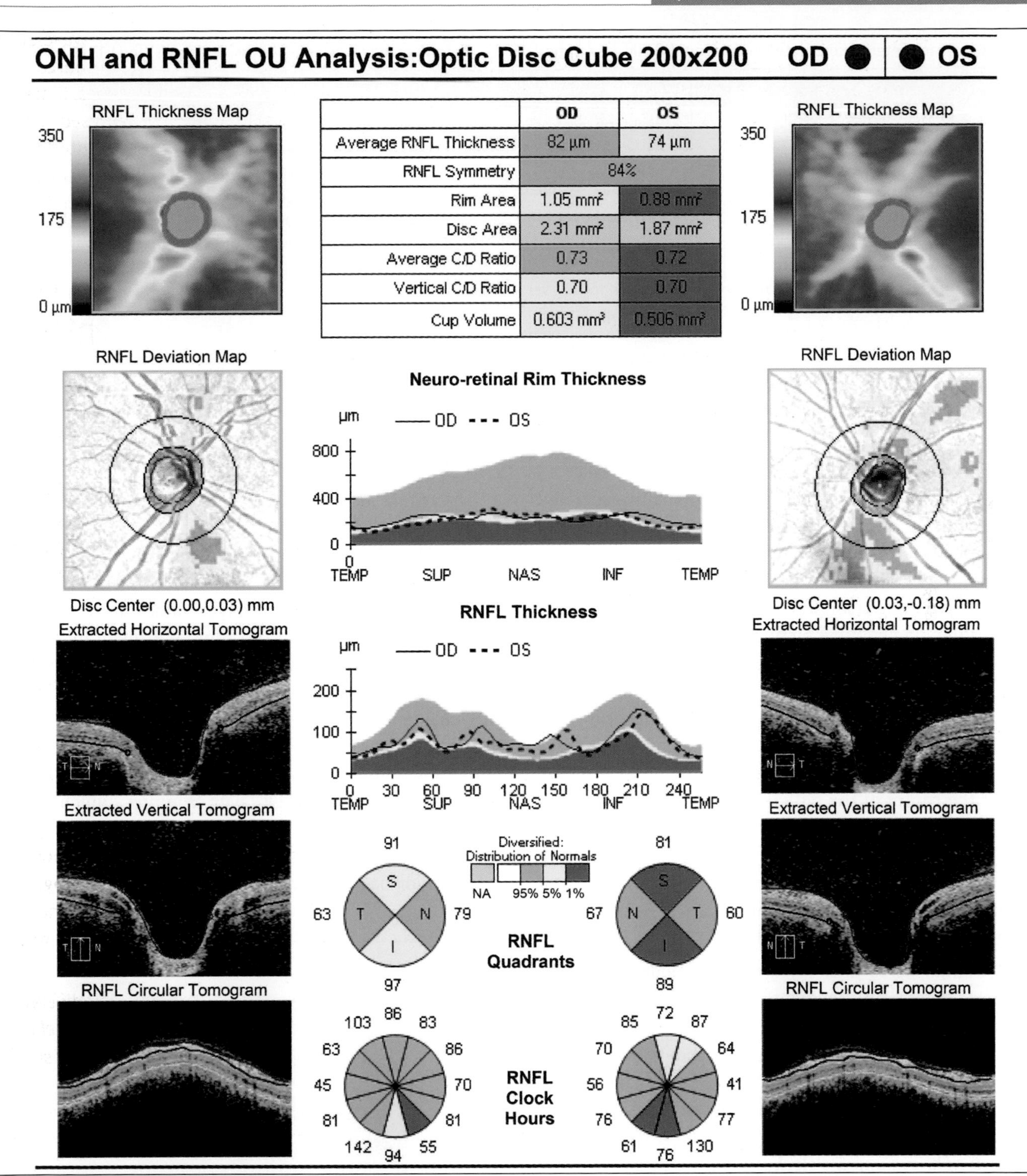

	OD	OS
Average RNFL Thickness	82 µm	74 µm
RNFL Symmetry	84%	
Rim Area	1.05 mm²	0.88 mm²
Disc Area	2.31 mm²	1.87 mm²
Average C/D Ratio	0.73	0.72
Vertical C/D Ratio	0.70	0.70
Cup Volume	0.603 mm³	0.506 mm³

Fig. 6.2 Reading an optical coherence tomography printout for glaucoma.

The most important parameters for glaucoma diagnosis in any spectral domain optical coherence tomography machine are thought to be:

- Retinal nerve fiber layer thickness.
- Macular ganglion cell complex (GCC) and ganglion cell layer + inner plexiform layer.
- Optic nerve head—rim area and vertical cup:disc ratio.

Retinal Nerve Fiber Layer Analysis

Clinically, retinal nerve fiber layer loss in the superior or inferior quadrant leads to the appearance of a wedge-shaped

Table 6.1 Parameters incorporated in three commonly used optical coherence tomography machines—Cirrus, Spectralis, and RTVue

Cirrus	Spectralis	RTVue
▪ Axial resolution – 5 µm ▪ RNFL: Average 84–94 µm +/– 13.68 ▪ Measure – pRNFL, GCL + IPL, ONH, macular thickness ▪ **Disc area:** 1.66 to 1.97 mm sq ▪ Outer retinal boundary: Outer RPE ▪ **Corrects for disc size** ▪ Well-centered scans with signal strength >7 and the absence of movement artifact	▪ Real-time eye tracking system that couples CSLO and SD-OCT scanners ▪ Resolution – 7 um ▪ RNFL: Average 89–97.3 µm +/– 9.6–15.87 µm ▪ **Centered over BMO** ▪ **Reference plane independent BMO – MRW** ▪ Outer retinal boundary: Bruch's membrane ▪ Thicker ppRNFL versus Cirrus in same eyes ▪ Image quality: Signal strength ≥5 dB and absence of movement artifact ▪ Posteror pole asymmetry analysis	▪ Resolution – 5 µm ▪ Average 107.9 +/– 10 µm ▪ RNFL, GCC, macular thickness ▪ GCC: NFL + GCL + IPL ▪ Disc area: Range 1.86–2.1 mmsq ▪ Outer retinal boundary: External RPE ▪ Signal strength index >30

Abbreviations: BMO-MRW, Bruch's membrane opening–minimum rim width; CSLO, confocal scanning laser ophthalmoscope; GCC, ganglion cell complex; GCL, ganglion cell layer; IPL, inner plexiform layer; ONH, optic nerve head; ppRNFL, peripapillary retinal nerve fiber layer; RNFL, retinal nerve fiber layer; RPE, retinal pigment epithelium; SD-OCT, spectral domain optical coherence tomography.

retinal nerve fiber layer defect, which is usually associated with a localized notch in the neuroretinal rim. Yet, retinal nerve fiber layer changes may often precede changes on the optic nerve head, and these are not visible clinically. Retinal nerve fiber layer scanning with optical coherence tomography may be done by two strategies. First, a three-dimensional construct of the retinal nerve fiber layer around the optic nerve is made in a cube comprised of A-scans, and reported as a retinal nerve fiber layer thickness map. Second, peripapillary retinal nerve fiber layer thickness is studied at a specific, commonly 3.46 mm, scan circle around the center of the optic disc. This circle is obtained from a 6 × 6 optic disc cube scan in Cirrus high-definition optical coherence tomography, whereas Heidelberg Spectralis optical coherence tomography measures retinal nerve fiber layer at a single circular scan of 3.5 mm or at three concentric circles of 3.5, 4.1, and 4.7 mm.

The retinal nerve fiber layer thickness map is depicted in pseudo-colors—blue being thin, while red and white are thicker areas. The normal retinal nerve fiber layer thickness map shows thicker areas as red–white areas in superotemporal and inferotemporal quadrants. *It has been noted that inferotemporal quadrants are commonly the first affected in glaucoma and are the best discriminants—7 o'clock right eye and 5 o'clock left eye, resulting in a color change from red–white to yellow or blue* (**Fig. 6.3**).

Retinal nerve fiber layer deviation map: This uses an enface retinal image highlighting cup, disc edge, and calculation circle upon which *any significant deviation from normal is superimposed in red.*

It is important to understand that the "hot" colors on the retinal nerve fiber layer thickness map represent thicker retinal nerve fiber layer, while red on the deviation map denotes a significant thinning of the retinal nerve fiber layer.

The *retinal nerve fiber layer calculation circle* is divided into quadrants—temporal, superior, nasal, and inferior (as the TSNIT plot)—reporting retinal nerve fiber layer thickness values along the scan circle versus normative data. The retinal nerve fiber layer values are reported as black lines, starting from the temporal quadrant in each eye, that is, clockwise starting from 9 o'clock in right eye and counter-clockwise starting from 3 o'clock in left eye. *A double hump pattern is seen in normal eyes, with peaks at superotemporal and inferotemporal areas.* This elevation or double hump is characteristically lost in glaucoma-related retinal nerve fiber layer thinning, which occurs predominantly in these areas. The probability levels for abnormality on the black TSNIT graph are shown against a four color backdrop, namely, white, green, yellow, and

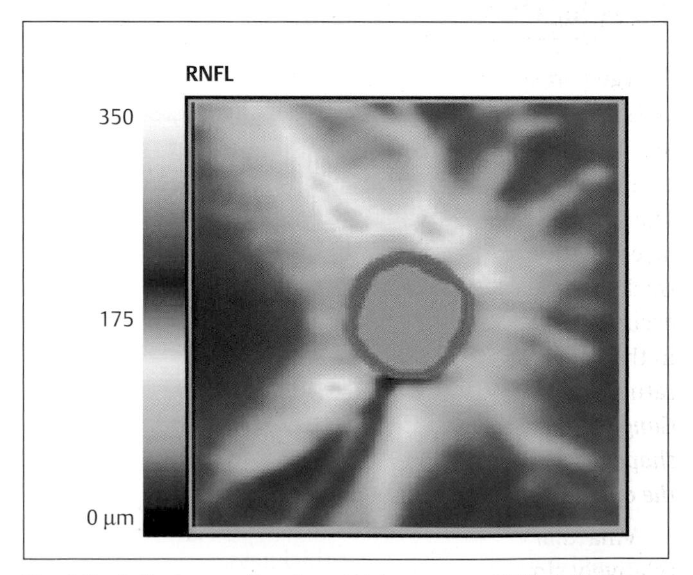

Fig. 6.3 Retinal nerve fiber layer thickness map. RNFL, retinal nerve fiber layer. Pseudo-colors—blue-yellow being thin, while red-white are thicker areas.

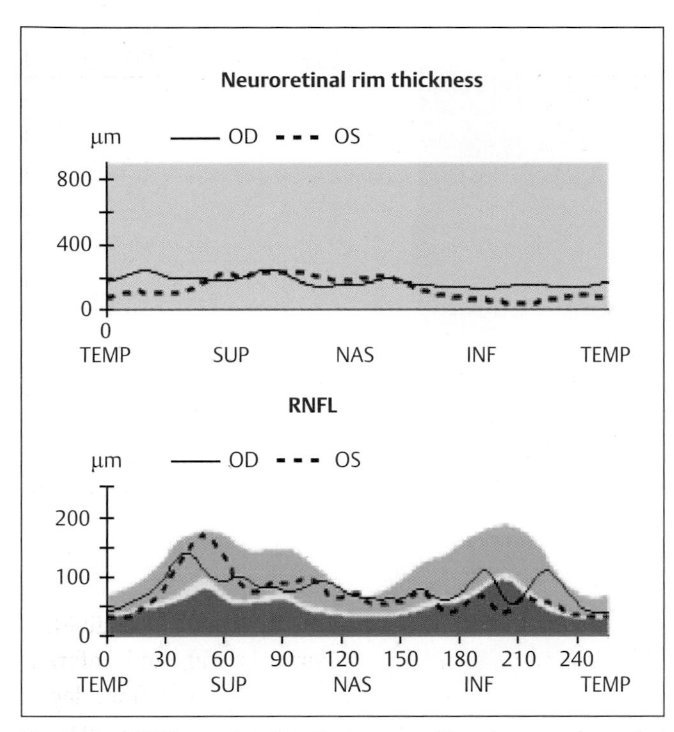

Fig. 6.4 TSNIT graph of retinal nerve fiber layer, color-coded compared to normative data. White being supranormal, green for normal, yellow for borderline, and red being definitely abnormal. INF, inferior; NAS, nasal; RNFL, retinal nerve fiber layer; SUP, superior; TEMP, temporal.

red, against age-matched normal individuals. *White being supranormal, green for normal (likely to be seen in 5–95th percentile of normal eyes), yellow for borderline (likely to be seen in 1–5th percentile of normals), and red being definitely abnormal (likely to be seen in <1st percentile of normal eyes)* (**Fig. 6.4**).

Macular Ganglion Cell Complex

A large percentage, approximately 50%, of retinal ganglion cells are located at the macula, and histologically, RGCs are seen 150 to 250 µm from the fovea up to 4.5 mm temporally, and up to the optic nerve head nasally. The ganglion call layer is made up of six to eight cell layers with RGC bodies forming 30 to 40% of the retinal thickness. Optical coherence tomography can now accurately delineate this layer, and diagnose any changes in the ganglion cell layer, loss of cell bodies and dendrites, rather than waiting to detect axonal loss that occurs later. *Ganglion cell loss and macular thinning seen in an arcuate shape, with corresponding areas of neuroretinal rim loss on the optic nerve head, are diagnostic.*

A macular cube centered on the fovea is scanned. Due to relatively similar reflectivity of the inner layers, the *RTVue optical coherence tomography calculates GCC* as combined retinal nerve fiber layer, ganglion cell, and inner plexiform, measured from the inner limiting membrane to the inner plexiform layer. *Cirrus optical coherence tomography uses ganglion cell analysis* which comprises the ganglion cell layer and inner plexiform layer and excludes retinal nerve fiber layer thickness. *Spectralis optical coherence tomography calculates each retinal layer separately* as well as provides total retinal thickness. Average macular layer thickness is useful in all spectral domain optical coherence tomography devices for diagnosing different severities of glaucoma (**Fig. 6.5**).

The current best GCC parameters for detecting early perimetric glaucoma are reported to be average GCC thickness and inferior GCC thickness. Both retinal nerve fiber layer and GCC thickness on optical coherence tomography are equally good at diagnosing moderate and severe glaucoma. GCC is increasingly accurate with more severe glaucomatous neuropathy. Advanced Imaging for Glaucoma Study (AIGS) found that inferior GCC thickness was significantly thinner in the fast progression group as compared to slow progressors. However, *artifacts caused by segmentation or acquisition errors are frequent, and the presence of many other age-related macular changes and diseases can affect the thickness measured*, making this more variable.

Optic Nerve Head Analysis

Optic nerve head analysis requires an optical coherence tomography machine to identify optic nerve head boundaries. Bruch's membrane opening (BMO) is taken as the optic nerve head boundary because it is easy to identify. The *distance from the BMO to the internal limiting membrane (ILM) is taken as the neuroretinal rim in that area.* The optic nerve head data is extracted from a 200 × 200 cube centered at optic disc and the data is again shown as an TSNIT graph. The Cirrus high-definition optical coherence tomography has corrected normative data for optic nerve changes like tilt or size. The Spectralis Glaucoma Premium Edition software can determine neuroretinal rim boundaries without input from the operator or a reference plane, thereby decreasing errors (**Fig. 6.6**).

How to Read a Retinal Nerve Fiber Layer Optical Coherence Tomography Report

1. **Patient information/details:** Patient information like date of birth, gender, and unique ID should be entered into the machine correctly for comparison with normative data base and further follow-up.

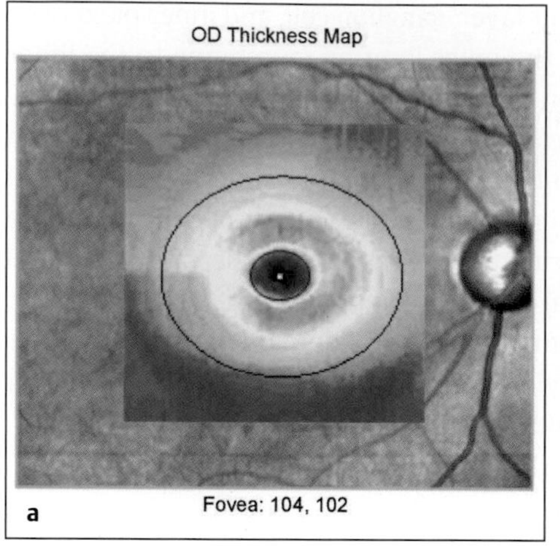

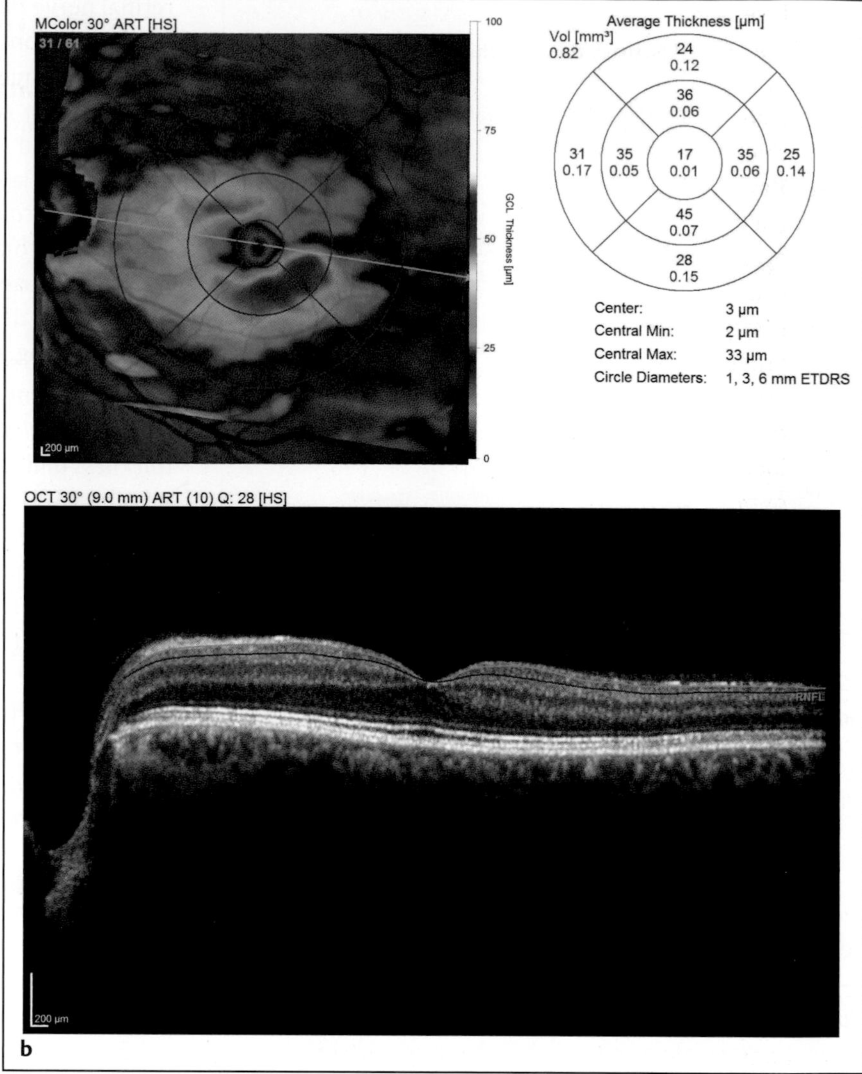

Fig. 6.5 (a, b) Macular thickness map—normal eye on Cirrus and glaucomatous eye on Spectralis optical coherence tomography.

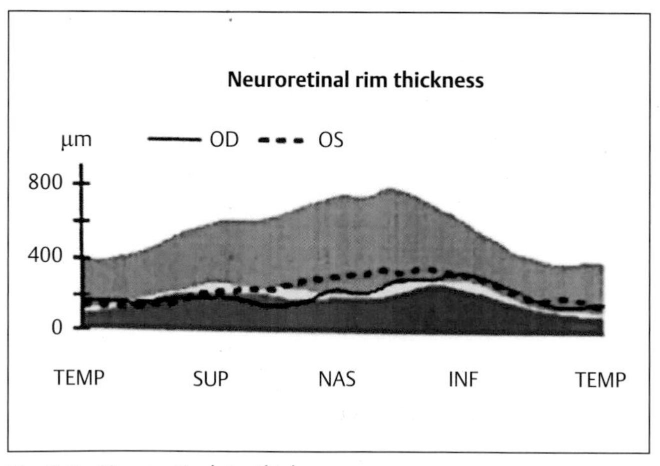

Fig. 6.6 Neuroretinal rim thickness map.

2. **Quality scores/signal strength:** The quality scores or signal strength of the optical coherence tomography scan obtained should be good, as a scan with poor quality will provide faulty results and may lead to an impression of false progression, as generally lower thickness of retinal nerve fiber layer would be recorded. *The acceptable quality scores are different for different machines: >6 for Cirrus optical coherence tomography (Range 1–10); Q-score >15 for Spectralis optical coherence tomography (Range 0–40); signal strength index (SSI) >45 for RTVue (Range 0–100).*
3. **Retinal nerve fiber layer thickness map:** This is the raw data of the thickness of retinal nerve fiber

layer around the optic nerve and is not correlated to normative data. Areas which are not scanned due to dry eye or excessive blinking may result in black-colored artifacts in the retinal nerve fiber layer thickness map, suggestive of a poor-quality scan.

4. **Key parameters table:** Summary of all the key parameters is made in one table comparing both eyes and providing color-coded squares after comparison with normative database.
5. **Retinal nerve fiber layer deviation map:** This graph shows a superimposed BMO, BMO boundary, and calculation circle on a gray scale fundus picture. This is important as proper/faulty BMO identification and centration of the scan around the optic nerve head is highlighted. Additionally, any deviation of the retinal nerve fiber layer thickness is shown color coded as yellow (likely to be seen in <5th percentile of the normal population) or red (likely to be seen in <1st percentile of the normal population). The region that is gray is within normal limits.
6. **Neuroretinal rim thickness plots and retinal nerve fiber layer thickness plots:** The neuroretinal rim thickness map and retinal nerve fiber layer thickness map are color-coded double-hump patterns with black lines showing the actual value of each eye in comparison to the underlying normal distribution shown in green (5–95th percentile of the normal population), borderline cases in yellow (likely to be seen in 1–5th percentile), and abnormal in red (likely to be seen <1st percentile of the normal), while white areas correspond to supranormal values (higher than seen in >95th percentile).
7. **Retinal nerve fiber layer quadrant and clock-hour maps:** These color-coded pie diagrams point out the exact quadrant and clock-hour of significant defects. Artifacts while taking the scan or poor scan quality may lead to deranged values.
8. **Extracted vertical and horizontal tomograms:** These are vertical and horizontal line diagrams depicting the cup configuration. Any artifacts such as a missing scan area, segmentation errors, and vitreoretinal interface problems can cause defects in these tomograms.
9. **Retinal nerve fiber layer circular tomogram:** This is a raw image of the retinal layers as reflected and pictured by the machine. It shows segmentation lines separating retinal nerve fiber layer from other layers. Sometimes segmentation errors may lead to abnormally low or high retinal nerve fiber layer values (**Fig. 6.7**).

How to Read a Macula Report

1. **Patient information/details and quality scores.**
2. **Thickness map:** This is a pseudocolor image of the raw values of macula thickness. *It is not compared to normative data.* The white, red, and yellow are thick areas whereas blue depicts thin areas. The range of thickness is from 0 to 225 µm.
3. **Deviation map:** This graph shows a superimposed macular picture, with super-pixels in areas where there is thinning as compared to normal. Additionally, any deviation of the macular thickness is shown color coded as yellow (<5th percentile) or red (<1st percentile). The region that is gray is within normal limits.
4. **The sector map:** It provides the sectoral thickness of macula in an oval of 4.8 × 4.0 mm in six sectors. The macular thickness is given in numerical values as well as color coded after comparison with normative data.
5. **Thickness table:** The table provides average and minimum thickness of ganglion cell layer, color coded after normative data comparison.
6. **Horizontal tomogram of the macula:** The horizontal tomogram gives a raw picture generated by the machine. This tomogram should pass from the center of fovea for proper centration of the sector map. Also, if there is any macular abnormality, it can be picked up by taking a quick look at this scan (**Fig. 6.8**).

Optic Nerve Head Analysis

Optic nerve head analysis is also useful in identifying the presence and extent of neuroretinal rim loss early. The best assessment is thought to be after identification of BMO, and then assessing minimum rim width (MRW).

Reading a printout of the Spectralis optical coherence tomography with BMO-MRW includes the following (**Fig. 6.9**):

- Patient details above.
- Images of the disc and neuroretinal rim have the BMO placement shown as red dots.
- Optic nerve head tomograph.
- TSNIT plot and sector analysis of the MRW.
- Retinal nerve fiber layer tomography.
- TSNIT plot and sector analysis of the retinal nerve fiber layer using the 3.5-mm circle.

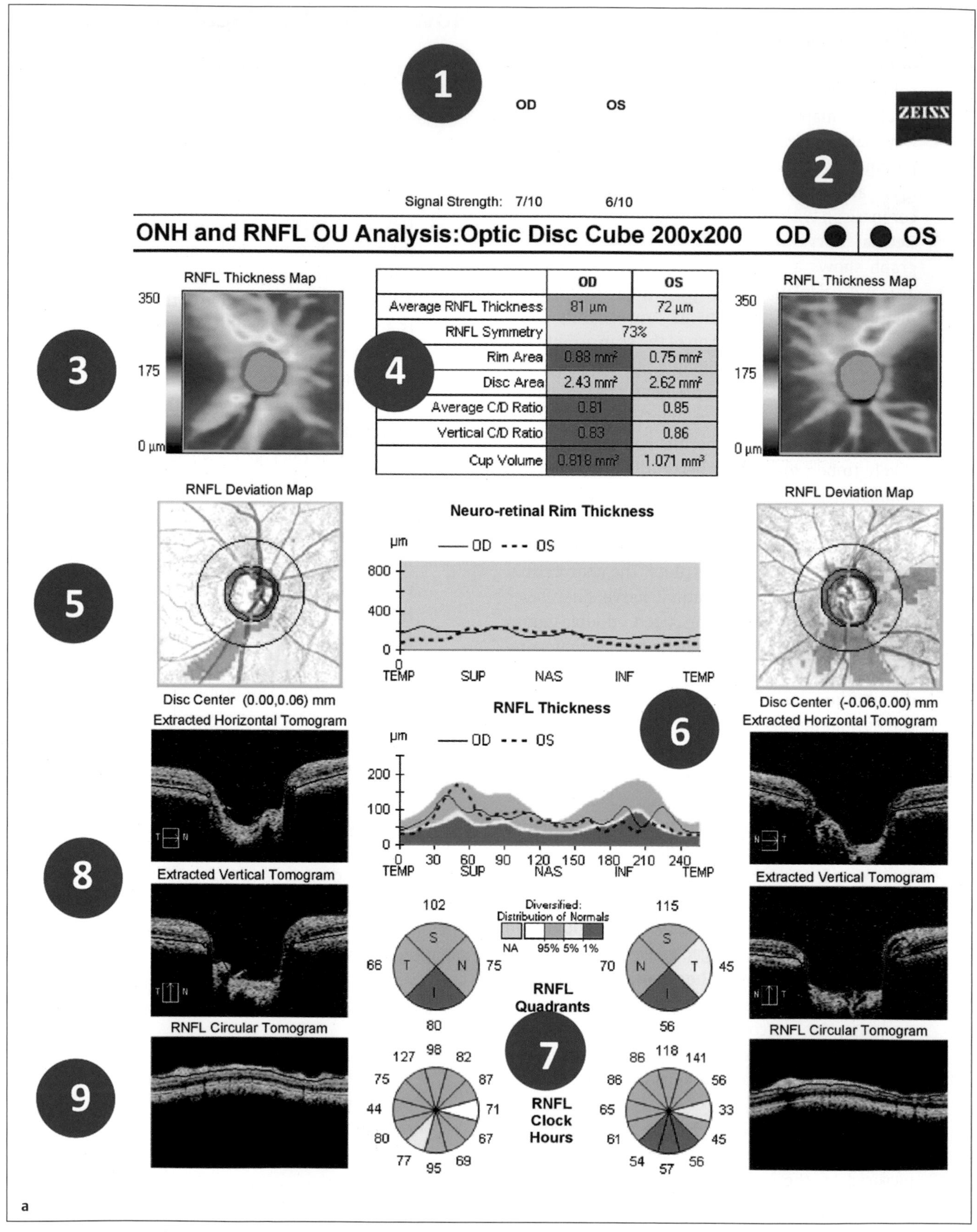

Fig. 6.7 **(a)** Sections of a retinal nerve fiber layer analysis printout report in Cirrus optical coherence tomography. *(Continued)*

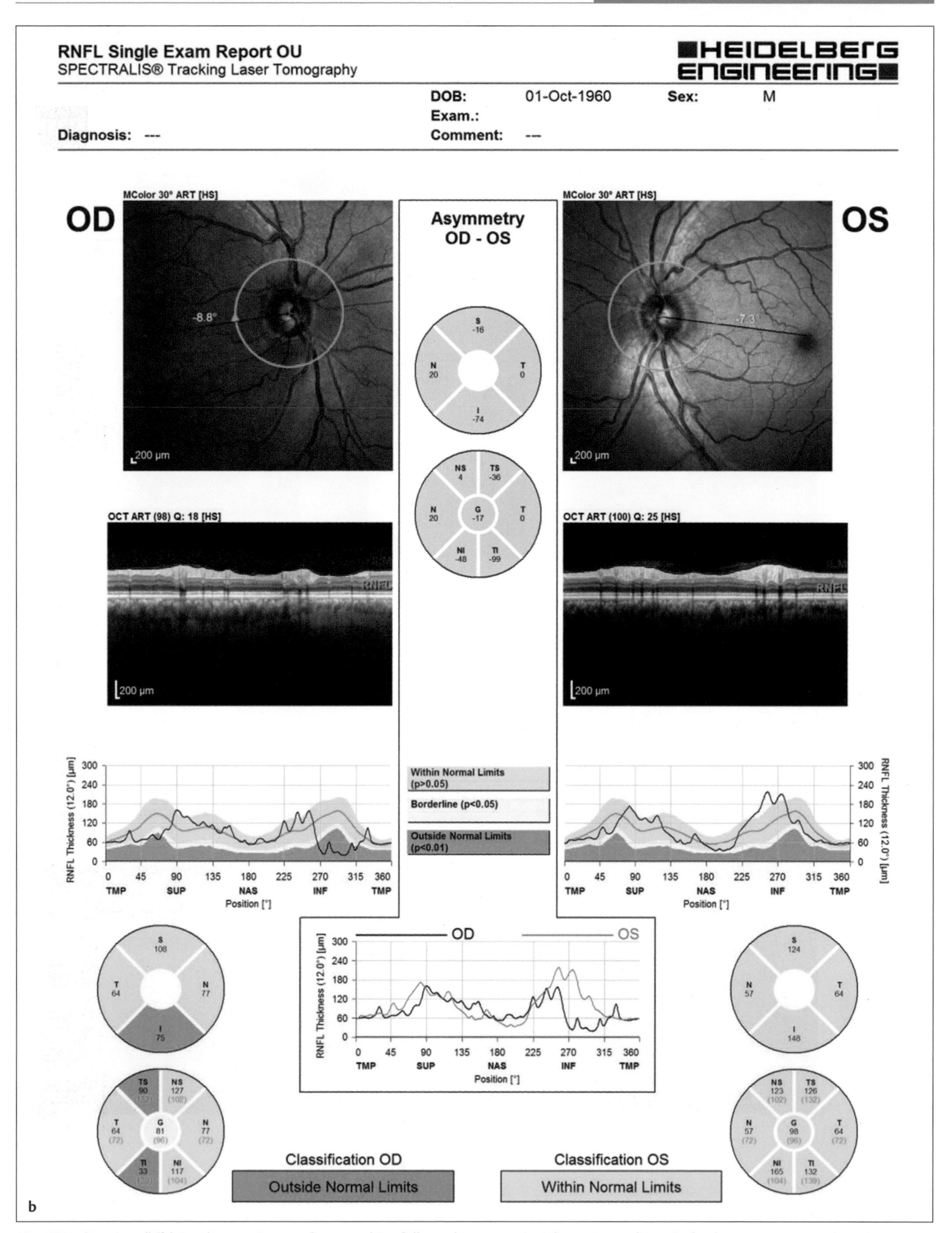

Fig. 6.7 *(Continued)* **(b)** Reading a printout of any machine follows the same principles; a Spectralis optical coherence tomography printout.

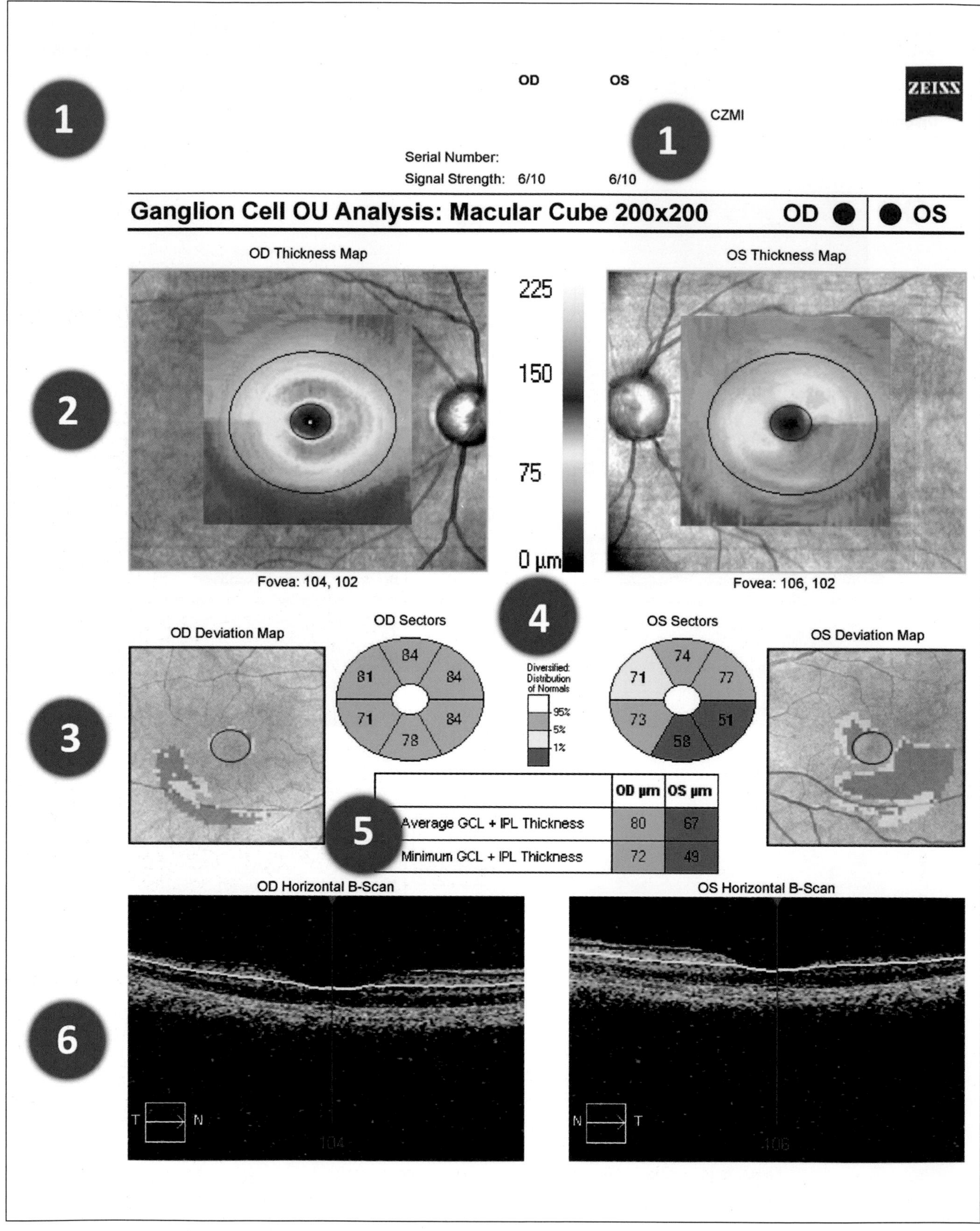

Fig. 6.8 Printout report of ganglion cell analysis.

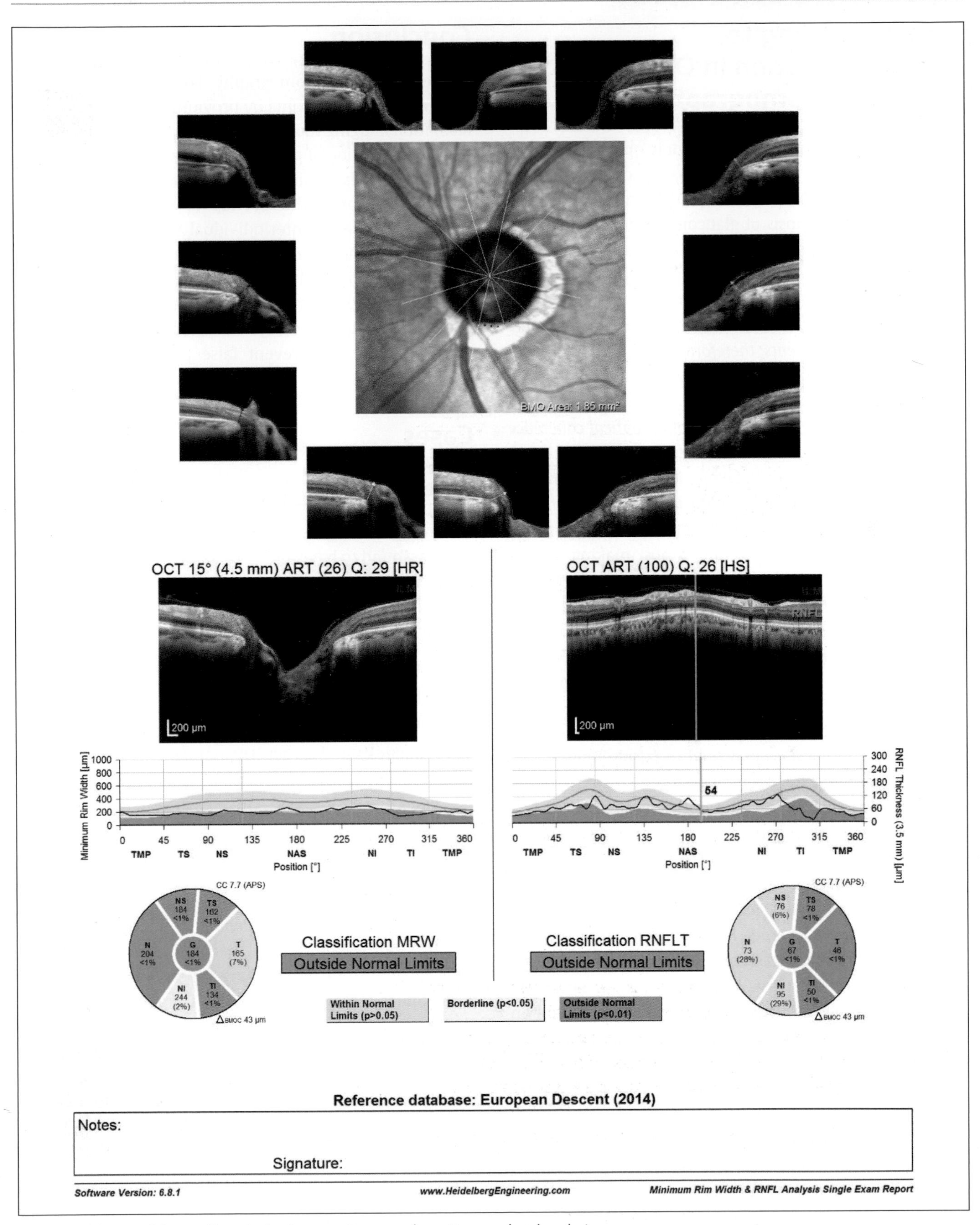

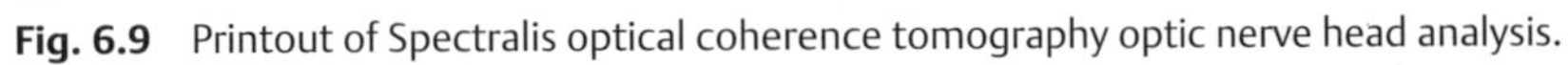
Fig. 6.9 Printout of Spectralis optical coherence tomography optic nerve head analysis.

Factors Leading to Misinterpretation in Optical Coherence Tomography

1. **Red green disease:** Green color in optical coherence tomography denotes normal and red denotes abnormal. "Red disease" is that in which a false positive diagnosis of glaucomatous defect is made in an otherwise normal eye. Green disease is a result of inability of the software to identify glaucomatous damage. *The red green color distribution depends upon a small normal data base which consists of only 300 to 500 patients; therefore, people with tilted discs or higher refractive errors may show either red/green disease.*
2. **Floor effect:** *The segmentation in optical coherence tomography can measure retinal nerve fiber layer thickness >30 µm; therefore, if a scan shows retinal nerve fiber layer of <30 µm it should be evaluated carefully.* In advanced glaucoma, progressive retinal nerve fiber layer thinning stops, making optical coherence tomography less useful for detecting progression. In such cases, GCC evaluation or visual field testing is better at diagnosing progression.
3. **Poor-quality scans:** The quality scores should be acceptable for studying the scans and commenting upon progression.
4. **Segmentation errors:** *Improper placement of segmentation lines* may lead to falsely high or low retinal nerve fiber layer values.
5. **Patient-related artifacts:** *Extremes of refractive error or a tilted optic nerve head* may show shifted retinal peaks compared to a standard double hump on optical coherence tomography. *Any media opacity such as a cataract/Weiss ring/vitreous membranes/ asteroid hyalosis may cause window defects and partial absence of scan areas, resulting in low retinal nerve fiber layer values.* Epiretinal membranes or vitreomacular traction may pull on the retina leading to falsely high retinal or retinal nerve fiber layer thickness values being recorded.

Diagnosing Progression

Imaging with optical coherence tomography is able to detect even small changes in the neuroretinal rim, retinal nerve fiber layer, and GCC over time.

These will be discussed in Chapter 21 on progression.

Conclusion

Optical coherence tomography has revolutionized the management of glaucoma by providing an objective, high-resolution imaging tool that is highly reproducible, making the early detection of progressive change possible. It is also useful in the diagnosis of moderate to severe glaucomas. In early glaucoma, the overlap of small glaucomatous abnormalities and interindividual variability of optic nerve head and retinal nerve fiber layer parameters makes definitive diagnosis more difficult. Optical coherence tomography has changed the way glaucoma is being managed, but always needs to be correlated with clinical findings to prevent false positive and negative interpretations.

Cases

Case 1

A 60-year-old male complained of banging into objects, and was found to have an IOP of 32/36 mm Hg in both eyes and a cup:disc ratio of 0.9 in both eyes with an open angle on gonioscopy. Despite a visual acuity of 6/12 in both eyes he was unable to do perimetry reliably.

Points to consider

- Elderly patients find it difficult to perform automated perimetry.
- Diagnosis and target IOP assessment needs to know the severity of glaucomatous optic neuropathy.
- An objective record of the glaucomatous neuropathy can be obtained by imaging, e.g., optical coherence tomography.

Diagnosis and Management

Optical coherence tomography signal strength was 6/10, which is borderline. Retinal nerve fiber layer deviation map showed extensive thinning superiorly and inferiorly, with similar red highlights in TSNIT graph and quadrant/ clockwise charts, signifying that these values are likely to be seen in <1% of normal. Neuroretinal rim TSNIT has the right eye in red, with the left eye as low normal or in the yellow band, likely to be seen in <5% of normal. In the table, average retinal nerve fiber layer is 45 µm with significant asymmetry. All values for the right eye are highlighted in red (**Case 1-1**). A diagnosis of severe primary open-angle glaucoma (POAG) was made, with a target IOP around 12 mm Hg to preserve remaining vision. Review with macular GCC evaluation would be best.

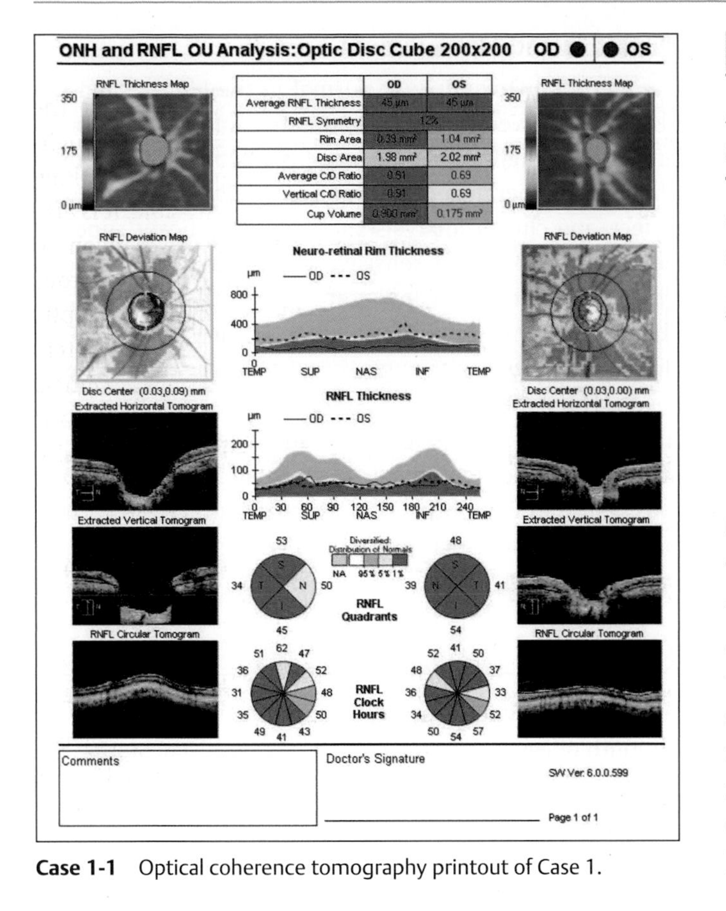

Case 1-1 Optical coherence tomography printout of Case 1.

Case 2

A 64-year-old male had been diagnosed to have POAG and prescribed medications. He sought a second opinion. The diagnosis appeared to have been made on the basis of an noncontact tonometer (NCT) of 20/21 and an optical coherence tomography he brought with him (**Case 2-1**).

Points to consider

- First assess scan quality.
- Rule out the presence of artifacts.
- Optical coherence tomography report should be correlated with clinical findings.

Diagnosis and Management

The optical coherence tomography printout signal strength was 5/10, which was unacceptable and many parameters are highlighted in white, a supranormal value. The left eye was not centered. On examination, gonioscopy showed an occludable angle, cup:disc ratio was 0.7/0.6, with a normal neuroretinal rim. Perimetry was normal in both eyes. A repeat optical coherence tomography of signal strength 6/10 showed a retinal nerve fiber layer within normal limits on all graphs, and possible anomaly of the right eye

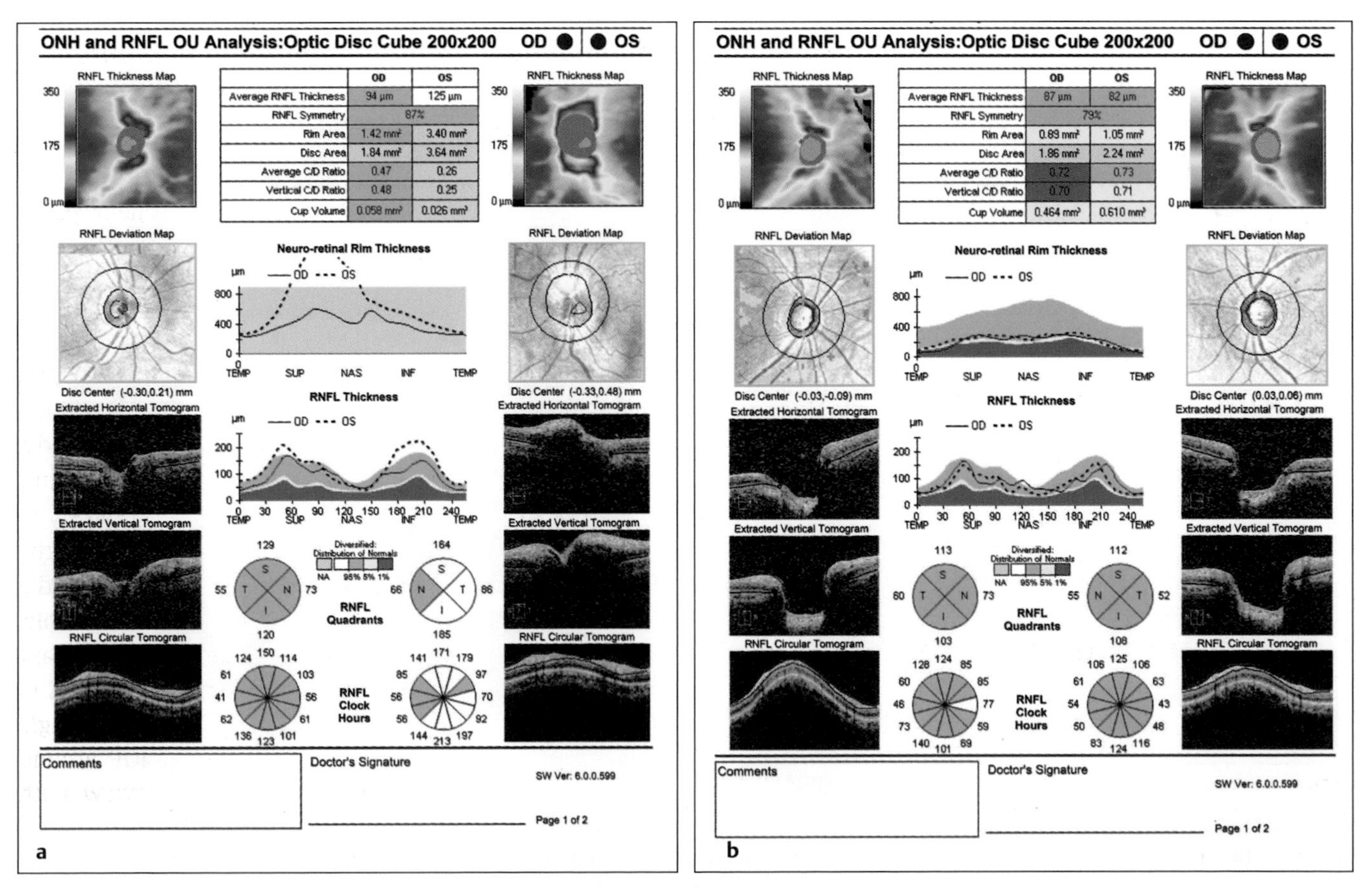

Case 2-1 **(a, b)** Initial and repeat optical coherence tomography scans of Case 2.

disc as it was small—disc area of 1.86 mm². A diagnosis of primary angle closure suspect was made, and a Nd:YAG laser iridotomy was done. Diurnal applanation tonometry after 3 weeks was advised with review.

Case 3

A 62-year-old male complained of noticing a diminution of vision in the right eye. On examination there was an immature senile cataract, open angles, cup:disc ratio of 0.9 in the right eye and 0.6 in the left eye and an IOP of 26 and 22 mm Hg. An optical coherence tomography was done; however, the signal strength was only 4/10 and 5/10.

Points to consider

- Media opacification can lead to artifacts.
- Severity of glaucomatous field loss determines target IOP.
- Significant asymmetry in POAG should be investigated.

Diagnosis and Management

Perimetry on Octopus was normal in the left eye and the right eye showed a superior arcuate scotoma, with polar analysis highlighting an inferior loss. Bebie's defect curve showed a general decrease of sensitivity with localized defect, and cluster analysis showed a significant superior hemifield decrease in sensitivity (**Case 3-1**). Gonioscopy revealed a quadrant of angle recession in the right eye and the patient remembered a childhood injury with a ball. A diagnosis of POAG with angle recession in the right eye was made. The patient was advised a combination of timolol and dorzolamide in both eyes, and phacoemulsification was done in the right eye. Optical coherence tomography was repeated 3 months after cataract surgery to form a baseline against which further assessment of progression can be made.

Case 4

A 14-year-old child operated for congenital glaucoma at 1 month of age was reviewed for current visual status. His

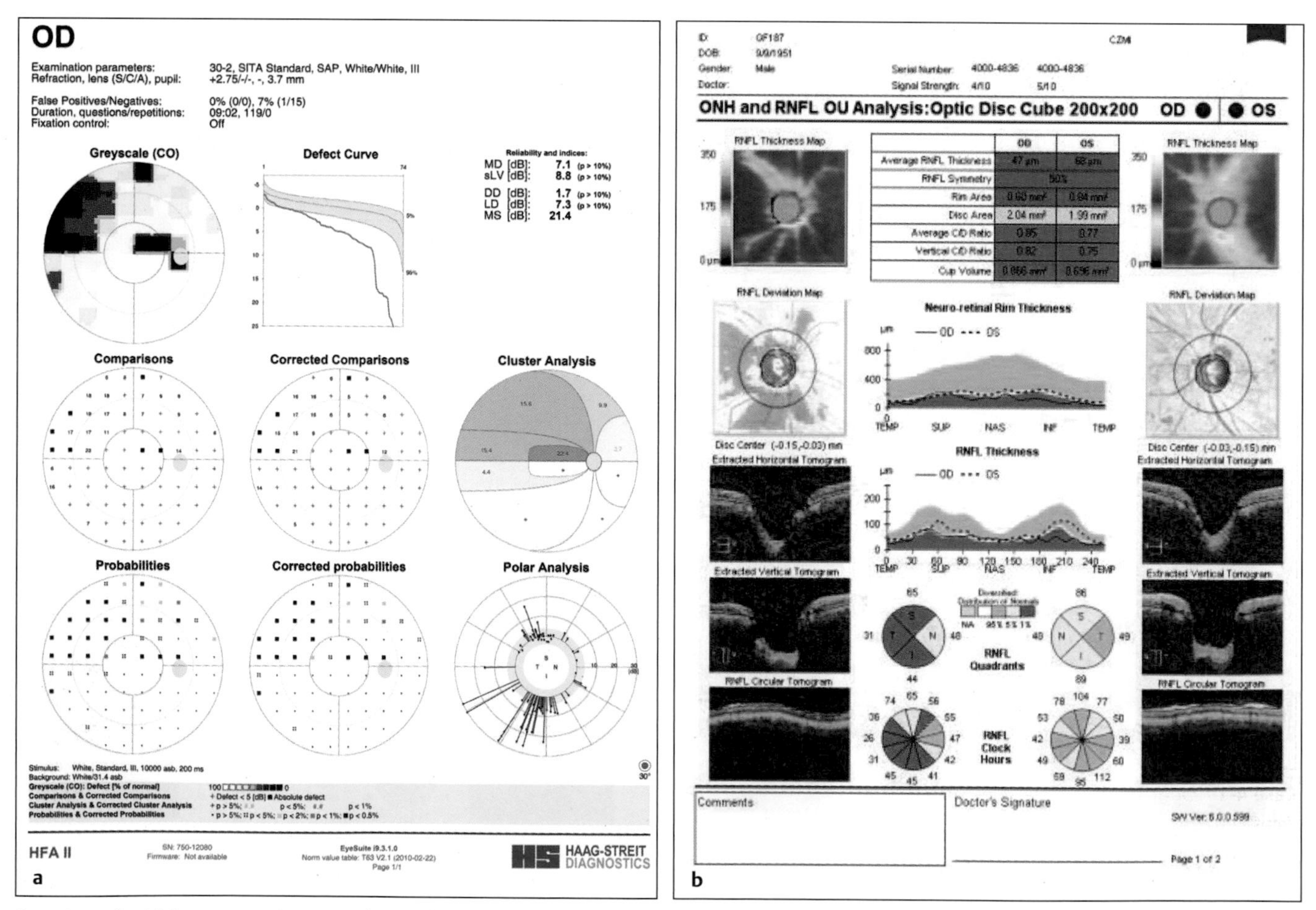

Case 3-1 **(a, b)** Octopus perimetry and optical coherence tomography printout for Case 3.

IOP was 12/14 mm Hg, and visual acuity was 6/6 in both eyes. Estimation of severity of glaucomatous damage was required for further management.

Points to consider

- IOP is within normal limits for his age.
- Perimetry does not have normative data for this age.
- Kinetic perimetry can identify only absolute scotomas.

Diagnosis and Management

An optical coherence tomography was done, which was well centered, but with a low signal strength (**Case 4-1**). The retinal nerve fiber layer thickness was 81/85 μm; however, no deviation from normal could be mapped as normative data for this age is not available. Absolute values may be followed over time. A Goldmann kinetic perimetry was recorded and was normal.

Case 5

A 54-year-old myopic lady with a visual acuity of 6/18 was found to have fluctuating scotomas in the superior nasal area, left eye > right eye. Her angles were wide open, and IOP was 20/18 mm Hg with a horizontally tilted disc and extensive peripapillary atrophy in the right eye.

Points to consider

- Refractive scotomas can be seen in myopes
- Imaging may better reflect glaucomatous neuropathy.

Diagnosis and Management

Spectralis optical coherence tomography report of a 54-year-old lady (**Case 5-1**). The scan is well centered and of good quality. Retinal nerve fiber layer thickness on TSNIT and quadrant or clock-hour analysis show a loss inferiorly, likely to be seen in <1% of age-matched normal. The scans

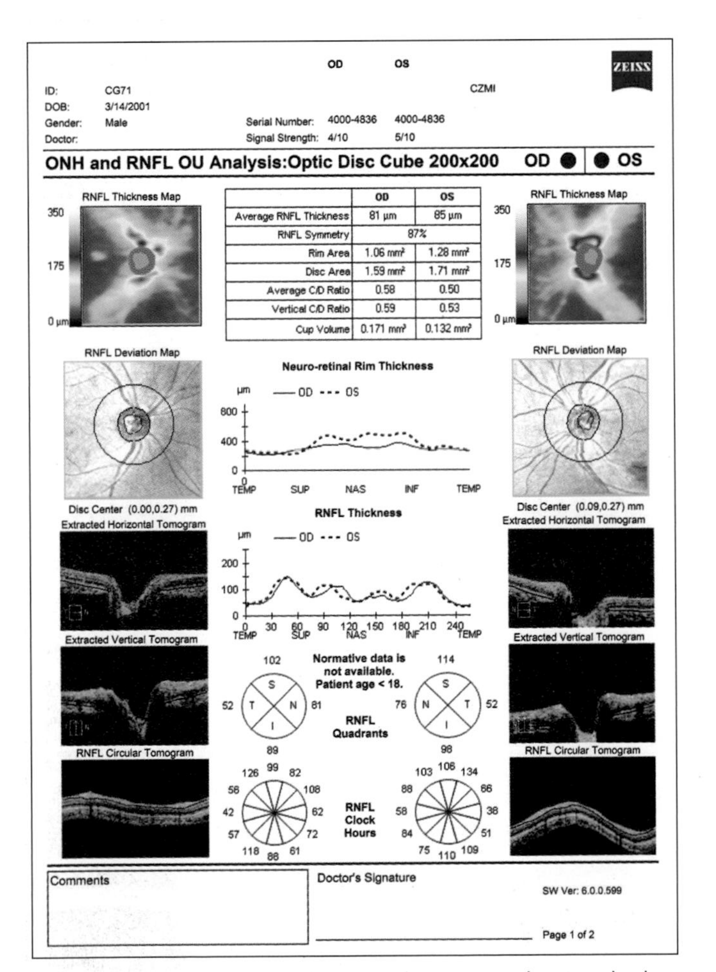

	OD	OS
Average RNFL Thickness	81 μm	85 μm
RNFL Symmetry	87%	
Rim Area	1.06 mm²	1.28 mm²
Disc Area	1.59 mm²	1.71 mm²
Average C/D Ratio	0.58	0.50
Vertical C/D Ratio	0.59	0.53
Cup Volume	0.171 mm³	0.132 mm³

Case 4-1 Optical coherence tomography printout showing absolute values recorded. No normative data for <18 years available.

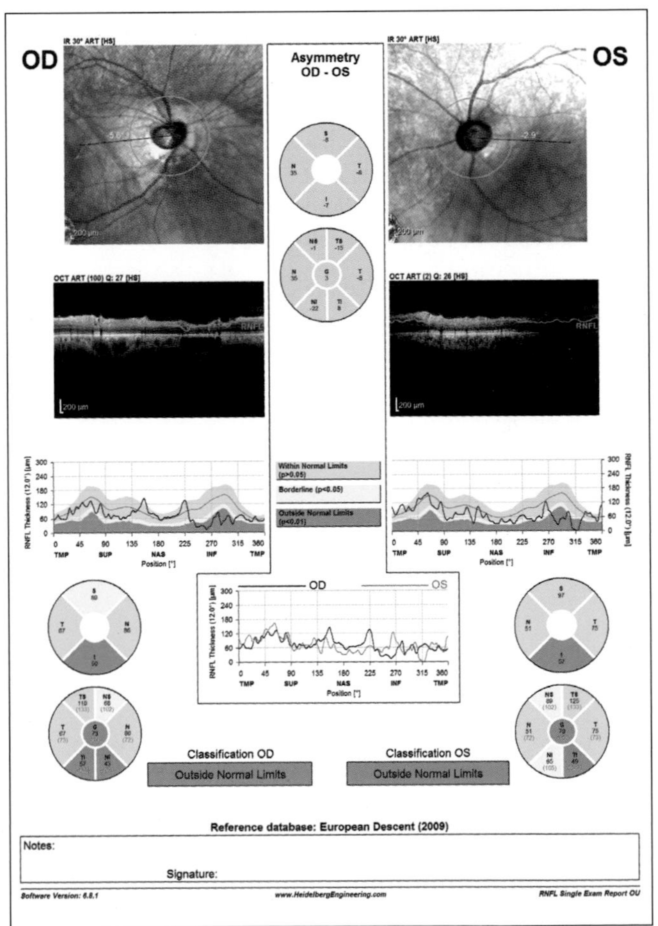

Case 5-1 Spectralis optical coherence tomography showing irregularity of the internal limiting membrane (ILM) and a dysplastic disc.

show a significant irregularity of the ILM, suggesting a retinal pathology as well. A definitive diagnosis of early POAG could be reached. Additionally, a possible epiretinal membrane was diagnosed.

Suggested Readings

Ahmed S, Khan Z, Si F, et al. Summary of glaucoma diagnostic testing accuracy: an evidence-based meta-analysis. J Clin Med Res 2016;8(9):641–649

Bekkers A, Borren N, Ederveen V, et al. Microvascular damage assessed by optical coherence tomography angiography for glaucoma diagnosis: a systematic review of the most discriminative regions. Acta Ophthalmol 2020;98(6):537–558

Bussel II, Wollstein G, Schuman JS. Optical coherence tomography for glaucoma diagnosis, screening and detection of glaucoma progression. Br J Ophthalmol 2014;98(Suppl 2):ii15–ii19

Chen TC, Hoguet A, Junk AK, et al. Spectral-domain optical coherence tomography: helping the clinician diagnose glaucoma: a report by the American Academy of Ophthalmology. Ophthalmology 2018; 125(11):1817–1827

Kansal V, Armstrong JJ, Pintwala R, Hutnik C. Optical coherence tomography for glaucoma diagnosis: an evidence based meta-analysis. PLoS One 2018;13(1):e0190621

Liu S, Yu M, Ye C, Lam DS, Leung CK. Anterior chamber angle imaging with swept-source optical coherence tomography: an investigation on variability of angle measurement. Invest Ophthalmol Vis Sci 2011;52(12):8598–8603

McKee H, Ye C, Yu M, Liu S, Lam DS, Leung CK. Anterior chamber angle imaging with swept-source optical coherence tomography: detecting the scleral spur, Schwalbe's line, and Schlemm's canal. J Glaucoma 2013;22(6):468–472

Michelessi M, Lucenteforte E, Oddone F, et al. Optic nerve head and fibre layer imaging for diagnosing glaucoma. Cochrane Database Syst Rev 2015;(11):CD008803

Oddone F, Lucenteforte E, Michelessi M, et al. Macular versus retinal nerve fiber layer parameters for diagnosing manifest glaucoma: a systematic review of diagnostic accuracy studies. Ophthalmology 2016;123(5):939–949

Onishi anterior chamber, Fawzi AA. An overview of optical coherence tomography angiography and the posterior pole. Ther Adv Ophthalmol 2019;11:2515841419840249

Scuderi G, Fragiotta S, Scuderi L, Iodice CM, Perdicchi A. Ganglion cell complex analysis in glaucoma patients: what can it tell us? Eye Brain 2020;12:33–44

Traber GL, Della Volpe-Waizel M, Maloca P, et al. New technologies for outcome measures in glaucoma: review by the European Vision Institute Special Interest Focus Group. Ophthalmic Res 2020;63(2):88–96

Triolo G, Rabiolo A. Optical coherence tomography and optical coherence tomography angiography in glaucoma: diagnosis, progression, and correlation with functional tests. Ther Adv Ophthalmol 2020;12:2515841419899822

Weinreb RN, Garway-Heath DF, Leung C, Mederios FA, Liebmann J. Diagnosis of primary open angle glaucoma. In: World Glaucoma association Consesus Series. Vol. 10. 2016. Amsterdam, The Netherlands.: Kugler Publications; 2016

CHAPTER 7 Target Intraocular Pressure in Different Types and Severities of Glaucoma

Overview

- Normal Intraocular Pressure
- Target Intraocular Pressure
- Factors Determining Target Intraocular Pressure
  - Importance of Baseline Intraocular Pressure
  - Clinical Staging of Glaucomatous Damage
- Methods of Determining Target Intraocular Pressure
  - Absolute/Threshold Values as Target Intraocular Pressure
  - Percentage Reduction in Intraocular Pressure
  - Formula-Based Values for Setting a Target Intraocular Pressure
- Clinical Recommendations of Absolute or Threshold Target IOP Range in Different Stages of POAG and PACG
- Limitations of Setting a Target Intraocular Pressure
- Reassessing Target Intraocular Pressure over Time
  - Regular Review of Target Intraocular Pressure over a Lifetime Is Essential
- Cases
- Suggested Readings

Introduction

Visual field (VF) loss due to glaucoma is irreversible, and therefore damage needs to be prevented or slowed down, so that the patient can continue his or her daily activities through life, without a problem. Intraocular pressure (IOP) is the primary risk factor for the development and progression of glaucoma, and studies have shown that IOP reduction can slow/prevent progression of glaucoma. Therefore, it is important to understand the derivation and know "target" IOP levels suggested for each individual patient, to stabilize glaucoma over the patient's lifetime.

In 1977, Chandler reviewed patients seen by him over the years, and noted that patients with increasing severity of glaucomatous neuropathy did better with IOPs in the mid-teens or lower. The American Academy of Ophthalmology introduced the term *"target" IOP for appropriate management based on existing glaucomatous damage and other risk factors.*

Normal Intraocular Pressure

The average IOP recorded in normal eyes during surveys around the world has been 14 to 17 mm Hg, associated with a normally functioning optic nerve. Once glaucomatous damage is present, the IOP recorded has been shown to be higher, and can vary from the normal range in normal tension glaucoma to over 40 mm Hg in primary angle-closure glaucoma (PACG) and secondary glaucomas.

Hollows and Graham conducted a survey in the United Kingdom in 1966, where they found the mean applanation IOP to be 15.9 mm Hg in males and 16.6 mm Hg in females. Two standard deviations above the mean, that is, the 97.5th percentile, were calculated to be 21 mm Hg; therefore, it is a myth that an IOP >21 mm Hg should be considered as abnormal and that below 21 mm Hg is normal. Hollows and Graham themselves noted that >21 mm Hg "should not be construed as meaning clinical abnormality, as the distribution is skewed and physiological variables need not necessarily follow a Gaussian distribution." It is therefore to be understood that *the so-called cutoff IOP <21 mm Hg is not clinical, or evidence-based proof of "normal," but only a statistical construct.*

Target Intraocular Pressure

The best definition of target IOP has been put forward by the *European Glaucoma Society* guidelines as "an estimate of the mean IOP obtained with treatment that is expected to prevent further glaucomatous damage." The *American Academy of Ophthalmology* relates target IOP to the mechanical theory for pathogenesis of glaucoma, and defines it as "a range of IOP adequate to stop progressive pressure induced injury."

Factors Determining Target Intraocular Pressure

These largely include assessment of baseline IOP and clinical staging of glaucomatous damage, with age and other systemic abnormalities.

Importance of Baseline Intraocular Pressure

It is important to know the *IOP at which the glaucomatous optic neuropathy occurred*, as it provides a yardstick against which the degree of IOP lowering can be ascertained. For example, if the patient presents with an IOP of 40 mm Hg with severe VF damage, dropping it to the normal range of IOP, around 15 mm Hg, would be a reduction of over 60%, which could be enough to prevent further optic nerve damage. In contrast, if the same patient had a baseline IOP of 24 mm Hg, a drop to 15 mm Hg would be 37% of baseline, but this may not be enough to prevent further damage.

At least three IOP measurements, taken at different times of the day, ideally with an applanation tonometer, help determine baseline IOP. Any single IOP measurement taken between 7 am and 9 pm has a more than 75% chance of missing the highest point of a diurnal curve. *In PACG, it is important that the baseline IOP be recorded after an iridotomy, as intermittent attacks of angle closure may lead to intermittent high IOP recordings, with an unwarranted increase in medications causing attendant side effects.*

Clinical Staging of Glaucomatous Damage

The extent of existing glaucomatous damage appears to significantly influence likely progression at a given IOP, and therefore is extremely important in determining "target" IOP. Staging of glaucomatous damage can be done on the basis of either, or both—the structural optic nerve head damage or functional loss on perimetry. Unfortunately, there is no universally accepted staging of either optic nerve head abnormalities or VF changes, with regard to their relevance in progression.

Optic Nerve Head Examination

Cup:disc ratio is more commonly employed in clinical practice and recommended by the Canadian Guidelines as a means of staging glaucomatous damage into mild with a cup:disc ratio of <0.65, moderate (0.7 to 0.85), and severe (>0.9) (refer to **Table 2.2**) (**Fig. 7.1**). Ocular Hypertension Treatment Study (OHTS) found baseline cup:disc ratio to be a predictor of further damage in ocular hypertensives. However, in patients with early primary open-angle glaucoma (POAG), Early Manifest Glaucoma Trial (EMGT) did not find baseline cup:disc ratio to be a significant risk factor for glaucomatous progression. In advanced POAG, Advanced Glaucoma Intervention Study (AGIS) reported that patients with more severe glaucomatous damage, as measured by larger cup:disc ratio, 0.81 + 0.13, were at a greater risk of progression. Sihota et al found baseline linear

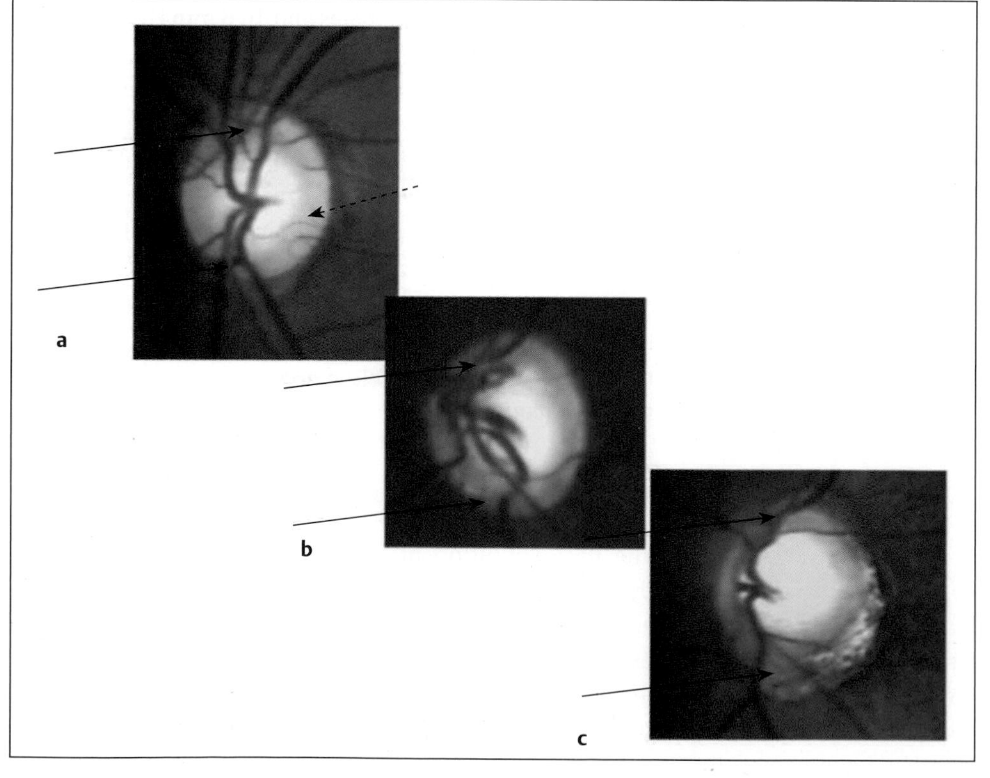

Fig. 7.1 **(a)** Left optic nerve head, cup:disc ratio 0.6, showing a thinning of the inferior neuroretinal rim, being almost similar to superior; *solid arrow* marking change in contour of blood vessels on the surface of the neuroretinal rim, with *baring of the circumlinear vessel inferiorly, dotted arrow, and alpha zone peripapillary atrophy*. **(b)** Cup:disc ratio 0.75, with neuroretinal rim thinning at both poles. **(c)** Cup:disc ratio 0.9, *loss of neuroretinal rim inferiorly* and superiorly and β-zone peripapillary atrophy from 3 to 7 o'clock.

cup:disc ratio on Heidelberg retina tomography (HRT) to be a significant risk factor for progression at all stages of glaucomatous neuropathy in both POAG and PACG eyes.

For example, a significant narrowing or loss of neuroretinal rim at both poles, with a cup:disc ratio of 0.8, would need a "target" IOP below the population average, which in Indians would mean <14 mm Hg.

Using the disc damage likelihood score, Stages 6 to 10 require aggressive glaucoma therapy (refer to Chapter 2 for details).

Perimetric Staging

Determination of baseline functional damage requires the defect to be reproduced on at least two occasions, to obviate a learning curve, perimetric noise, etc. All perimeters with normative data provide global indices and contain a plot highlighting localized loss in the VF that is definitive of glaucoma, similar to the pattern deviation plot on Humphrey field analyzer (HFA). These can be easily used to ascertain the pattern of loss, involvement of one/both hemispheres, and proximity to fixation, to stage glaucoma in each eye (**Fig. 7.2**).

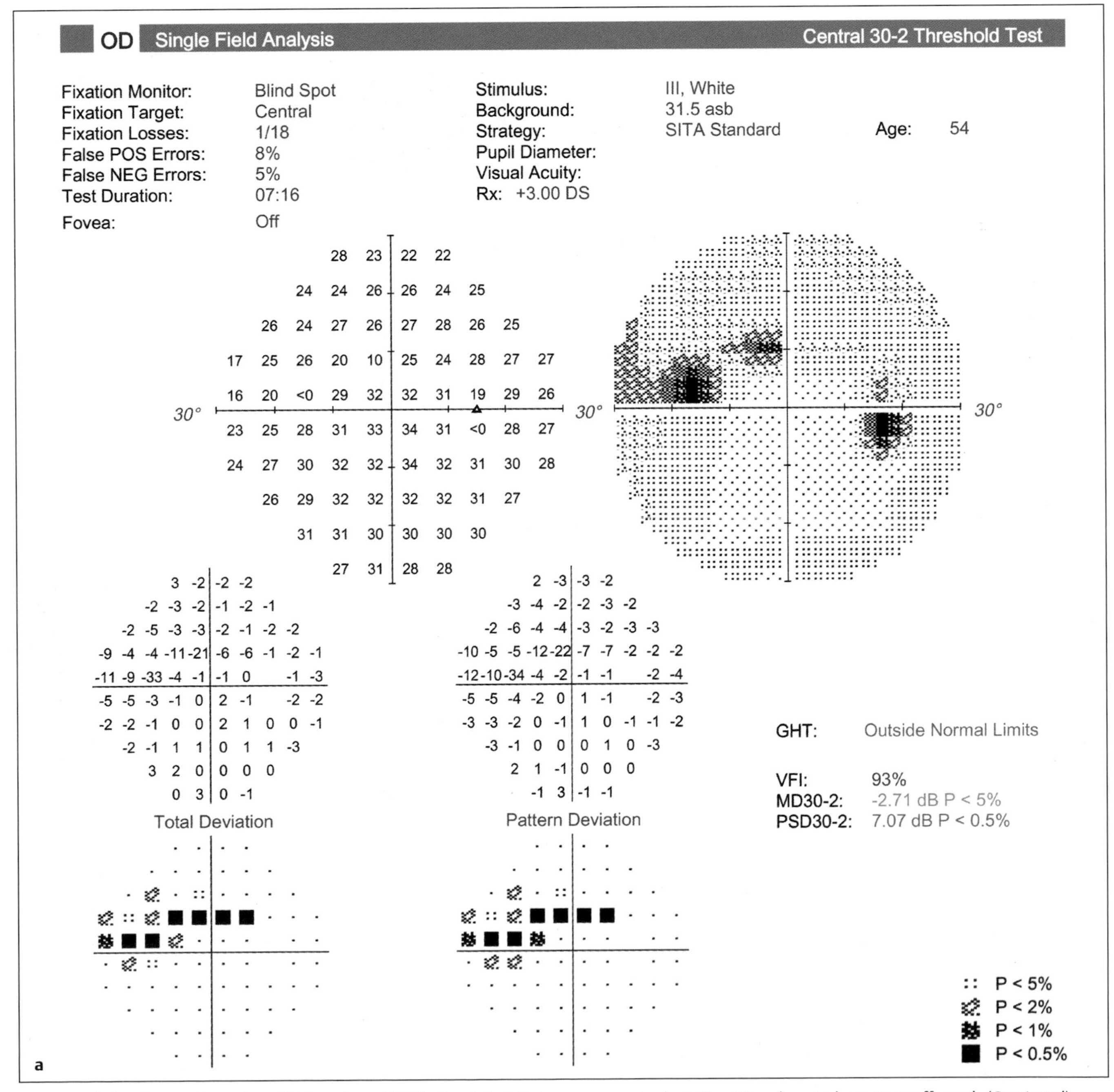

Fig. 7.2 **(a)** Right eye Humphrey field analyzer (HFA) of early/mild glaucoma; mean deviation ≥6 and central points unaffected. *(Continued)*

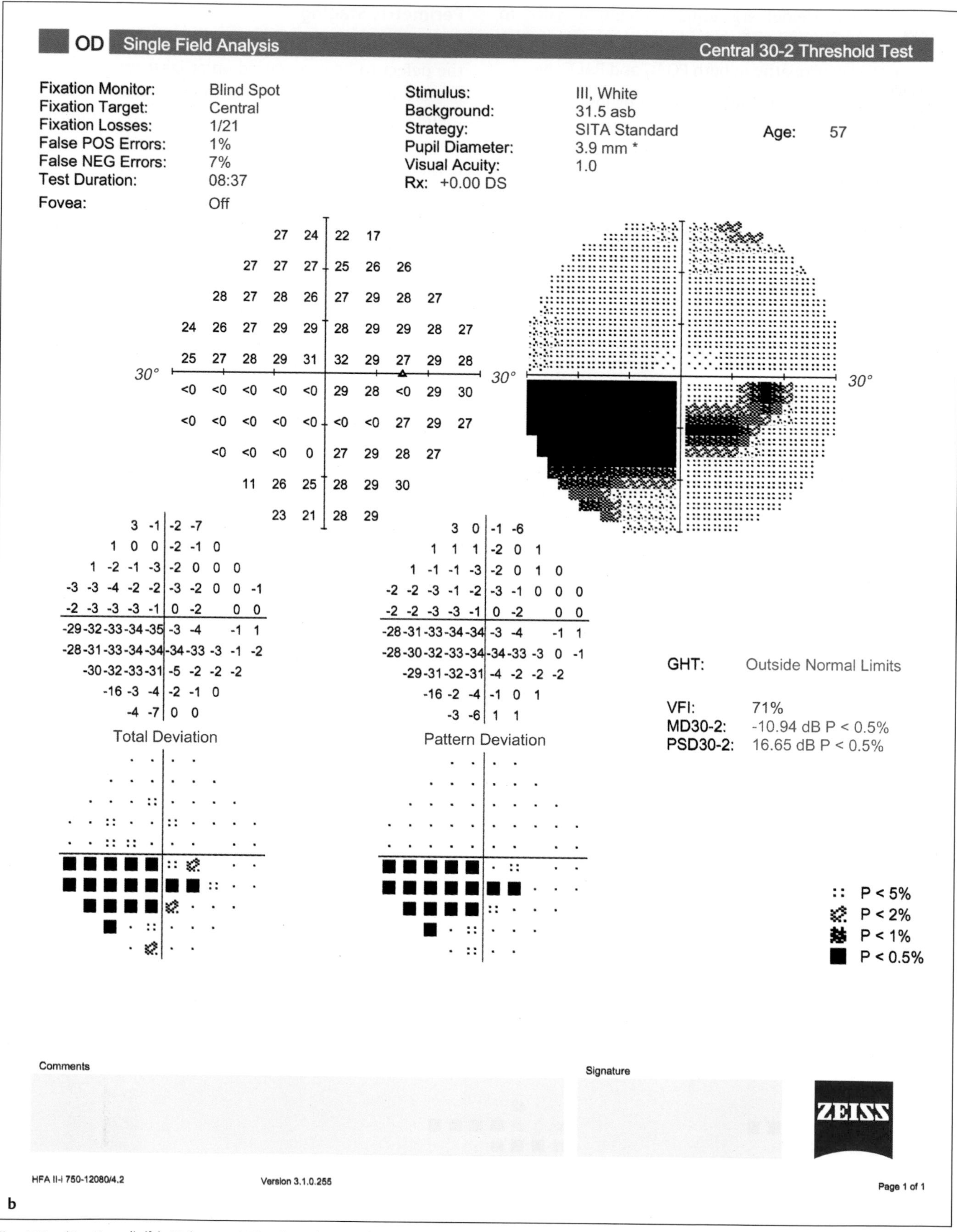

Fig. 7.2 *(Continued)* **(b)** Right eye HFA of moderate glaucoma; mean deviation −6 to −12 dB and <50% of points depressed, central points unaffected in one hemisphere.

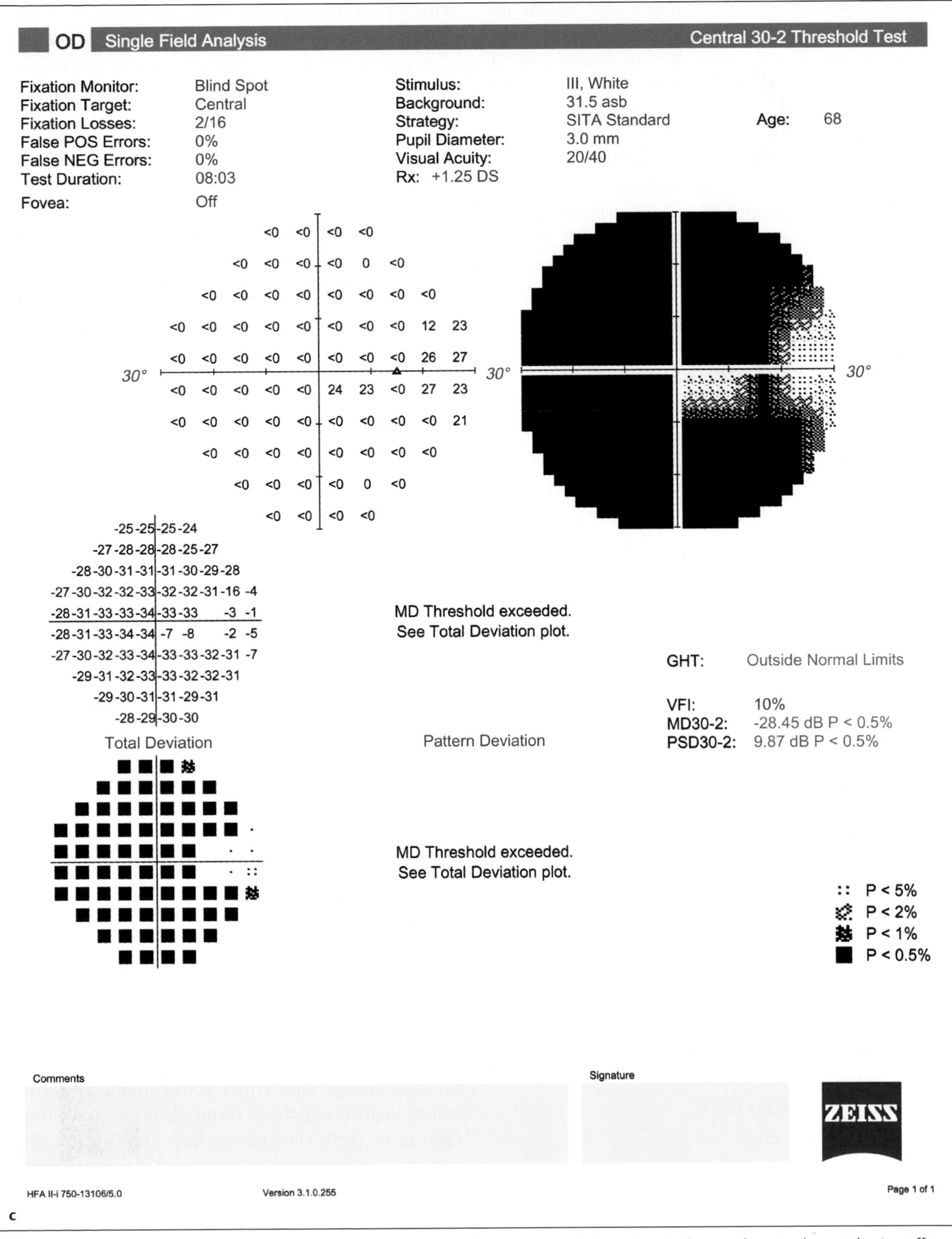

Fig. 7.2 *(Continued)* **(c)** Right eye HFA of severe glaucoma; mean deviation less than −12 dB and >50% of points depressed, central points affected in both hemispheres.

There are many suggested classifications of the severity of glaucomatous damage: Hodapp, Parrish, and Anderson (HPA) classification, glaucoma severity staging system (GSS), and enhanced glaucoma severity staging system (eGSS) (refer Chapter 5). These need time and effort to analyze and stage a patient's perimetric loss, and are largely used for research purposes at present and are difficult to apply clinically, by most ophthalmologists.

EMGT found that a *greater mean deviation loss at baseline was a risk factor for greater progression*. In the AGIS, patients with greater baseline damage, as evidenced by perimetric mean deviation values of −11.4 ± 5.5 dB were more likely to progress rapidly. The odds of VF progression increased by 11% for every 1-dB worsening in baseline mean deviation.

Other Significant Risk Factors to Consider

- Ocular:
  - Central corneal pachymetry—thin suggesting greater risk and thick a lower risk.
  - Disc hemorrhages are biomarkers for ongoing damage.
- Systemic:
  - Age—older more likely to progress, but longevity would be less.
  - Family history of severe glaucoma or glaucoma blindness could have a genetic predisposition to damage.
  - Vascular perfusion abnormalities—cerebrovascular spasm/plaques, hypotension.

Methods of Determining Target Intraocular Pressure

Having ascertained the degree of VF damage, baseline IOP, and risk factors, an IOP that would prevent further damage needs to be set. There should to be *a balance between setting an appropriate target to prevent optic nerve damage and being overaggressive*, so as to avoid side effects and economic burden.

Various approaches for setting a target IOP include:

- Threshold/absolute cutoff value.
- Percentage reduction in IOP.
- Formula-based values.

Absolute/Threshold Values as Target Intraocular Pressure

Threshold or absolute values of target IOP are those that are relatively fixed, and can be applied to a large number of, if not all, patients having a similar degree of glaucomatous damage. These can be applied easily in busy clinics.

In the AGIS a post hoc analysis showed that eyes with an average IOP of 12.3 mm Hg had no progression, while eyes that had a mean IOP in the mid-teens progressed by 2.5 dB and eyes with a mean IOP of 20 mm Hg progressed by 3.5 dB. There was a 30% chance of progression at an IOP in the mid-teens and 70% chance of progression at 20 mm Hg.

On analyzing POAG and PACG eyes over 5 years in India, with a "target" IOP of <18 mm Hg in eyes having mild or moderate VF loss, and 12 to 14 mm Hg in severe glaucoma, 12.1 and 15.5% of POAG and PACG eyes showed progression over 5 years. Moderate glaucomas progressed more frequently suggesting that a target IOP of <18 mm Hg was not low enough in these eyes. Eyes with severe glaucoma rarely progressed at an IOP of 10 to 12 mm Hg. After that analysis, "target" IOPs in the same population for moderate glaucoma was revised to 15 mm Hg, and a later evaluation of moderate POAG and PACG eyes over 10 years showed a progression in only 11% of eyes, over 10 years of review.

In general, for mild, moderate, and severe stages of glaucoma, the initial target for absolute IOP cutoffs could be kept as IOP equal to or below 18, 15, and 12 mm Hg, respectively.

Percentage Reduction in Intraocular Pressure

Some randomized controlled trials (RCTs) aimed for percentage reduction in IOP in the long-term management of different severities of POAG, but reported progression in many eyes.

In *ocular hypertensives*, OHTS found that an IOP reduction of 20% or an IOP of 24 mm Hg lead to progression in 19% of high-risk eyes over 8 to 10 years, suggesting that a greater reduction is necessary. Patients having early glaucoma, an mean deviation <5 dB, were studied in EMGT, with a 72% progression off treatment, as compared with 45% on therapy, when IOP was lowered by a mean of 5.1 mm Hg or 25%. In Collaborative Initial Glaucoma Treatment Study (CIGTS), similar patients had a calculated lowering of IOP based on damage, with a mean IOP of around 17 mm Hg, a reduction of 38 and 46% in medically or surgically treated eyes, respectively. Progression was seen in 15% of the eyes and 15% improved. When peak IOP was >16 mm Hg, progression was significant. *Early glaucoma, therefore, appears to need an IOP in the mid-teens.*

An Indian study found perimetric progression in 21.3% of POAG and PACG eyes with *moderate glaucomatous damage* over 5 years when the target IOP was <18 mm Hg.

For a patient with moderate glaucomatous optic neuropathy, it appears that lower IOPs, with an upper limit of 15 mm Hg, would be required to stabilize VFs.

The AGIS found that despite an average reduction in IOP of 40% there were significant rates of progression. *An Indian study recorded progression in just 2.3% of POAG and PACG eyes with advanced glaucoma over 5 years when the target IOP was 10 to 12 mm Hg.*

Literature regarding the analysis of mean IOP and percentage reduction in IOP with progression in different stages of POAG and PACG are collated in **Table 7.1**.

Formula-Based Values for Setting a Target Intraocular Pressure

Formulas attempt to incorporate baseline and risk factors when determining "target" IOP. Jampel first calculated target IOP by taking into account several attributes of the patient—initial pretreatment IOP, Z score (an indicator of disease severity), and Y factor (burden of therapy):

$$\text{Target IOP} = [\text{Initial IOP} \times (1 - \text{Initial Pressure} / 100) - Z \pm 1 \text{ mm Hg}]$$

Modified equations increased the range of Z score, 0 to 7. The CIGTS formula for target IOP was based on a patient's baseline IOP (mean of six IOP measurements taken over two visits) and its reference VF score (the mean of VF scores from at least two Humphrey 24–2 VF tests).

Clinical Recommendations of Absolute or Threshold Target IOP Range in Different Stages of POAG and PACG

Setting and achieving a "target" IOP range provides an algorithm for management. Quality of life may be affected by the medications used, but progressive glaucomatous optic neuropathy will affect it much more. Therefore, adequate IOP control for all glaucomatous eyes is a must. It is not VF defects only that influence quality of vision, but contrast sensitivity, mobility, night vision, driving, etc., that are significantly affected. *After an iridotomy, PACD eyes appear to respond similarly to IOP control, as in POAG.*

To assess the efficacy of therapy on baseline IOP, one should be aware of the average effect of each. An average

Table 7.1 Analysis of mean IOP and percentage reduction in IOP with progression in different stages of POAG and PACG

Study	Type of glaucoma	Baseline IOP (mm Hg)	Therapy	Percentage IOP reduction	Progression	Mean IOP level
Ocular hypertension treatment study	OHT	24.9	Topical medications	20	4.4/9.5%	19.3 mm Hg
Early manifest glaucoma trial	POAG	20.6	Topical medications + laser	25	45/62%	Mean fall 5.2 mm Hg
Collaborative normal tension glaucoma study	NTG	<21	Medications + surgery No adrenergic drugs	30	12/35%	10.6 mm Hg
Collaborative initial glaucoma treatment study	POAG	27	Medical	35	21% progressed at 8 years	17–18 mm Hg
		27	Surgical	48	25% progressed at 8 years	14–15 mm Hg
European glaucoma prevention study	OHT	22–29	Dorzolamide	22	13.4% treated 14.1% placebo	
Advanced glaucoma intervention study	POAG	23.7–24.8	ATT or TAT		Mean IOP 12.3 mm Hg did not progress overall, one-third progressed	
Stewart et al	POAG	19.5 ± 3.8			0% 6% 26%	≤12 mm Hg ≤17 mm Hg ≥18 mm Hg
Sihota et al ▪ Early ▪ Moderate ▪ Advanced	POAG and PACG	24.9 ± 8 28.3 ± 5 27.7 ± 9		32–43 44 50	18.7% 21.3% 2.3%	<18 mm Hg <18 mm Hg 12 mm Hg

Abbreviations: ALT, argon laser trabeculoplasty; ATT, ALT-trabeculectomy-trabeculectomy; IOP, intraocular pressure; NTG, normal tension glaucoma; OHT, ocular hypertension; PACG, primary angle-closure glaucoma; POAG, primary open-angle glaucoma; TAT, trabeculectomy-ALT-trabeculectomy.

reduction of IOP by 20 to 25% can be seen with monotherapy using selective β-blockers, α-agonists, or topical carbonic anhydrase inhibitors. A reduction of 30% or more may rarely be seen after the use of prostaglandin (PG) analogs, but more often requires multiple topical medications, or even filtering surgery. Laser trabeculoplasty and minimally invasive surgeries commonly lead to an IOP reduction of 20 to 25% (**Table 7.2**). Medical therapy is the norm to start with, and the choice of drugs could be based on baseline IOP, with addition of drugs only when efficacy of the first has been documented. (**Flowchart 7.1**).

In ***ocular hypertension or primary angle closure with ocular hypertension***, the decision to treat should depend on the presence of high risk factors—family history of glaucomatous field loss, high baseline cup:disc ratio, high baseline IOP, high baseline pattern standard deviation (PSD), low central corneal thickness (CCT), and older age. The suggested upper limit of the initial target IOP range should be 18 mm Hg in such patients.

In ***early POAG/PACG after iridotomy***, an IOP in the mid-teens, with an upper limit of 17 mm Hg, should be initially aimed for, and modified after a review, looking at changes on imaging or perimetry.

In ***moderate POAG and PACG after iridotomy***, an initial upper limit of ≤15 mm Hg should be tried to stabilize VFs, and later readjusted.

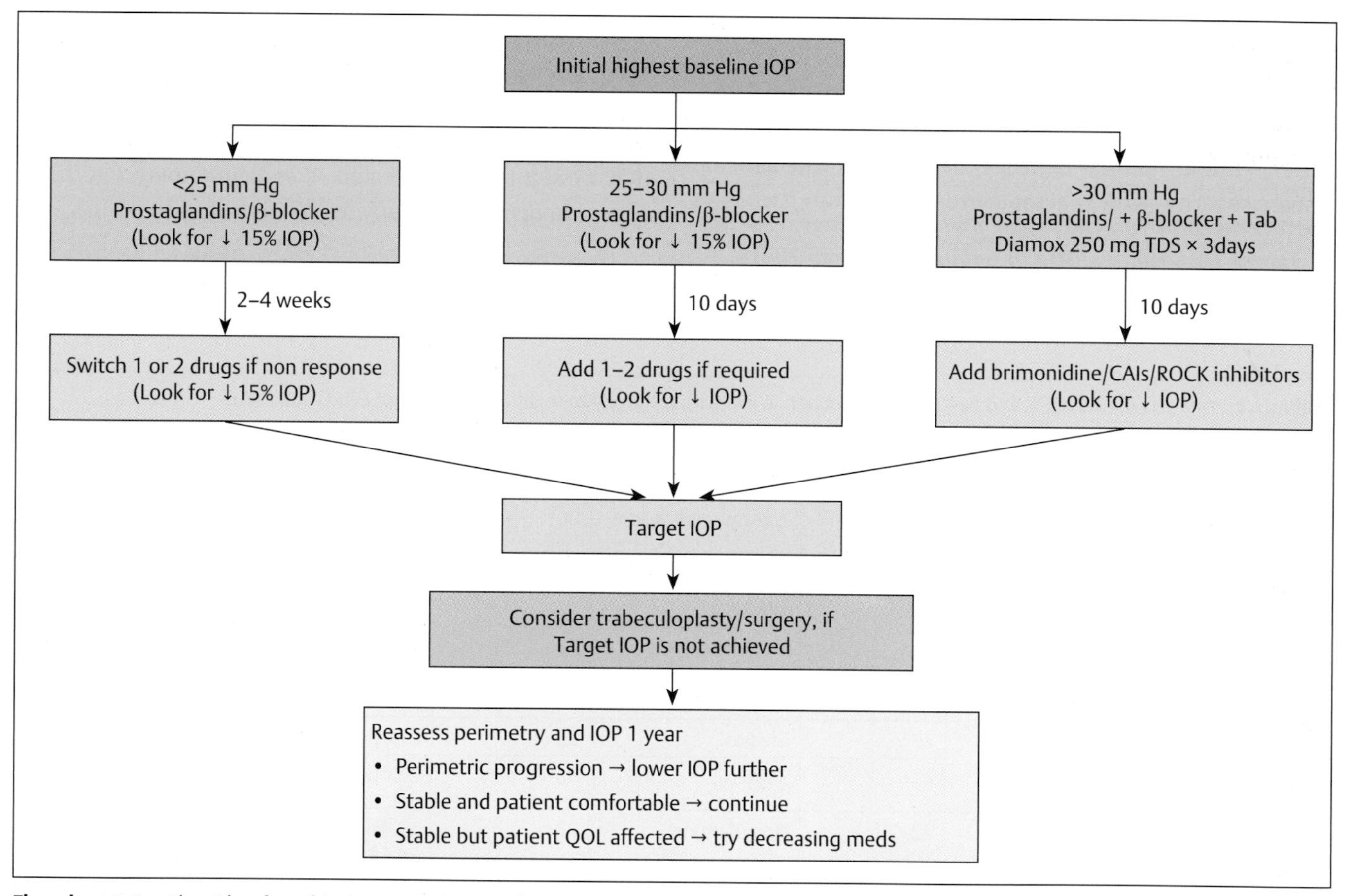

Flowchart 7.1 Algorithm for achieving target intraocular pressure. CAIs, carbonic anhydrase inhibitors; IOP, intraocular pressure; QOL, quality of life; ROCK inhibitors, Rho kinase inhibitors.

Table 7.2 Suggested therapies based on the reduction in IOP required

IOP reduction (%)	Topical medications	Laser trabeculoplasty	Filtering surgery	Drainage devices
20–25	Monotherapy—β-blockers, α-agonists, or topical carbonic anhydrase inhibitors	SLT ALT	Not required	Not required
30	PG analogs or combinations of drugs	Rarely with high baseline IOP	May be required	May be required
40	More than four medications	No	Required	Required

Abbreviations: ALT, argon laser trabeculoplasty; IOP, intraocular pressure; PG, prostaglandin; SLT, selective laser trabeculoplasty.

In ***advanced POAG and PACG after iridotomy***, an IOP in the low teens should be first tried to reduce progression, preferably a mean of 12 mm Hg with minimal fluctuations over time.

After resolution of ***acute PACG***, patients need long-term review as optic nerve head damage and a chronic rise in IOP occurs in many patients, depending upon the duration of the attack. IOP should be kept to at least the population normal.

In ***secondary glaucomas*** such as one following trauma, it may be presumed that the optic nerve head is not predisposed to glaucoma as in POAG, and the height of the IOP is what will damage the optic nerve head. Many of these are related to inflammation, steroid use, etc., which may resolve with time. Also, most such patients are younger than POAG or PACG patients and may tolerate a borderline high IOP for a few days. Therefore, the aim is to lower the IOP to within the population normal with topical and oral glaucoma medications, and taper the medications over time depending on the optic nerve head status, perimetry and IOP recorded. Chronically, raised IOP in the presence of glaucomatous optic neuropathy would need a target IOP similar to POAG/PACG eyes.

Determination of a target IOP is an important step in the management of glaucoma but it cannot be determined with any certainty and achieving the set target IOP does not give complete assurance that disease progression will be prevented, as many other factors also play a part in glaucoma progression.

EMGT concluded that mean elevated IOP is a major risk factor for progression in POAG, while fluctuations are not. A change in IOP by 1 mm Hg resulted in about a 10% change in the risk of progression. De Moraes et al found mean IOP, peak IOP, and IOP fluctuation to be significant risk factors for progression in POAG. Sihota et al found that an intervisit fluctuation in IOP of >4 mm Hg over a median of three visits was associated with progression in POAG and chronic PACG eyes.

The question frequently raised is whether such low IOPs should be aimed for as soon as therapy is instituted, or whether a graded lowering of IOP should be done. Van Gestel et al studied a mathematical model of stepped reduction of IOP 21 to 18 mm Hg, then further to 15 mm Hg, or directly <15 mm Hg, and found that an initially low target IOP gave better quality adjusted life years, as compared with a gradual reduction over time. These lower target IOPs, however, required more medications, laser trabeculoplasty, trabeculectomies, and drainage implants. From a cost-effectiveness and quality of life point of view, it seems advantageous to aim for a low IOP in all glaucoma patients.

Limitations of Setting a Target Intraocular Pressure

Corneal thickness and hysteresis changes can influence IOP measurements, so that a baseline IOP and later IOPs should be evaluated keeping these fallacies in mind. For example, an IOP of 16 mm Hg in a patient with moderate damage and a CCT of 420 microns would actually have a higher corrected IOP, which is not appropriate for this eye.

Aiming for low IOPs in all glaucoma patients needs aggressive IOP reduction and may lead to a reduction in quality of life due to the medications necessary to achieve this, or the risks of glaucoma surgery, if not done carefully and step wise. Adherence to therapy is difficult to ascertain on review and may lead to unnecessary increases in therapy when a patient does not disclose forgetfulness or economic problems with drug application and an IOP appears to be above the target. In addition once a "target" IOP is set, patients could be stressed and unhappy if it is not achieved at every visit. There may be possible medicolegal consequences if despite "target" IOP progression continues.

To date, there is inadequate data available to show that if an individual patient exceeds this target, he or she will progress, or enough evidence-based studies to determine absolute IOP levels in each individual. It is also difficult to definitively diagnose early progression by perimetry or objective monitoring, so that resetting target IOP may be delayed, allowing some loss of VF.

However, setting a "target" IOP range has been shown to help prevent progression, and should be discussed thoroughly with the patient.

Reassessing Target Intraocular Pressure over Time

There is no single, safe level of IOP that is appropriate for all patients at all times, and in spite of achieving target IOP, a few patients show progression of the disease, probably because of other pathological factors. A "target" IOP requires further lowering when the patient continues to progress or develops a systemic disease such as transient ischemic attack (TIA). Conversely, in the event of a very elderly or sick patient with stable nerve and VF over time, the target IOP could be raised and medications reduced.

An example: A 35-year-old male presented at a routine evaluation with a focal narrowing of the inferior neuroretinal rim, associated retinal nerve fiber layer loss and a corresponding superior arcuate defect. The mean baseline IOP, after three readings at different points of time, was 32 mm Hg, and on gonioscopy the angle was open (**Fig. 7.3**).

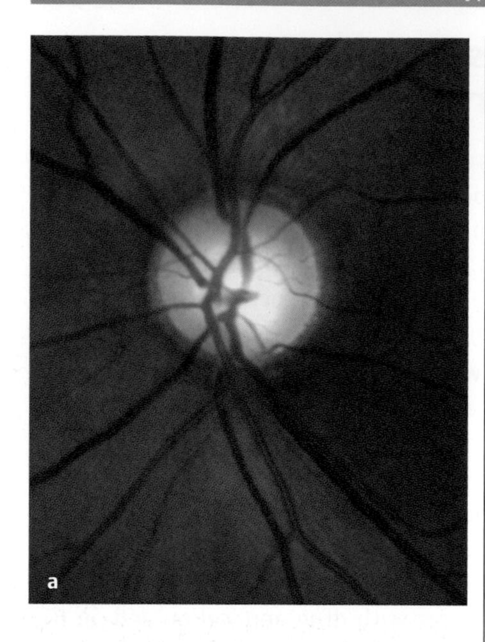

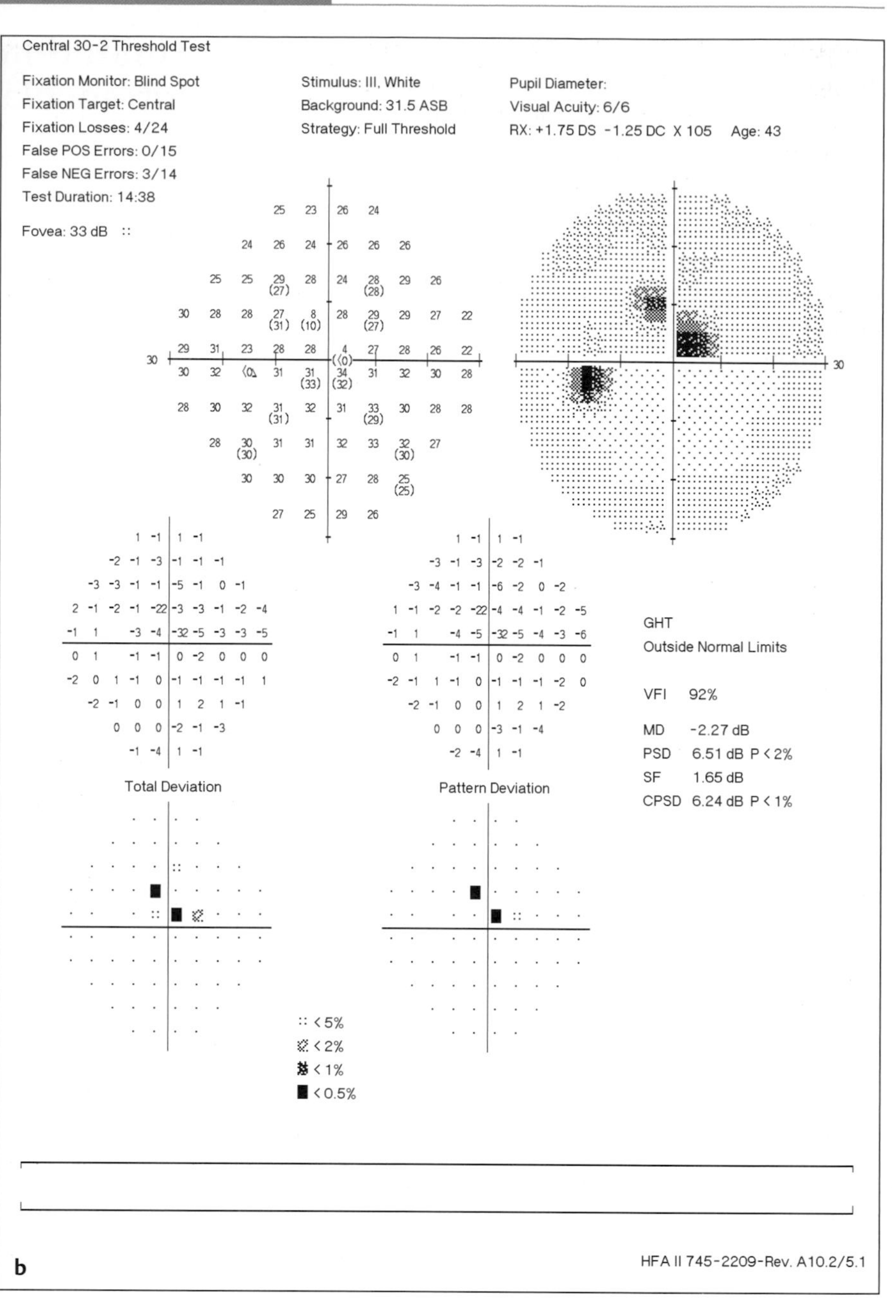

Fig. 7.3 (a, b) Optic nerve head with an inferotemporal notch and retinal nerve fiber layer defect having a corresponding superior arcuate scotoma on Humphrey field analyzer (HFA).

These clinical features and the field can be interpreted as being a moderate glaucoma, and the patient would be expected to live for the next 50 to 60 years. The "target" IOP should therefore be 12 to 15 mm Hg by the absolute/threshold method of target determination. For percentage reduction, using Collaborative Initial Glaucoma Treatment Study (CIGHTS), a reduction in IOP of around 40% could be tried initially, again 12.8 mm Hg.

Perimetry and optic nerve head/retinal imaging should be repeated every 6 months, and applanation tonometry every 3 months.

If perimetry over time shows progression Target IOP would need to be reduced further, for example, if on Humphrey perimetry Guided progression analysis any of the following are seen:

- Decrease in mean deviation by >1 dB/year.
- Rate of progression, of >1% per year.
- Event analysis highlighting deepening/expansion of the existing scotoma or a new scotoma.

Also, if he develops any cardiovascular problems like TIAs, ischemic heart disease, or a stroke, the "target" IOP may be further lowered. *On the other hand, if imaging and perimetry remains stable over a year or more, the "target" IOP could be raised and one medication withdrawn.*

Regular Review of Target Intraocular Pressure over a Lifetime Is Essential

A change in mean deviation of more than 1 dB/year, any reproducible change in two to three loci—deepening, expansion, or new scotomas on perimetry or in known risk factors, should alert the treating ophthalmologist to the possibility of progression, and hence a closer review for perimetry and a change in medications. A change of >2 dB/year signifies a "fast" progress or who warrants aggressive IOP lowering.

Imaging of the optic nerve by optical coherence tomography or HRT may help pick up progression earlier than perimetry in certain patients. Therefore, patients with progression on imaging need to be reviewed more closely and target IOP revised, so that there is no further VF loss.

Conclusion

Target IOP is a useful concept to formulate broad guidelines in the treatment of all glaucomas, however, it should not be "written in stone." Long-term serial objective recording of the optic disc, macula, and retinal nerve fiber layer together with perimetry can highlight early progression and therefore modification of glaucoma therapy when required. There is significant individual variability in anatomical and physiological parameters, and numerous other coexisting systemic diseases and medications. However, it is apparent that with an appropriate target IOP range, and continuous reassessment, glaucoma progression can be considerably slowed down, so that at most, only a few loci show a change.

For both POAG and PACG after an iridotomy, in mild glaucoma the initial target IOP range could be kept as 15 to 17 mm Hg, for moderate glaucoma as 12 to 15 mm Hg, and in the severe stage of glaucomatous damage as 10 to 12 mm Hg. For chronic secondary glaucomas also the glaucomatous loss would determine target similarly, while an acute, transient secondary IOP rise would only need to be reduced to average normal IOPs for the duration of the insult. A yearly diurnal IOP should be to look for IOP fluctuations to re-evaluate target IOP.

Cases

Case 1

A 49-year-old lady was diagnosed as a POAG suspect based on optic nerve head evaluation (**Case 1-1a**). Perimetry of right eye showed a superior arcuate scotoma close to fixation (**Case 1-1b**).

Points to consider

- This is a moderate glaucoma with a life expectancy of at least another 20 years.
- To maintain her quality of life and stabilize VF a target IOP of 12 to 15 mm Hg is required.

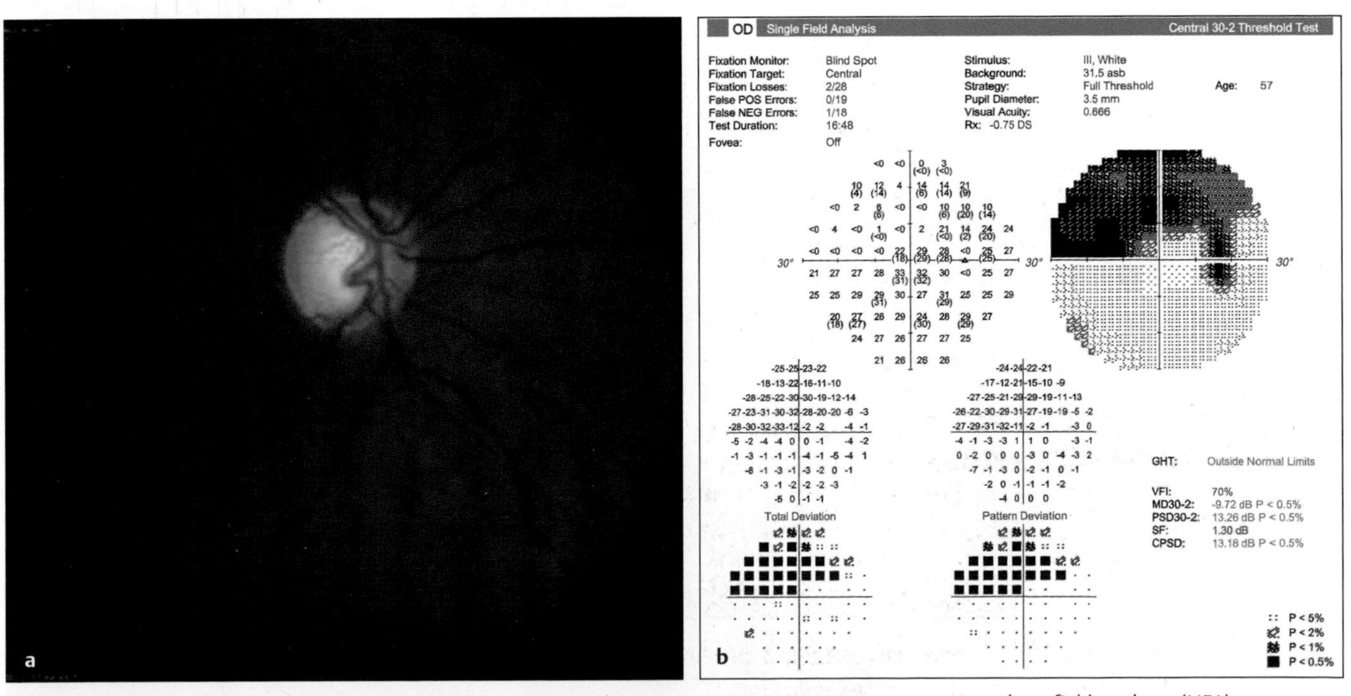

Case 1-1 **(a, b)** Inferotemporal neuroretinal rim loss corresponding to a superior arcuate scotoma on Humphrey field analyzer (HFA).

Diagnosis and Management

This was achieved in the long term with a PG analog hs and timolol bd. A review after a year showed an IOP range of 12 to 16 mm Hg, stable perimetry, with no side effects from the medications.

Case 2

A 14-year-old boy with a firecracker injury presented 2 days later with a clot and fresh bleed in the anterior chamber, and an IOP of 44 mm Hg. With timolol, brimonidine, oral acetazolamide, and glycerol medication, the IOP fell to 26 mm Hg (**Case 2-1**).

Point to consider

- This is a young patient with a secondary, traumatic glaucoma, and not predisposed to optic nerve damage, as is thought to happen in POAG. Therefore, a borderline high IOP may be tolerated for a few days to weeks, till the hyphema resolves and IOP begins to subside. However, an IOP approaching 28/30 mm Hg on maximum medications after 1 week needs a trabeculectomy to prevent vascular blocks as the retinal venous pressure is approximately 23 mm Hg.

Diagnosis and Management

The patient was reviewed every 2 weeks and IOP kept below 22 mm Hg. The hyphema resolved to show a cup:disc ratio of 0.4 having a regular neuroretinal rim with normal color. Medications were slowly tapered off, leaving him on a combination of timolol and brimonidine at 3 months with an IOP of 14 to 18 mm Hg. Angle recession of 100 degrees was seen, and a long-term review advised in view of the possibility of a rise in IOP years later.

Case 3

A 30-year-old female was noted to have an IOP of 28/32 mm Hg and investigated. Her anterior segment was within normal limits. Gonioscopy showed an open angle having many iris processes. Perimetry was reliable and showed biarcuate scotoma breaking into the periphery **Case 3-1**.

Point to consider

- Currently there is severe glaucomatous loss, and the patient has a life expectancy of over 50 years.

Diagnosis and Management

A target IOP of 10 to 12 mm Hg was set. The patient was advised to use Travoprost drops hs, and her diurnal after 2 weeks showed an IOP range of 22 to 24 mm Hg, highest at 7 am. Timolol was added bd and the IOP was rechecked at 7 am after a further 2 weeks to be 10 to 14 mm Hg. She was advised a review and repeat perimetry every 4 months for reassessment of target IOP.

Case 4

A 50-year-old lady complained of diminution of vision in the left eye. On examination, both eyes were van Herick grade 1; pupillary ruff atrophy was seen. A laser iridotomy done 4 years earlier was patent. Her IOPs were 28/34 mm Hg. Gonioscopy showed an angle recess of less than 15 degrees with peripheral anterior synechiae >180 degrees. She had small optic nerves, with a cup:disc ratio of 0.6/0.8 and left optic nerve head showing a very thin and pale neuroretinal rim. Perimetry showed biarcuate scotomas in the left eye (**Case 4-1a–c**).

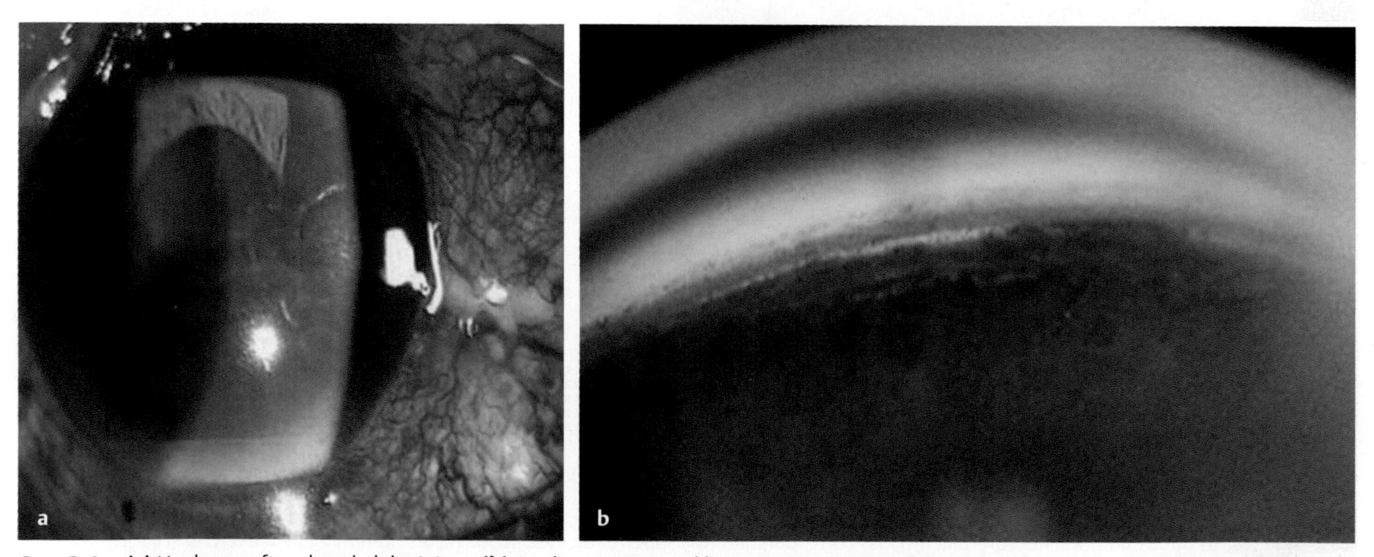

Case 2-1 **(a)** Hyphema after closed globe injury. **(b)** Angle recession and heavy pigmentation of the trabecular meshwork, both causing a rise in intraocular pressure (IOP).

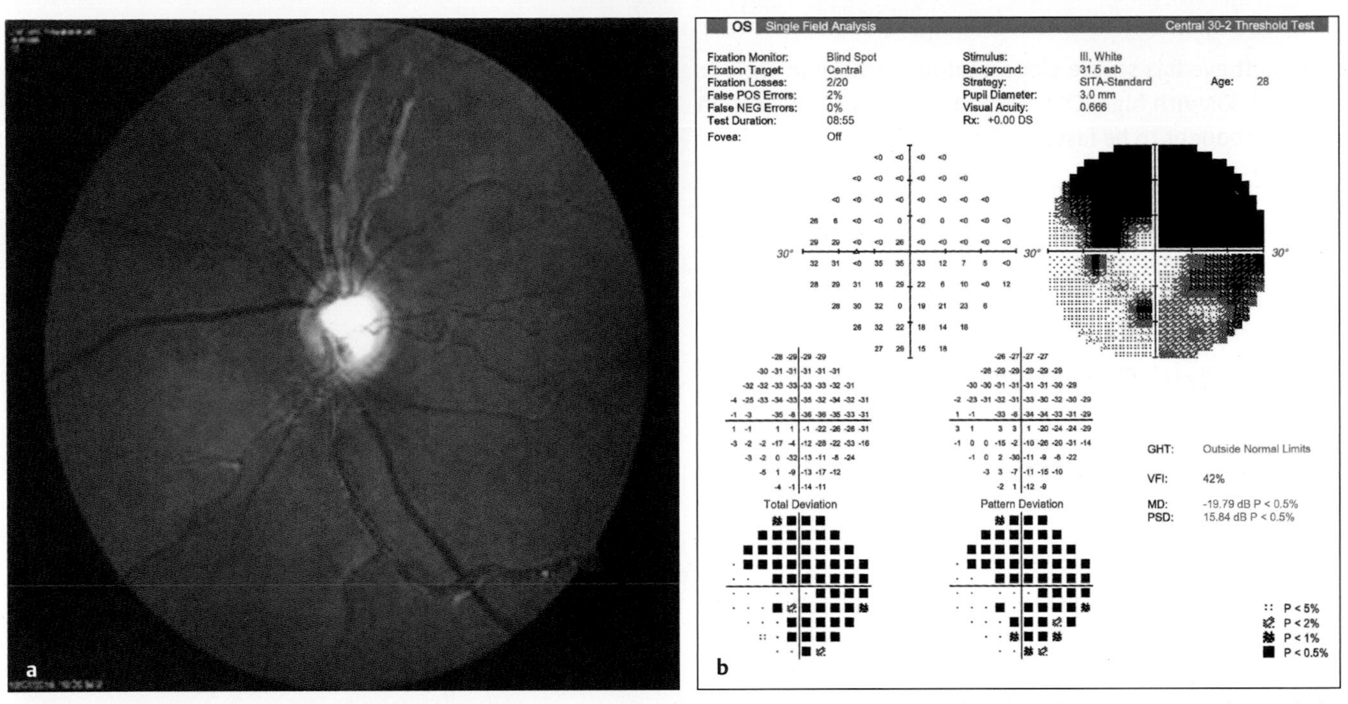

Case 3-1 **(a, b)** Large optic nerve heads with cup:disc ratio of 0.9 and 0.8, neuroretinal rim loss inferiorly in the right eye, corresponding with the arcuate scotoma seen on Humphrey field analyzer (HFA).

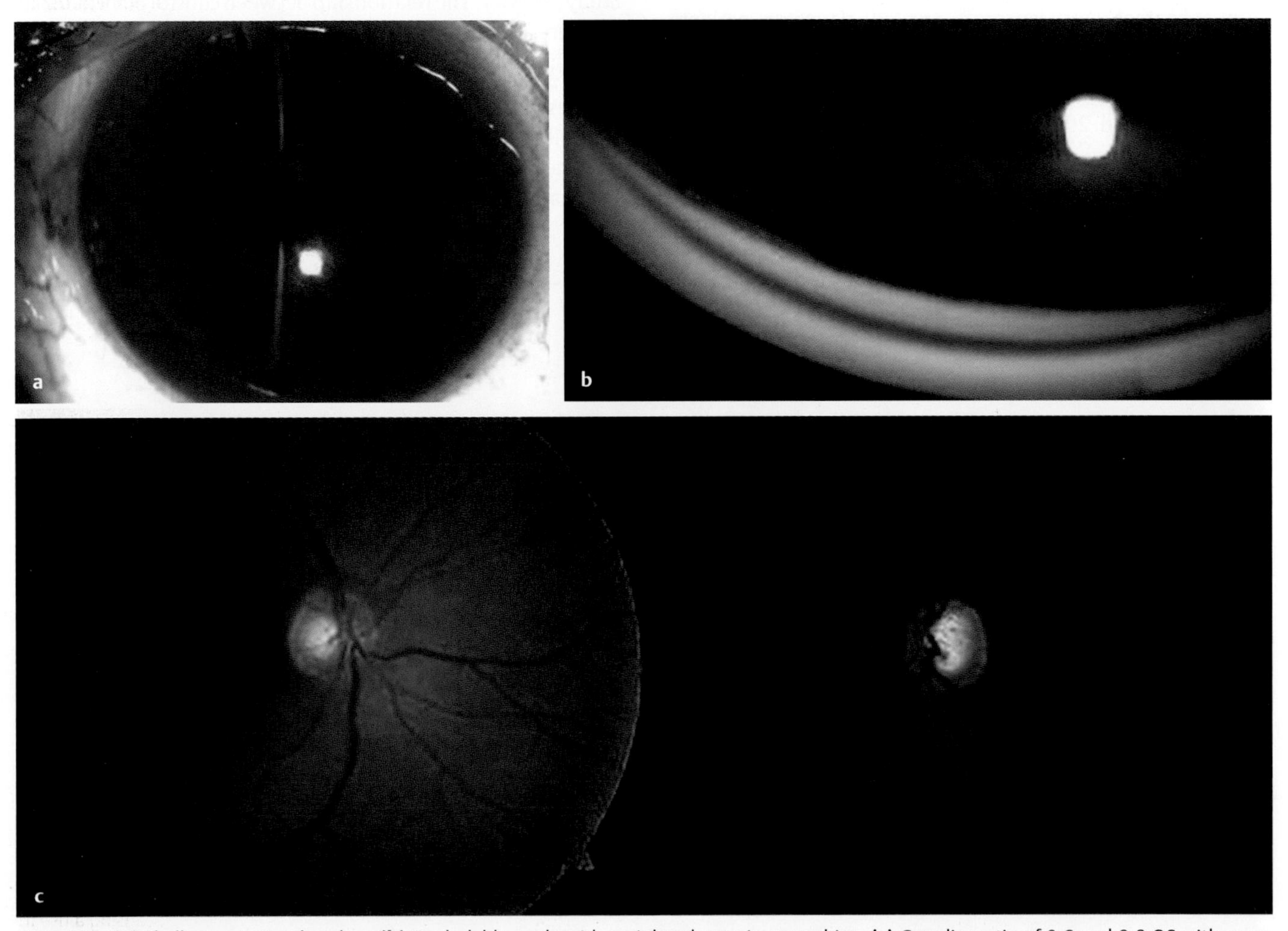

Case 4-1 **(a)** Shallow anterior chamber. **(b)** Occludable angle with peripheral anterior synechiae. **(c)** Cup:disc ratio of 0.6 and 0.8 OS with some neuroretinal rim pallor.

Point to consider

- Left eye has severe glaucomatous damage in chronic PACG, with high IOPs after an iridotomy. Progression is thought to be faster in PACG.

Diagnosis and Management

The target IOP in the left eye was 10 to 12 mm Hg, and was achieved with a PG analog hs, and a combination of timolol and brimonidine bd.

Suggested Readings

Chandler PA. Progress in the treatment of glaucoma in my lifetime. Surv Ophthalmol 1977;21:412–28

Clement CI, Bhartiya S, Shaarawy T. New perspectives on target intraocular pressure. Surv Ophthalmol 2014;59(6):615–626

Damji KF, Behki R, Wang L; Target IOP Workshop participants. Canadian perspectives in glaucoma management: setting target intraocular pressure range. Can J Ophthalmol 2003; 38(3):189–197

De Moraes CG, Jasien JV, Simon-Zoula S, Liebmann JM, Ritch R. Visual field change and 24-hour IOP-related profile with a contact lens sensor in treated glaucoma patients. Ophthalmology 2016;123:744–53

European Glaucoma Society Terminology and Guidelines. For Glaucoma, 4th ed. 2017

European Glaucoma Society Terminology and Guidelines for Glaucoma, 4th Edition, Chapter 2: Classification and terminology Supported by the EGS Foundation: Br J Ophthalmol. 2017 May;101(5):73–127

European Glaucoma Society Terminology and Guidelines for Glaucoma, 4th Edition, Chapter 2: Classification and terminology Supported by the EGS Foundation: Br J Ophthalmol. 2017 Jun;101(6):130–195

Hollows FC, Graham PA. Intra-ocular pressure, glaucoma, and glaucoma suspects in a defined population. Br J Ophthalmol. 1966 Oct;50(10):570-586

Jampel HD. Target pressure in glaucoma therapy. J Glaucoma 1997;6:133–8

Kazemian P, Lavieri MS, Van Oyen MP, Andrews C, Stein JD. Personalized prediction of glaucoma progression under different target intraocular pressure levels using filtered forecasting methods. Ophthalmology 2018;125(4):569–577

Sihota R, Angmo D, Ramaswamy D, Dada T. Simplifying “target” intraocular pressure for different stages of primary open-angle glaucoma and primary angle-closure glaucoma. Indian J Ophthalmol 2018;66(4):495–505

Stewart WC, Kolker AE, Sharpe ED, et al. Factors associated with long-term progression or stability in primary open-angle glaucoma. Am J Ophthalmol 2000;130(3):274–279

The AGIS Investigators. The Advanced Glaucoma Intervention Study (AGIS): 7. The relationship between control of intraocular pressure and visual field deterioration. Am J Ophthalmol 2000; 130(4):429–440

van Gestel A, Webers CA, Severens JL, Beckers HJ, Jansonius NM, Hendrikse F, et al. The long-term outcomes of four alternative treatment strategies for primary open-angle glaucoma. Acta Ophthalmol 2012;90:20–31

CHAPTER 8 Glaucoma Suspect Management—Open Angle

Overview

- Suspicion on the Basis of Raised Intraocular pressure: Ocular Hypertension
- Suspicion on the Basis of Optic Nerve Head Abnormalities: POAG/JOAG Suspect
- Cases
- Suggested Readings

Introduction

In patients with a deep anterior chamber and open angle, the basis of suspicion could be one of the following:

- Suspicion on the basis of raised intraocular pressure (IOP): *Ocular hypertension* (OHT).
- Suspicion on the basis of optic nerve head abnormalities: *Primary open-angle glaucoma (POAG) suspect.*

Suspicion on the Basis of Raised Intraocular pressure: Ocular Hypertension

IOP in individuals varies like most other physiological parameters, and the distribution is not Gaussian. It shows a distinct skewing of the curve toward higher pressure levels, ranging from 10 to 26 mm Hg. Most surveys in India have shown an average IOP of 13 to 16 mm Hg.

Perkins *defined ocular hypertension as an IOP equal to or greater than 22 mm Hg in one or both eyes as measured by applanation tonometry on two or more occasions with no glaucomatous field defects, an open angle, and no history suggestive of closed-angle glaucoma.* Ocular hypertension should be diagnosed if the IOP is two standard deviations beyond the mean for the population, and this is taken to be an IOP of >21 mm Hg, in the presence of a normal optic nerve and normal visual field (**Fig. 8.1**). The prevalence of OHT is around 1 to 3% of individuals over 40 years.

The *Ocular Hypertension Treatment Study* (OHTS) defined OHT as an IOP of 24 to 32 mm Hg with no visual field loss or glaucomatous optic nerve damage, and set a target IOP of <24 mm Hg or a 20% reduction, for treatment of half the randomized participants. OHTS diagnosed progression on perimetry when three consecutive fields showed abnormal loci at the same location. After 5 years, 4.4% of treated and 9.5% of untreated eyes developed POAG. Only 41.7 and 32.6% of eyes progressing to POAG were diagnosed on perimetry alone, 35 and 55% of patients on perimetry and optic nerve head photographs, and the rest based on changes on the optic nerve head alone. After this, medication was provided to the untreated cohort, and at 13 years the incidence of POAG was reported to be similar in both groups—22% of initially untreated and 16% of initially treated eyes—suggesting that delayed treatment may not be overly detrimental. The median time to progression was 6 and 8.7 years, respectively. *Older patients, those with higher IOPs, greater cup:disc ratio, thinner corneas, and of*

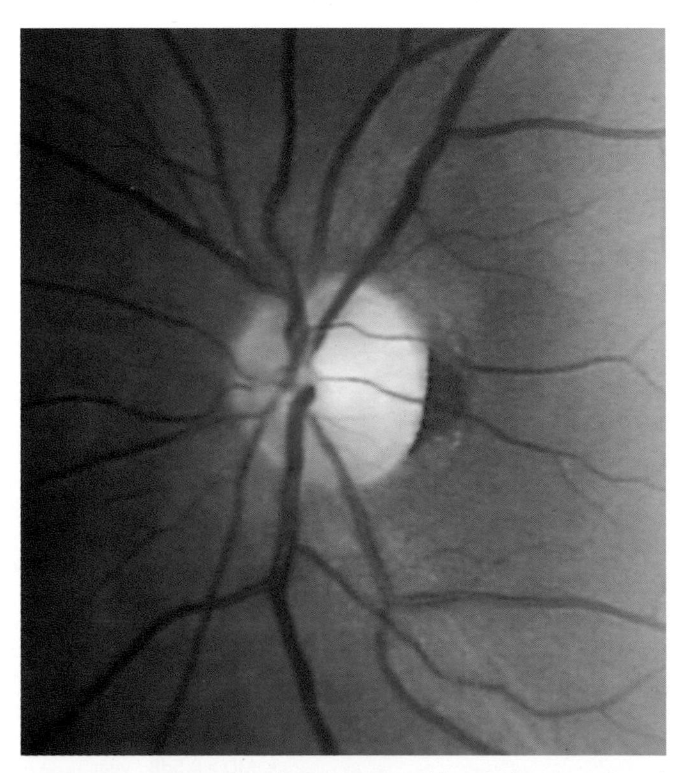

Fig. 8.1 Optic nerve head of a 30-year-old male having a diurnal phasing intraocular pressure (IOP) of 18 to 26 mm Hg. The optic nerve head has a cup:disc ratio of 0.3, the neuroretinal rim is regular with a good color, and the inferior, superior, nasal, temporal (ISNT) rule is followed.

African descent were more likely to progress. It was also suggested that a 20% reduction may not be adequate, and a greater reduction could have further reduced progression. It is now also understood that measurement of IOP is significantly affected by the thickness of the central cornea, corneal hysteresis, and scleral rigidity.

The OHTS led to the development of risk calculators for the progression from OHT to POAG, using these risk factors. Unfortunately these do not hold true for Indians, as a central corneal thickness (CCT) of <555 microns is considered a high-risk factor, and almost all Indians have this pachymetry.

It is thought that raised IOP is the major precursor of glaucoma, with the risk increasing rising IOP, being approximately ten times greater in eyes having an IOP of >21 mm Hg, than individuals with an IOP of less than 21 mm Hg.

Risk factors for OHT converting to POAG can be summarized as follows:

- Thin corneas: <500 μm in Indians.
- Baseline IOP >26/28 mm Hg.
- Older age.
- optic nerve head cup:disc ratio > 0.6 or inferior neuroretinal rim thinning.
- Increased pattern standard deviation (PSD).
- Pseudoexfoliation.
- Family history of glaucoma.
- Systemic hypotension.

Differential diagnoses to keep in mind are thicker corneas, inaccuracy in tonometry, especially noncontact tonometry, and a steroid-induced IOP rise.

Management

Management of OHT is based upon the perceived or
Management of OHT is based upon the perceived or
calculated risk of progression. Diurnal phasing, perimetry, retinal nerve fiber layer, optic nerve head and macular optical coherence tomography, and photography are essential to form a complete baseline picture. As long as *the IOP is at 26 mm Hg or less, individuals can be reviewed periodically with imaging, twice a year* initially followed by an annual review. In the presence of an *IOP >28 mm Hg, there is a risk of retinal vein occlusion, and medications may be used to reduce this to the normal range*. Despite this reduction, some eyes may show preperimetric progression on optical coherence tomography, in which situation the IOP should be further lowered, after discussions with the high-risk patient. A reduction of 20% is not ideal as shown by OHTS.

An Indian study lowered IOP to <18 mm Hg and reported OHT progression to POAG in 2.63% cases. The risk factors being older age, coronary artery disease, use of ≥2 drugs, and systemic use of steroids. CCT was not found to be a significant risk factor (**Flowchart 8.1**).

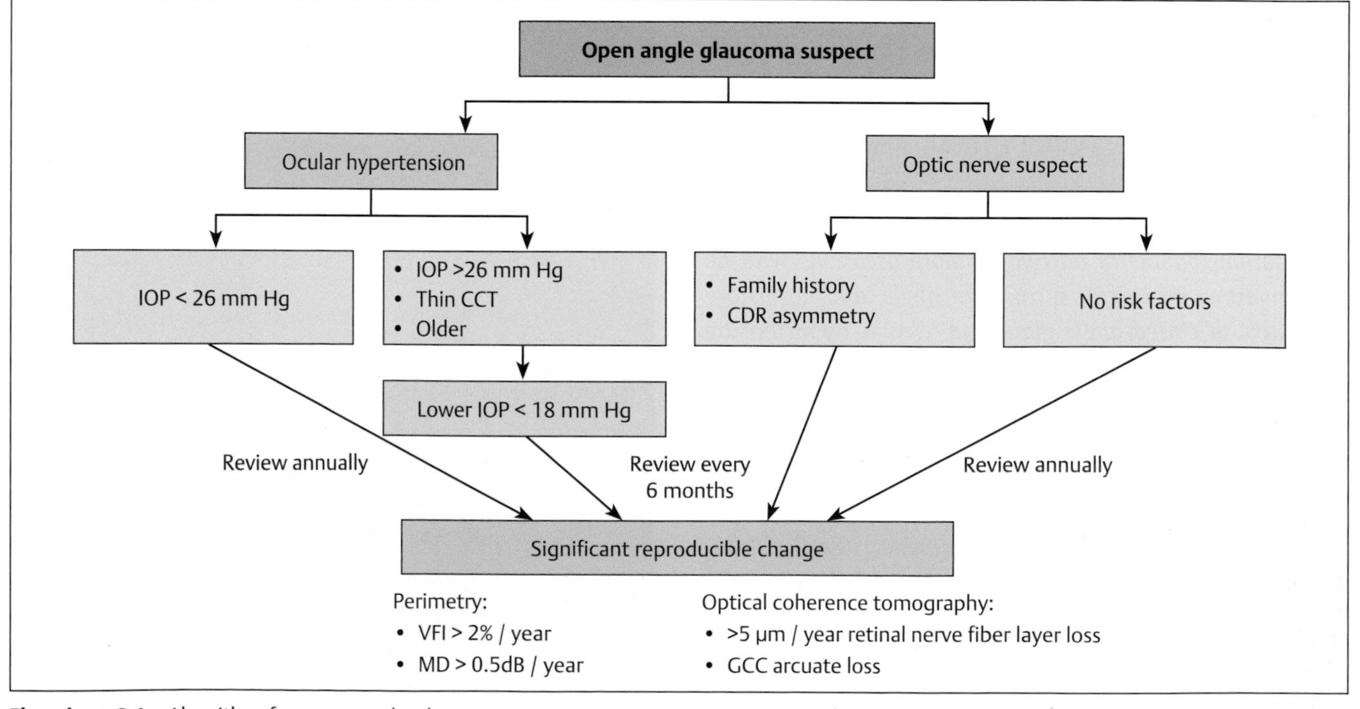

Flowchart 8.1 Algorithm for open angle glaucoma suspect management. CDR, cup:disc ratio; GCC, ganglion cell complex; IOP, intraocular pressure; MD, mean deviation; VFI, visual field index.

Suspicion on the Basis of Optic Nerve Head Abnormalities: POAG/ JOAG Suspect

Optic nerve head changes are suggestive of glaucomatous neuropathy, without visual field loss or raised IOP, in the presence of an open angle. This is a group of individuals who again may be predisposed to POAG, if followed up long enough. The clinical feature commonly seen is a vertical cup:disc ratio of >0.5, with thinning of the inferior neuroretinal rim, (**Fig. 8.2**). This may often occur in eyes with a large disc size, or it may be an inherited familial large physiological cup. The features not present in such eyes would be disc hemorrhages and retinal nerve fiber layer defects, which are considered to be definitive signs of glaucoma. The IOP may or may not be borderline or normal.

Differential diagnoses to keep in mind are a large optic nerve head as in myopes, physiological larger cup, resolved steroid-induced rise in IOP, neurological causes of optic nerve head cupping, and optic nerve head dysplasias.

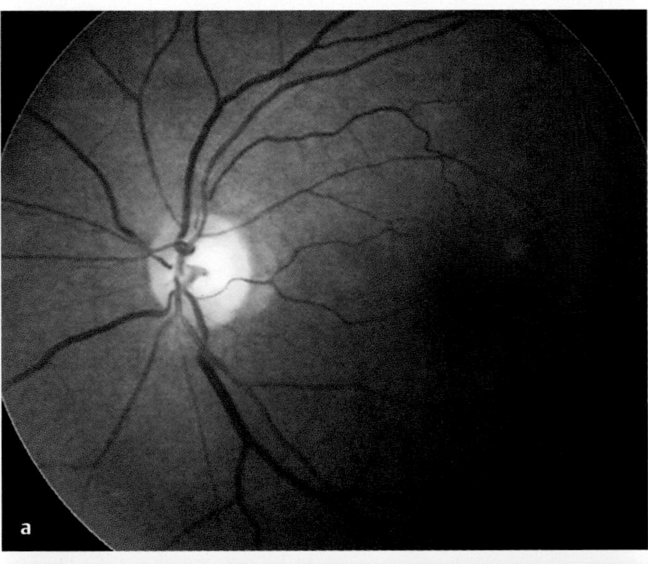

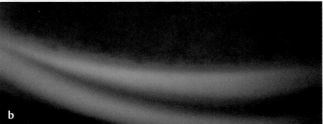

Fig. 8.2 (a) Primary open angle glaucoma (POAG) suspect. Optic nerve head appearance of a 25-year-old male with no family history or elevated intraocular pressure (IOP). The optic nerve head has a cup:disc ratio of 0.6 with early baring of the circumlinear vessel, a thin inferior neuroretinal rim and corresponding possible retinal nerve fiber layer defects. Perimetry was within normal limits. **(b)** Wide open angle on gonioscopy with no evidence of any other pathology.

Risk factors for progression in POAG suspects are:

- Localized thinning of the neuroretinal rim, especially inferotemporally.
- Intereye asymmetry.
- High PSD.
- Older age.
- Family history of glaucoma.
- Thin pachymetry.

Management

Management of an optic nerve head suspect needs a battery of baseline tests, optic nerve head photographs, imaging with optical coherence tomography or Heidelberg retina tomography (HRT), perimetry, and diurnal phasing. If all these are normal, the patients should be reviewed for a repetition of these tests every 6 months, two to three times, to form a good baseline. Thereafter, annual reviews may be undertaken, unless the patient develops vascular problems or the need to use steroids for some other disease.

The European Glaucoma Prevention Study (EGPS) found similar risk factors as OHTS, wherein the presence of optic nerve head defects lead to a greater progression to POAG. These risk factors are as follows:

- Age (risk increased by 26% per decade).
- IOP (risk increased by 9% per 1 mm Hg).
- Vertical and horizontal cup:disc ratio (risk increased by 19% for every 0.1 increase).
- PSD in the visual field (risk increased by 13% for every 0.2 dB increase).
- CCT (risk increased by 2.04-fold for every decrease in thickness by 40 mm).

Other studies have also named intereye asymmetry, family history of glaucomatous loss, coronary disease, and steroid use as risk factors. Each patient should be assessed individually when deciding whether to treat or not.

Cases

Case 1

A 32-year-old male was found to have an IOP of 24/22 mm Hg on routine examination, with a cup:disc ratio of 0.5 in both eyes, regular neuroretinal rim of good color, and open, normal angles on gonioscopy. Diurnal phasing showed an IOP range of 22 to 24 mm Hg in both eyes (**Case 1-1**).

Points to consider

- Is the patient an ocular hypertensive?
- Is there a steroid response?

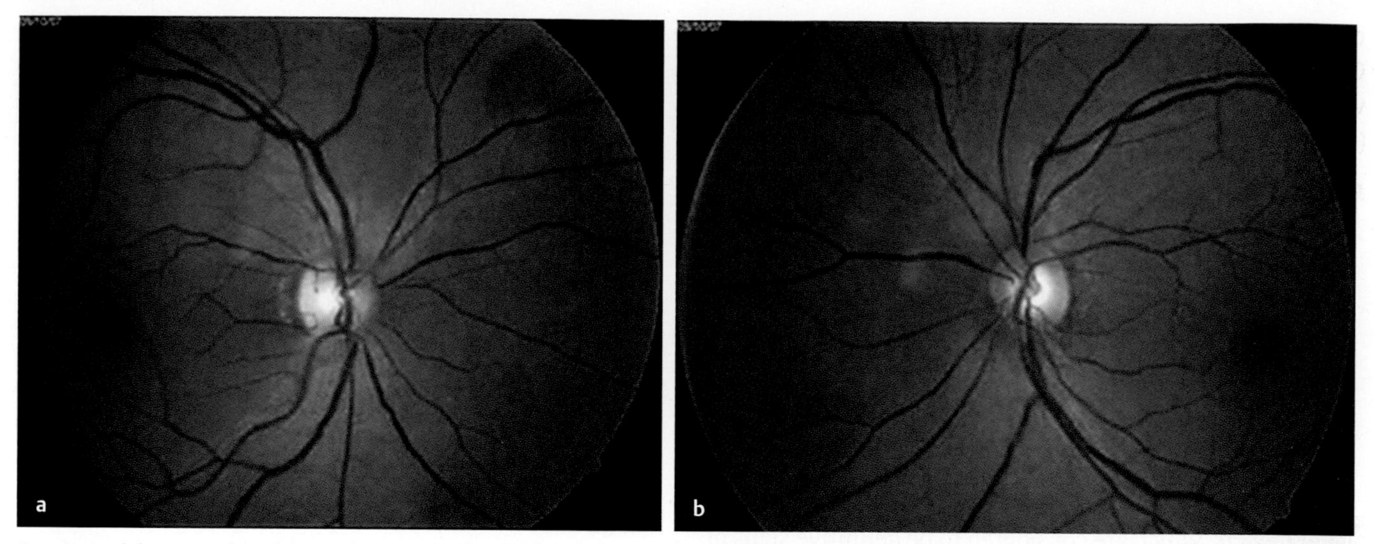

Case 1-1 **(a)** Asymmetry of the optic nerve head. Cup:disc ratio of 0.7 with thinning of neuroretinal rim at both poles, and mild pallor. No retinal nerve fiber layer loss present. **(b)** Left eye cup:disc ratio of 0.6, with some thinning of neuroretinal rim inferiorly, and good color of neuroretinal rim.

- Does the patient have a thicker CCT than the normal for Indians, i.e., 520 µm?

Diagnosis and Management

The patient's CCT was 580 µm in both eyes, perimetry normal, and there was no history of steroid use. He underwent optical coherence tomography for retinal nerve fiber layer and ganglion cell complex (GCC) which were within normal limits, and he was asked to repeat them in 3 months. Thereafter diagnosis of ocular hypertension was made and a review every 6 months was recommended.

Case 2

A 54-year-old male had undergone a renal transplant 2 years ago, and was recently referred as a glaucoma suspect. The patient had a family history of glaucoma. On examination, a deep anterior chamber, with cup:disc ratio of 0.7 and 0.5, thinning of the neuroretinal rim on right eye more than left with no retinal nerve fiber layer defects, and an open, normal angle, was seen. Diurnal phasing showed IOPs of 18 to 24 mm Hg in both eyes, CCT was 520 µm, and his perimetry was within normal limits (**Case 2-1**).

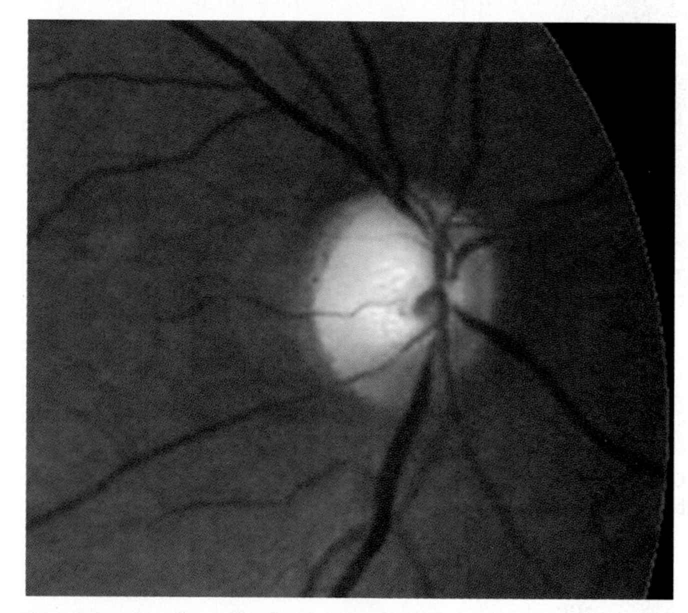

Case 2-1 Cup:disc ratio of 0.6 with a thin but regular neuroretinal rim of good color.

Points to consider

- Is this a steroid-induced glaucoma as the patient is on long-term oral steroids?
- In the absence of a posterior subcapsular cataract, is it more likely to be an early POAG?
- Is he an ocular hypertensive?

Diagnosis and Management

As there was no definitive glaucomatous neuropathy or visual field defect, repeat 6 monthly tonometry and optic nerve head imaging was advised to look for any change over time. A lifelong review was emphasized.

Case 3

A 10-year-old boy was brought to the hospital due to problems in seeing the blackboard in school. On examination, his visual acuity was 6/24 and 6/36 with a compound myopic refractive error. His anterior segment showed posterior embryotoxon, iris hypoplasia, ectopic pupils, and iris holes. His optic nerve head was large with a cup:disc ratio of 0.7 in the right eye and 0.6 in the left, with baring of the circumlinear vessels, but a regular neuroretinal rim of good color, IOP of 22 to 24 mm Hg and CCT of 600 µm. A diagnosis of Axenfeld–Rieger anomaly was made as no systemic abnormalities were present (**Case 3-1**).

Points to consider

- Highest corrected IOP was approximately 19/20 mm Hg, with cup:disc ratio of 0.6 in a large optic nerve head having a regular, orange neuroretinal rim, and a thicker cornea.
- Automated perimetry does not have normative data below 18 years of age.
- The possibility of JOAG should be kept in mind.

Diagnosis and Management

Goldmann kinetic perimetry was within normal limits (WNL). As the patient lived nearby, optic nerve head imaging was advised to look for any change over time. A regular biannual review was emphasized.

Case 4

A 42-year-old patient was thought to be a glaucoma suspect when he came for presbyopic correction. The anterior segment was normal and fundus showed a large optic nerve head in both eyes, with a cup:disc ratio of 0.7, and regular but thinner neuroretinal rim of good color (**Case 4-1**).

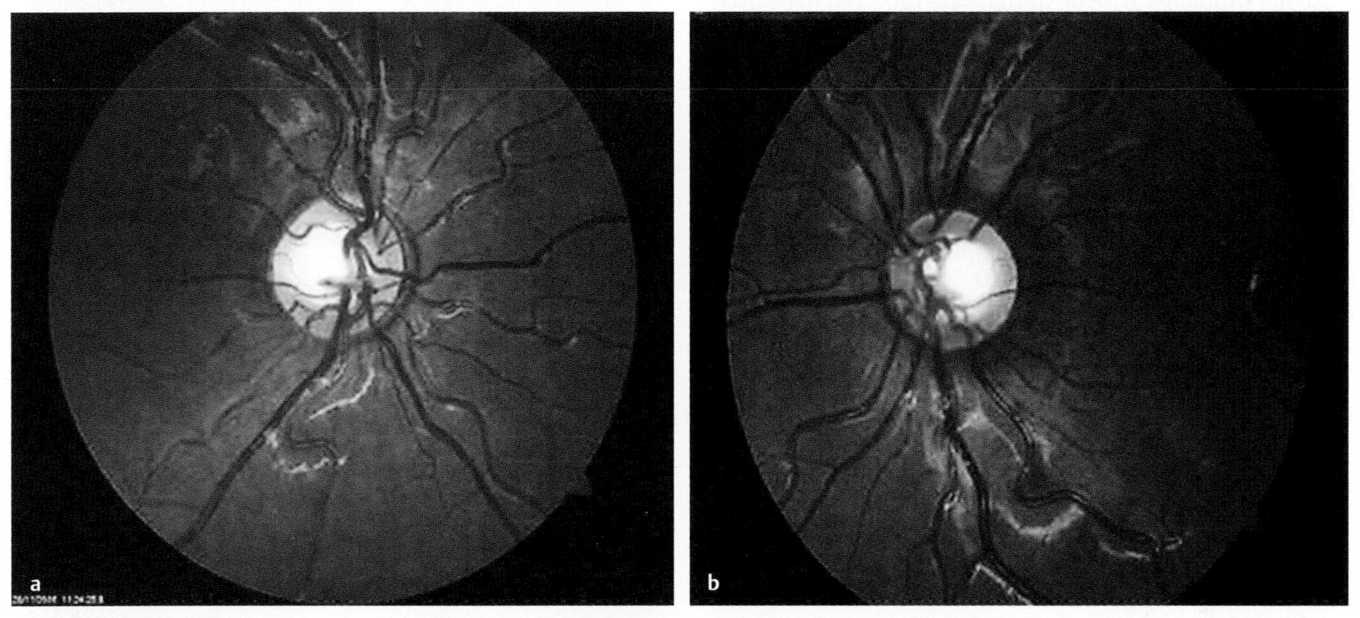

Case 3-1 (a, b) Large optic nerve head, cup:disc ratio of 0.7 with baring of the circumlinear vessels and regular neuroretinal rim of good color in both the eyes.

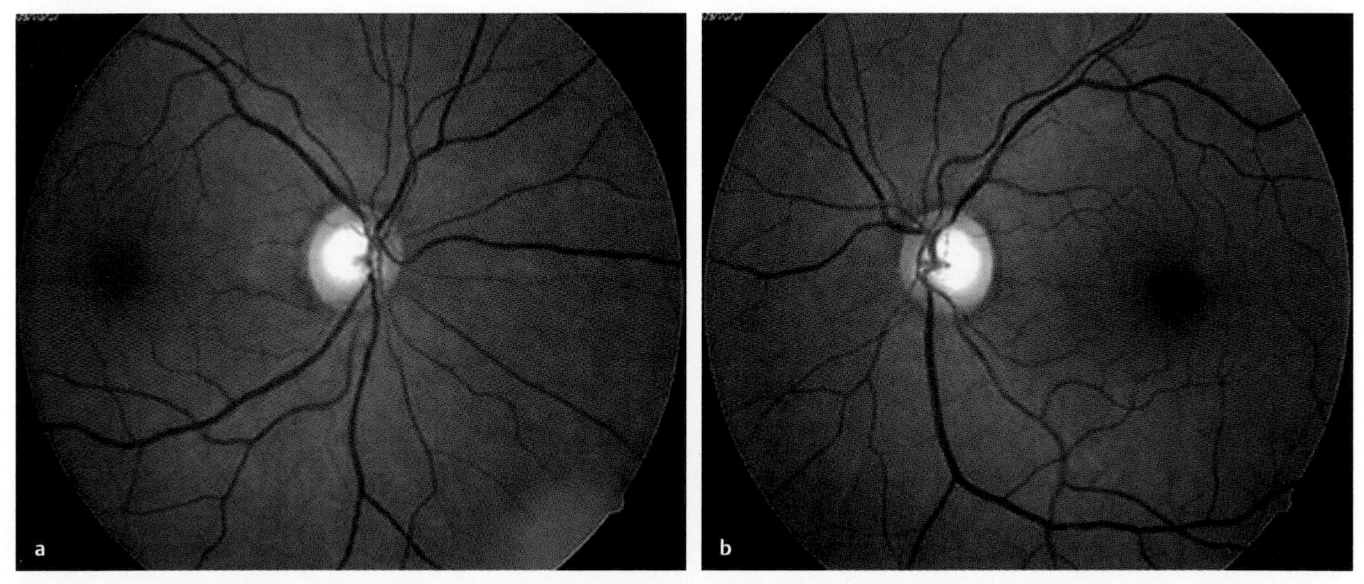

Case 4-1 (a, b) Large optic nerve head with a similar cup:disc ratio of 0.7 in both eyes. Neuroretinal rim is thin but regular.

Diurnal phasing showed an IOP range of 14 to 18 mm Hg. Perimetry was normal in both eyes. There was no family history of glaucoma.

Points to consider

- A large cup can be seen in a larger optic nerve head.
- No asymmetry is present.

Diagnosis and Management

A diagnosis of possibly a large physiological cup or POAG suspect was entertained. Optic nerve head imaging was performed every 6 months over 2 years. As there was no change, an annual review was advised, which if stable would allow a review once in 2-3 years, or if systemic vascular problems arise or steroids are required to be used.

Suggested Readings

Anderson DR. Glaucoma: the damage caused by pressure. XLVI Edward Jackson memorial lecture. Am J Ophthalmol 1989;108(5):485–495

Cheng EM, Giaconi JA, Coleman AL, et al; Appropriateness of Treating Glaucoma Suspects RAND Study Group. For which glaucoma suspects is it appropriate to initiate treatment? Ophthalmology 2009;116(4):710–716e1–716.e82

Gordon MO, Beiser JA, Brandt JD, et al. The Ocular Hypertension Treatment Study: baseline factors that predict the onset of primary open-angle glaucoma. Arch Ophthalmol 2002;120(6):714–720, discussion 829–830

Gordon MO, Torri V, Miglior S, et al; Ocular Hypertension Treatment Study Group; European Glaucoma Prevention Study Group. Validated prediction model for the development of primary open-angle glaucoma in individuals with ocular hypertension. Ophthalmology 2007;114(1):10–19

Kass MA, Heuer DK, Higginbotham EJ, et al. The Ocular Hypertension Treatment Study: a randomized trial determines that topical ocular hypotensive medication delays or prevents the onset of primary open-angle glaucoma. Arch Ophthalmol 2002;120(6):701–713, discussion 829–830

Miglior S, Zeyen T, Pfeiffer N, Cunha-Vaz J, Torri V, Adamsons I; European Glaucoma Prevention Study (EGPS) Group. Results of the European Glaucoma Prevention Study. Ophthalmology 2005;112(3):366–375

Miglior S, Torri V, Zeyen T, Pfeiffer N, Vaz JC, Adamsons I; EGPS Group. Intercurrent factors associated with the development of open-angle glaucoma in the European glaucoma prevention study. Am J Ophthalmol 2007;144(2): 266–275

Öhnell H, Bengtsson B, Heijl A. Making a correct diagnosis of glaucoma: data from the EMGT. J Glaucoma 2019;28(10): 859–864

CHAPTER 9

Glaucoma Suspect Management—Shallow Anterior Chamber with Narrow Angles

Overview

- Diagnosing a Shallow Anterior Chamber
  - Clinical Features
  - Further Evaluation
  - Gonioscopy
  - Anterior Segment Imaging
  - Management of Eyes with Shallow Anterior Chambers
- Primary Angle-Closure Disease
  - Primary Angle-Closure Suspect
  - Primary Angle Closure
  - PAC with Ocular Hypertension
  - Plateau Iris Syndrome
  - Exaggerated Lens Vault
  - Secondary Angle Closure
- Cases
- Suggested Readings

Introduction

A greater prevalence of shallow anterior chambers (ACs) and angles is found in Indians, making the recognition of early signs of angle closure important, so as to prevent needless morbidity. Anterior chamber depth is recorded as the distance between the posterior surface of the cornea and anterior surface of the lens, and is normally 2.5 to 3.0 mm deep. It is seen to be shallow in infancy and in older patients, and in certain races.

Diagnosing a Shallow Anterior Chamber

Diagnosing a shallow anterior chamber is the first step in suspecting any form of angle closure, and can be easily done using a torch or slit lamp. These are noncontact and subjective assessments, but are easily applied in a busy outpatient clinic.

- *Torch light*: The depth of the anterior chamber can be clinically evaluated by flashing a beam of light from the temporal limbus, parallel to the surface of the iris. In a normal or deep anterior chamber the beam will pass across, illuminating the entire iris and the opposite limbus. In eyes with a shallow anterior chamber, the forward convexity or bowing of the iris on either side of the pupil obstructs the beam, and a crescentic shadow is observed on the nasal iris and limbus (**Figs. 9.1a** and **9.2a**).
- The *van Herick test* employs a comparison of the depth of the most peripheral anterior chamber to the peripheral corneal thickness in a dark room. The slit-lamp illumination and viewing arms are placed at 60 degrees to each other, with the viewing arm

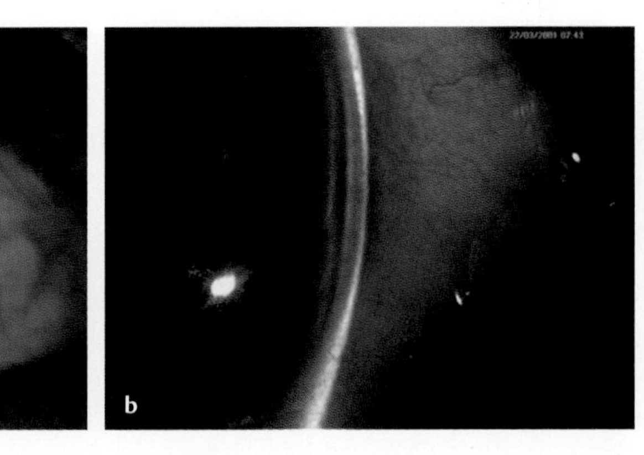

Fig. 9.1 **(a)** A focused torch shone parallel to the iris from the temporal limbus should illuminate the entire iris and a glow should be visible at the nasal limbus in a deep anterior chamber with an open angle. **(b)** The van Herick test shows an anterior chamber of grade 4, with peripheral anterior chamber more than half the width of the cornea.

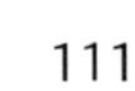

in primary position, using a magnification of 16×, and the patient fixating straight ahead (**Fig. 9.1b**). A *fine slit is placed just inside and perpendicular to the temporal limbus*: peripheral anterior chamber depth equal to or greater than the corneal thickness is recorded as grade 4, half corneal thickness as grade 3, quarter thickness of cornea as grade 2, and less than a quarter as grade 1 (**Table 9.1** and **Figs. 9.2** and **9.3**). Grade 1 anterior chamber depth suggests that angle closure is possible, while in grade 4, closure is unlikely. Thomas et al found the sensitivity and specificity on the flashlight test were 45.5 and 82.7%, respectively, and for the van Herick test these were 61.9 and 89.3%.

- A further modification, *van Herick plus*, is performed at the inferior limbus with slit-lamp illumination and viewing arms placed at 30 degrees to each other. A short, thin, vertical slit-lamp beam evaluation straddling the inferior angle is an easy and relatively accurate method for evaluating both peripheral anterior chamber depth and an estimation of the anterior chamber (**Fig. 9.4**).
- The anterior chamber can be *objectively measured* by all anterior segment imaging systems such as Pentacam, IOL Master, LenStar, and anterior segment optical coherence tomography, and ultrasonic biomicroscopy with similar accuracy.

Table 9.1 van Herick test grading

Grade	Limbal depth relative to corneal thickness
4	≥ corneal thickness
3	>½ corneal thickness
2	½ to ¼ corneal thickness
1	<¼ corneal thickness

Clinical Features

The presence of a shallow anterior chamber of grade 2 should immediately alert the ophthalmologist to the possibility of angle-closure glaucoma—primary or secondary—or anterior segment dysgenesis. Therefore, further evaluation should be directed at identifying the various causes of a shallow anterior chamber, which can present in many forms such as:

- Peripherally shallow anterior chamber with convex or flat iris.
- Centrally shallow anterior chamber.
- Very shallow anterior chamber, both central and peripheral.
- Irregularly shallow anterior chamber.

A peripherally shallow anterior chamber with a convex iris configuration is the hallmark of *primary angle-closure disease*, caused by a relative pupillary block. With increased iridolenticular apposition at the pupil, the flow of aqueous

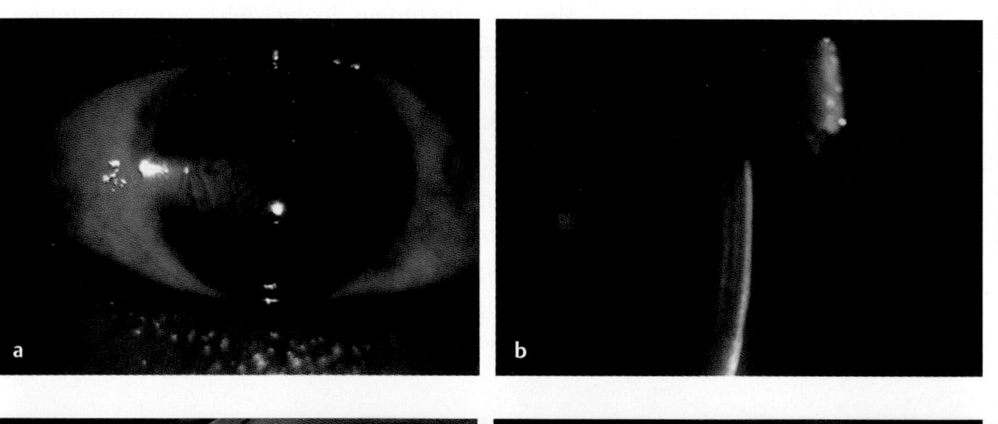

Fig. 9.2 **(a, b)** In a shallow anterior chamber with a narrow anterior chamber angle, a crescentic shadow at the nasal iris with a dark nasal limbus is seen on torch light. The van Herick test shows an anterior chamber of grade 2, with peripheral anterior chamber less than one-fourth the width of the cornea.

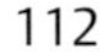

Fig. 9.3 **(a)** van Herick grade 4, with anterior chamber more than the thickness of the cornea. **(b)** Grade 3, anterior chamber width more than half the corneal thickness.

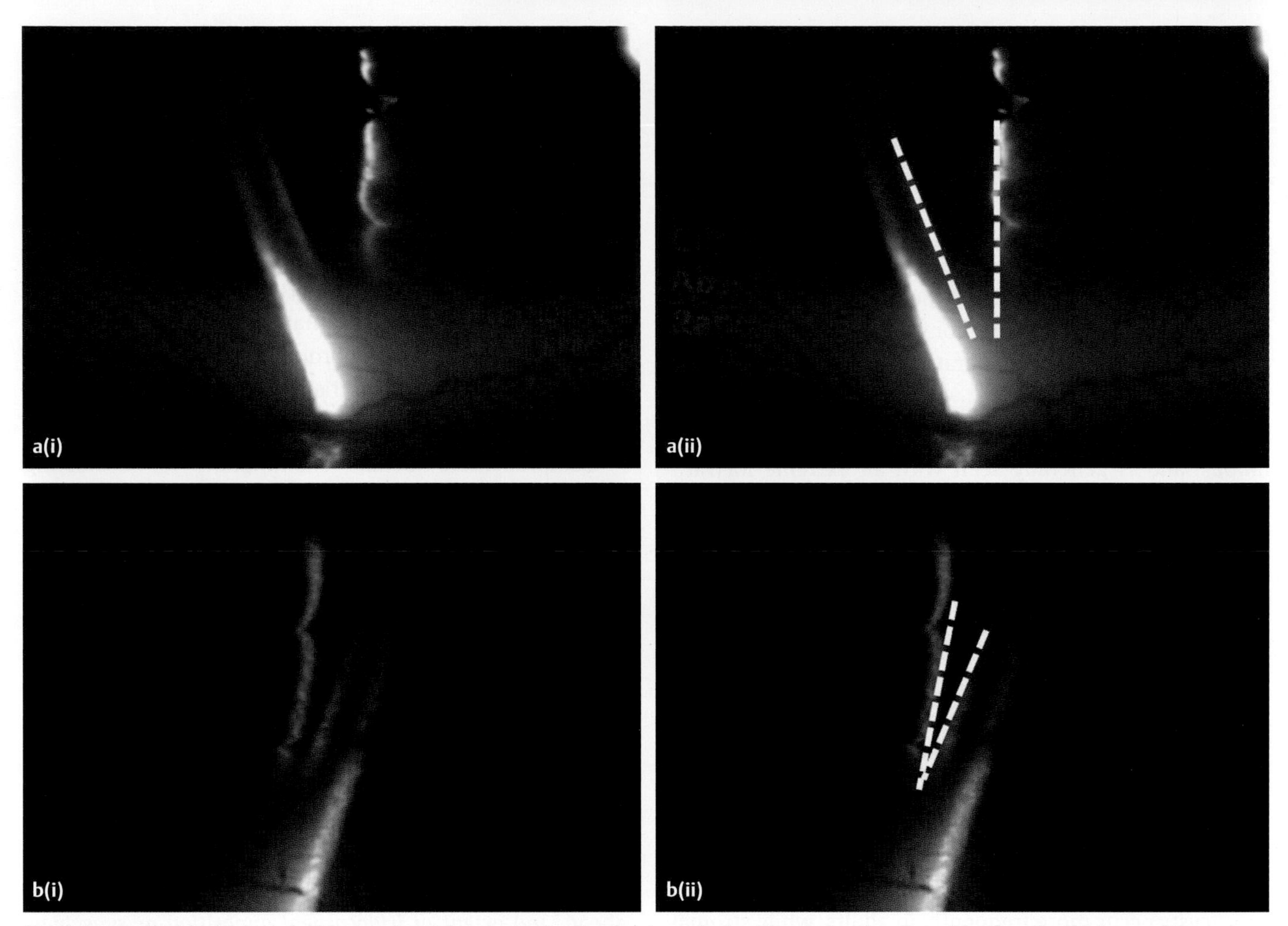

Fig. 9.4 van Herick plus test. **(a)** The most peripheral anterior chamber is grade 4, with anterior chamber wider than the thickness of the cornea. **(b)** Grade 1, less than one-fourth the corneal thickness, with an estimated iridocorneal angle of about 10 degrees. *Dashed lines* depict the angle recess in both the figures.

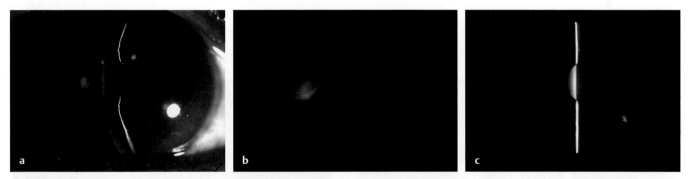

Fig. 9.5 **(a)** A shallow anterior chamber, centrally and peripherally. **(b)** Narrow angle with a relatively normal central anterior chamber, as in plateau iris configuration. **(c)** Very shallow central and peripheral anterior chamber.

from the posterior to anterior chamber is impeded, and pushes the iris forward, forming iris bombe. A similar appearance with associated features of iridocyclitis, such as posterior synechiae or occlusion pupillae, causes uveitic secondary angle-closure glaucoma (**Fig. 9.5a**).

An *anterior chamber that is shallow in the extreme periphery, with a flat iris and a relatively normal central depth*, is characteristically due to *plateau iris*. This iris configuration is thought to be caused by anteriorly rotated ciliary processes that push up the peripheral iris by at least 180 degrees. The iris then falls back toward the pupil (**Fig. 9.5b**).

A *peripherally shallow anterior chamber* may also be caused by a *thick iris, with prominent, peripheral circumferential folds* adjacent to the angle. On dilation of the pupil, these become more pronounced and could oppose the trabecular meshwork.

A *centrally shallow anterior chamber, relatively deeper in the periphery*, is seen in eyes with a significant lens vault. An exaggerated lens vault is caused by a normal or large lens pushing the iris forward and resulting in a small anterior chamber volume and markedly reduced space between the iris and the cornea, especially when the pupil dilates. The iris appears to drape the anterior surface of the lens, giving rise to a "volcano-like configuration" (**Fig. 9.5c**).

A *very shallow anterior chamber, central and peripheral* would have a similarly shallow appearance limbus to limbus, and is generally seen with an extreme forward displacement of the lens as in *malignant glaucoma*.

An irregularly shallow anterior chamber is associated with other ocular pathologies of the anterior segment (**Figs. 9.6** and **9.7**):

- Angle recession in closed globe injury leads to a deeper anterior chamber in the affected quadrants, generally the inferotemporal area.
- Subluxation of the lens, as seen in Marfan syndrome, trauma, etc., may lead to either a localized deepening or shallowing of the anterior chamber and may have associated glaucoma.
- Iris or ciliary body cysts. Primary pigment epithelial cysts occur more frequently in adults, while stromal cysts are common in children. Acquired cysts are often seen after trauma. These can lead to angle closure, a plateau iris configuration, and pigment dispersal.
- Developmental anomalies such as Axenfeld syndrome, Rieger anomaly, Peters anomaly, and iridocorneal endothelial (ICE) syndrome also have an irregular anterior chamber and may be associated with glaucoma.

Further Evaluation

Systemic history is evaluated for the use of sulfa-based drugs such as topiramate in migraines and weight loss; hydrochlorothiazide for hypertension and congestive cardiac failure; and promethazine for allergies. These drugs may lead to cilio-choroidal effusions in otherwise normal eyes, pushing the iris lens diaphragm leading to angle closure.

Comprehensive ocular examination for coexisting pathologies is essential to identify uveitis, signs of trauma, developmental anomalies, etc., that may be contributing to the shallowing of the anterior chamber. Evaluation of the optic nerve head to identify and record changes at the neuroretinal rim is also essential. It is important to take an applanation tonometry thrice at preferably different times of the day.

Gonioscopy

It is necessary to determine the presence of an *occludable angle*, where >180 degrees of the posterior trabecular meshwork is not visualized with the patient looking straight ahead, and *extent of iridocorneal apposition or synechiae*. This provides an approximate estimate of trabecular meshwork damage and can alert the ophthalmologist to a possible elevation in intraocular pressure (IOP). Identifying Schwalbe's line as the point where a fine light beam from the anterior and posterior surfaces of the cornea meets, the corneal wedge is the first step for orientation (**Fig. 9.8 a, b**).

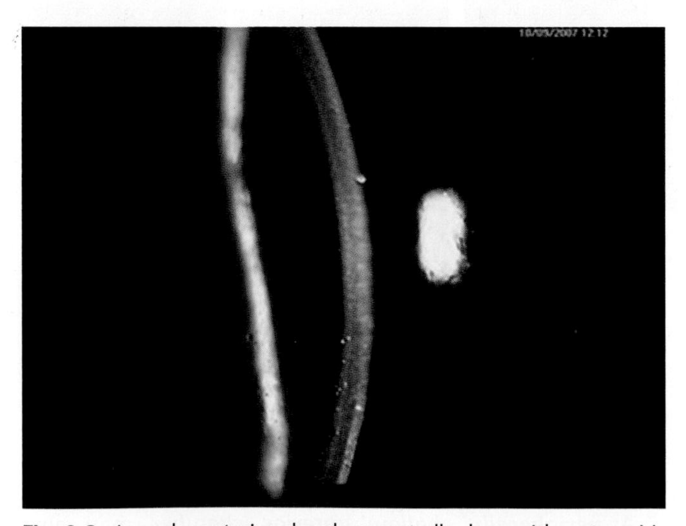

Fig. 9.6 Irregular anterior chamber, centrally deep with a steep iris due to occlusio pupillae after uveitis, keratic precipitates seen.

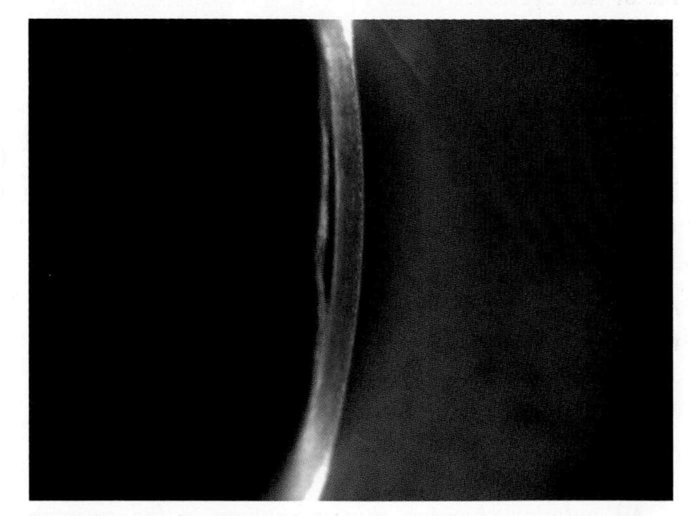

Fig. 9.7 Irregular anterior chamber due to iris cysts.

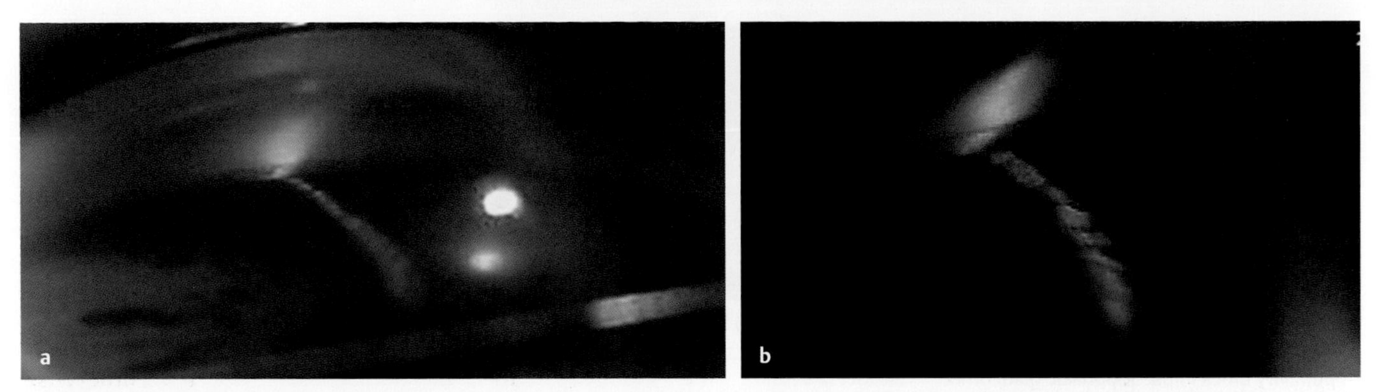

Fig. 9.8 (a) The corneal wedge, marking the position of Schwalbe's line, is seen to be very close to the peripheral iris and the angle recess is narrow, with a flat iris configuration as in plateau iris configuration. **(b)** The corneal wedge, marking the position of Schwalbe's line, is seen to be very close to the peripheral iris and the angle recess is narrow, with a steep iris configuration.

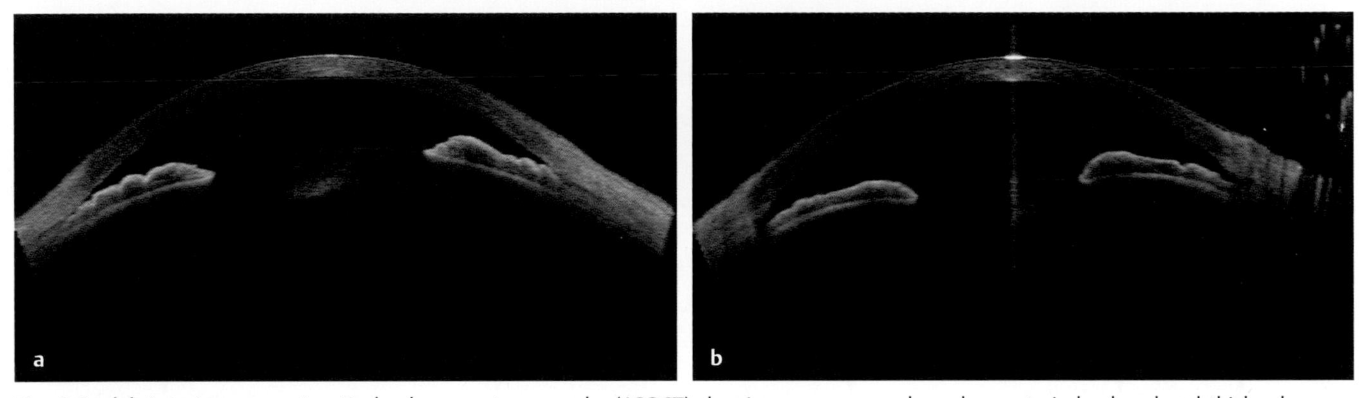

Fig. 9.9 (a) Anterior segment optical coherence tomography (ASOCT) showing a narrow angle and an anteriorly placed and thicker lens, an exaggerated lens vault. **(b)** ASOCT showing a narrow angle with a convex iris configuration.

Posterior to this is the nonpigmented anterior trabecular meshwork and further posteriorly the pigmented posterior trabecular meshwork. Looking for apposition or synechiae needs a view of the depth of the angle recess, which is difficult in narrow angles. When using a two-mirror gonioscope, manipulation—asking the patient to rotate his or her eye toward the mirror being used, or moving the mirror toward the angle being viewed—will permit a view over iris convexity. A four-mirror gonioscope having a smaller base of about 7 mm permits indentation, depression of the central cornea, which displaces central aqueous peripherally, and opens up the angle recess.

Anterior Segment Imaging

Anterior segment imaging is done using optical coherence tomography and ultrasound biomicroscopy (UBM).

- *Anterior segment optical coherence tomography* (ASOCT) provides a noncontact, semiautomatic, reproducible, and objective record of the anterior segment for diagnosing reasons for a shallow anterior chamber, anterior to the iris pigment epithelium. This is especially useful in identifying primary angle-closure disease, lens vault, iris configuration, and angle recession. CASIA ASOCT can give a quantitative evaluation of the extent of iridotrabecular contact (ITC) (**Figs. 9.9a, b** and **9.10b**).
- *UBM* can image structures posterior to the iris as well as anterior segment structures through media opacification. It has helped in determining the various causes of a shallow anterior chamber—plateau iris, angle recession, ciliary effusion syndrome, lens subluxation, ciliary body cyst, or tumor. Eyes with plateau iris syndrome have anteriorly situated ciliary processes on UBM, and in malignant glaucoma ciliary bodies are thinner and more anteriorly rotated (**Fig. 9.10**).

Management of Eyes with Shallow Anterior Chambers

A gonioscopy is necessary to record the extent of abnormalities at the angle and trabecular meshwork, to identify a possible cause and its resolution. *Treatment for the cause may prevent progression of the angle closure and further glaucomatous neuropathy*, as in stopping topiramate,

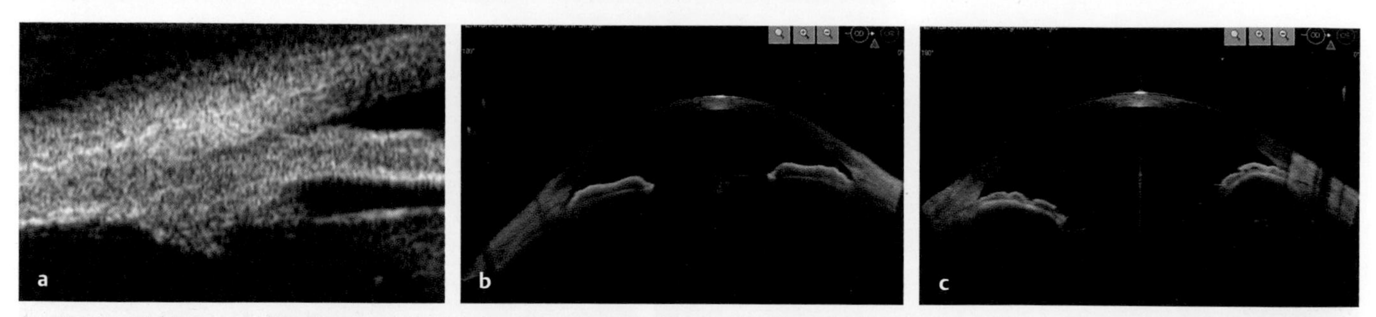

Fig. 9.10 **(a)** Ultrasound biomicroscopy (UBM) showing a narrow angle with a flat iris configuration. The peripheral iris is being pushed from behind by ciliary processes. **(b)** Anterior segment optical coherence tomography (ASOCT) of a patient with a plateau iris configuration. **(c)** ASOCT of pupillary block in pseudophakic glaucoma.

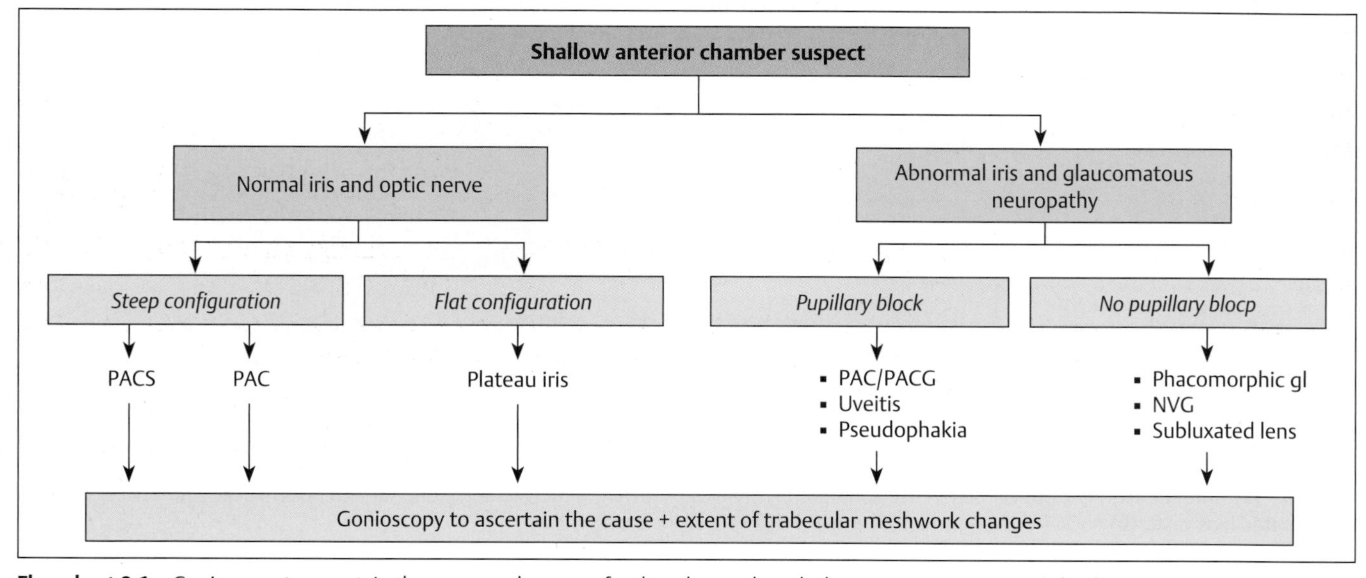

Flowchart 9.1 Gonioscopy to ascertain the cause and extent of trabecular meshwork changes. PAC, primary angle-closure; PACG, primary angle-closure glaucoma; PACS, primary angle-closure suspect; NVG, neovascular glaucoma.

treating uveitis, etc. Medical control of IOP is required in the interim to prevent further glaucomatous neuropathy. An algorithm for identifying a possible causative diagnosis, based on examination and gonioscopy, is provided in **Flowchart 9.1**.

Common diseases associated with a shallow anterior chamber and narrow angle are discussed below.

Primary Angle-Closure Disease

Primary angle-closure disease needs an initial laser iridotomy and also therapy to attain an appropriate target IOP proportionate to the extent of visual field damage present.

Primary Angle-Closure Suspect

Foster et al defined this as an eye in which appositional contact between the peripheral iris and posterior trabecular meshwork is considered possible. On gonioscopy, this occludable angle is one in which ≥270 degrees of the posterior trabecular meshwork (the part which is often pigmented) cannot be seen, with the patient looking in primary position. The World Glaucoma Association (WGA) and the preferred practice patterns of the American Academy of Ophthalmology have defined it as an angle with 180 degrees or more of ITC on dark-room gonioscopy, no peripheral anterior synechiae (PAS), and normal IOP without disc and field changes. The second criteria appears to overlap with features of PAC, and is probably best avoided. It is essential to do an indentation gonioscopy in such cases. If an indentation gonio lens is not available, one must do a manipulative gonioscopy. This should be followed by a complete baseline glaucoma evaluation to exclude a raised IOP or optic neuropathy, and confirm the diagnosis of a PACS.

Primary Angle Closure

Primary angle closure (PAC) is traditionally diagnosed in eyes with >180 degrees of occludable angle with evidence of ITC: PAS, blotchy pigment on the trabecular meshwork with pigment deposition on the superior trabecular meshwork, ischemic sequelae of acutely raised IOP (distortion of the radially orientated iris musculature, iris stromal atrophy, or glaucomfleken), or a definite history of symptoms consistent with sudden IOP rise and evidence of an iridotomy. However, the optic disc and visual field are not glaucomatous. A darkroom-prone provocation test (DRPPT) giving a rise in IOP of greater than or equal to 8 mm Hg from baseline could also be used to diagnose PAC.

PAC with Ocular Hypertension

This has all the angle features described above, with an IOP elevated >21 mm Hg on at least three occasions. This is more likely to progress to an optic neuropathy and needs long-term review and therapy if IOP rises over 18 mm Hg.

Clinical Features

The following are characteristic clinical features of primary angle-closure disease:

- Cornea: Usually has a smaller white-to-white diameter and is steeper.
- anterior chamber is shallow (**Figs. 9.2a** and **9.5a**).
- Iris generally shows a convex configuration, pupillary ruff atrophy may be seen in PAC, distortion of the radially orientated iris musculature, "whorling" and sector iris stromal atrophy after acute primary angle-closure glaucoma (PACG).
- Lens—anterior subcapsular opacities, "glaucomfleken" after acute attacks.
- Fundus examination:
  - Optic disc is usually smaller in size.
  - Therefore, even a small loss of neuroretinal rim or cup:disc ratio of even 0.5 becomes significant for glaucoma.

Management

Observational studies suggest that the majority of PACS patients will not develop either PAC or PACG. In a population-based study of PACS, 22% of PACS, over a 5-year period, converted to PAC and no PACS patients developed functional damage. Therefore, an iridotomy needs to be done only in patients who have a family history of PACG, those requiring frequent dilation, and those who cannot be reviewed regularly.

Functional evaluation of laser iridotomy in early PAC eyes showed a significant reduction in the pupillary block component of IOP response to provocative testing, possibly decreasing IOP fluctuations over time. Patients will, however, live for 30+ years and may develop PAC with ocular hypertension. Therefore, early identification and iridotomy is essential.

Following are the indications for Nd-YAG laser iridotomy with an Abraham lens (Fig. 9.11):

- All cases of PAC. PACS with risk factors:
  - Family history of PACG.
  - Frequent dilation required, as in retinal pathologies, for example, diabetic retinopathy.
  - Positive provocative tests: Dark room or mydriatic.
  - Difficult to follow up or poor access to laser: Patients coming from rural areas with limited socio-economic resources.
- Fellow eyes of patients having PAC/PACG: An untreated fellow eye of acute PACG has a 40 to 50%

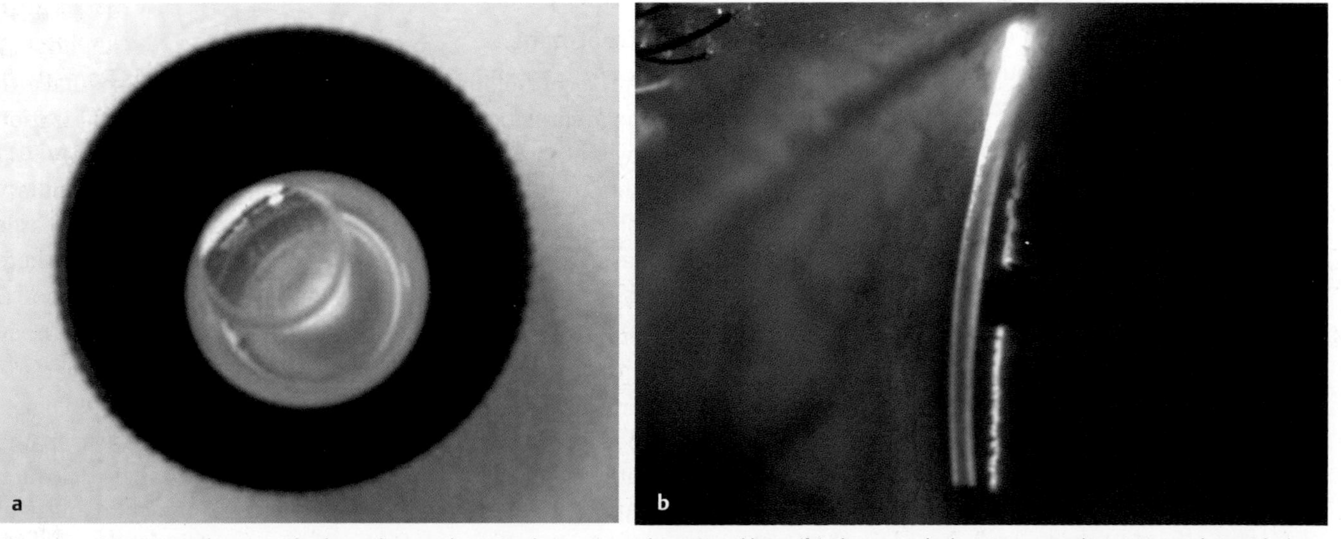

Fig. 9.11 **(a)** Picture showing Abrahams lens with +66D planoconvex decentered lens. **(b)** Photograph showing a good position and size of a laser iridotomy.

chance of developing an acute attack over a period of 5 to 10 years. Performing laser iridotomy in these eyes decreases such a risk.

- Patients requiring systemic medication which may provoke pupillary block (nebulized bronchodilators like ipratropium bromide, salbutamol, selective serotonin reuptake inhibitors, tricyclic antidepressants, proprietary cold and flu medicines, muscle relaxants, topiramate, and other agents with parasympatholytic and sympathomimetic action).

Goals of Treatment

- Prevent the angle-closure process by modifying anterior segment configurations that damage trabecular meshwork.
- Prevent IOP fluctuations which could damage the optic nerve.

Laaser peripheral iridotomy (LPI) is a relatively innocuous procedure when done with accurate focus of an Nd–YAG laser, and could be used prophylactically for PACS. Some eyes, especially where iris crypts are not seen, may require more than one session at weekly intervals. PAC/PACG patients may exhibit a rise in IOP and require IOP-lowering agents after laser iridotomy.

Continued observation for progression even after a successful laser iridotomy is always warranted as some existing trabecular damage is later compounded by age-related changes at the trabecular meshwork.

Plateau Iris Syndrome

The peripheral iris is forced into the angle by anterior rotation of the ciliary body or anteriorly positioned ciliary processes. Therefore, angle-closure attacks may be precipitated after dilatation of pupil even in the presence of patent iridotomy. Plateau iris syndrome is also first treated with an iridotomy first, and may be followed up, if required, with peripheral iridoplasty. Iridoplasty leads to significant pigment release and needs periodic review. Low dose miotics may be tried.

Exaggerated Lens Vault

Such eyes can also undergo an iridotomy first, and only if extensive ITC persists, a lens extraction may be considered.

Long-Term Follow-up

Patients with PACS who have not had an iridotomy should be counseled that they are at risk for an acute angle-closure crisis. They should be educated regarding the symptoms of an acute attack and instructed to seek ophthalmic care immediately. Such patients should be aware that anti allergic and cold medications could induce angle closure.

Follow-up intervals depend on severity of glaucomatous neuropathy and appropriate IOP control. All PACS/PAC patients should be explained the need for periodic follow-up.

Secondary Angle Closure

Common Reasons for Secondary Angle Closure

Primary angle closure tends to be bilateral, so that angle closure in one eye and a wide-open angle in the fellow eye suggests a diagnosis other than PAC. In secondary angle closure iris and pupil abnormalities, an irregularly shallow anterior chamber, other ocular pathology, IOP chronically >21 mm Hg, and optic nerve head features compatible with glaucoma are common. Clinical features will also depend on whether the angle closure is due to or without pupillary block.

Secondary angle closure with pupillary block may be due to the following reasons:

- Inflammatory causes of angle closure, occlusion/seclusion pupillae causing iris bombé.
- Lens-induced angle closure—phacomorphic, subluxated, and microspherophakia.
- Associated with intraocular lenses—pseudophakic, phakic, or dislocated lenses.

Secondary angle closure without pupillary block may be due to iris being pulled up to the trabecular meshwork, for example, neovascular glaucoma and ICE syndromes, or due to a pathology pushing from behind, for example, ciliochoroidal effusion caused by systemic medications such as topiramate, sulfonamides, phenothiazines, or aqueous misdirection syndrome.

Treatment

After controlling IOP, the causative mechanisms have to be identified and treated, for example, neovascularization by anti-vascular endothelial growth factor (anti-VEGF) therapy, discontinuation of topiramate, etc. Any papillary block element will need to be resolved by multiple large laser iridotomies or even a surgical iridectomy if there is decreased corneal clarity or no space between the iris and cornea.

The early diagnosis of a shallow anterior chamber and angle closure is frequently overlooked, as ophthalmologists become concerned about a glaucomatous optic neuropathy or the disease causing a secondary angle closure. Appropriate therapy initiated before significant damage to the trabecular meshwork occurs can prevent a rise in IOP, optic neuropathy and irreversible visual loss.

Cases

Case 1

A 40-year-old lady from a village had lost one eye due to trauma from a buffalo's tail. On examination of the good eye, she had a shallow anterior chamber, van Herick grade 1, with a normal iris pattern and pupillary reaction. Fundus examination was normal. Gonioscopy revealed a narrow angle recess of <10 degrees, which could be opened to show the posterior trabecular meshwork, without any pigmentation or PAS (**Case 1-1**).

Points to consider

- This is the patient's only seeing eye.
- There is a very narrow and occludable angle.
- The lady has poor access to eye care.

Diagnosis and Management

An Nd-YAG iridotomy was done, and 1 week later the angle was seen to have opened to around 20 degrees during repeat gonioscopy. After 2 weeks, a diurnal phasing was within normal limits, 14 to 18 mm Hg. In the absence of any other risk factors, she was advised to review at 6 months, and then annually.

Case 2

A 40-year-old lady was diagnosed to have possible glaucoma during a routine evaluation. On examination, there was an extremely shallow anterior chamber, van Herick grade 1, and iridocorneal touch could be seen. Her IOP was 12 mm Hg and the optic nerve head was within normal limits. Gonioscopy showed a very narrow recess with iridocorneal apposition (**Case 2-1**).

Points to consider

- Extremely narrow angle recess.
- There is definitive evidence of iridocorneal apposition.
- She is a young individual with a long life ahead.

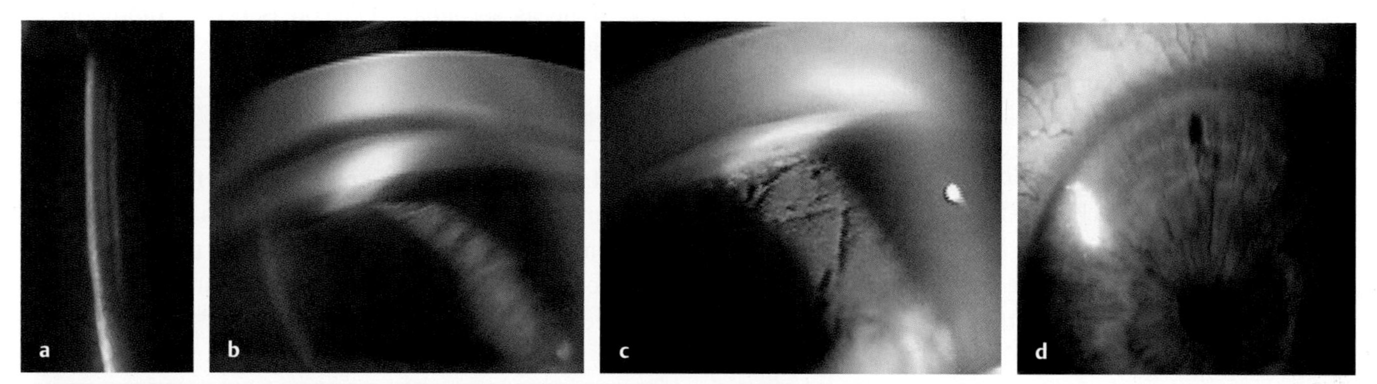

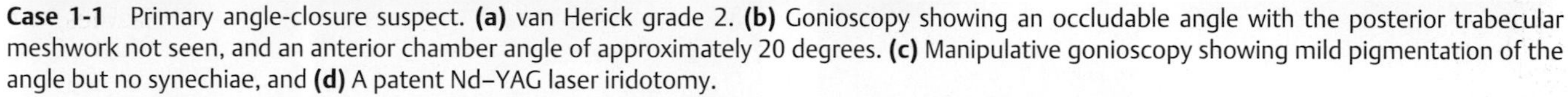

Case 1-1 Primary angle-closure suspect. **(a)** van Herick grade 2. **(b)** Gonioscopy showing an occludable angle with the posterior trabecular meshwork not seen, and an anterior chamber angle of approximately 20 degrees. **(c)** Manipulative gonioscopy showing mild pigmentation of the angle but no synechiae, and **(d)** A patent Nd–YAG laser iridotomy.

Case 2-1 **(a)** van Herick grade 1. **(b)** van Herick plus test showing peripheral iridocorneal apposition.

Diagnosis and Management

The lady was not keen on a laser, so a DRPPT was done, during which her IOP rose to 24 mm Hg. On counseling, she understood the cause of the rise in IOP and agreed to bilateral iridotomy. After 10 years, no rise in IOP or neuropathy occurred.

Case 3

A 36-year-old lady with a history of recurrent redness and pain in both eyes, diagnosed to have anterior uveitis, was found to have an IOP of 26 mm Hg in the left eye. On examination the left eye had an irregular anterior chamber, shallow in the periphery and deep centrally, with posterior synechiae involving almost 360 degrees of the pupil, and iris bombe. A complicated cataract and a hazily seen cup:disc ratio of 0.4 were noted. Angle structures could not be visualized on gonioscopy due to the highly convex iris (**Case 3-1**).

Points to consider

- Is it only a narrow angle recess or are there synechiae?
- Is it secondary angle closure?
- Is it a steroid response?

Diagnosis and Management

Two large, midperipheral iridotomies were done, after which the iris fell back. On gonioscopy a week after iridotomy, there were only a few pigments on the trabecular meshwork, while the IOP reduced to 20 mm Hg with timolol. Perimetry was within normal limits.

A diagnosis of secondary angle closure was made, and the IOP was 12 mm Hg, off therapy 3 months later. Keeping in mind the possibility of further uveitic attacks blocking the iridotomy or causing further trabecular meshwork damage, a regular review of IOP was advised.

Case 4

An 18-year-old highly myopic girl underwent an implantable collamer lens (ICL) in the left eye, following which she had persistent blurring of vision and redness. On examination there was mild corneal edema, anterior chamber was very shallow, and there was no visible iridotomy. IOP was 24 mm Hg (**Case 4-1**).

Points to consider

- Pseudophacomorphic glaucoma may be caused by pupillary block or pigment dispersion.
- anterior chamber depth should be evaluated and gonioscopy done in the fellow eye to determine preoperative shallow anterior chamber.
- Glaucoma evaluation of the fellow eye should be done as secondary glaucomas occur commonly in eyes predisposed to glaucoma.

Diagnosis and Management

The ICL did not have a hole present, therefore, an Nd-YAG iridotomy was performed in two sittings under cover of glaucoma medications. One month later, the IOP without any medication was 14 mm Hg, and the anterior chamber had deepened.

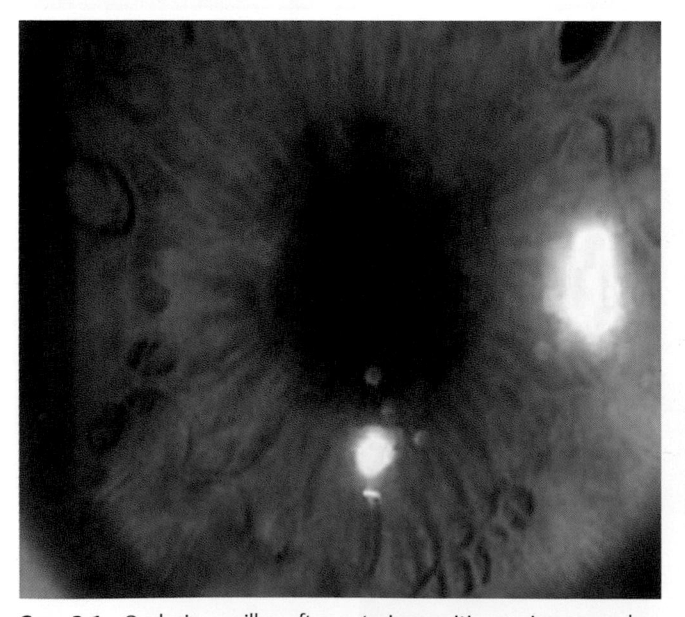

Case 3-1 Occlusio pupillae after anterior uveitis causing secondary angle closure, relieved by an early, large laser iridotomy.

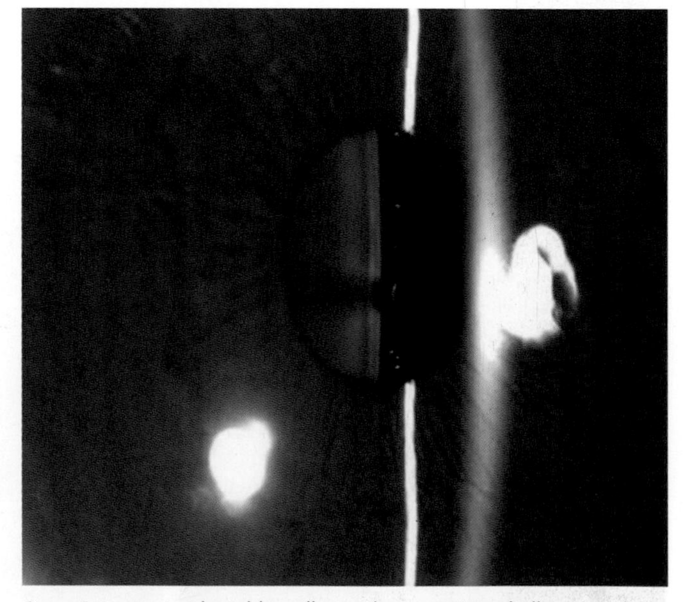

Case 4-1 An implantable collamer lens causing shallowing of the anterior chamber and peripheral iridocorneal apposition.

Case 5

A 46-year-old male presented after noticing a gradual diminution of vision in his right eye for 4 to 5 years. On examination, the right eye had a shallow anterior chamber, an ectopic pupil, iris stromal atrophy, and polycoria. Gonioscopy showed extensive iridocorneal adhesions more temporally. No pigment release was seen. The left eye was normal. Cup:disc ratio was 0.8 OD and 0.3 OS (**Case 5-1**).

Points to consider

- Unilateral iris atrophy.
- Extensive angle closure with no pigmentation.
- Mild corneal edema.

Diagnosis and Management

Specular microscopy revealed ICE cells and pleomorphic dark endothelial, with a highlighted center and light intercellular borders. A diagnosis of iridocorneal endothelial syndrome was made, even though it rarely affects male. Topical medications reduced the IOP to only 26 mm Hg and a trabeculectomy was done. The patient is being reviewed for corneal and glaucoma status.

Case 6

A 50-year-old female was referred to the glaucoma clinic as an angle-closure suspect. Her IOP was: OD: 20 mm Hg, OS: 20 mm Hg. The anterior chamber was van Herick grade 3 and gonioscopy showed an occludable angle with pigmentation anterior to Schwalbe's line and after manipulation goniosynechiae to posterior trabecular meshwork **(Case 6-1)**. There was no family history of glaucoma. The optic nerve head showed a cup:disc ratio of 0.5 and 0.6 with healthy neuroretinal rim. Diurnal IOP showed pressure ranging from 18 to 26 mm Hg.

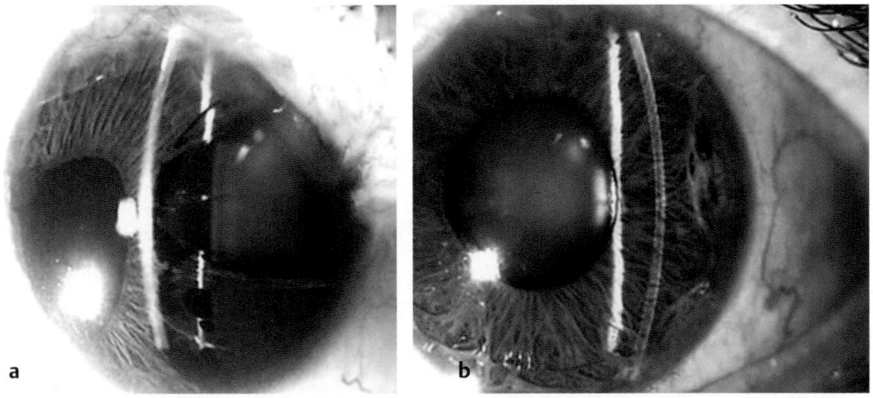

Case 5-1 **(a)** Shallow anterior chamber with ectopic pupil and multiple holes. **(b)** Left eye with normal appearance.

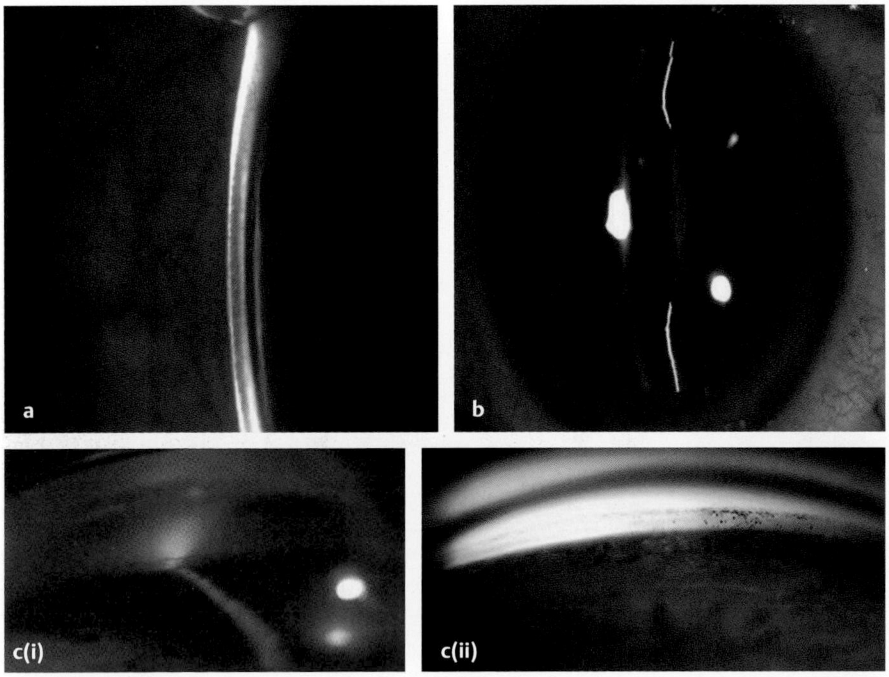

Case 6-1 **(a)** van Herick grade 3. **(b)** Shallow anterior chamber with a steep iris configuration. **(c)** Occludable angles with ≥90 degrees of iridotrabecular contact (ITC) in dark room and visualization of goniosynechiae on posterior trabecular meshwork as the illumination is increased by widening of slit beam allowing llight to touch the pupil and flatten the iris.

Points to consider

- Definite ITC was seen.
- IOP is higher than average.
- cup:disc ratio is suspicious of glaucoma.

Diagnosis and Management

A diagnosis of PAC was made and laser iridotomy was performed on both eyes. At 4 weeks a diurnal phasing showed IOP ranging from 16 to 20 mm Hg. Perimetry was within normal limits. Optic nerve head imaging was done with optical coherence tomography for retinal nerve fiber layer and ganglion cell complex. Patient was advised a review every 6 months.

Suggested Readings

Emanuel ME, Parrish RK II, Gedde SJ. Evidence-based management of primary angle closure glaucoma. Curr Opin Ophthalmol 2014;25(2):89–92

Foster PJ, Buhrmann R, Quigley HA, Johnson GJ. The definition and classification of glaucoma in prevalence surveys. Br J Ophthalmol 2002;86(2):238–242

Jindal A, Ctori I, Virgili G, Lucenteforte E, Lawrenson JG. Non-contact methods for the detection of people at risk of primary angle closure glaucoma. Cochrane Database Syst Rev 2018;(2):CD012947

Nolan WP, Foster PJ, Devereux JG, Uranchimeg D, Johnson GJ, Baasanhu J. YAG laser iridotomy treatment for primary angle closure in east Asian eyes. Br J Ophthalmol 2000;84(11):1255–1259

Preferred Practice patterns 2016 by the American Academy of Ophthalmology. www.aao.org

Ritch R. Plateau iris is caused by abnormally positioned ciliary processes. J Glaucoma 1992;1:23–26

Radhakrishnan S, Chen PP, Junk AK, Nouri-Mahdavi K, Chen TC. Laser peripheral iridotomy in primary angle closure: a report by the American Academy of Ophthalmology. Ophthalmology 2018;125(7):1110–1120

Sihota R, Rishi K, Srinivasan G, Gupta V, Dada T, Singh K. Functional evaluation of an iridotomy in primary angle closure eyes. Graefes Arch Clin Exp Ophthalmol 2016;254(6):1141–1149

Thomas R, George R, Parikh R, Muliyil J, Jacob A. Five year risk of progression of primary angle closure suspects to primary angle closure: a population based study. Br J Ophthalmol 2003;87(4):450–454

Van Herick W, Shaffer RN, Schwartz A. Estimation of width of angle of anterior chamber. Incidence and significance of the narrow angle. Am J Ophthalmol 1969;68(4):626–629

Weinreb RN, Friedman DS, eds. Angle Closure and Angle Closure Glaucoma: Reports and Consensus Statements of the 3rd Global AIGS Consensus Meeting on Angle Closure Glaucoma. The Netherlands: Kugler Publications; 2006

Wilensky JT, Kaufman PL, Frohlichstein D, et al. Follow-up of angle-closure glaucoma suspects. Am J Ophthalmol 1993;115(3):338–346

CHAPTER 10

Primary Open-Angle Glaucoma

Overview

- Pathophysiology of Glaucomatous Neuropathy
  - Pressure Dependent or Mechanical Factors
  - Vascular Perfusion Factors
  - Neurodegeneration
  - Cerebral Spinal Fluid Hydrodynamics
  - Genetics
- Pathophysiology of Raised Intraocular Pressure
- Predisposing and Risk Factors for Developing Primary Open-Angle Glaucoma
  - History
  - Clinical Features
  - Perimetry
- Clinical Features
  - Presenting Symptoms
- Investigations
  - Gonioscopy
  - Perimetry and Imaging
  - Pachymetry
- Normal Tension Glaucoma
- Management in Primary Open-Angle Glaucoma
  - Setting a Target Intraocular Pressure
  - Medical Management
  - Trabeculoplasty
  - Surgery
- Follow-up
- Prognosis
- Cases
- Suggested Readings

Introduction

Primary open-angle glaucoma (POAG) is a chronic, progressive, multifactorial optic neuropathy with characteristic optic nerve head and visual field loss in an eye with an open angle, in the absence of other ocular disease or congenital anomalies. A raised intraocular pressure (IOP) is the major risk factor. Normal tension glaucoma (NTG), a variant of POAG, is diagnosed when the features of POAG are seen, but the IOP is constantly below 21 mm Hg. NTG is a diagnosis of exclusion, after investigating for other causes of optic neuropathy such as ischemia and central nervous system (CNS) pathologies.

Pathophysiology of Glaucomatous Neuropathy

There are many suggested hypotheses for the onset of POAG, for example, genetic, trophic factor withdrawal, altered axon transport, vascular perfusion deficiency, reactive oxygen species, and excitotoxicity by glutamate among many others as depicted in **Fig. 10.1.**

Pressure Dependent or Mechanical Factors

A significant mechanical effect on the optic nerve head by an increased IOP that is not commensurate with the structure and function of the ON could lead *to changes in axoplasmic flow, blood flow, as well as compression and backward bowing of the lamina cribrosa*. Elevated IOP may also damage retinal ganglion cell (RGC) axons, which are unmyelinated and therefore more vulnerable, especially at their exit through the lamina cribrosa. Retrograde and anterograde neuronal transport in glaucomatous eyes can be disturbed or even interrupted by increased IOP.

Vascular Perfusion Factors

Ocular perfusion pressure is the difference between systolic ophthalmic artery pressure and IOP. It can therefore be seen that alterations in either, due to abnormal autoregulation, systemic hypotension, microvasculopathies, etc., could result in reduced perfusion to the optic nerve head.

Neurodegeneration

Any deficit of retrograde transport of brain-derived neurotrophic factor (BDNF) from superior colliculus to

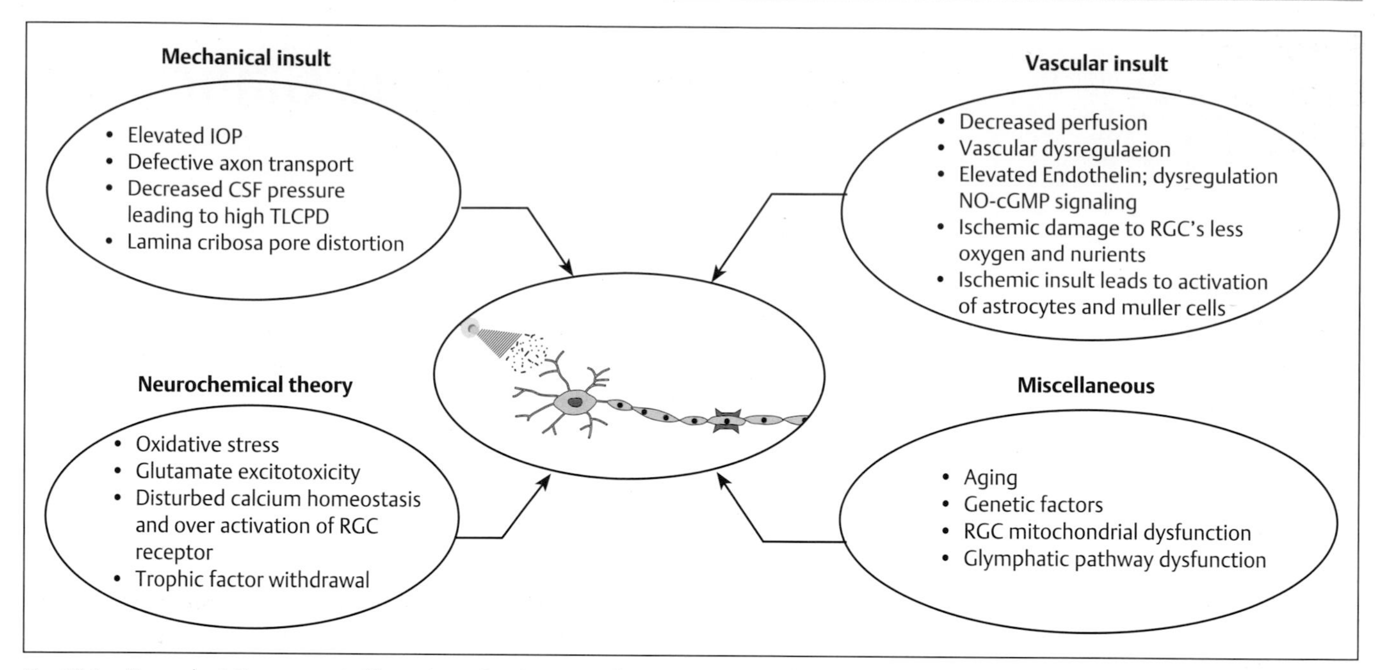

Fig. 10.1 Figure depicting suggested hypotheses for the onset of primary open-angle glaucoma. CSF, cerebrospinal fluid; IOP; intraocular pressure; NO-cGMP, nitric oxide-cyclic guanosine-3′,5′-monophosphate; RGC, retinal ganglion cell; TLCPD, trans-lamina cribrosa pressure difference.

RGCs, results in retrograde neuronal degeneration and the onset of apoptosis. RGCs may also be damaged by glutamate release, which interacts with cell receptors and leads to an increase in intracellular calcium levels, cell death, and further release of glutamate, in a vicious cycle.

Cerebral Spinal Fluid Hydrodynamics

A lower intracranial pressure leads to an imbalance in translaminar pressure, causing a shearing force at the lamina cribrosa, that leads to neuronal and microvascular changes. An elevated CSF pressure could also result in RGC damage as metabolic toxic substances may accumulate in axons at the lamina cribrosa.

Genetics

Many genes have been reported to contribute to POAG, and many more will probably be found in due time. Known genes are seen in only about 5% of POAG patients, with some being MYOC, WDR36, OPTN, TBK1, NTF4, ASB10, EFEMP1, and IL20RB. Genome-wide association studies have found many contributory loci, MYOC, WDR36, OPTN, TBK1, NTF4, ASB10, EFEMP1, and IL20RB, specifically affecting structural elements of the eye, transforming growth factor-β (TGF-β) pathway, and IOP. It is more prevalent in families, with *first-degree relatives having a nine times increased risk.* Early onset may be associated with a MYOC mutation, while later onset is associated with polymorphisms in different genes. *Genetic analysis in a POAG patient is probably only of use to family members if an index patient has severe POAG at a younger age, or there is an autosomal-dominant pedigree.* A specific mutation, if identified, can help in early diagnosis of POAG in individuals at risk, and therefore help in controlling progression.

Pathophysiology of Raised Intraocular Pressure

The trabecular meshwork in POAG shows age-related changes, together with a significant increase in sheath-derived plaques, which are thought to be thickened sheaths of elastic fibers. These plaques form due to the adherence of fine fibrils and other extracellular matrix (ECM) components to the elastic fibers at the endothelium. There is also a greater loss of trabecular meshwork endothelial cells, allowing fusion of trabecular beams, and narrowing of spaces available for aqueous outflow. In addition, a number of studies have shown that fibrous granular material deposition contributed to increasing outflow system resistance in eyes with glaucoma.

Mutations in TMCO1 have been associated with IOP in POAG, and are possibly predictors of progression from ocular hypertension to POAG.

Predisposing and Risk Factors for Developing Primary Open-Angle Glaucoma

History

- Family history: Siblings are affected more often than children.
- Older age.
- Steroid use.
- Reduction in perfusion pressure: Systemic hypotension, nocturnal hypotension, sleep apnea.
- Thyroid disorders.

Clinical Features

- Thin corneas.
- Large optic disc diameter.
- Pseudoexfoliation.
- Myopia.

Perimetry

- Increased pattern standard deviation on perimetry.

Clinical Features

Patients generally have no symptoms, and the glaucomatous optic neuropathy or raised IOP is detected on routine review for presbyopic or refractive evaluation. A family history of glaucoma in parents, grandparents, or siblings should be asked for. A systemic history is important as there are many possible risk factors for progression of POAG, especially vascular pathologies such as cerebrovascular accidents—transient ischemic attack (TIA), stroke, systemic hypotension, excessive or nocturnal antihypertensive therapy.

Presenting Symptoms

As the central vision is affected last, most patients only notice visual loss when glaucoma is very advanced, and patients then *complain of bumping into objects*, or have difficulty negotiating stairs. POAG patients also have *delayed dark/light adaptation, loss of contrast, and often complain of glare.* Some perceptive patients may notice an inferior scotoma. It has been suggested that POAG patients need more frequent changes in presbyopic correction as compared to normal individuals.

Clinical examination reveals a normal depth of the anterior chamber, with a sluggish pupillary reaction or relative afferent pupillary defect (RAPD) in eyes with more advanced POAG. The presence of pseudoexfoliative material at the pupil or on the lens is important as this makes therapy difficult and progression frequent.

The optic nerve head in early POAG would show a *thinning of the inferior neuroretinal rim*, going against the ISNT rule, which states that most eyes have a graded neuroretinal rim thickness with thickest being Inferior→Superior→Nasal →Temporal. There may also be an irregular neuroretinal rim, focal notching, and disc hemorrhages, generally asymmetric, affecting one eye more than the other. This asymmetry or any glaucomatous abnormality is noticed when both ONHs are evaluated carefully (**Figs. 10.2** and **10.3**). Moderate and severe neuropathy would present as neuroretinal rim thinning at both poles associated with retinal nerve fiber layer loss (**Figs. 10.4** and **10.5**). Peripapillary atrophy in the area of the neuroretinal rim loss is a feature of POAG, with a prominent beta-zone peripapillary atrophy, hypopigmented crescentic area at the disc margin, with retinal pigment epithelium atrophy and visibility of large choroidal vessels and sclera (**Fig. 10.6**). Baring of circumlinear vessels is considered to be a sign of acquired loss of the neuroretinal rim, highly sensitive and specific in the diagnosis of glaucoma (**Figs. 10.7** and **10.8**). Optic disc hemorrhages are splinter shaped when present over the neuroretinal rim, but may be more rounded when present within the cup, preceding visual field loss by months or years (**Fig. 10.9**).

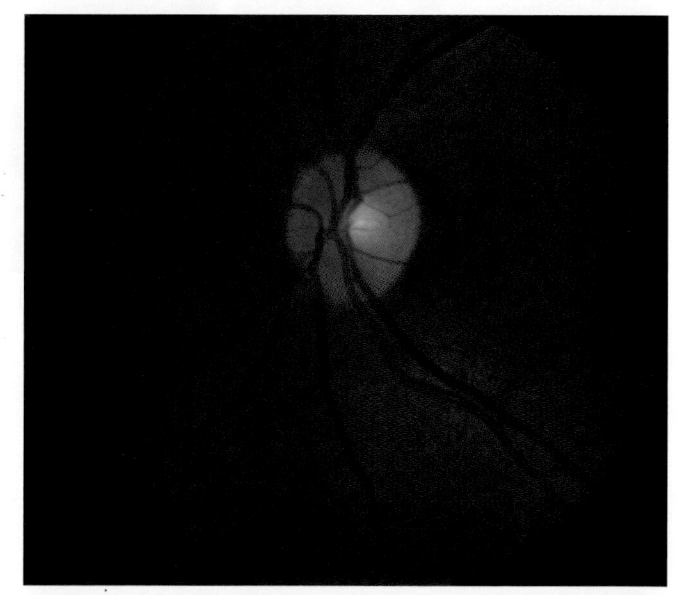

Fig. 10.2 A normal optic nerve head of average size, cup:disc ratio of 0.3:1, where the inferior neuroretinal rim is the broadest followed by superior, nasal, and temporal, the inferior, superior, nasal, temporal (ISNT) rule.

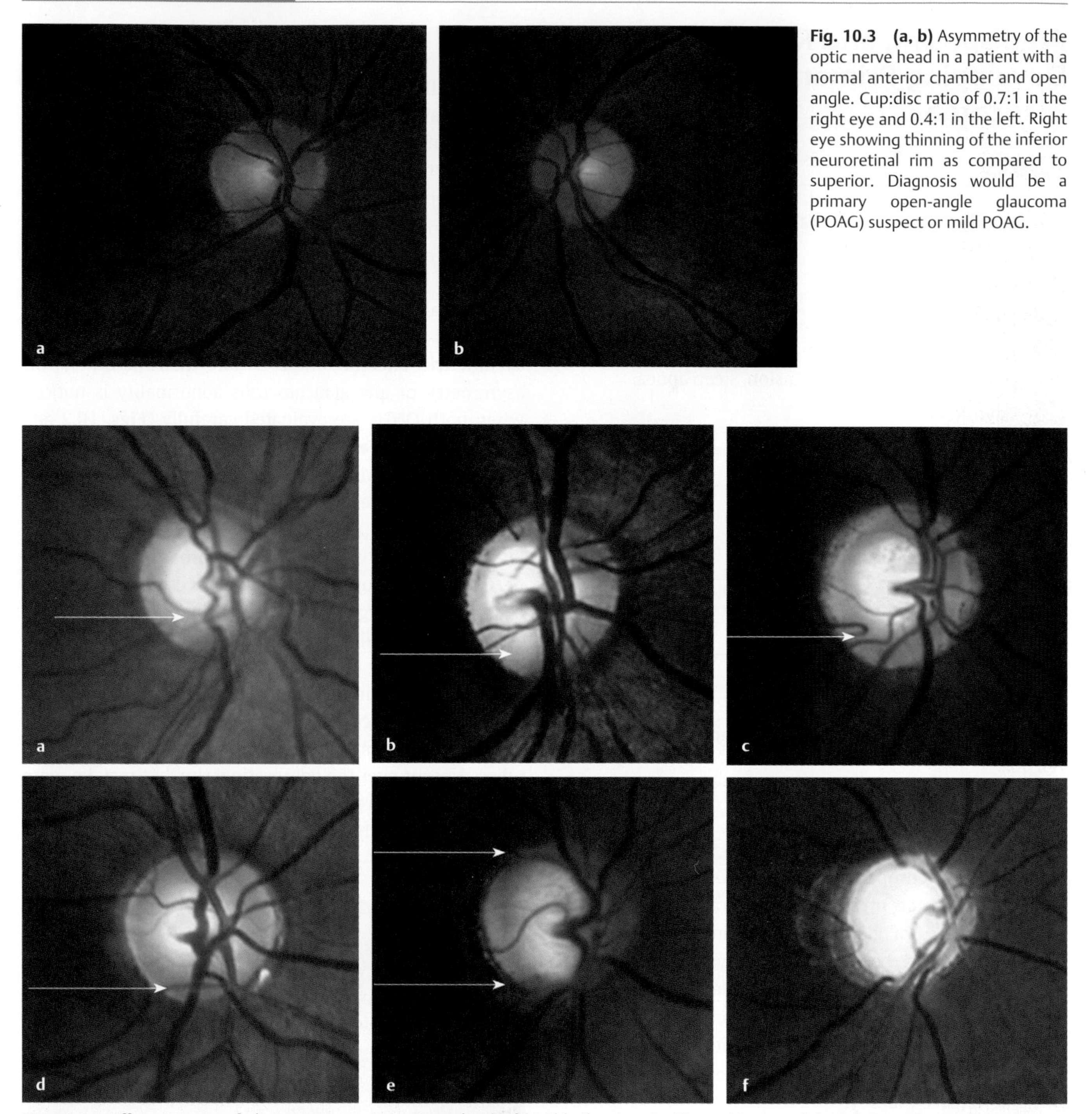

Fig. 10.3 **(a, b)** Asymmetry of the optic nerve head in a patient with a normal anterior chamber and open angle. Cup:disc ratio of 0.7:1 in the right eye and 0.4:1 in the left. Right eye showing thinning of the inferior neuroretinal rim as compared to superior. Diagnosis would be a primary open-angle glaucoma (POAG) suspect or mild POAG.

Fig. 10.4 Different stages of glaucomatous optic neuropathy. **(a, b)** Mild—showing significant thinning of the inferior pole. **(c, d)** Moderate—showing thinning of both poles. **(e, f)** Severe glaucomatous optic neuropathy (GON)—with pallor and extensive loss of neuroretinal rim. Edge of the cup marked by *arrows*.

Applanation tonometry may show an initial IOP of 16 to 21 mm Hg, and on diurnal phasing up to 24 to 28 mm Hg is commonly recorded. Tonometry needs to be repeated at least two to three times, ideally at different times of the day before a baseline IOP can be ascertained. *Diurnal phasing done every 3 to 4 hours provides more data relevant to future management, e.g., the highest IOP requiring treatment, the time of peak rise in IOP, and the range of IOP fluctuations.* A tonometry done as early as possible, around 7 am and one at 7 pm, would provide more information than recordings during office hours, as the peaks are generally toward the night or early morning.

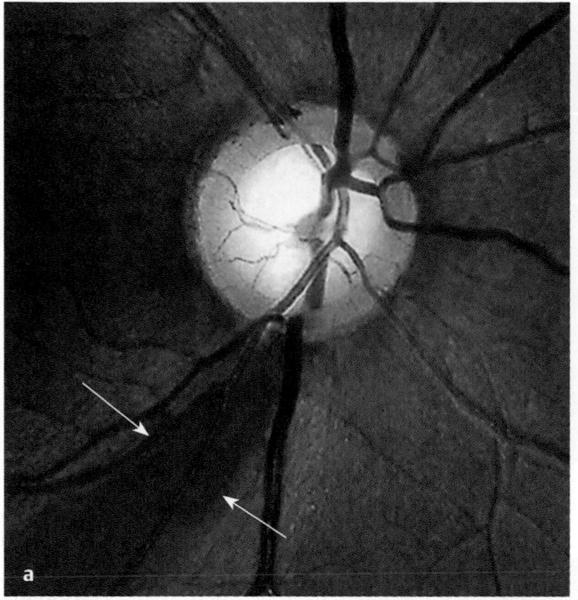

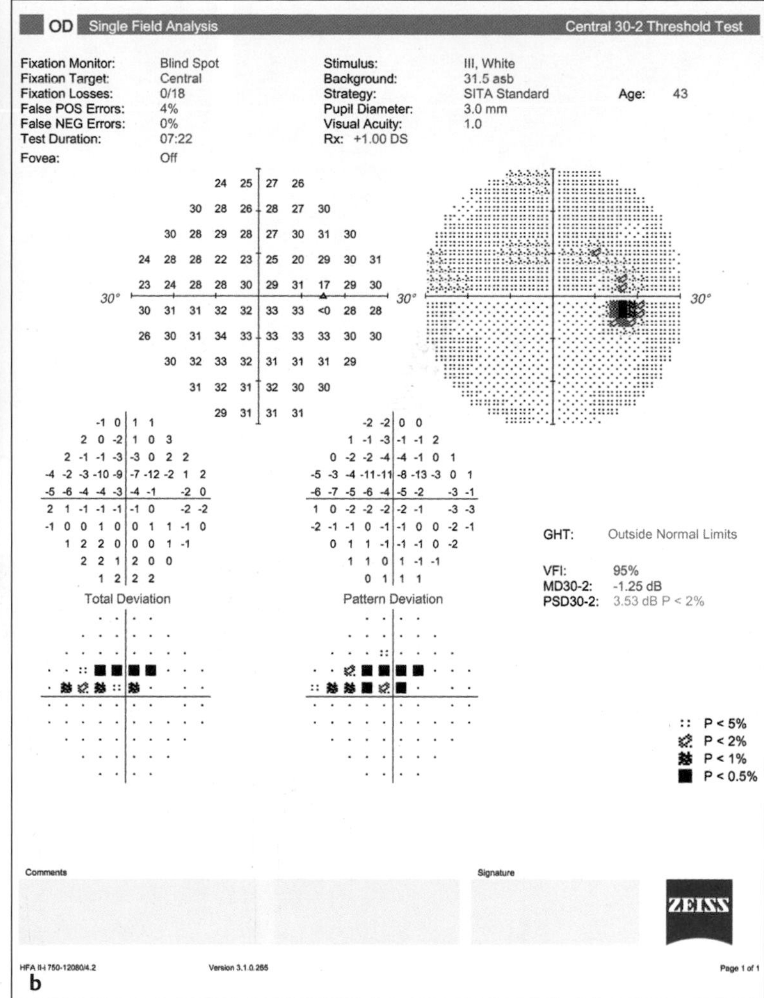

Fig. 10.5 (a, b) *White arrows* showing retinal nerve fiber layer defect and corresponding visual field defect seen on Humphrey field analyzer (HFA).

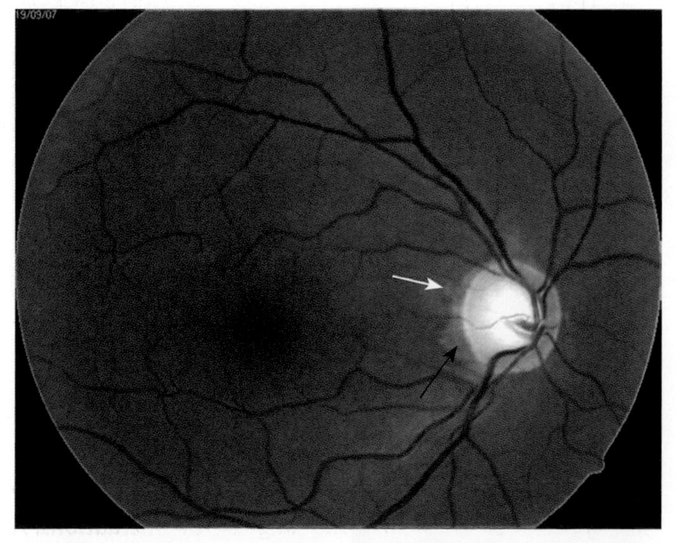

Fig. 10.6 Peripapillary atrophy seen as alpha zone, with irregular hyperpimentation and hypopigmention (*white arrow*). The hypopigmented beta zone, adjacent to the disc margin showing sclera and large choroidal vessels (*black arrow*), corresponds to areas of neuroretinal rim loss, 7 to 12 o'clock.

Investigations

Gonioscopy

In POAG gonioscopy shows an open angle with a recess wider than 20 degrees and rarely there may be some iris processes seen. Iris processes are identified by the fact that they arise from the iris and follow the contour of the angle, unlike peripheral anterior synechiae that tent up from the peripheral iris and cross the angle (**Fig. 10.10**; also refer to **Fig. 3.3a**). There may be mild pigmentation of the trabecular meshwork seen in the inferior angle of older Indians.

Perimetry and Imaging

Perimetry determines the extent of functional visual field loss, which with imaging of the optic nerve head and retina, is the main criterion for determining target IOP, prognosis, and further management.

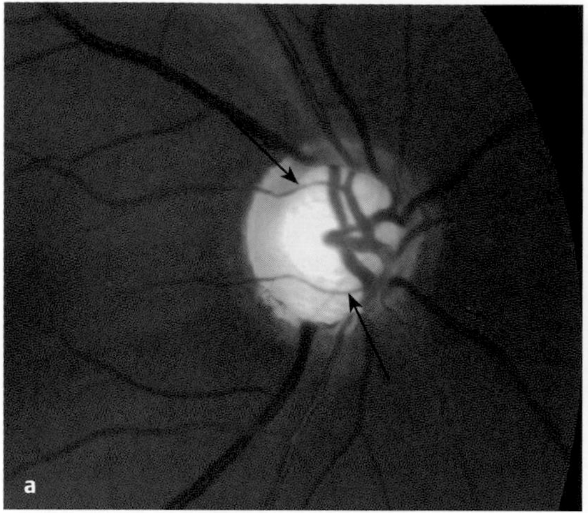

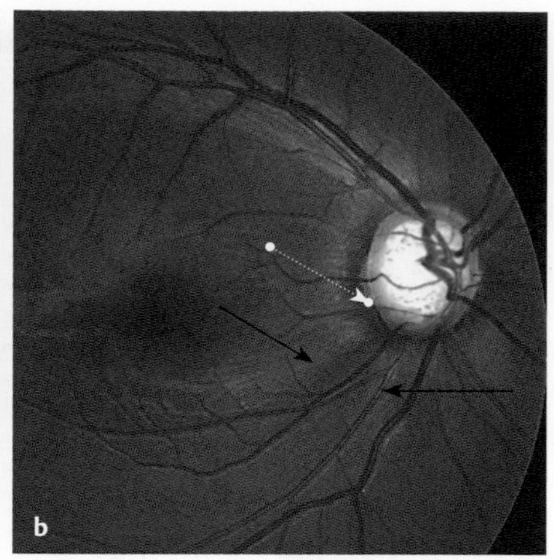

Fig. 10.7 **(a)** Baring of both circumlinear vessels (*black arrows*), with pallor and thinning of the inferior neuroretinal rim. Alpha-zone peripapillary atrophy is from 6 to 10 o'clock and beta zone from 6 to 8 o'clock. Beta zone corresponds to the area of neuroretinal rim loss. **(b)** Inferotemporal notch, having no neuroretinal rim (*dotted arrow*), with corresponding retinal nerve fiber layer defect (*black arrows*). In addition to baring of both circumlinear vessels, nasalization of the larger vessels and laminar dot sign are seen.

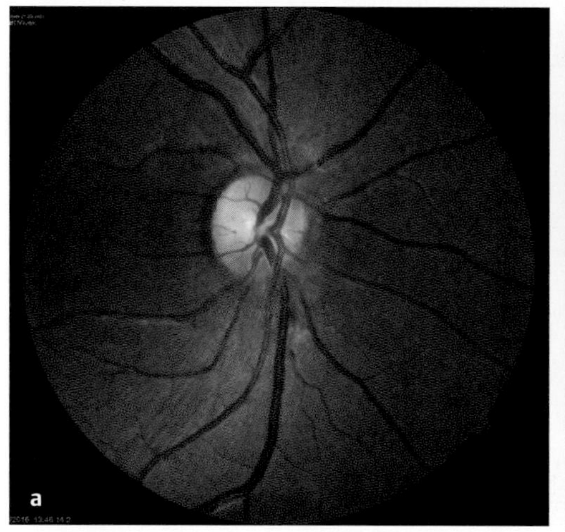

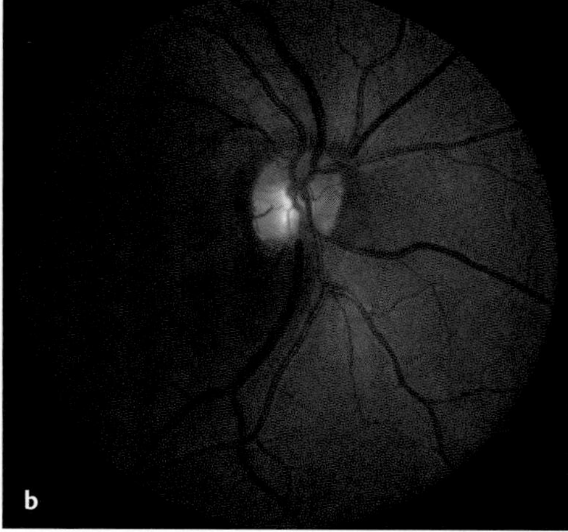

Fig. 10.8 **(a)** A small optic nerve head showing a smaller cup:disc ratio of 0.2:1. **(b)** In such eyes even a 0.5 cup:disc ratio becomes significant, having neuroretinal rim thinning with associated baring of the circumlinear vessel and a retinal nerve fiber layer defect.

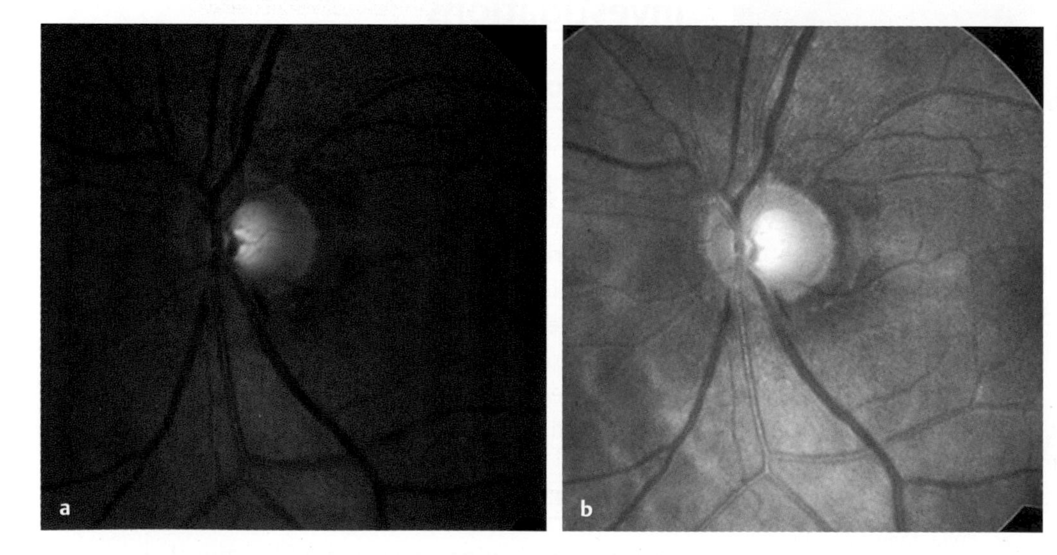

Fig. 10.9 **(a, b)** Splinter optic disc hemorrhage on color and red-free photographs.

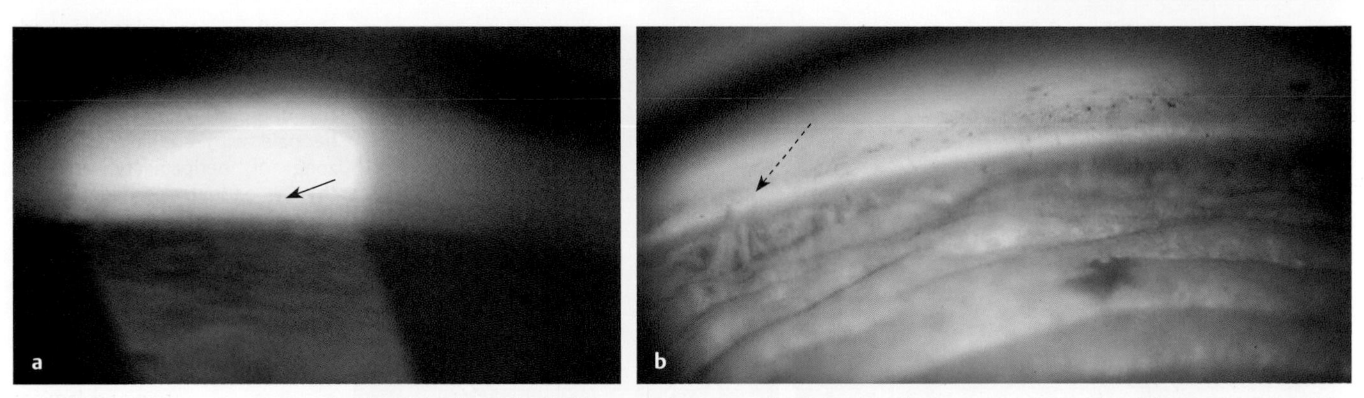

Fig. 10.10 **(a)** Primary open-angle glaucoma (POAG): 40-degree angle recess, showing all angle structures, but with mild pigmentation of the posterior trabecular meshwork. The *black arrow* is on Schwalbe's line, which appears white because it is elevated and pigment does not lodge on it. **(b)** POAG: Wide open angle with few iris processes that follow the contour of the angle (*dotted arrow*).

Pachymetry

The average normal corneal thickness in Indians is around 525 µm. There are no accepted nomograms for conversion of the IOP recorded based on pachymetry. An approximate correction of 0.7 mm Hg for each increase or decrease of pachymetry by 10 µm may be applied. Patients diagnosed with NTG may have a thinner cornea leading to a mistaken recording of lower IOPs. On the other hand, a thicker cornea leads to a recording of higher IOP, and may lead to unnecessary treatment, especially in ocular hypertension. A baseline measurement of central corneal thickness (CCT) is important because *if it is thinner than normal, it provides a possible biomarker for progression from ocular hypertension to glaucoma, and also for a greater predisposition to progression in POAG.*

Normal Tension Glaucoma

It is diagnosed in the presence of an open angle, glaucomatous neuropathy and corresponding visual field loss as in POAG, but occurring at the normal range of IOP, generally less than 21 mm Hg when measured at any time of the day. Therefore, IOP-independent factors, *decreased optic nerve head perfusion, low CSF pressure, lamina cribrosa abnormalities, and predisposition to apoptosis*, are thought to be the cause of optic neuropathy. The perfusion abnormalities are often sustained nocturnal dips in blood pressure (BP), or associated vasospastic disorders or endothelial dysfunction. Reduced blood flow velocity in the retrobulbar and cerebral vessels has been found. Cerebral microinfarcts may be seen. Mutations of optineurin, myocillin, and optic atrophy type 1 genes have been seen. It is therefore thought to be the result of poor optic nerve head perfusion, probably caused by vascular dysregulation in the eye or an optic nerve head more susceptible to damage at low IOPs (**Figs. 10.11** and **10.12**).

NTG patients have associated primary vascular dysfunction, or vasospastic diseases such as migraine, Raynaud's phenomenon, obstructive sleep apnea, etc. The optic nerve head is generally larger, with beta-zone peripapillary atrophy, and is more likely to have splinter disc hemorrhages. Visual field defects in NTG have been reported to be denser and closer to fixation. *The Collaborative Normal Tension Glaucoma Study (CNTGS) has shown a 50% reduction in progression with a reduction in IOP of 30%* (**Flowchart 10.1**).

NTG should be a diagnosis by exclusion, especially looking out for:

- "Burnt-out" glaucomas, such as a past steroid response or resolved post-traumatic or uveitic IOP rise.
- Ischemic optic neuropathy.
- Optic pathway compression—pituitary adenomas, meningiomas, aneurysms, arachnoiditis.
- optic nerve head dysplasia—optic nerve head pits, colobomas.

Management in Primary Open-Angle Glaucoma

The decision to start therapy is taken after glaucomatous neuropathy, with a corresponding visual field loss, is definitively recorded, and baseline IOP rechecked at least twice, at different times of the day. A target IOP is set based upon the optic nerve head and visual field loss, with mild glaucomatous neuropathy requiring 15 to 17 mm Hg, moderate loss 12 to 15 mm Hg, and severe neuropathy 10 to 12 mm Hg.

Risk factors for progression also need to be kept in mind, for example, older age causes an increasing probability of progression by about 30% every 5 to 10 years. The presence of pseudoexfoliation, thinner cornea, and disc hemorrhages

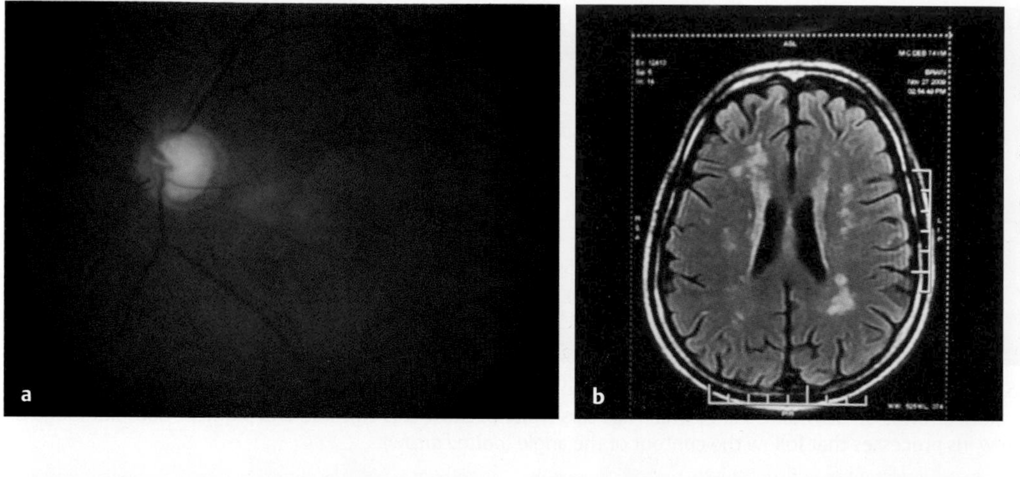

Fig. 10.11 **(a)** Normal tension glaucoma: In the presence of generalized chorioretinal atrophy, the neuroretinal rim is seen to be pale with an extensive beta zone of peripapillary atrophy. **(b)** The patient also had areas of cortical microinfarcts on magnetic resonance imaging (MRI).

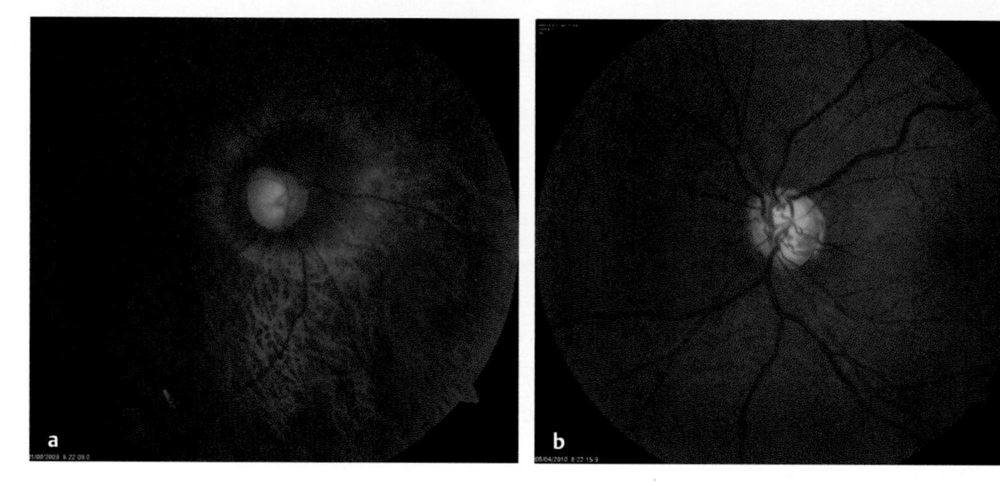

Fig. 10.12 **(a)** Normal tension glaucoma with extensive choroidal sclerosis and severe glaucomatous neuropathy. **(b)** Fundus picture showing an inferotemporal retinal vein occlusion, cup:disc ratio of 0.8:1, and significant neuroretinal rim thinning all over with pallor. Collateral vessels are seen on the disc.

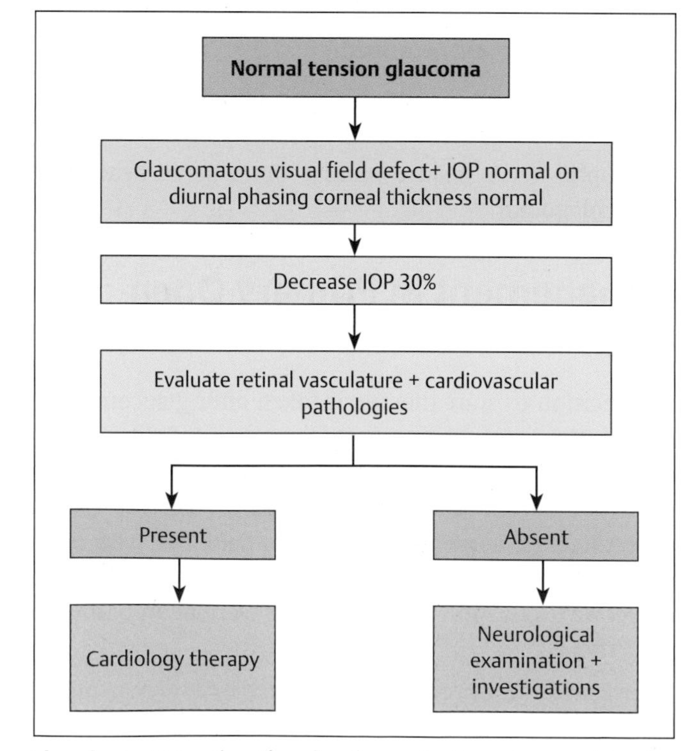

Flowchart 10.1 Algorithm for the evaluation of normal tension glaucoma. IOP, intraocular pressure.

increases the chances of progression significantly, and should alert the ophthalmologist to keep a closer follow-up, and at the first evidence of progression to lower target IOP further (**Table 10.1**).

Therapy is started with medications, followed, if required, by laser trabeculoplasty and finally surgery. The advent of selective laser trabeculoplasty has provided an alternative first-line therapy in mild POAG. Minimally invasive glaucoma surgeries are also being evaluated in mild POAG.

Setting a Target Intraocular Pressure

A target IOP range has to be set based on the optic nerve head and perimetric damage in each patient. Simplified ways of doing this are by looking at the mean deviation on Humphrey fields, > −6 being mild glaucomatous loss, −6 to −12 being moderate, and <−12 being severe. A look at the pattern deviation plot gives additional information about the percentage of loci having a significantly low sensitivity, <25% seen in mild, 25 to 50% in moderate glaucoma, and >50% in severe. Proximity to fixation also needs to be evaluated, that is, points within central 5 degrees: mild

Table 10.1 Risk factors for progression reported in randomized control studies of POAG

Study	EMGT	CNTGS	AGIS	OHTS	EGPS
Criteria					
IOP	√	–	√	√	√
Baseline optic nerve damage	√	–	√	No data	No data
Age	√	–	√	√	√
Pseudoexfoliation	√	x	x	x	√
Disc hemorrhages	√	√	x	√	X

Abbreviations: AGIS, Advanced Glaucoma Intervention Study; CNTGS, Collaborative Normal Tension Glaucoma Study; EGPS, European Glaucoma Prevention Study; EMGT, Early Manifest Glaucoma Trial; OHTS, Ocular Hypertension Treatment Study, POAG, primary open-angle glaucoma.

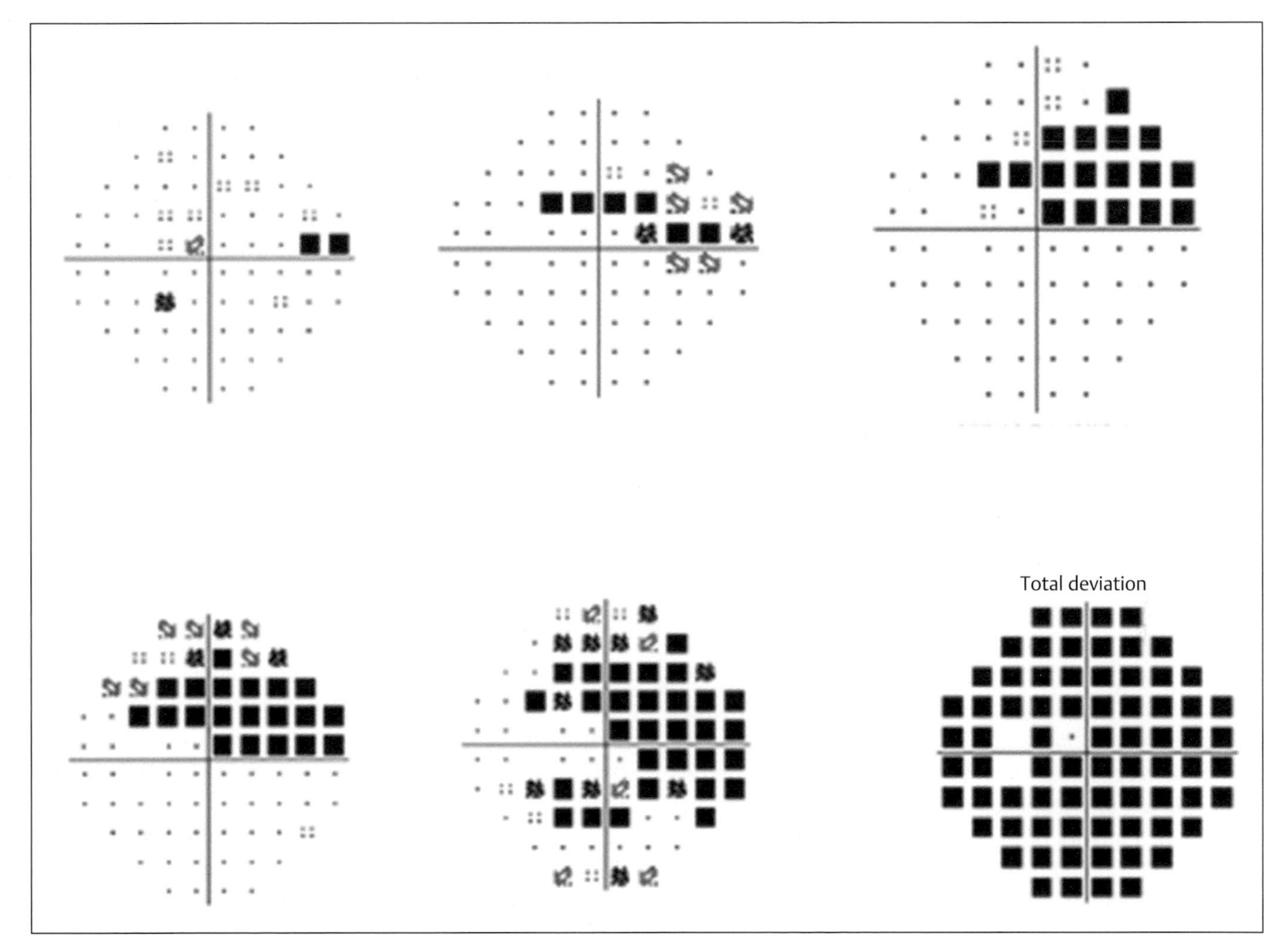

Fig. 10.13 Pattern deviation plots for easy clinical assessment: 1 and 2 are eyes with mild glaucoma, 3 and 4 with moderate, and 5 and 6 with severe glaucomatous damage.

glaucoma has no affected central points, moderate has some loci in one hemisphere, and severe has a significant number of affected loci in both hemispheres with one point recording 0 dB (**Fig. 10.13**).

The IOP should be reviewed every 6 months and assessed the patient for changes in the optic nerve head and on perimetry periodically, at least once a year (**Flowchart 10.2**).

Medical Management

After an assessment of the systemic status of the patient, especially for asthma, heart block, and Parkinsonism, his/her *socioeconomic circumstances need to be ascertained, as well as the ability to instill drops.*

First-line therapy for POAG should be one of the most effective medications available—prostaglandin (PG)

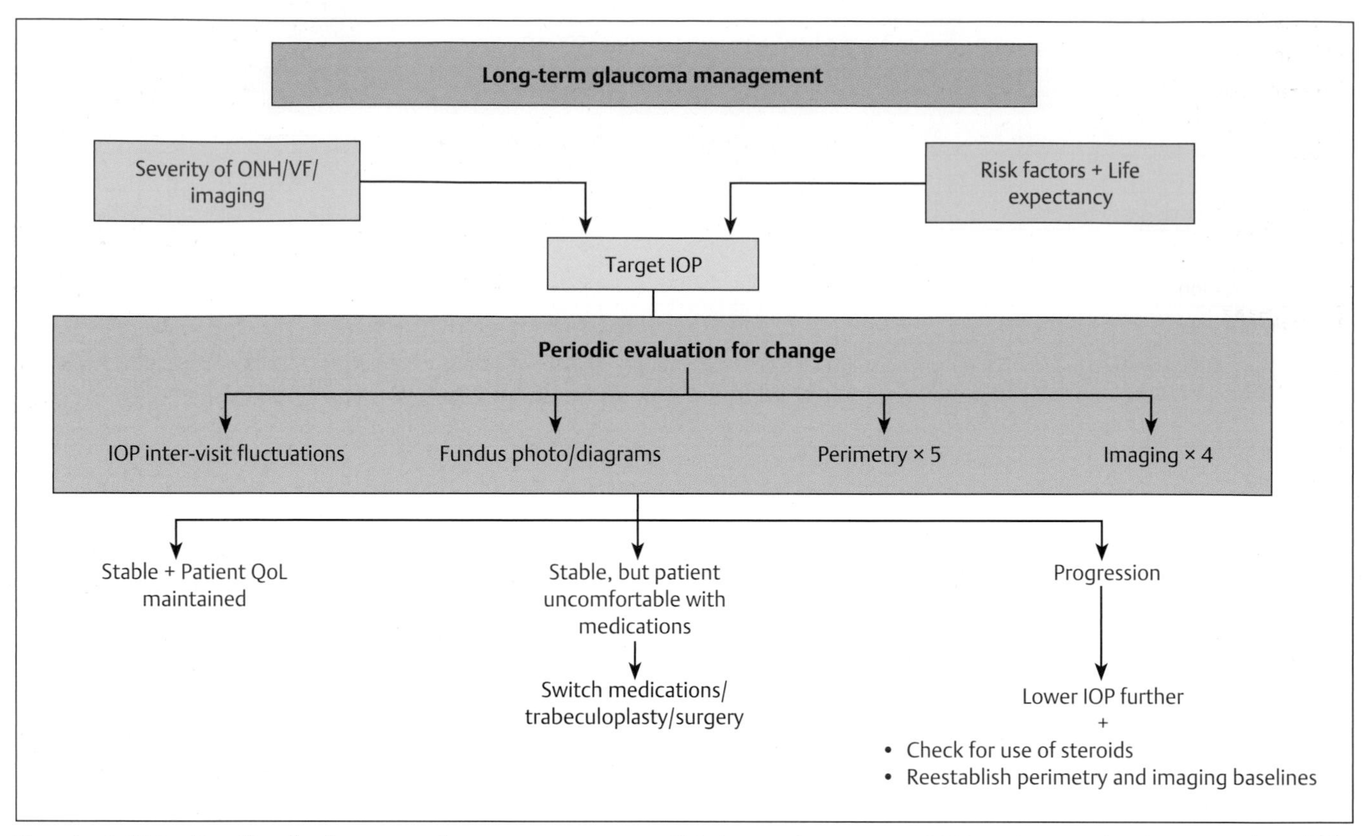

Flowchart 10.2 Algorithm for long-term glaucoma management. IOP, intraocular pressure; ONH, optic nerve head; QoL, quality of life; VF, visual field.

analogs or β-blockers at present. *A fall in IOP of at least 15% would suggest continuation of the drug*, but if this is not seen after 1 to 2 weeks, another drug may be substituted and the first stopped. The second drug should be similarly assessed for at least a 15% IOP fall, and if this drop is seen but target IOP is not reached, a third drug may be added. The additional drug should be one that works by a different IOP-lowering mechanism and should be noted to have further lowered the IOP. *A maximum of four drugs in two bottles should be tried*, keeping in mind both efficacy and the patient's quality of life. Any further additions are not likely to substantially affect IOP, but would add to drug-induced side effects in the patient.

In NTG the use of PG analogs is suggested, as they are seen to lower IOPs even in the normal range. Brimonidine is thought to have probable neuroprotective properties, and is the other drug commonly used for NTG (**Flowchart 7.1**). Neuroprotection has still not been proven; however, the additional use of antioxidants, vitamin B3, etc., has been suggested.

Trabeculoplasty

Laser trabeculoplasty provides about a 20% drop in IOP in about 30 to 50% of Indian eyes, but the effect wanes over months. Iridocyclitis, and sometimes a raised IOP, may be seen after selective laser trabeculoplasty (SLT). The *Laser in Glaucoma and Ocular Hypertension (LIGHT) trial* compared SLT to medications as first-line therapy in ocular hypertension and early POAG, and found SLT to be better in terms of cost efficacy and quality of life over 3 years in these patients. Argon and diode laser trabeculoplasty also produce a similar effect, but coagulate the trabecular meshwork.

Surgery

If target IOP is not achieved with maximal tolerable medications and/or trabeculoplasty, there is noncompliance or allergies, or patients cannot afford medications, surgery may be considered.

Trabeculectomy is the most commonly performed first surgery in POAG, with the use of low-dose, low-duration antifibroblastic agents, if required. The Primary Tube versus Trabeculectomy (PTVT) Study has shown a better efficacy of trabeculectomy for IOP lowering. A drainage implant could be considered in POAG eyes, where one to two trabeculectomies have failed. Cataract surgery alone reduces IOP by only 1 to 2 mm Hg, if at all.

Many randomized control trials have looked at treatment options and their efficacy in POAG (**Table 10.2**).

Follow-up

Follow-up intervals depend upon the stage of the disease and on the rate of change seen, with an examination and recording of the optic nerve head, perimetry, and IOP being essential. Imaging of the optic nerve head, retinal nerve fiber layer, or macula should be done if available, especially for patients with a risk of progression or those with advanced glaucoma.

At first it is important to find medications that suit the patient, or use other therapies to lower IOP to the target set so that the neuropathy can be stabilized. For this, an evaluation every 3 to 4 months may be required. Also, *repeated perimetry, at least five fields in the first 2 years, to identify both a learning curve and a rate of change is required,* which can help determine long-term therapy and chances of progression.

The target IOP may then be altered downwards if progression has occurred, with a fresh baseline perimetry and imaging instituted, and the patient recalled for a review in 3 months. The target IOP could also be revised upwards if the neuropathy is stable, and reviews thereafter may be every 6 months or even once a year.

Lifestyle modifications are also thought to improve the outcome in POAG.

Table 10.2 Summary of randomized control trials in POAG

Study	Inclusion criteria	Methodology	Duration	Results	Conclusions
Ocular Hypertension Treatment Study (OHTS)	IOP 24–32 mm Hg; normal disc and fields	Medical treatment to 20% reduction/ 24 mm Hg vs. observation	5/8 years	Progression in controls 9.5% vs. 4.4% in treatment group	Therapy reduces progression especially in high-risk patients—baseline age, IOP, CCT, vertical cup:disc ratio, and pattern standard deviation
OHTS phase II	As above	Treatment for earlier observation group after 7 years of observation	13 years	Progression 8% in early treatment vs. 7% in late overall	High-risk OHTs need early therapy
European Glaucoma Prevention Study (EGPS)	IOP 22–29 mm Hg; normal disc and fields	Dorzolamide vs. placebo	5 years	Progression 13.4 vs. 14.1%	Dorzolamide and placebo effect similar
Early Manifest Glaucoma Trial (EMGT)	IOP <30 mm Hg	Betaxolol + ALT vs. observation	4 years	Less progression in treatment group (45% vs. 62%) Average IOP reduction 5.1 mm Hg or 25%	Risk of progression decreased 10% with each 1 mm Hg IOP reduction from baseline to the first follow-up visit
Collaborative Initial Glaucoma Treatment Study (CIGTS)	IOP >20 mm Hg	Medical treatment vs. trabeculectomy	5 years	Both groups had similar perimetric outcomes Trabeculectomy had lower IOP, but more cataractogenesis	Medical and surgical therapy have similar efficacy in early glaucoma
Glaucoma Laser Trial Study and Follow-Up Study (GLT and GLTFUS)	IOP >/= 22 mm Hg, optic nerve damage in at least one eye	ALT vs. Timolol	7 years	ALT had lower IOP, better fields, and optic disc	Initial ALT is a good option
Advanced Glaucoma Intervention Study (AGIS)	Uncontrolled on maximal therapy	Trab-ALT-Trab vs. ALT-Trab-Trab	7/11 years	TAT had lower IOP than ATT	Lower IOP lead to slower progression
Collaborative Normal Tension Glaucoma Study (CNTGS)	NTG Disc and visual field changes Median IOP not more than 20 mm Hg	Medical treatment ± surgery to reduce IOP by 30% vs. observation	7 years	Progression 12% in treated group vs. 35% in controls	Faster progression in NTG in females, with migraine and disc hemorrhages

Abbreviations: ALT, Argon laser trabeculoplasty; ATT, ALT-trabeculectomy-trabeculectomy; CCT, central corneal thickness; IOP, intraocular pressure; NTG, normal tension glaucoma; OHT, ocular hypertension; POAG, primary open-angle glaucoma; TAT, trabeculectomy-ALT-trabeculectomy.

Prognosis

The prognosis for POAG is extremely good with current medications, laser, and surgery available, if an appropriate target IOP can be maintained. *Stabilization of the remaining field can be achieved in almost 90% of such patients.* NTG is more difficult to control, and needs concurrent cardiovascular and neurological management. The availability of “over-the-counter” steroids and their use in such patients is commonly responsible for a sudden rise in IOP on review, and *patients should be asked to avoid steroids in any form,* inhalers, skin creams, etc., as most POAG patients have a high steroid response.

Cases

Case 1

A 62-year-old lady of asthenic build and a history of migraine presented with high myopia and advanced glaucoma in the left eye with a superior arcuate scotoma in the right, and recorded IOPs between 10 and 12 mm Hg over the last 6 months. Diurnal phasing showed an IOP of 10 to 16 mm Hg on a β-blocker, and a CCT of 500 µm. There was extensive chorioretinal degeneration, and tilted optic nerve head with a cup:disc ratio of 0.7 in the right eye with a loss of inferior neuroretinal rim and 0.8 cupping with neuroretinal rim pallor in the left. Peripapillary atrophy was seen in both eyes. Gonioscopy showed a wide open angle. On review, the patient continued to progress despite lowering the IOP to 8 to 10 mm Hg with an additional PG analog (**Case 1-1**).

Points to consider

- IOPs <21 mm Hg even in early morning and night.
- Thin corneas.
- History of migraine.

Diagnosis and Management

A diagnosis of normal tension glaucoma was made. The patient underwent a carotid Doppler, cardiac Holter, sleep apnea test, and magnetic resonance imaging (MRI) of the brain. All were within normal limits. She was advised to use a PG analog and brimonidine drops instead of timolol, and oral antioxidant therapy.

Case 2

A 45-year-old male was referred to the glaucoma clinic. His highest baseline IOPs were 18 mm Hg (OD) and 24 mm Hg (OS). On performing gonioscopy, angles were found to be open. Fundus showed a cup:disc ratio of 0.6:1 in the right eye and 0.7:1 in the left eye, with vertically oval cup. CCT was 510 and 499 µm. Humphrey field analyzer (HFA) 30-2 showed a possible nasal step defect in the left eye. A diagnosis of mild POAG or ocular hypertension was made (**Cases 2-1** and **2-2**).

Points to consider

- Inferior neuroretinal rim thinning in the left eye.
- Significantly depressed loci on the pattern deviation plot are inferior and adjacent to an area of supranormal responses.
- Significantly depressed loci are not abutting the horizontal meridian.
- Disc and field changes do not correlate.

Diagnosis and Management

On repeat perimetry there was no defect seen. The patient was counseled for regular review in view of the raised IOP and optic nerve head asymmetry.

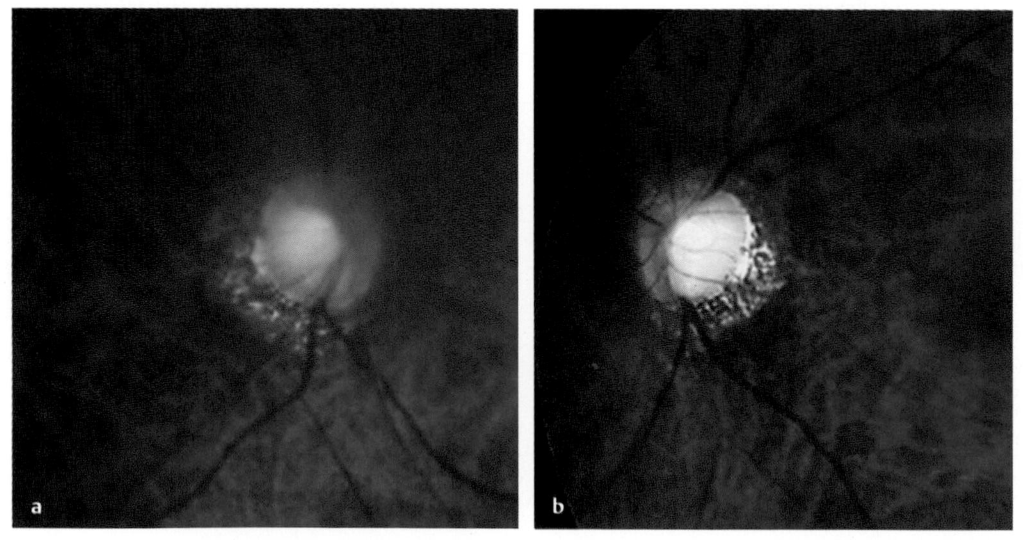

Case 1-1 (a, b) Tilted discs in both eyes. Extensive chorioretinal atrophy with a cup:disc ratio of 0.8 in the right eye, loss of neuroretinal rim from 5 to 9 o’clock with corresponding peripapillary atrophy. The left eye has more extensive loss of neuroretinal rim from 1 to 7 o’clock with concentric peripapillary atrophy.

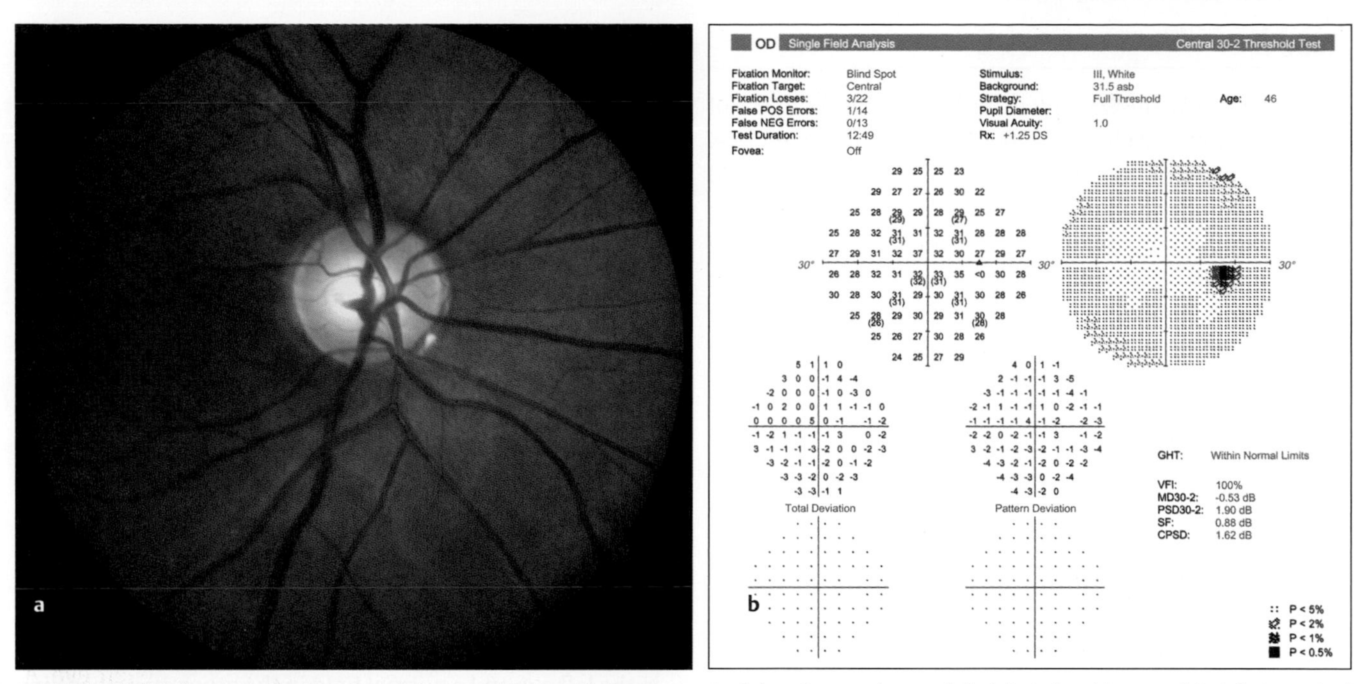

Case 2-1 **(a)** Right eye optic nerve head showing thinning of the neuroretinal rim all around, especially inferiorly with a possible inferior retinal nerve fiber layer defect. **(b)** Humphrey field analyzer (HFA) 30-2 has three points above the nasal meridian, having a likelihood of being seen in a normal population of only <5%.

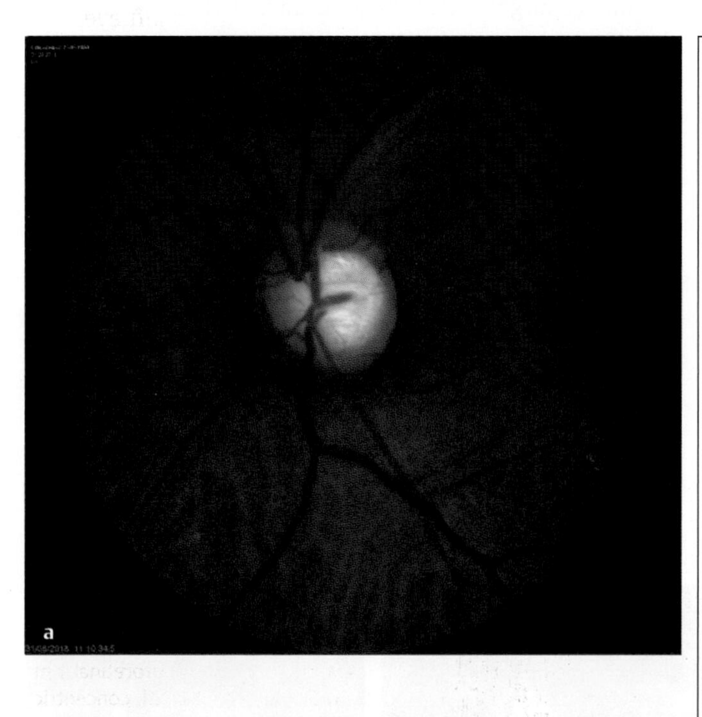

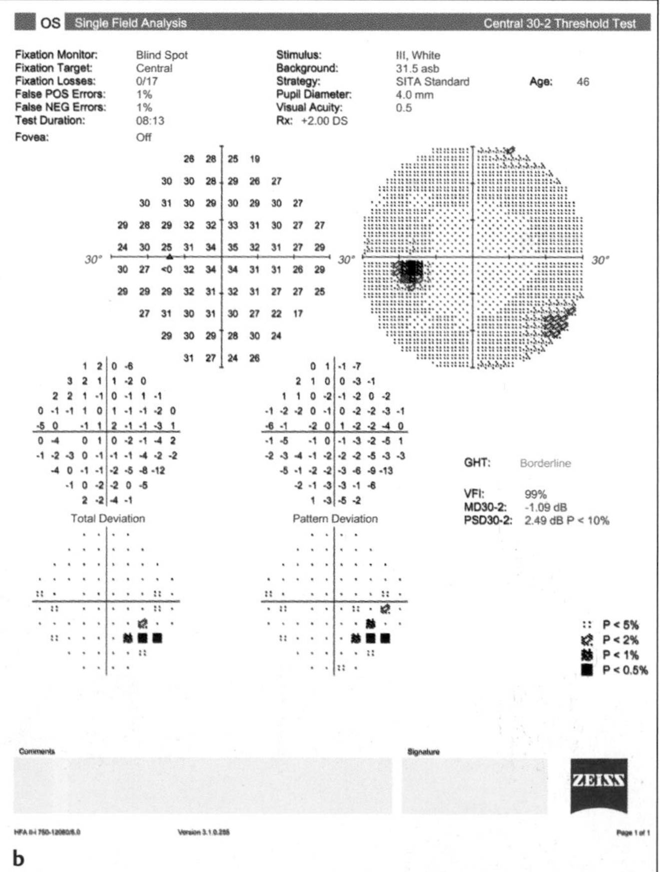

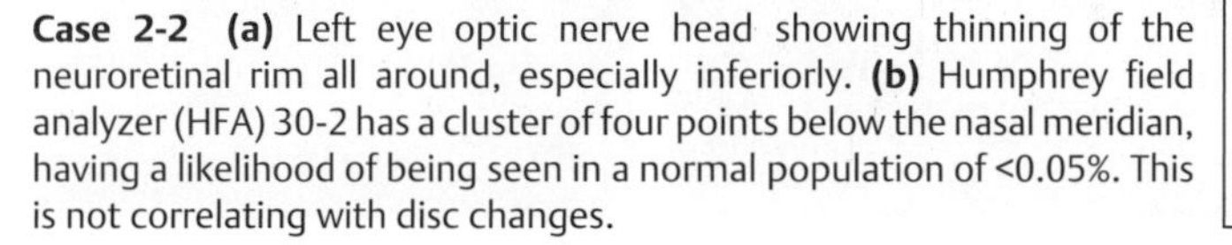

Case 2-2 **(a)** Left eye optic nerve head showing thinning of the neuroretinal rim all around, especially inferiorly. **(b)** Humphrey field analyzer (HFA) 30-2 has a cluster of four points below the nasal meridian, having a likelihood of being seen in a normal population of <0.05%. This is not correlating with disc changes.

Case 3

A 59-year-old male was found to have a baseline IOP of 40 mm Hg in the right eye and 36 mm Hg in the left eye. Anterior segment examination was unremarkable, and on gonioscopy, the angles were found to be open. Fundus showed near-total cupping with laminar dot sign in the right eye and 0.7:1 with neuroretinal rim pallor in the left. CCT was 510 and 516 µm. A diagnosis of POAG with OD advanced glaucomatous optic neuropathy was made (**Case 3-1**).

Points to consider

- Very significant neuroretinal rim pallor in both eyes.
- Such high IOPs are unusual in POAG.
- Pallor exceeding cupping is a marker for neurological abnormalities.

Diagnosis and Management

His MRI showed a pituitary macroadenoma with high plasma cortisol, which was then resected. The patient was started on a PG analog bedtime, β-blocker–dorzolamide combination, and brimonidine drops twice a day. An IOP of 22 to 24 mm Hg was recorded over 2 weeks, as against a target IOP of low teens, both for the thin neuroretinal rim as well as the neurological changes visible which may make the optic nerve more susceptible to damage. Both eyes underwent a trabeculectomy, and an IOP of 12 to 14 mm Hg was achieved in both eyes, and his cup:disc ratio and field has been stable over the last 3 years.

Case 4

A 56-year-old male had a baseline IOP of 26/28 mm Hg 18 years earlier, for which he was treated with a PG analog. However, progression was seen over the last 2 years, at IOPs of 20/22 mm Hg. A β-blocker–brimonidine combination was added twice a day and the IOP reduced to 14/14 mm Hg with stable fields for the next few years on the same medicines. A routine review a year later again found raised IOPs of 24/26 mm Hg (**Case 4-1**).

Points to consider

- Was the patient compliant?
- Had tolerance to medications developed?
- Was there any concomitant steroid use?

Diagnosis and Management

After repeated questioning the patient gave a history of dermatitis treated with Betnovate N cream on and off. He was advised to stop steroids, while Ripasudil drops were added, with close follow-up till IOP returned to 14/14 mm Hg. He was made aware of this steroid response, and advised to avoid steroids.

Case 5

A 60-year-old lady with POAG, having an arcuate scotoma in the left eye and a normal field in the other, had a baseline IOP of 24/28. She had an IOP of 14/16 mm Hg on three glaucoma medications. Her vision was 6/9 and 6/9p, with nuclear sclerosis grade 2. An ophthalmologist advised her a cataract surgery with the assurance that she would then be off her glaucoma medicines (**Case 5-1**).

Points to consider

- The total and pattern deviation plots are similar, suggesting clear media.
- Average lowering of IOP after cataract surgery in POAG is 1 to 1.5 mm Hg.
- Moderate glaucoma would need an IOP <15 mm Hg.

Diagnosis and Management

A refraction brought her visual acuity to 6/6 and 6/9, and the very small IOP fall after cataract surgery and continued need for subsequent glaucoma medications were explained to her. She chose to continue with medications and review regularly.

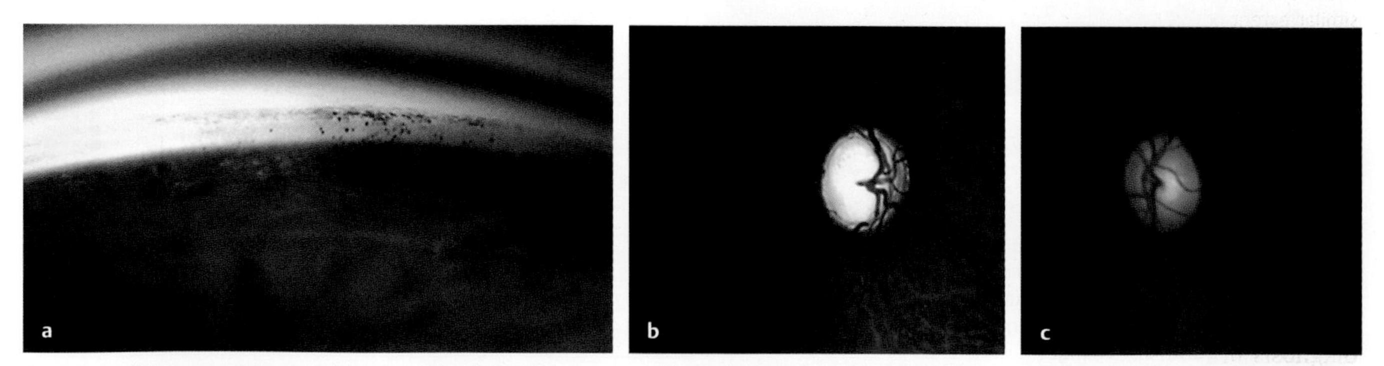

Case 3-1 **(a)** Open angle on gonioscopy. **(b, c)** Right optic nerve head showing an almost total cup and left a cup:disc ratio of 0.6, with a generalized significant pallor of the neuroretinal rim in both eyes. (The images are provided courtesy of Dr Dewang Angmo, AIIMS, New Delhi, India.)

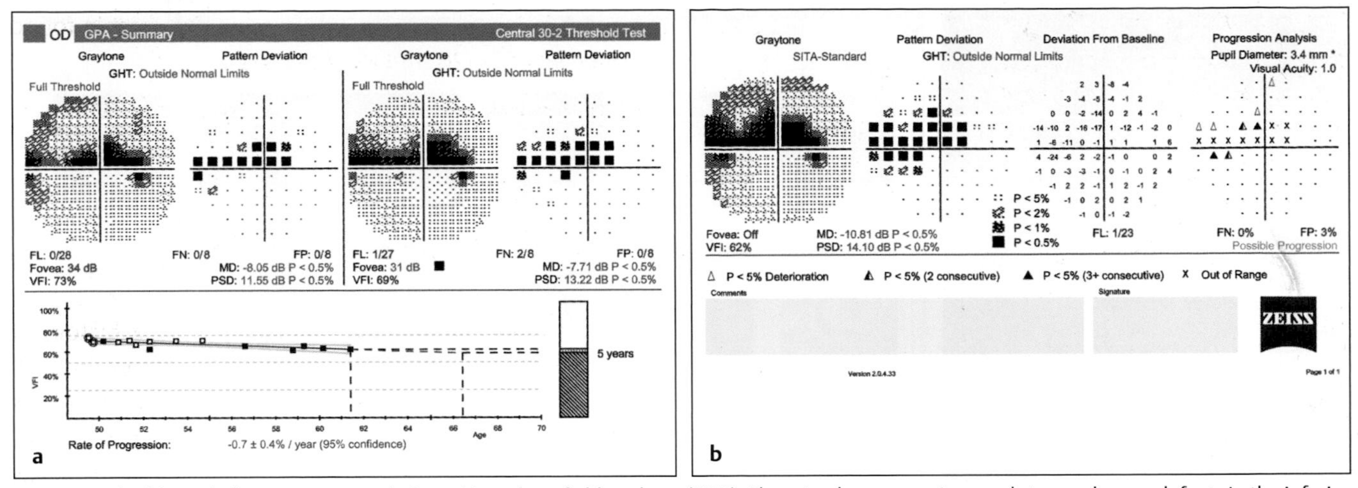

Case 4-1 (a, b) Guided progression analysis on Humphrey field analyzer (HFA). There is a large superior nasal step and some defects in the inferior nasal area at baseline. Over 18 years fields were relatively stable, till the steroid response seen in 2018 when likely progression was highlighted on two consecutive fields by fully black triangles.

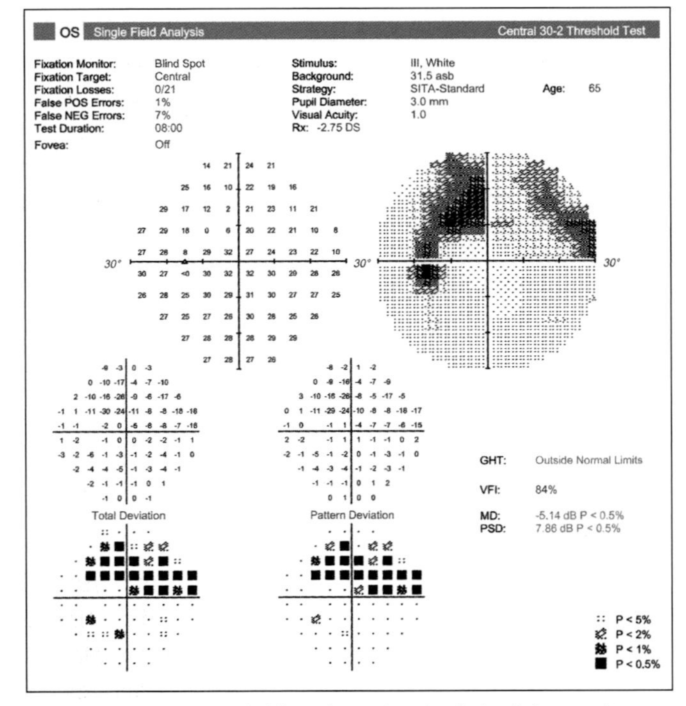

Case 5-1 Humphrey field analyzer (HFA) of the left eye showing mean deviation of less than −6 dB, and a superior arcuate scotoma of similar extent on both total and pattern deviation plots suggesting a moderate glaucoma with no significant lens opacification.

Case 6

A 63-year-old hypertensive male presented with a baseline IOP of 16/18 mm Hg, a normal anterior segment, and an open angle on gonioscopy. There was a left superior arcuate scotoma, and right perimetry was normal at baseline. A diagnosis of NTG was made and he was advised the use of a PG analog and timolol drops with which the IOP was 12 to 14 mm Hg. Over 1 year progression was noted on perimetry and serial Heidelberg retinal tomography even though the IOP was in the low teens (**Case 6-1**).

Points to consider

- Overtreated systemic hypertension or specifically nocturnal hypotension could decrease vascular perfusion of the optic nerve.
- Carotid plaques could decrease ocular perfusion.
- Was the patient compliant overall or only when coming to the clinic?

Diagnosis and Management

Hypertension was found to be adequately controlled. A carotid Doppler showed significant blockage on both sides and his MRI showed areas of cerebral ischemia. A carotid endarterectomy was done and the patient is on close review for his glaucoma.

Case 7

A 61-year-old lady was diagnosed with POAG and advised the use of a PG analog. She came for a second opinion. On examination, the anterior segment was within normal limits, cup:disc ratio was 0.5 in both eyes with a regular neuroretinal rim of good color (**Case 7-1**).

Points to consider

- There was no neuroretinal rim loss or pallor in either eye.
- Visual field defects were not in Bjerrum's area.
- The defects respected the vertical meridian.

Diagnosis and Management

As the field defects respected the vertical meridian, but were not congruous, damage to the optic radiations was

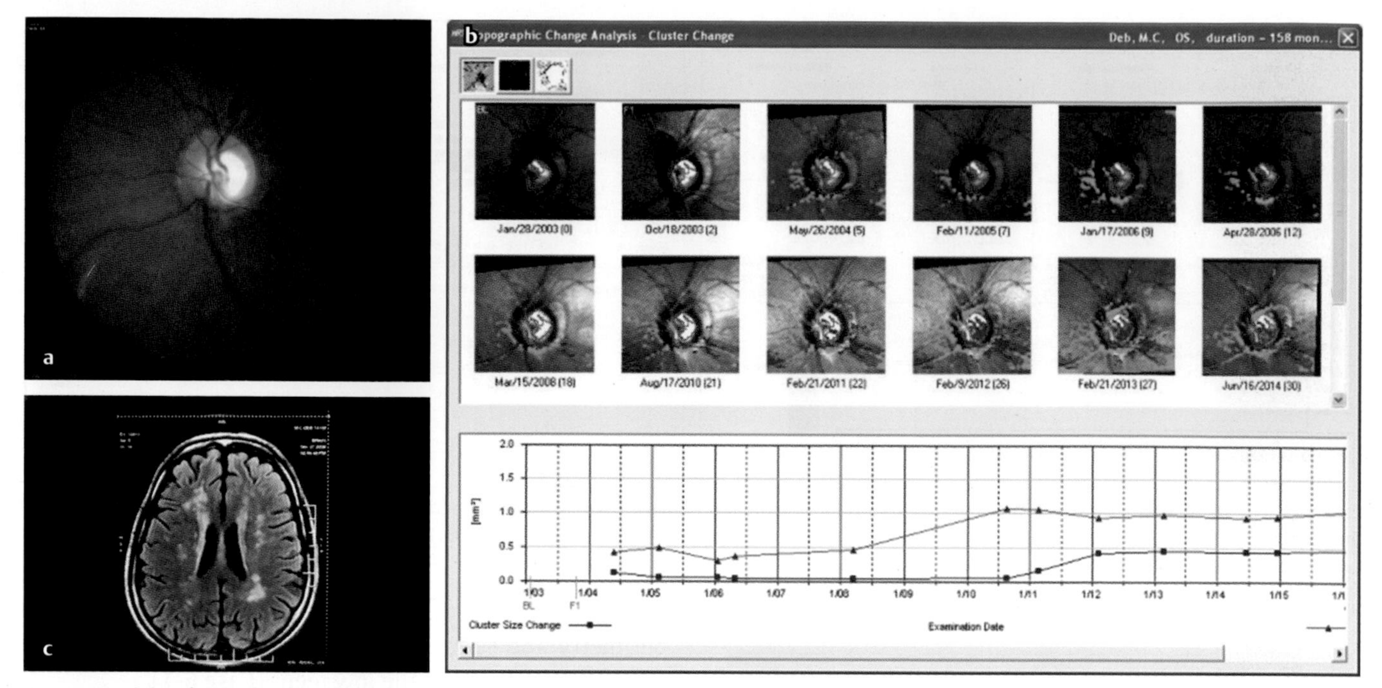

Case 6-1 **(a)** Left eye fundus picture showing loss of neuroretinal rim from 4 to 6 o'clock and gray peripapillary halo. **(b)** Scanning laser ophthalmoscopy showing a progressive loss of inferotemporal neuroretinal rim seen as increasing number of red pixels on the neuroretinal rim. **(c)** Magnetic resonance imaging (MRI) showing infarcted areas.

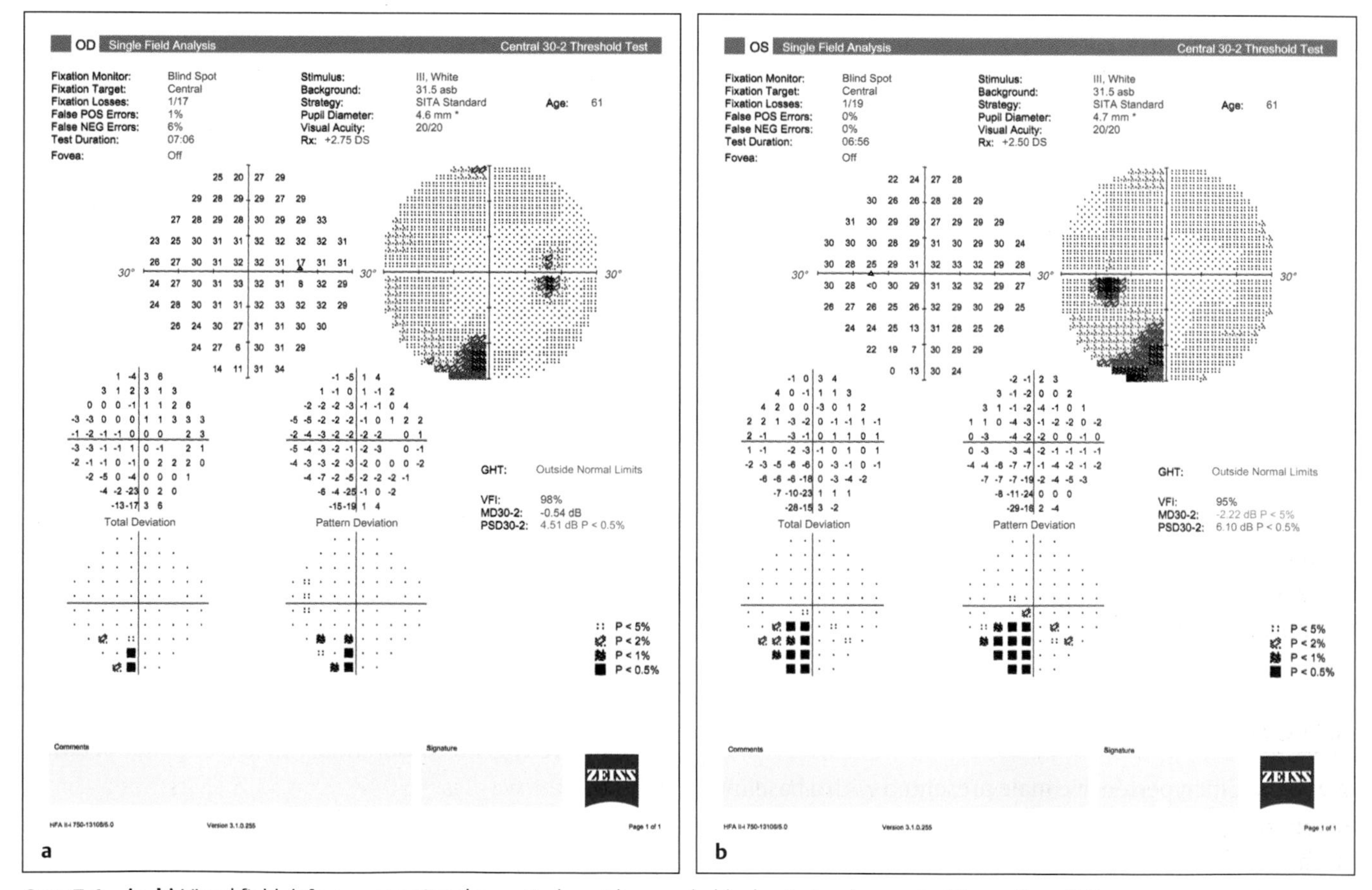

Case 7-1 **(a, b)** Visual field defects respecting the vertical meridian, probably due to involvement of the optic radiations.

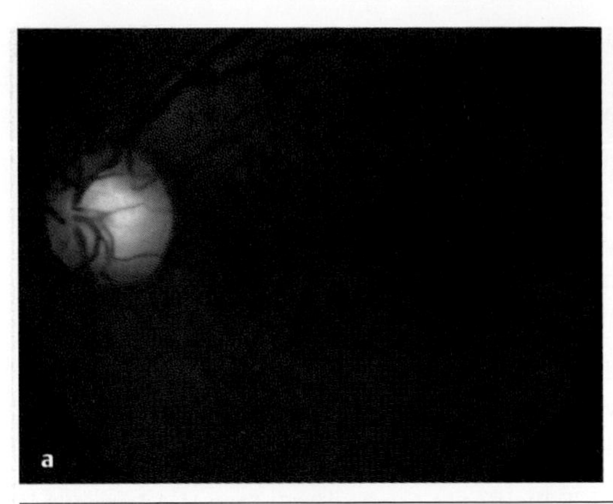

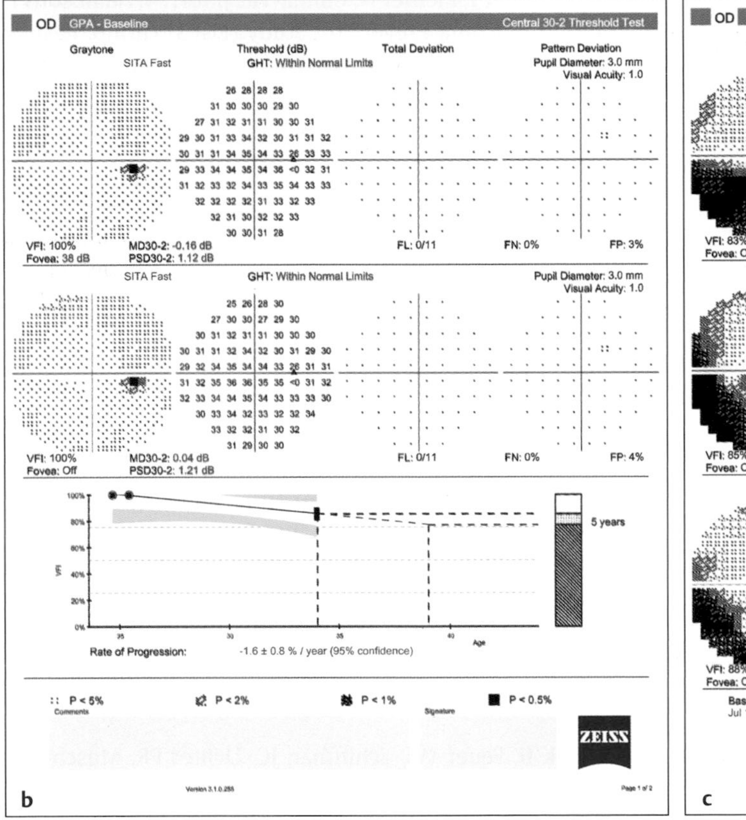

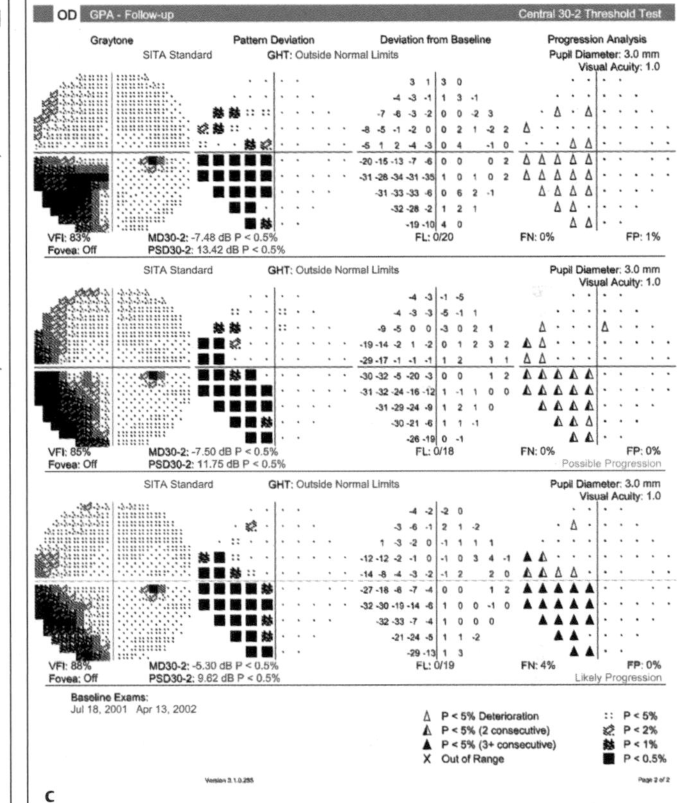

Case 8-1 **(a)** Right eye fundus photograph showing an inferior notch and possible retinal nerve fiber layer defect. **(b, c)** Guided progression analysis showing normal baseline fields, a loss to review, and later progressing to superior and inferior nasal steps in the repeated fields labeled as: Outside normal limits, possible progression, and likely progression.

suspected. An MRI revealed a cerebral infarct. The glaucoma medications were discontinued and a diurnal a month later showed an IOP range of 10 to 14 mm Hg. She was found to have hypertension and evidence of a past cardiovascular episode, for which therapy was instituted.

Case 8

A 25-year-old doctor presented with conjunctivitis and was diagnosed as a POAG suspect. His anterior chamber was normal, cup:disc ratio was 0.7 with superior and inferior neuroretinal rim thinning, and a possible retinal nerve fiber layer defect. Pachymetry was 512 and 520 µm and IOP diurnal range was 12 to 22 mm Hg. As his perimetry was normal but disc suspicious, he was advised fundus photography, five fields and repeat optical coherence tomography over 2 years, and a regular review (**Case 8-1**).

Points to consider

- Young patient with significant neuroretinal rim loss.
- Large range of diurnal IOP.

Diagnosis and Management

The patient was lost to follow-up for 8 years and returned with visual field defects, superior and inferior nasal areas in both eyes, with an IOP now of 20 to 24 mm Hg. He was started on a PG analog to lower his IOP. In view of vertical edges of the visual field defect, an MRI was done, but was within normal limits. Compliance for medications and review was emphasized.

Suggested Readings

AGIS Investigators. The Advanced Glaucoma Intervention Study (AGIS): 11. Risk factors for failure of trabeculectomy and argon laser trabeculoplasty. Am J Ophthalmol 2002; 134(4):481–498

Caprioli J, Coleman AL. Intraocular pressure fluctuation a risk factor for visual field progression at low intraocular pressures in the advanced glaucoma intervention study. Ophthalmology 2008;115(7):1123–1129.e3

Collaborative Normal-Tension Glaucoma Study Group. Comparison of glaucomatous progression between untreated patients with normal-tension glaucoma and patients with therapeutically reduced intraocular pressures. Am J Ophthalmol 1998;126(4):487–497

Damji KF, Behki R, Wang L; Target IOP Workshop participants. Canadian perspectives in glaucoma management: setting target intraocular pressure range. Can J Ophthalmol 2003; 38(3):189–197

Grant WM, Burke JF Jr. Why do some people go blind from glaucoma? Ophthalmology 1982;89(9):991–998

Grzybowski A, Och M, Kanclerz P, Leffler C, Moraes CG. Primary open angle glaucoma and vascular risk factors: a review of population based studies from 1990 to 2019. J Clin Med 2020;9(3):E761

Hecht I, Achiron A, Man V, Burgansky-Eliash Z. Modifiable factors in the management of glaucoma: a systematic review of current evidence. Graefes Arch Clin Exp Ophthalmol 2017;255(4):789–796

Heijl A, Leske MC, Bengtsson B, Hyman L, Bengtsson B, Hussein M; Early Manifest Glaucoma Trial Group. Reduction of intraocular pressure and glaucoma progression: results from the Early Manifest Glaucoma Trial. Arch Ophthalmol 2002;120(10):1268–1279

Hyman L, Heijl A, Leske MC, Bengtsson B, Yang Z; Early Manifest Glaucoma Trial Group. Natural history of intraocular pressure in the early manifest glaucoma trial: a 6-year follow-up. Arch Ophthalmol 2010;128(5):601–607

Kass MA, Heuer DK, Higginbotham EJ, et al. The Ocular Hypertension Treatment Study: a randomized trial determines that topical ocular hypotensive medication delays or prevents the onset of primary open-angle glaucoma. Arch Ophthalmol 2002;120(6):701–713, discussion 829–830

Leske MC, Heijl A, Hyman L, Bengtsson B, Komaroff E. Factors for progression and glaucoma treatment: the Early Manifest Glaucoma Trial. CurrOpinOphthalmol 2004;15(2):102–106

Li F, Huang W, Zhang X. Efficacy and safety of different regimens for primary open-angle glaucoma or ocular hypertension: a systematic review and network meta-analysis. Acta Ophthalmol 2018;96(3):e277–e284

Li T, Lindsley K, Rouse B, et al. Comparative effectiveness of first-line medications for primary open-angle glaucoma: a systematic review and network meta-analysis. Ophthalmology 2016;123(1):129–140

Miglior S, Zeyen T, Pfeiffer N, Cunha-Vaz J, Torri V, Adamsons I; European Glaucoma Prevention Study (EGPS) Group. Results of the European Glaucoma Prevention Study. Ophthalmology 2005;112(3):366–375

Musch DC, Gillespie BW, Niziol LM, Cashwell LF, Lichter PR; Collaborative Initial Glaucoma Treatment Study Group. Factors associated with intraocular pressure before and during 9 years of treatment in the Collaborative Initial Glaucoma Treatment Study. Ophthalmology 2008;115(6):927–933

Musch DC, Gillespie BW, Lichter PR, Niziol LM, Janz NK; CIGTS Study Investigators. Visual field progression in the Collaborative Initial Glaucoma Treatment Study the impact of treatment and other baseline factors. Ophthalmology 2009;116(2):200–207

Musch DC, Gillespie BW, Niziol LM, Lichter PR, Varma R; CIGTS Study Group. Intraocular pressure control and long-term visual field loss in the Collaborative Initial Glaucoma Treatment Study. Ophthalmology 2011;118(9):1766–1773

Nouri-Mahdavi K, Hoffman D, Coleman AL, et al; Advanced Glaucoma Intervention Study. Predictive factors for glaucomatous visual field progression in the Advanced Glaucoma Intervention Study. Ophthalmology 2004;111(9):1627–1635

Parrish RK II, Feuer WJ, Schiffman JC, Lichter PR, Musch DC; CIGTS Optic Disc Study Group. Five-year follow-up optic disc findings of the Collaborative Initial Glaucoma Treatment Study. Am J Ophthalmol 2009;147(4):717–724.e1

Parrish RK II. The European Glaucoma Prevention Study and the Ocular Hypertension Treatment Study: why do two studies have different results? CurrOpinOphthalmol 2006;17(2): 138–141

Razeghinejad MR, Lee D. Managing normal tension glaucoma by lowering the intraocular pressure. SurvOphthalmol 2019; 64(1):111–116

CHAPTER 11 Primary Angle-Closure Disease

Overview

- Classification
- Pathophysiology
  - Anatomic Features of PACD Eyes
  - Physiological Factors that Precipitate Angle Closure
  - Current Hypothesis
  - Genetics
- Provocative Tests
- Clinical Features
  - Primary Angle Closure
  - Primary Angle Closure with Hypertension
  - Primary Acute Angle-Closure Glaucoma
  - Primary Angle-Closure Glaucoma
- Cases
- Suggested Readings

Introduction

Primary angle-closure disease (PACD) is common in India, affecting almost 3 to 5% of individuals over 40 years of age in many different forms. ***PACD is characterized as occurring in an anatomically predisposed eye, when it undergoes a physiological change in the configuration of the iris, allowing it to become apposed/adherent to the trabecular meshwork.*** The iridotrabecular contact (ITC) itself prevents aqueous outflow, producing a rise in intraocular pressure (IOP) proportionate to the extent of circumference closed and the speed of this closure. In addition, single or repeated episodes may lead to gradually progressive trabecular dysfunction and damage and thereby a chronically raised IOP, leading to glaucomatous neuropathy and visual field loss.

Classification

Over the years, studies have shown that the International Society of Geographical and Epidemiological Ophthalmology (**ISGEO**) **classification of primary angle closure** that was meant to be used in surveys may not reflect the myriad forms of the disease seen in clinics, so common clinical stages as discussed are more practical (**Table 11.1**). The **ISGEO** classification did not take into account different

Table 11.1 Primary angle-closure disease—clinical staging, ISGEO classification for surveys and summary of management

Clinical stages	ISGEO for survey	Diagnostic criteria	Management and prognosis
PACS	PACS	**Occludable angle**—posterior trabecular meshwork not seen in primary position	Iridotomy in high-risk patients Low-risk review
PAC	PAC	**Occludable angle—+Evidence of angle closure–** pigmentation, PAS, goniosynechiae No ↑ IOP, no disc/field changes	**Iridotomy** Review 6 monthly Baseline trabecular meshwork damage + age 33% develop OHT—5 years
PAC + OHT	PAC	+ **Chronically raised IOP** No disc/field changes	**Iridotomy** **Meds: Target <18** Review 6 months 19% progress to PACG 5 years
PACG	PACG	+ **Disc/field changes**	Iridotomy → Meds/Trab Target <16 Review every 3 to 4 months 11–15% progress

Abbreviations: IOP, intraocular pressure; ISGEO, International Society of Geographical & Epidemiological Ophthalmology; OHT, ocular hypertension; PAC, primary angle closure; PACG, primary acute angle-closure glaucoma; PACS, primary angle-closure suspect; PAS, peripheral anterior synechiae.

grades of damage to the trabecular meshwork or optic nerve head, or acknowledge the importance of ocular hypertension (OHT) in primary angle closure.

Pathophysiology

All PACD eyes have an anatomic predisposition. Significant biometric parameters are: a shallow anterior chamber, a shorter axial length, thicker lens, an anterior position of the lens, and a smaller corneal diameter. These features lead to a crowding of the anterior chamber, bringing the peripheral iris closer to the peripheral cornea, therefore predisposing to episodes of iris contact over the cameral face of the trabecular meshwork (**Fig. 11.1**).

There is a *graded difference in the biometry of PACD subtypes, with acute primary angle-closure glaucoma (PACG) eyes being most significantly smaller*, suggesting an anatomical role in the varying presentations of PACD. Ultrasound biomicroscopy (UBM) and anterior segment optical coherence tomography (ASOCT) studies have further shown a narrower trabecular iris angle, shorter angle opening distance, and trabecular ciliary process distance, with acute PACG eyes again having the lowest measurements.

Other anatomic factors thought to predispose to peripheral iridotrabecular contact are a thicker iris, a prominent last roll of iris, a more anterior origin of the iris, and a plateau iris.

Anatomic Features of PACD Eyes

The following are common anatomic features seen in eyes predisposed to developing PACD:

- Shallow anterior chamber.
- Thicker lens.
- Anteriorly positioned lens.
- Shorter axial length.
- Exaggerated lens vault.

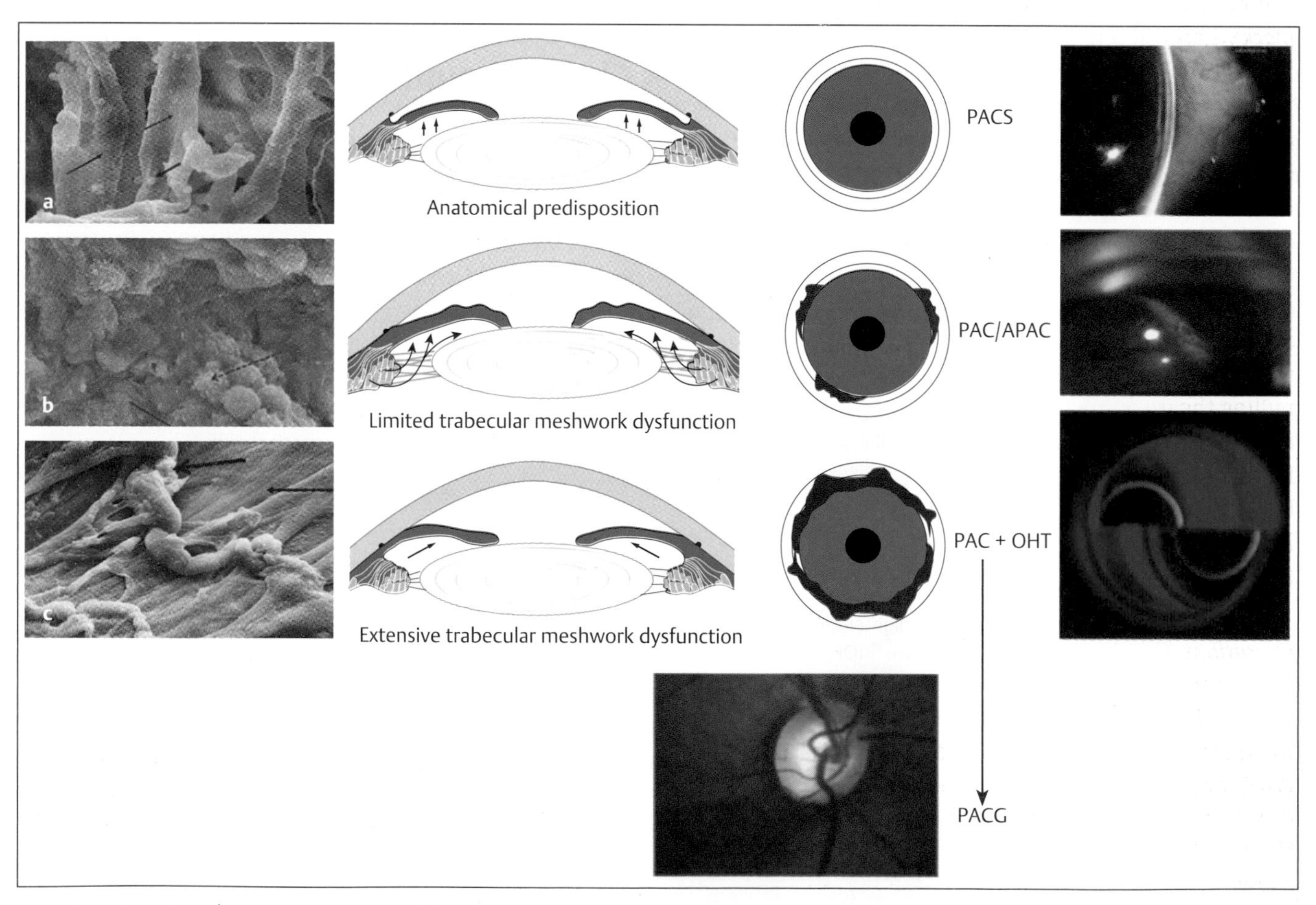

Fig. 11.1 Scanning electron microsopy, and diagrammatic representation of extent of iridotrabecular contact in the stages of primary angle-closure disease. **(a)** In primary angle-closure suspect (PACS), there is a narrow angle, but the trabecular meshwork is normal. **(b)** In primary angle-closure/acute primary angle-closure (APAC), a large portion of the trabecular meshwork is blocked by iris suddenly leading to edema of the trabecular endothelial cells and the presence of inflammatory cells. **(c)** In PACG eyes, there are extensive synechiae, with trabecular meshwork showing loss of endothelial cells, fusion of beams, and very few trabecular meshwork spaces. OHT, ocular hypertension; PAC, primary angle-closure.

- Small corneas.
- Anterior insertion of iris.
- Steeper cornea.

As not all primary angle-closure suspect (PACS) eyes develop PACG or primary angle closure (PAC). There are obviously other physiological changes that add to the underlying anatomy, causing iridocorneal contact.

Physiological Factors that Precipitate Angle Closure

Following are some of the common physiological factors which are implicated in the development of PACD:

- Mid-dilated pupil, as at twilight or in a cinema.
- Accommodation and near work.
- Stress.
- Uveal expansion.

Current Hypothesis

The most prevalent hypothesis is that of relative pupillary block wherein a mid-dilated pupil leads to a larger area of iris lying in contact with the anterior lens surface, preventing the normal movement of aqueous from the posterior to the anterior chamber. Aqueous accumulates behind the iris, leading to a pressure differential between the posterior and anterior chamber. As the iris is not a rigid structure, this billows forward, causing peripheral iridotrabecular contact. Relative pupillary block is seen in almost all PACD eyes to a greater or lesser extent. Mapstone had proposed an explanation using vectors of force generated, by the iris sphincter and dilator. The horizontal vectors—sphincter pulling the iris toward the pupil and the dilator away from the pupil—cancel each other to an extent. On the other hand, in the mid-dilated position, the posterior vectors of both sphincter and dilator muscles are synergistic and the iris is held against the lens capsule, blocking aqueous flow through the pupil, and leading to relative pupillary block.

Other suggested physiological changes are *uveal volume alterations* such as expansion of both iris and choroid, leading to narrowing of the angle. Quigley et al proposed that choroidal expansion may cause the anterior chamber to suddenly become shallow; however, a study of acute PACG eyes showed no change in anterior chamber depth or lens position at the time of an attack and 2 weeks later. Uveal congestion during a Valsalva maneuver has been shown to alter the volume and position of the ciliary body and iris, causing further narrowing of a predisposed angle recess and a significantly raised IOP. A uveal effusion has been thought to contribute to angle closure, and has been demonstrated in a small percentage of PACD eyes.

Stress is also thought to increase adrenergic responses and cause a dilation of the pupil.

Genetics

There is great interest in the genetics of PACD. Although no heritable disease-causing genes have been found, genetic loci have been identified that are associated with the risk of PACG. Some loci are PLEKHA7, COL11A1, PCMTD1, ST18, MMP9, MTHFR, MFRP, CHX10, and HGF, with more being added with ongoing studies.

PACD is a familial disease, around one-third of family members were found to have primary angle closure, and about one in five was PAC suspect.

The pathomechanisms for primary angle closure described above are thought to occur with different frequency, as recognized by ASOCT and UBM (**Figs. 11.2–11.4**):

- Relative pupillary block is thought to occur to a varying degree in all PACD eyes.
- Plateau iris has been reported in different races ranging from 8 to 23%.
- Exaggerated lens vault as a primary cause of PACD is reported in 7 to 24%.

Permutations of these mechanisms initially cause iridotrabecular contact, known as appositional or functional angle closure. *Proportionality of angle closure*, both circumferential extent and the time duration over which it occurs, is thought to determine the height of raised IOP. The IOP may return to normal when the iris falls back spontaneously or after therapy. Irreversible adhesions between the peripheral iris and trabecular surface or peripheral cornea hinder aqueous outflow permanently, and are known as *peripheral anterior synechiae (PAS).*

Iridotrabecular apposition and PAS both may alter the trabecular meshwork itself. Histopathology of the trabecular meshwork in PACG eyes has shown a significant loss of endothelial cells and fusion of trabecular beams around synechiae and even in areas without visible synechiae.

Iatrogenic PACD can be precipitated in anatomically predisposed eyes by the use of numerous *drugs that cause pupillary dilation, antipsychotics such as phenothiazines, anticonvulsants like topiramate, antidepressants, antihistaminics, sympathomimetics, and possibly botulinum toxin.*

Provocative Tests

Provocative tests are used to help ascertain which PACS eyes are likely to progress to PAC, so that a prophylactic laser iridotomy can be done. These are:

- *Dark-room prone provocative test*: Baseline IOP is measured by applanation tonometry and the

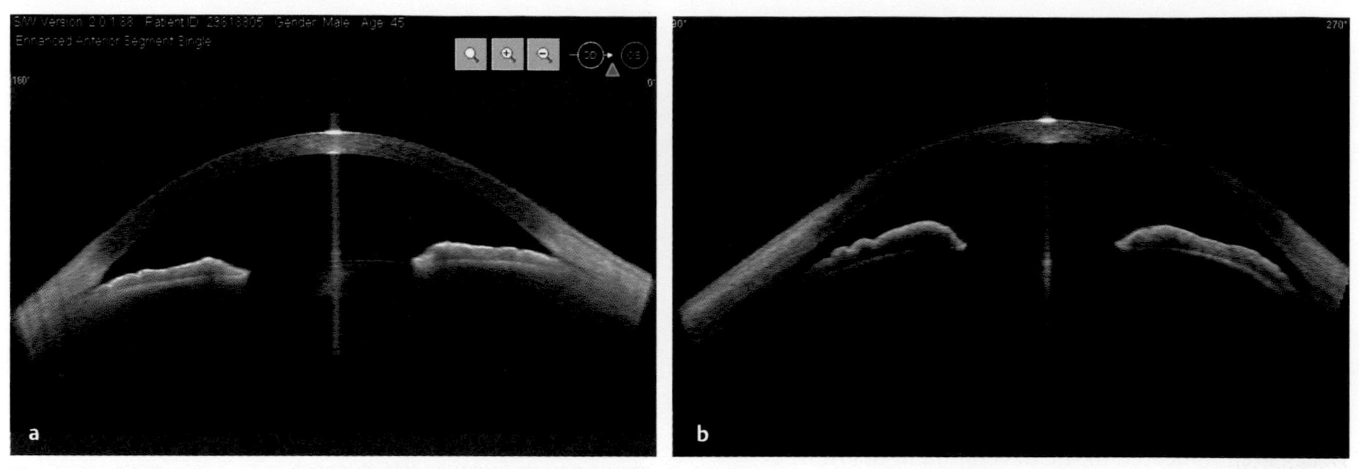

Fig. 11.2 **(a)** Anterior segment optical coherence tomography (ASOCT) showing an open angle, and regular configuration of the iris. **(b)** ASOCT showing a narrow but open angle, steep iris, and relatively anterior lens.

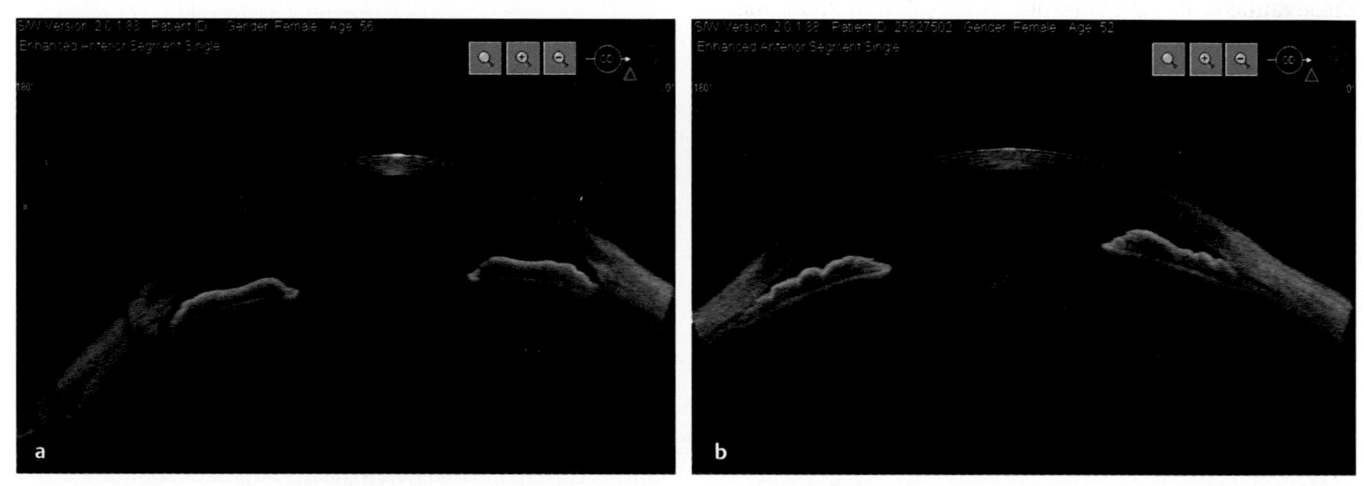

Fig. 11.3 **(a)** Plateau iris configuration: Flat iris contour dipping steeply in the periphery to narrow the angle recess. **(b)** Exaggerated lens vault: Very anteriorly placed lens with iris pushed forward by the anterior capsule, leading to a closed angle.

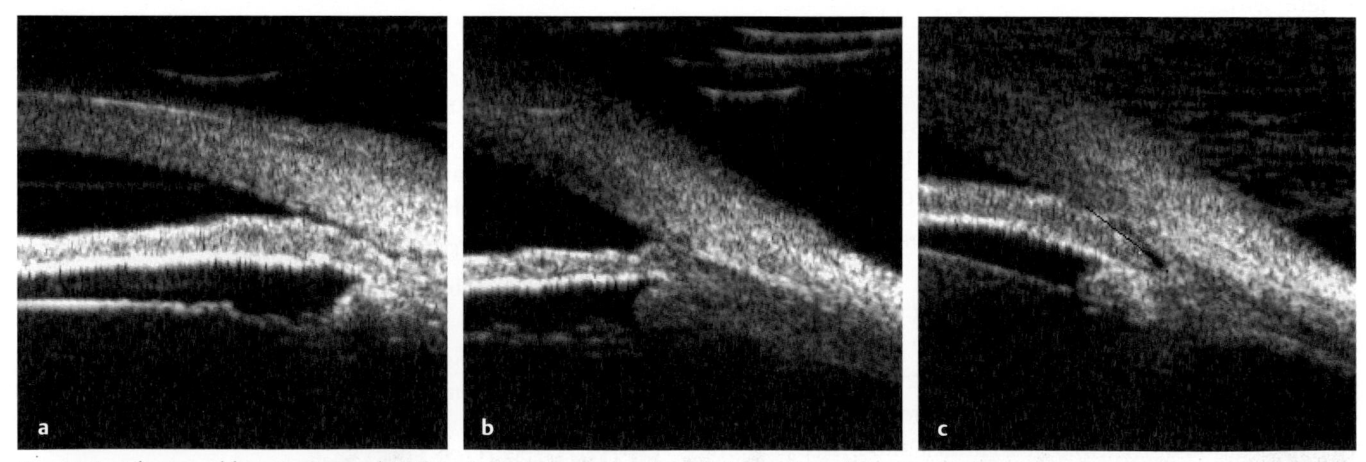

Fig. 11.4 Ultrasound biomicroscopy (UBM)—anterior chamber angle. **(a)** Steep iris configuration and a very narrow angle recess. **(b)** Flat iris configuration with a prominent last roll leading to narrowing of the angle. **(c)** Centrally flat iris with ciliary processes pushing up the peripheral iris causing a narrow angle recess, plateau iris.

patient placed in prone position in a dark room for 45 minutes. Head down position on a slit-lamp table is convenient. The patients are spoken to every 5 minutes to keep them awake. After 45 minutes, the IOP is re-measured using only the blue light of the tonometer in the dark room itself. A gonioscopy is repeated.

- *Mydriatic test:* Applanation tonometry is performed before instilling two drops of tropicamide 0.5%, and tonometry repeated every 15 minutes for 1 hour. A gonioscopy is repeated at 45 minutes.

An *increase in IOP of ≥6 to 8 mm Hg from baseline is considered a positive result* on both tests. The dark-room test is considered to be more physiological and therefore more clinically relevant. The mydriatic test has the disadvantage of not being physiological, and additionally sometimes results in chronic angle closure.

Clinical Features

Females are more likely to develop PACD, especially acute angle closure. Asymptomatic primary chronic angle closure is seen almost equally in both sexes.

Patients may complain of colored haloes and blurring of vision in twilight when the pupil is larger, or while doing near work in the evening, when a combination of a mid-dilated pupil with accommodation leads to a thicker and more anteriorly placed lens, shallowing the anterior chamber. However, *in India 80% of PACD cases are asymptomatic.*

An *"occludable" angle* is defined on gonioscopy as one where with the patient looking *in primary position, the posterior trabecular meshwork is not visible over at least 180/270 degrees, without indentation, while using the thinnest slit beam of 2-mm height.* The World Glaucoma Association (WGA) advocates the need to see the presence of iridotrabecular contact in PACS eyes. Stage 1 or 2 of Shaffer's grading, that is, an angle of <20 degrees, may help pick up eyes prone to PAS.

Primary Angle Closure

In PAC eyes there is a shallow anterior chamber (**Fig. 11.5**), and the ISGEO classification describes an occludable angle (**Fig. 11.6a**) with features suggestive of prior iridotrabecular contact, and/or raised IOP but without glaucomatous neuropathy. *Suggested features of iridotrabecular contact are PAS, iris whorling, blotchy pigment deposition on the trabecular surface, or even associated "glaucomflecken."* Repetition of such attacks could lead to a portion of the angle developing PAS, or the trabecular meshwork may be damaged by the episodes of iridotrabecular contact (**Fig. 11.6b**).

The anterior chamber in PAC eyes is shallow, less than grade 2 on *van Herick test* (**Fig. 11.7**). Observing the distance between the most peripheral corneal endothelium and iris at the inferior limbus using a short, thin, and bright slit allows better visualization of angular status. PAC eyes may also show evidence of *pupillary ruff atrophy*, seen as sectoral loss (**Fig. 11.8**). *Sphincter atrophy* causes a loss of circular appearance of the pupil with mild sectoral iris atrophy at the border of the pupil. A steep configuration of the iris is present (**Figs. 11.9** and **11.10**).

The *optic nerve head in such eyes is smaller* and therefore particular attention must be paid to the examination of the neuroretinal rim, to look for regularity and color. In PACD eyes, due to a smaller optic nerve head, focal thinning of the neuroretinal rim, or significant neuroretinal rim loss, may be observed, even if the cup:disc ratio appears to be 0.2 or 0.4 (**Fig. 11.11**).

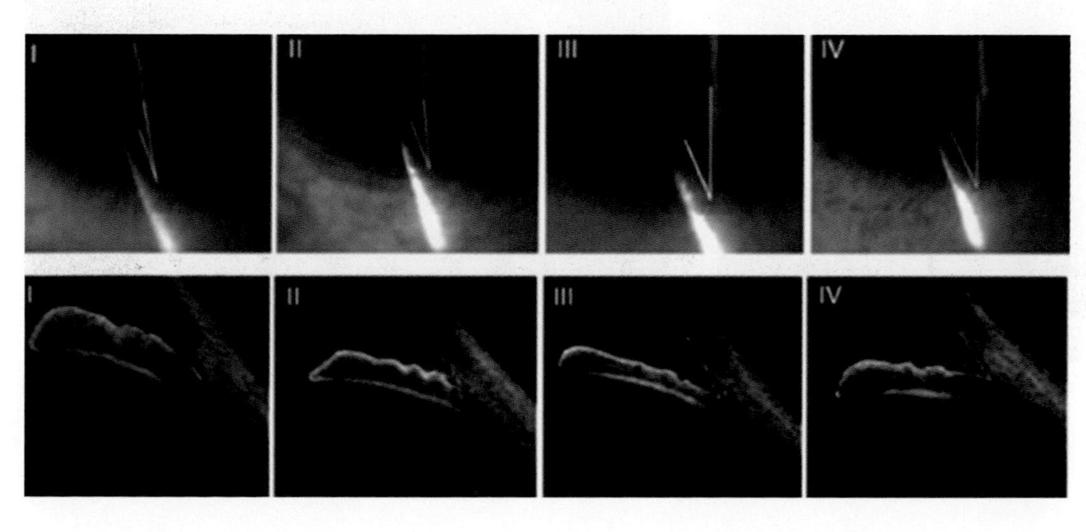

Fig. 11.5 Correlating grades of anterior chamber angle with anterior segment optical coherence tomography (ASOCT).

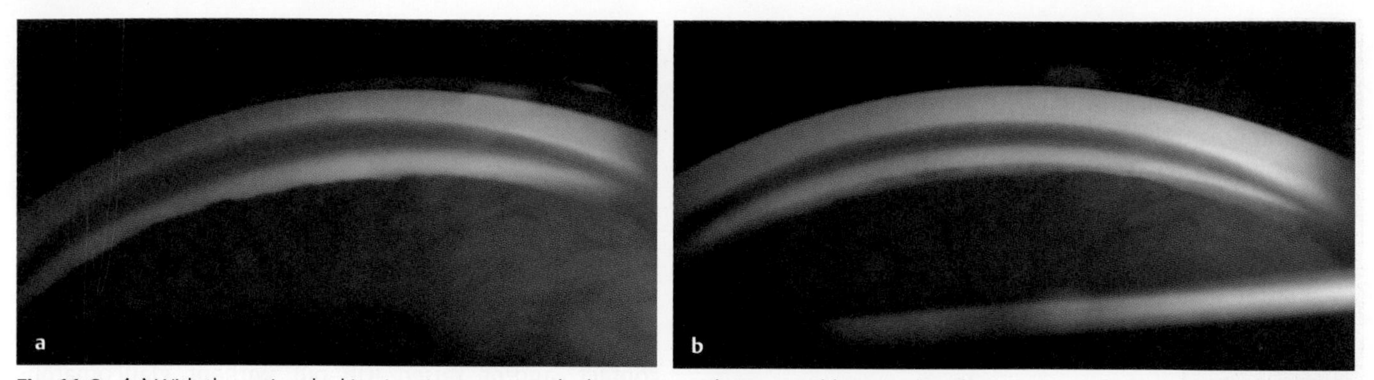

Fig. 11.6 **(a)** With the patient looking in primary gaze only the cornea and iris are visible, no trabecular structures. **(b)** On asking the patient to look toward the mirror being observed, trabecular meshwork with blotchy pigmentation and few areas of iridotrabecular synechiae can be seen.

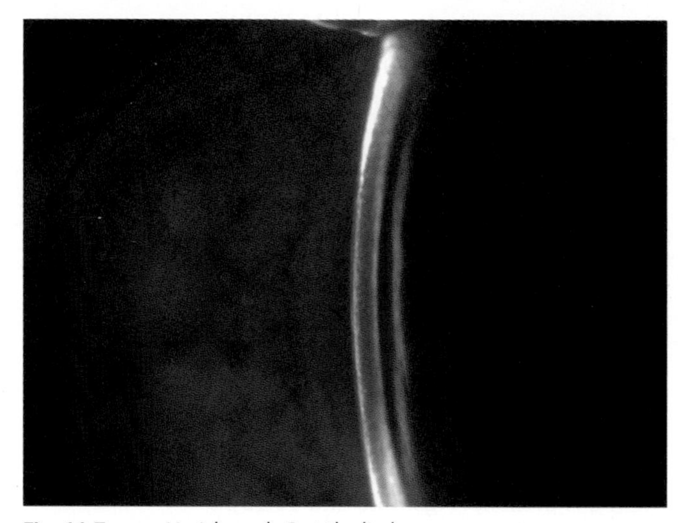

Fig. 11.7 van Herick grade 2 at the limbus.

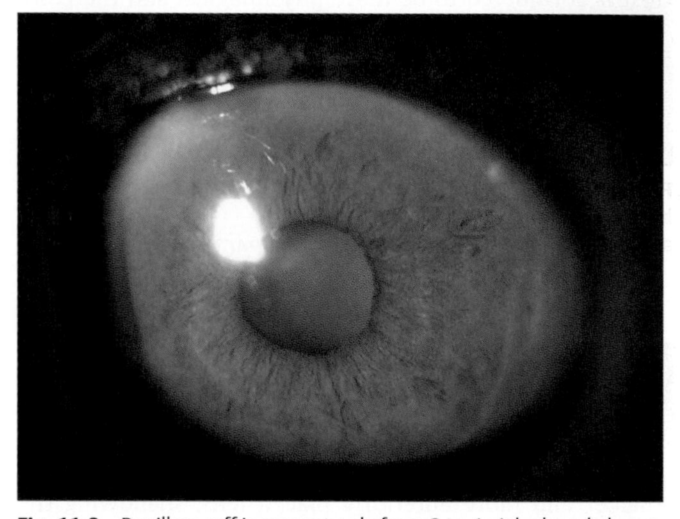

Fig. 11.8 Pupillary ruff is present only from 2 to 4 o'clock and absent over the rest of the pupil circumference. Sphincter atrophy is present at 4 and 6 o'clock.

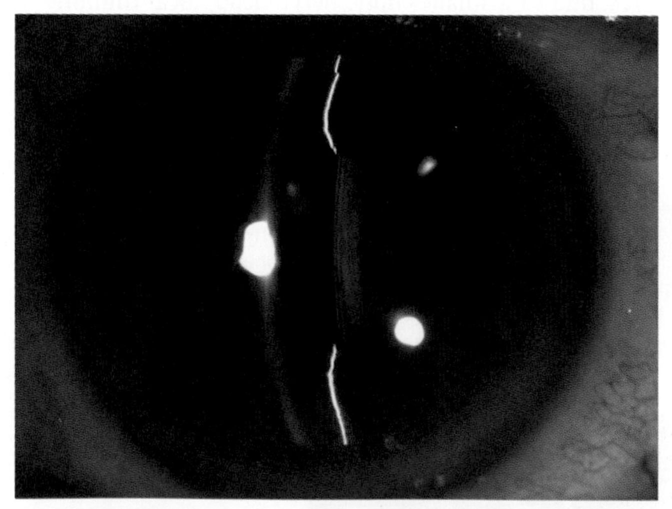

Fig. 11.9 Convex iris configuration.

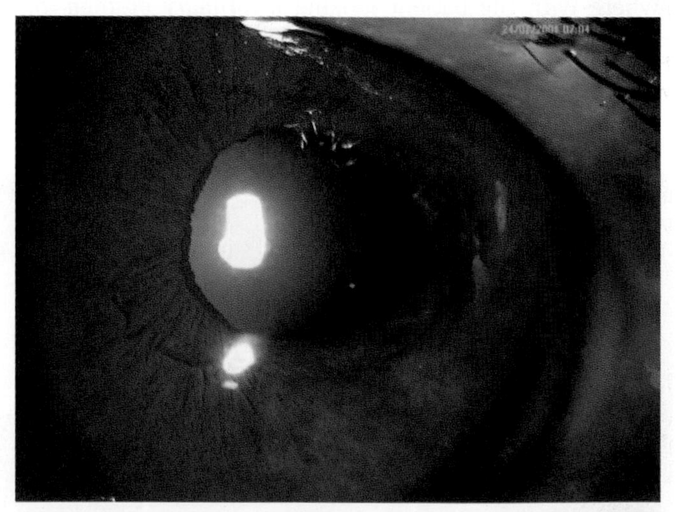

Fig. 11.10 Sectoral iris atrophy with "whorling" of radial iris folds after spontaneous resolution of angle-closure episode.

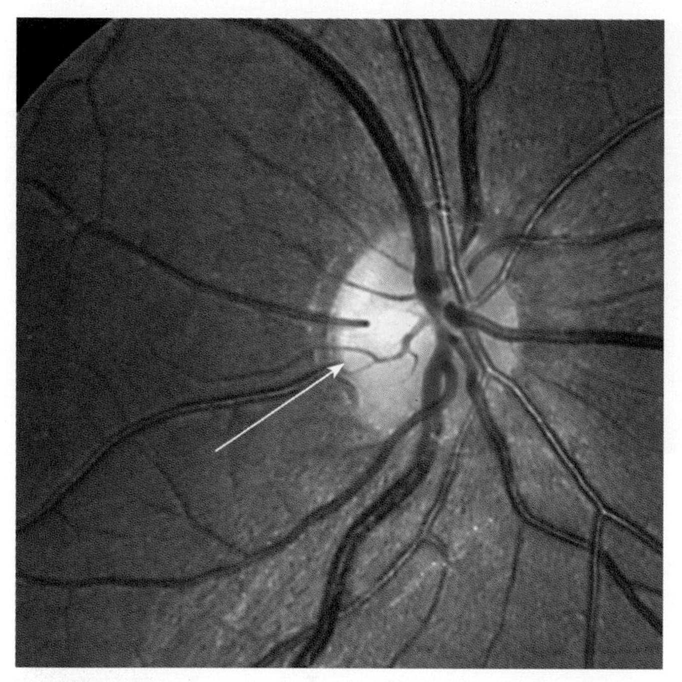

Fig. 11.11 Primary angle-closure (PAC) eyes have small optic nerve heads with commensurately small cup:disc ratio. *Arrow* pointing to area of neuroretinal rim thinning despite the cup:disc ratio being 0.5.

Gonioscopy in such eyes shows an occludable angle, with no angle structures visible in primary position, only the cornea and iris. On *indentation* with a four-mirror gonioscope or manipulation with a two- or single-mirror gonioscope, one can look over the convexity of the iris into the angle recess (**Fig. 11.12**). For *manipulation*, the patient should be asked to look toward the mirror being observed or the Goldmann gonioscope mirror can be slid toward the angle being seen. In PAC eyes, indentation or manipulation would allow visualization of the presence of blotchy pigment deposition from prior iridotrabecular contact, or any PAS (**Figs. 11.13** and **11.14**).

Thomas et al re-examined 37 patients diagnosed as PAC during a population-based study, after 5 years. A progression to PACG was noted in 28.5%, based on optic disc damage and field defects on automated perimetry. *Progression was significantly more frequent, 36.8% in patients who had refused an iridotomy, and only 11.1% who underwent iridotomy.*

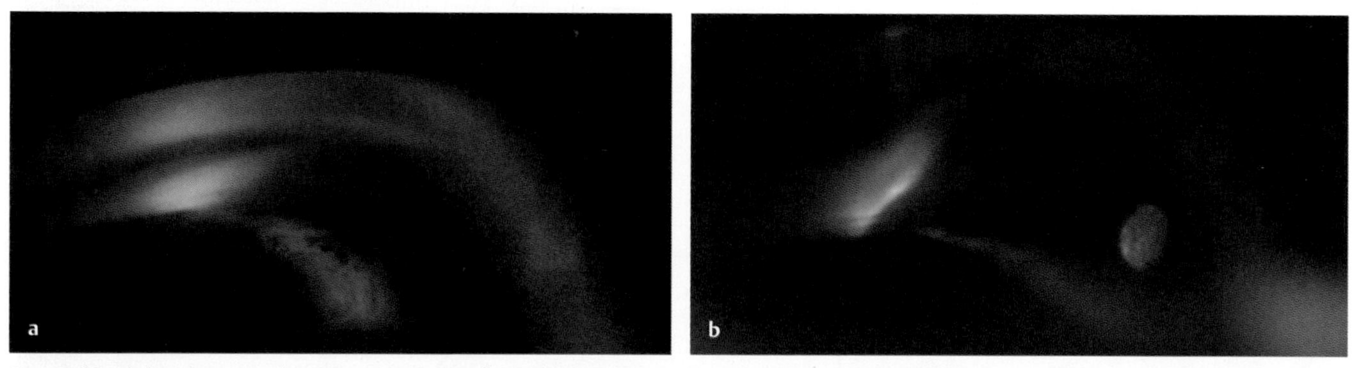

Fig. 11.12 **(a)** Gonioscopy shows a convex iris configuration preventing the visualization of any angle structures. **(b)** On manipulation, the corneal wedge, Schwalbe's line, and anterior and posterior pigmented trabecular meshwork can be seen. The angle recess is around 20 degrees.

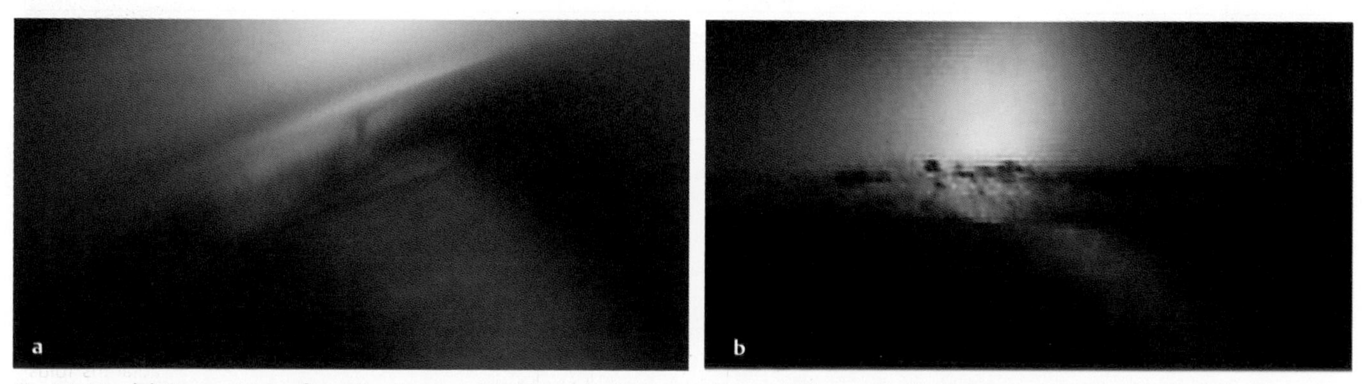

Fig. 11.13 **(a)** Convex iris configuration in an occludable angle. On manipulation a filiform synechia is seen in a 35-year-old daughter of a patient with primary angle-closure glaucoma (PACG). **(b)** Blotchy pigment above Schwalbe's line and on trabecular meshwork.

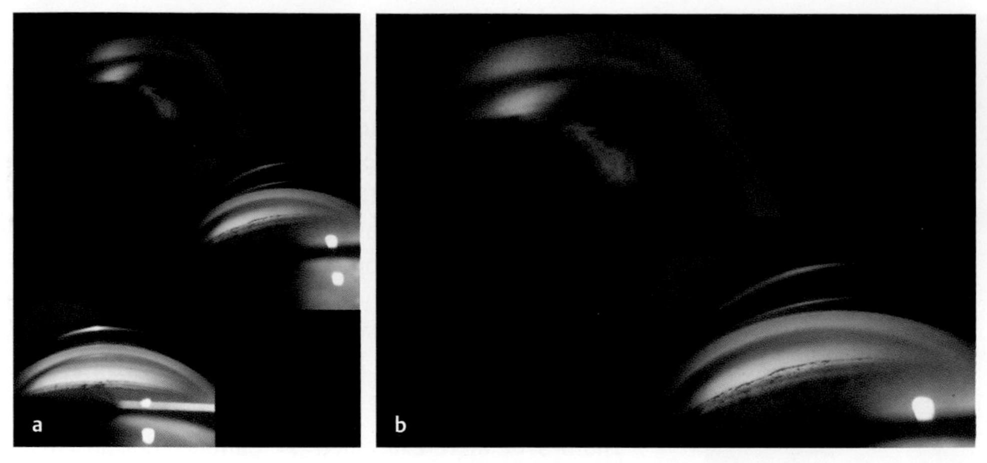

Fig. 11.14 **(a)** Trabecular structures seen after manipulation in an occludable angle—diffuse pigmentation of trabecular meshwork and two large blotches of pigment. **(b)** Irregular pigmentation of the trabecular meshwork and anterior to Schwalbe's line. Tenting of the peripheral iris forming peripheral anterior synechiae.

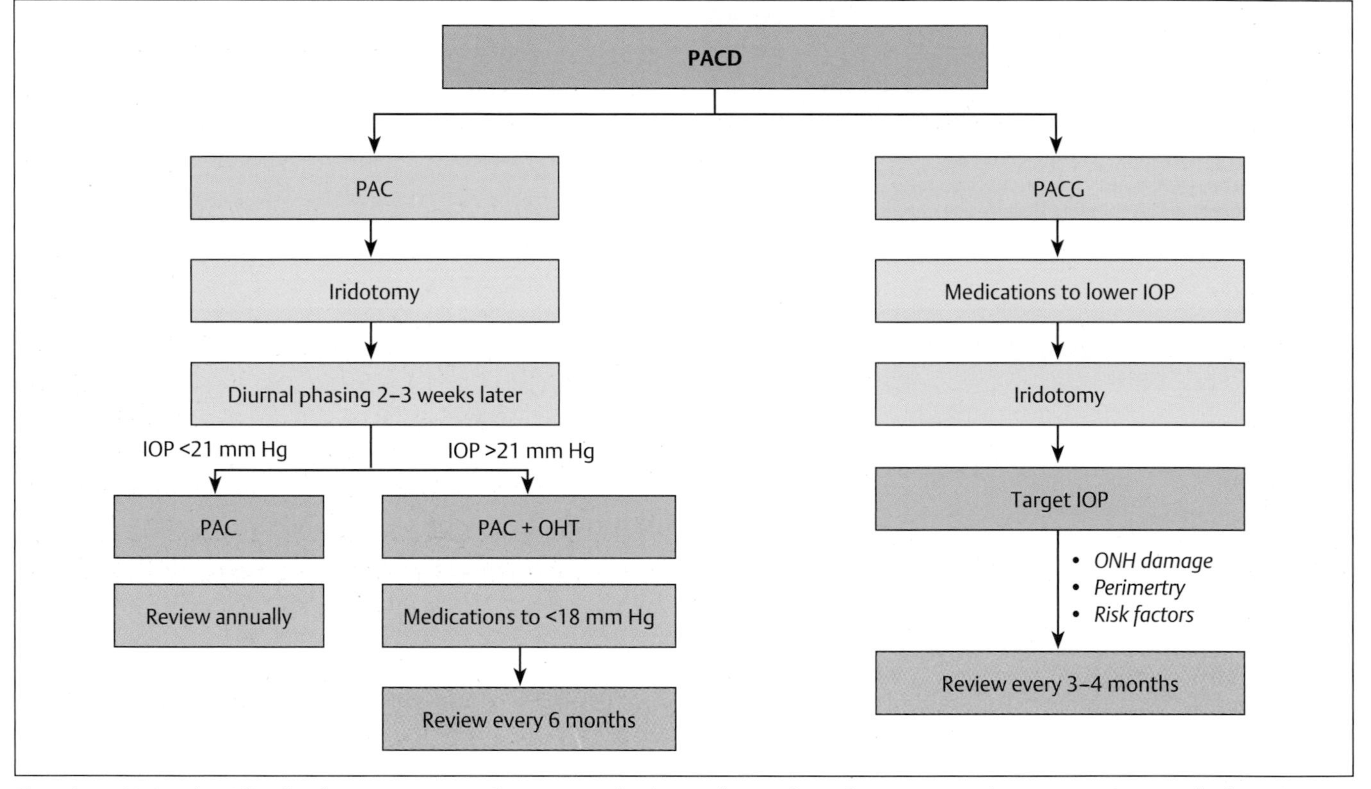

Flowchart 11.1 Algorithm for the management of primary angle-closure disease (PACD). IOP, intraocular pressure; OHT, ocular hypertension; ONH, optic nerve head; PAC, primary angle closure; PACG, primary angle-closure glaucoma.

Management

The management of PAC eyes would be a laser iridotomy in both eyes followed 6 weeks later by gonioscopy to look for residual angle closure and a chronically raised IOP.

Iridotomy

All PAC/PAC with OHT/PACG eyes should undergo an iridotomy, as relative pupillary block is seen to a smaller or greater extent in all these eyes (**Flowchart 11.1**). A Nd:YAG (neodymium:yttrium aluminum garnet) iridotomy of about 200 to 250 µm has been shown to be safe in the long term (**Fig. 11.15**). An Nd:YAG iridotomy is performed at a mid-peripheral crypt/site in the superonasal quadrant. Two to eight laser spots with energy of 4 to 6 mJ in one to three pulses are delivered quickly to penetrate the iris till a gush of aqueous with pigments is noticed. *After the iridotomy, one additional glaucoma medication should be added to any glaucoma medications the patient may already be using, and a topical steroid given for 5 days.* After 6 weeks slit-lamp examination for visualization of the lens surface and transillumination through the iridotomy should be done to ensure a patent iridotomy of at least 200 mm, and

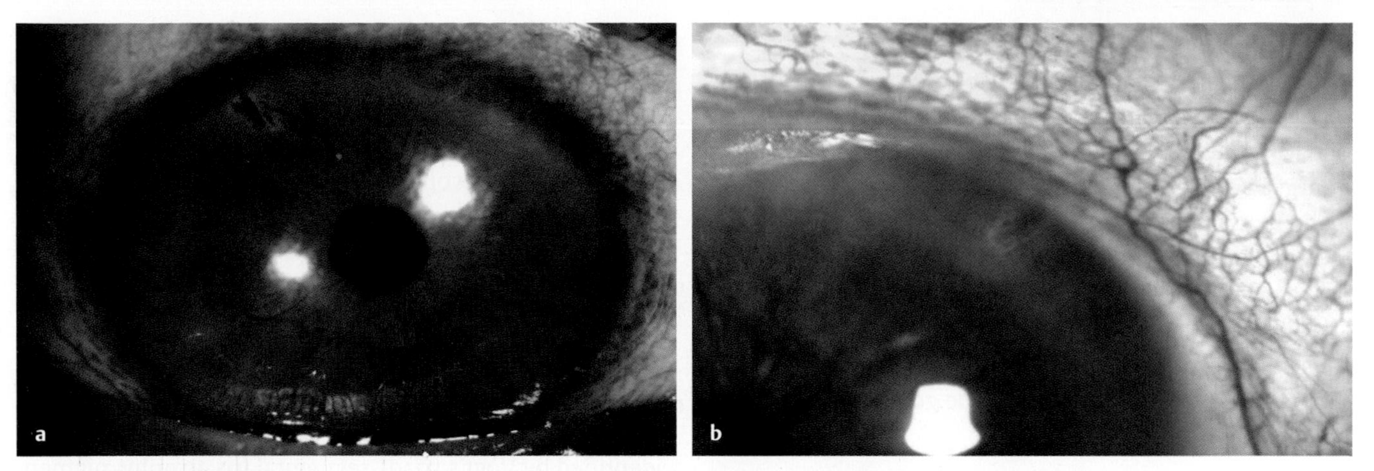

Fig. 11.15 **(a)** An iridotomy of appropriate size and placement. **(b)** An iridotomy of appropriate size but too peripherally placed, liable to get blocked with pupillary dilation.

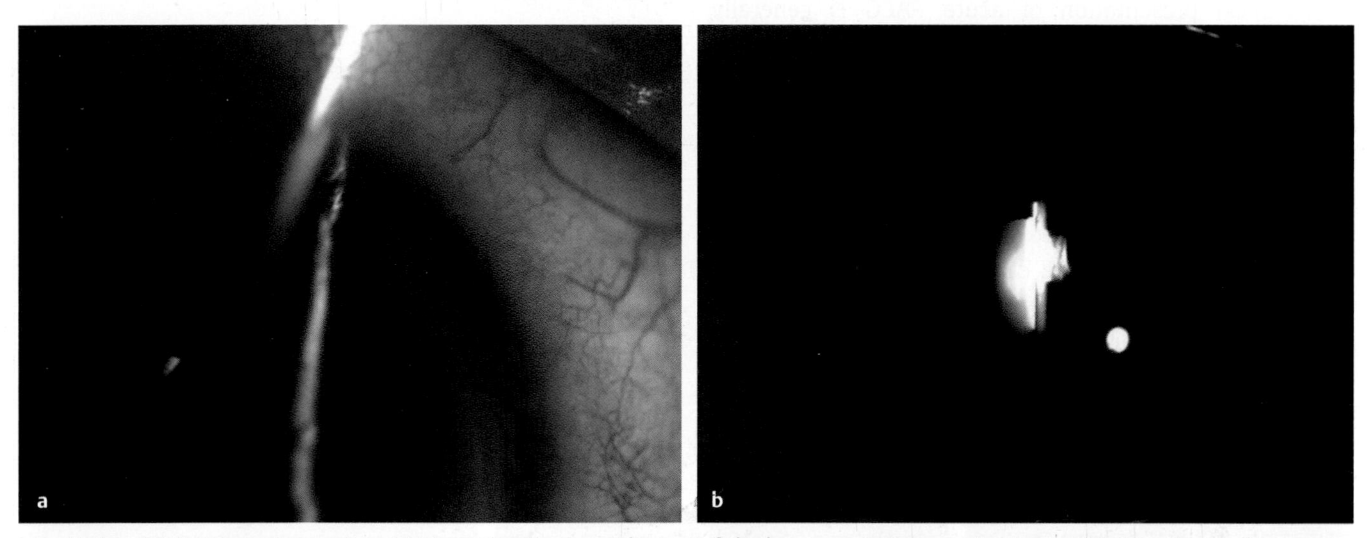

Fig. 11.16 **(a)** Judging patency of an iridotomy by direct visualization of the lens capsule through the defect. **(b)** Retroillumination may be fallacious if thinned tissue remains.

gonioscopy should be repeated to look for residual angle closure and its possible causes, plateau iris, or lens vault that may occur in some individuals (**Fig. 11.16**).

Iridotomy prevents further attacks of angle closure, but cannot change trabecular outflow status. A diurnal phasing should be done 3 weeks after iridotomy and any raised IOP has to be controlled to an appropriate target IOP. There may be continued positivity on provocative tests in eyes having PAS or an anteriorly rotated ciliary body, smaller anterior chamber angle dimensions, and a thicker iris.

Corneal decompensation reported after iridotomy was seen only when argon laser was used, alone or after sequential argon and YAG laser iridotomy.

Lifelong review, once in 6 months, is important, as *about a third are likely to develop a raised IOP over 4 to 5 years.* A baseline objective record of the IOP and optic nerve head or retinal nerve fiber layer would facilitate the diagnosis of change over time. *This is a stage at which it is possible to prevent the development of glaucomatous optic neuropathy.*

Primary Angle Closure with Hypertension

An eye with an occludable angle showing evidence of iridotrabecular contact, and chronically raised IOP after an iridotomy, should be considered PAC with OHT. *The corrected IOP should be above 97.5th percentile of a population, or >21 mm Hg. A suspicion of glaucomatous optic neuropathy could be expected in some eyes; no visual field defects should be present.*

This change over time to a chronically raised IOP may be caused by increasing trabecular meshwork dysfunction due to iridotrabecular contact or additional age-related changes in due course.

Management

Therapy should be started if the IOP rises to >26 mm Hg or there is evidence of progression on imaging or perimetry. The IOP could be lowered to "normal" range. Maintaining a target IOP of <18 mm Hg in Indian PAC with OHT eyes leads to about 20% progressing to PACG over more than 7 years. *Patients having a small disc area or requiring two or more drugs*, coronary artery disease, and using systemic steroids were more likely to progress and should have their IOP lowered further, with frequent review. The prognosis in such eyes appears to be good on therapy and lifelong review.

Primary Acute Angle-Closure Glaucoma

The clinical presentation of acute PACG is generally unmistakable: a congested, painful eye with a history of colored halos, intermittent blurring, and sudden diminution of vision. This is accompanied by severe unilateral headache and even nausea.

On examination, ciliary congestion, corneal edema, a vertically oval, mid-dilated pupil with a very high IOP, generally 40 mm Hg or more, can be seen (**Fig. 11.17a**). The anterior chamber is generally very shallow, and there may be pigment dispersion on the cornea and lens (**Fig. 11.17b, c**). Occasionally, posterior synechiae can be present.

Gonioscopy, if possible, initially will show a totally closed angle in most such eyes. After early resolution of the attack some PAS may be seen; however, if the attack persists for more than 2 to 3 days, extensive PAS extending up to the Schwalbe's line can be seen (**Fig. 11.17d, e**).

On fundus examination soon after resolution of the attack, the eye would have disc edema with possibly some retinal hemorrhages, similar to decompression retinopathy. The disc edema in the immediate aftermath of the attack resolves with control of IOP, to leave optic nerve head pallor in many eyes. Anterior ischemic neuropathy and retinal vascular occlusions have been described with an acute angle-closure attack.

Past attacks of primary acute angle closure can be identified by Vogt's triad—segmental iris atrophy, pigment dispersion, and glaucomflecken (**Fig. 11.17f**).

Management

Management requires lowering the IOP as quickly as possible with systemic and topical glaucoma medications. *After checking systemic history and blood pressure* intravenous (IV) mannitol should be given. Acetazolamide 500 mg and 1 oz of glycerol should also be given orally stat. All possible topical drugs like timolol, brimonidine, and brinzolamide/dorzolamide should be instilled to lower the IOP as much as possible. Once the IOP begins to settle down, within about 30 minutes, pilocarpine 2% should be instilled two to three times at half hour intervals to constrict the pupil and pull the iris out of the angle. Pilocarpine cannot work in an eye with high IOPs, such as 40 mm Hg. *Pilocarpine should be instilled 8 hourly in the fellow eye.*

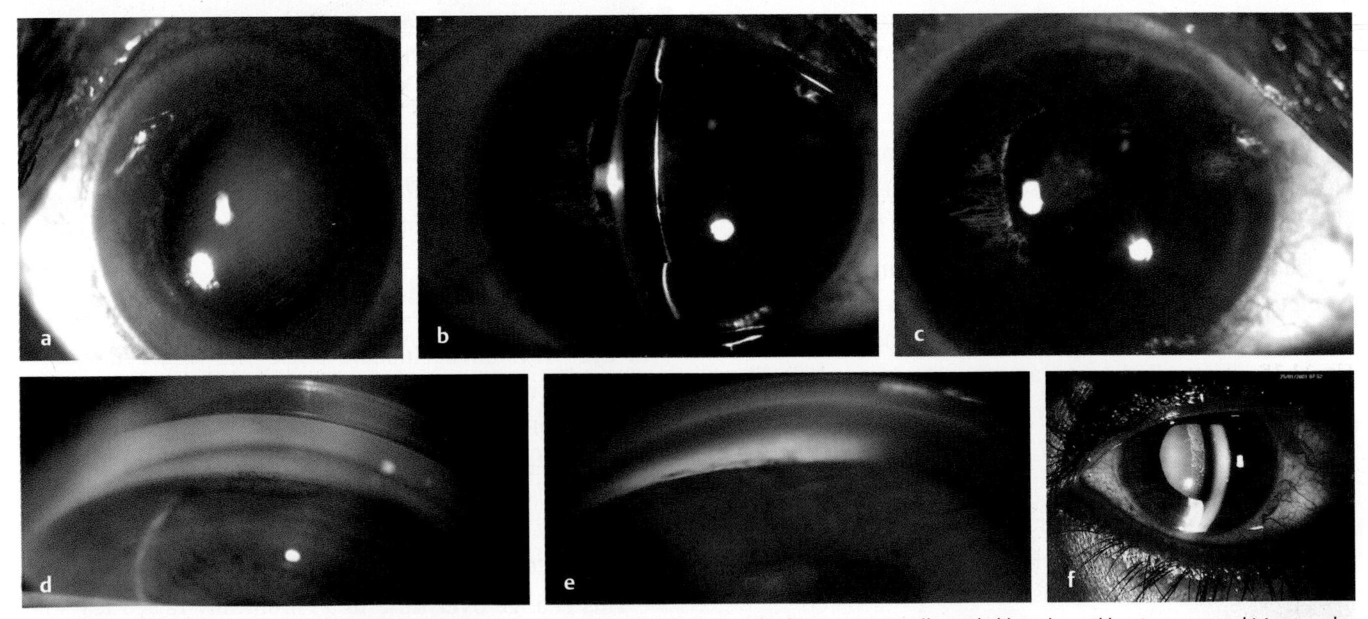

Fig. 11.17 **(a)** Eye with resolving acute angle closure. Ciliary congestion, corneal edema, a vertically mid-dilated pupil having sectoral iris atrophy from 6 to 11 o'clock. **(b, c)** Shallow anterior chamber, mid-dilated vertically oval pupil, steep iris configuration, sector iris atrophy, and anterior subcapsular cataract after resolution of primary acute angle-closure glaucoma. **(d)** Extensive peripheral anterior synechiae seen after resolution of an acute attack and iridotomy. **(e)** Convex iris configuration and completely closed angle with pigmentation seen anterior to Schwalbe's line, giving a misleading appearance of trabecular meshwork—"false" angle. **(f)** Primary acute angle-closure glaucoma. Eight hours after lowering of intraocular pressure (IOP) from 60 to 20 mm Hg, corneal edema and Descemet's folds are seen with anterior subcapsular cataract.

In the event that the attack doesn't resolve, pressure with a cotton tip in the center of the cornea can sometimes help direct aqueous toward the periphery and push the iris back, away from the cornea. Other measures suggested are laser peripheral iridoplasty to pull the peripheral iris away from the trabecular meshwork. This has been shown to work as well as medical therapy, but causes significant pigment release, diffuse corneal endothelial burns, and inflammation in the eye.

Once the eye quietens down, a laser peripheral iridotomy should be done in both eyes, and may require more than one sitting at an interval of 2 to 3 days. Following this, systemic glaucoma medications should be tapered, and then topical medications should be continued. Iridotomy alone may control the IOP if the attack is aborted within 1 to 2 days. If the symptoms have lasted longer, over 5 to 7 days, the chances of a chronically raised IOP are higher due to sustained trabecular damage. Glaucoma medicines can be gradually tapered off, with a careful review over 3 to 4 months. About 20 to 50% of the eyes may require continued therapy, or even a trabeculectomy, which in an inflamed eye would need to be augmented with mitomycin C 0.02% for 1 minute subconjunctival application, and releasable sutures to prevent a postoperative shallow anterior chamber.

Prognosis

Most acute PACG eyes show an IOP control with iridotomy alone or with additional medications, but show evidence of some optic neuropathy, after the attack resolves. Target IOP would depend on the severity of glaucomatous visual field loss and should stabilize the eye.

Primary Angle-Closure Glaucoma

PACG eyes have an occludable angle, PAS over more than 180 degrees, and a definitive glaucomatous optic neuropathy, with a chronically raised IOP after iridotomy. More than 80% can be asymptomatic.

Clinically, a shallow anterior chamber, with often a *featureless iris with no iris crypts and significant pupillary ruff atrophy*, is seen (**Fig. 11.18**). On gonioscopy, extensive PAS and trabecular pigmentation are present (**Fig. 11.19**). Fundus examination shows a small optic nerve head in which loss of neuroretinal rim has to be carefully looked for, as crowding of the optic nerve fibers makes the cup appear small even with an neuroretinal rim notch or loss of neuroretinal rim (**Figs. 11.20** and **11.21**). The untreated IOP is generally higher than that seen in POAG eyes, a mean of 32 to 34 mm Hg.

Management

All PACG eyes should undergo an *iridotomy as it allows the iris to fall back as aqueous passes through the patent iridotomy, and areas of the trabecular meshwork without synechiae are exposed and may begin to function to the extent possible.* The iridotomy also prevents further episodes of the angle closure that have caused trabecular meshwork dysfunction.

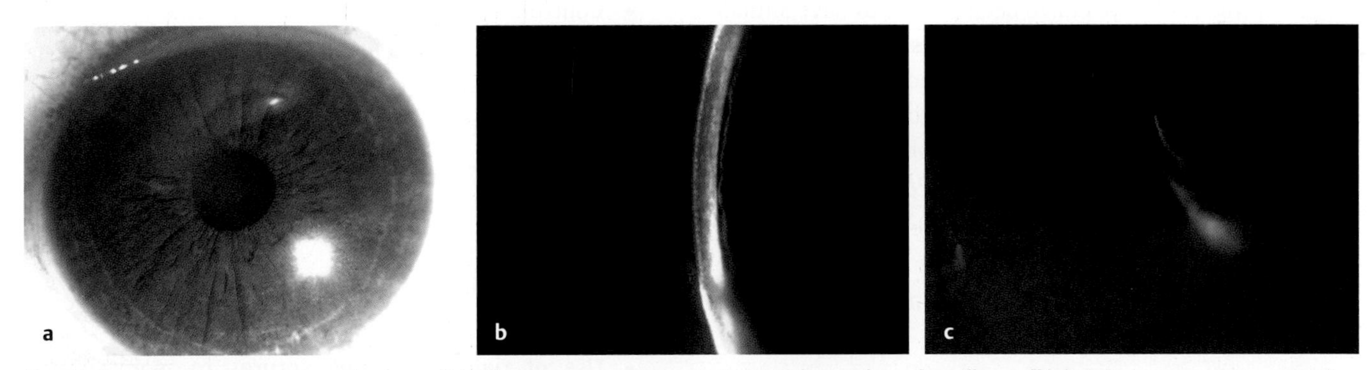

Fig. 11.18 Primary angle-closure glaucoma (PACG). Anterior segment examination shows a loss of pupillary ruff **(a)**. Anterior segment examination shows a loss of pupillary ruff and sphincter atrophy between 9 and 12 o'clock leading to a loss of radial folds **(b, c)**, van Herick grade 1.

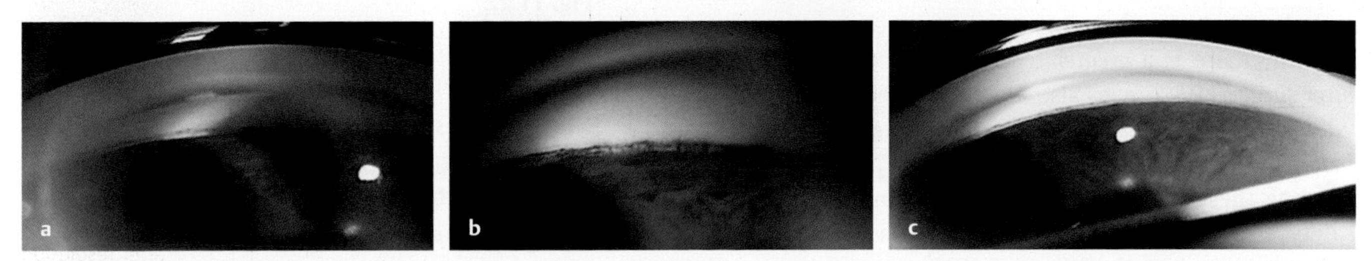

Fig. 11.19 Primary angle-closure glaucoma (PACG). **(a)** Occludable angle on primary gaze, with pigment seen anterior to Schwalbe's line. **(b)** Extensive peripheral anterior synechiae present. **(c)** PACG. "False" angle. Completely closed angle on manipulation, convex iris configuration with iris seen adherent to just behind Schwalbe's line, and pigmentation anterior to Schwalbe's line give a false impression of an open angle.

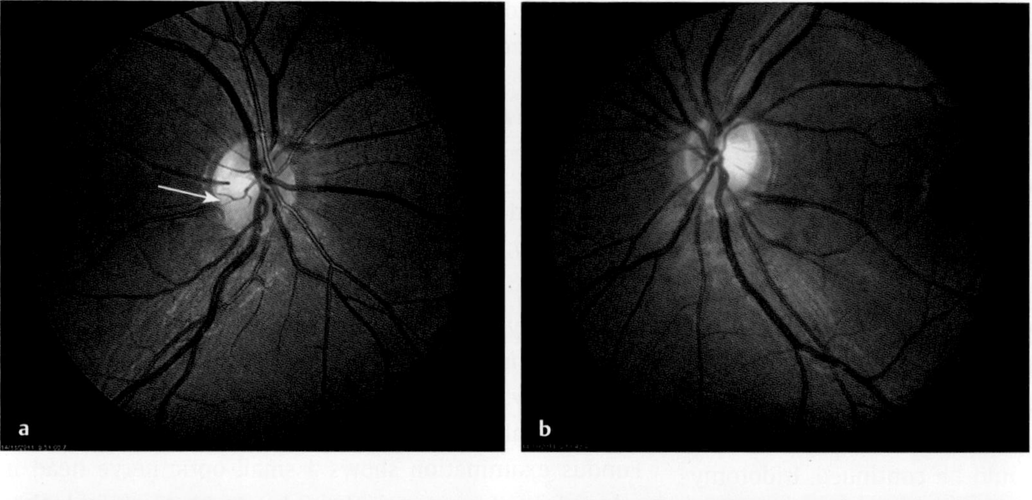

Fig. 11.20 (a, b) Chronic primary angle-closure glaucoma (CPACG)—small optic nerve heads, with asymmetry between the two eyes (*white arrow*). Right eye has a thin neuroretinal rim from 7 to 11 o'clock, with a cup:disc ratio of 0.5. Left eye shows a retinal nerve fiber layer defect at 4 to 5 o'clock despite a cup:disc ratio of only 0.6. The cup is not deep, but saucer like.

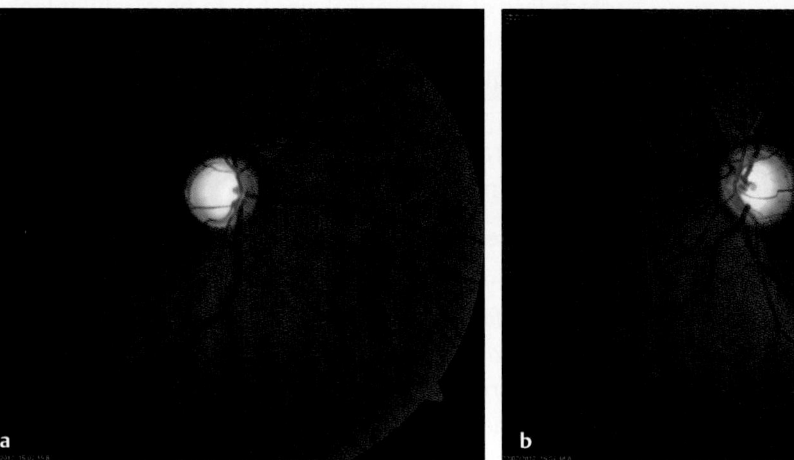

Fig. 11.21 (a, b) Primary angle-closure glaucoma (PACG). Small optic nerve heads showing cup:disc ratio of 0.9 and 0.8 with associated retinal nerve fiber layer defects. The cups are shelving, not deep.

As chronic PACG eyes have been shown to have similar factors associated with progression as POAG, setting a similar "target" IOP based on early, moderate, or severe visual field loss of <18, 15 to 17, and 12 to 14 mm Hg would help stabilize the neuropathy. *Fluctuations in IOP over visits should be minimized.* It is thought that PACG eyes progress faster than POAG, and a closer review may be required.

About 10% of such eyes may progress in 10 years due to age-related trabecular meshwork dysfunction, compliance issues, or the use of steroids.

Trabeculectomy in PACG

As all PACG have a shallower anterior chamber than normal, and the aim of trabeculectomy is to increase aqueous outflow, there is a *greater tendency to have shallow ACs after surgery*. PACG eyes also have high preoperative IOPs, which *may predispose to suprachoroidal hemorrhage, and malignant glaucoma intraoperatively and postoperatively*. Keeping these historically known problems in mind, the safety and efficacy of trabeculectomy in PACG can be enhanced by taking the following steps:

- Laser iridotomy prior to surgery.
- Controlling IOP to near-normal levels with systemic glaucoma medications preoperatively.
- IV mannitol half an hour prior to surgery to deturgesce the vitreous.
- Paracentesis after making a superficial sclera flap to reduce IOP and maintaining the anterior chamber with air.
- Stromal ostium to be removed only when the eye is soft.
- Use of tight releasable sutures to maintain the anterior chamber in the early postoperative period (**Fig. 11.22**).
- Use of short-acting cycloplegics to keep the iris mobile, not opposed to the sclera ostium.
- Release sutures after a couple of days when (i) anterior chamber is formed, (ii) bleb is not overfiltering, and (iii) IOP is on the higher side of target.

Cataract surgery in PACD is difficult, as the anterior chamber volume is less than 1 mL, making the corneal endothelium just millimeters away from a phacoemulsification probe.

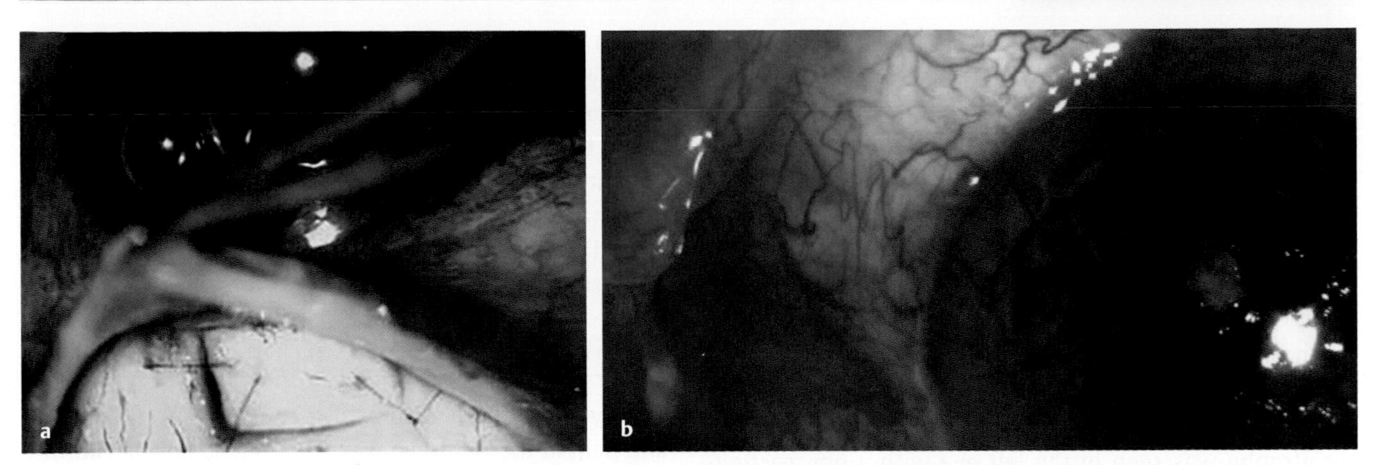

Fig. 11.22 **(a)** Two fixed sutures at the corners and two releasable sutures at the limbus are used to maintain the anterior chamber in the early postoperative period. **(b)** Box-type suture seen on the cornea.

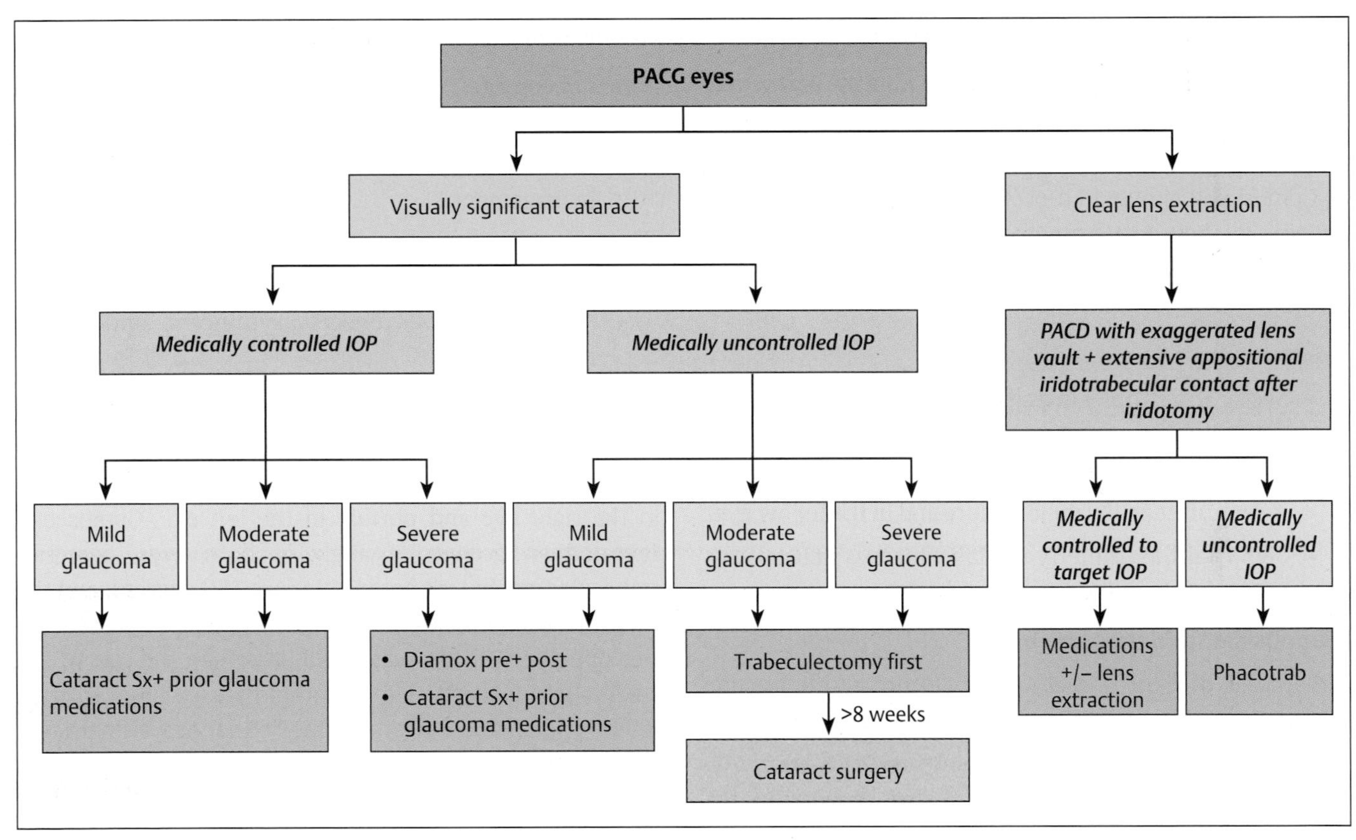

Flowchart 11.2 Algorithm for proper management and review of patients after cataract surgery. IOP, intraocular pressure; PACD, primary angle-closure disease; PACG, primary angle-closure glaucoma.

An atonic and atrophic iris in such eyes further leads to poor dilation and repeated prolapse of the iris. Capsulorhexis is difficult in these conditions, with poor maneuverability and a steep anterior lens capsule. The postoperative course is often stormy with a rise in IOP seen. Expulsive hemorrhage and malignant glaucoma are dreaded complications seen more often in PACG eyes. *In the EAGLE study, the difference in IOP between iridotomy or cataract surgery in PAC or PACG eyes was 1.15 mm Hg only after 3 years.*

As cataract surgery cannot alter/reverse trabecular damage, patient with chronically raised IOP and a glaucomatous neuropathy need close review and often continued glaucoma medications after cataract surgery **(Flowchart 11.2)**.

PACG and its blindness are preventable. If diagnosed early, an iridotomy performed, and target IOP maintained with lifelong review, prognosis is good.

Cases

Case 1

A 63-year-old lady complained of diminution of vision in the left eye. There was a past history of severe pain and redness of the left eye with a left-sided unilateral headache a year ago. She also complained of frequent unilateral headaches.

On examination, the corneas were on the smaller side of normal, with very shallow ACs in both eyes, the iris in the right eye was within normal limits, while extensive sectoral iris atrophy was seen in the left eye with a nonreacting pupil. There was a senile cataract in the left eye. Optic nerves in both eyes were small, and had a cup:disc ratio of 0.9:1 with a very thin and pale neuroretinal rim in the left eye, while the right eye had cup:disc ratio of 0.3:1. Applanation tonometry was 16 and 38 mm Hg, and vision was 6/6 in the right eye and counting fingers close to face in the left eye (**Case 1-1**).

Gonioscopy showed an occludable angle in both eyes, opening to show just a few blotchy pigments in the right eye, and a totally closed angle in the left eye with only Schwalbe's line visible.

Points to consider

- Sector iris atrophy in a shallow anterior chamber is a common sign of past acute angle closure.
- Asymmetry in extent of PAS and trabecular damage is seen after acute angle closure and in the fellow eye.
- Significant asymmetry of glaucomatous neuropathy is often seen in PACD.

Diagnosis and Management

A diagnosis of right primary angle closure and left acute angle closure progressing to chronic PACG was made.

The patient was started on pilocarpine 2% 8 hourly in both eyes, and bimatoprost, timolol, and brimonidine in the left eye. An Nd:YAG iridotomy was done in both eyes. After 1 week the IOP was 14 mm Hg in the right eye and 22 mm Hg in the left eye. On repeat gonioscopy, the angle was seen to have opened significantly in the right eye, but not in the left eye. Poor visual prognosis was explained to the patient for the left eye and a combined phacoemulsification with trabeculectomy was done. After 1 year her IOPs were 14 and 16 mm Hg in the right eye and left eye, respectively using timolol bd in the left eye.

Case 2

A 50-year-old lady with a history of occasional redness and pain in the right eye was recorded to have a cup:disc ratio of 0.5 and an IOP of 26 mm Hg in the right eye, and a cup:disc ratio of 0.3 and an IOP of 12 mm Hg in the left eye. She was referred for further evaluation with a diagnosis of chronic simple glaucoma.

Points to consider

- There was no record of anterior chamber depth or gonioscopy, which are imperative in glaucoma management.
- A cup:disc ratio of even 0.5 becomes significant in a small optic nerve head present in PACD.
- Asymmetric IOP reflects asymmetric optic nerve head damage.

Diagnosis and Management

On examination, her anterior chamber was van Herick grade 1 in both eyes, and pupillary ruff was completely absent in the right eye and normal in the left eye. Gonioscopy revealed an occludable angle in both eyes, posterior trabecular meshwork not visible for >180 degrees, and the right eye had PAS extending over 180 degrees (**Case 2-1**). Her optic nerve head was small, less than the size of the small spot on the Welch Allyn ophthalmoscope, with an inferior notch and corresponding retinal nerve fiber layer defect in the right eye. On perimetry a superior nasal step was present in the right eye, while the left was within normal limits.

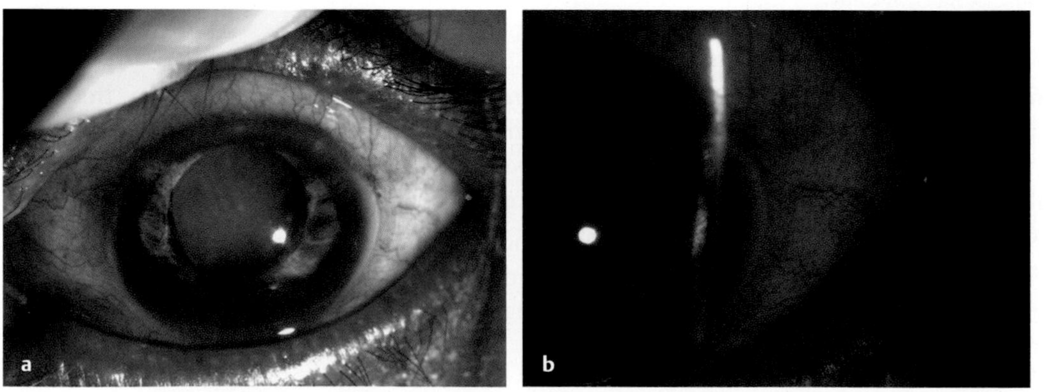

Case 1-1 **(a)** Sector iris atrophy with a vertically dilated, nonreactive pupil, and **(b)** grade 1 anterior chamber.

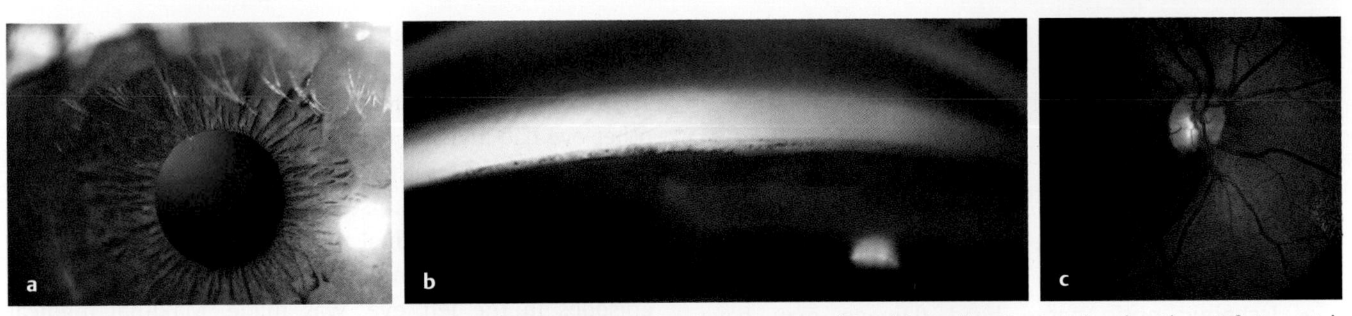

Case 2-1 Right eye. **(a)** Absence of pupillary ruff. **(b)** Extensive peripheral anterior synechiae. **(c)** Small optic nerve head, with an inferior notch and corresponding wedge-shaped retinal nerve fiber layer defect.

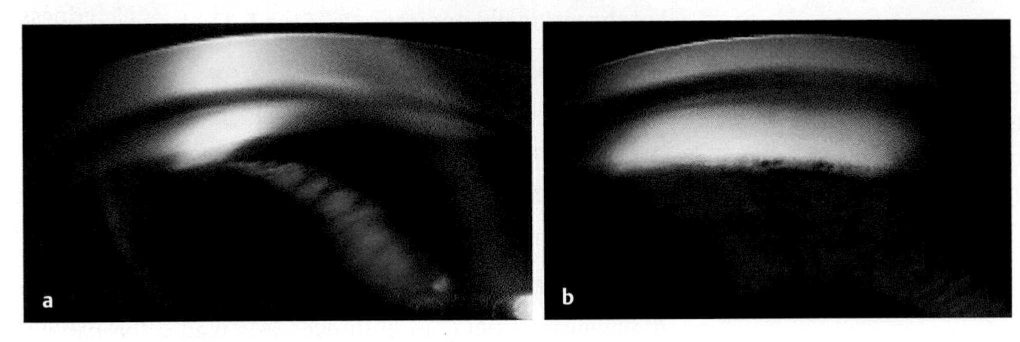

Case 3-1 **(a)** Occludable angle in which the posterior pigmented trabecular meshwork is not visible. **(b)** On manipulation clumps of iris pigment are seen attached to the trabecular meshwork.

A diagnosis of PACG in the right eye and left eye fellow eye was made, and an iridotomy done in both eyes to prevent further attacks. Diurnal phasing 2 weeks later recorded IOPs of 18 to 26 mm Hg in the right eye and 12 to 14 mm Hg in the left eye. She was advised to use a prostaglandin (PG) analog once a day in the right eye. On review 3 weeks later the peak IOP in the right eye was 20 mm Hg, still higher than the target IOP of 15 to 17 mm Hg, and timolol twice a day was added, after checking her pulse for regularity and rate and for a history of breathlessness/ asthma. Her IOP reduced to 16 mm Hg and she was advised a review every 4 months initially.

Case 3

The 30-year-old daughter of a patient having PACG was examined. There was a shallow anterior chamber, van Herick grade 2, with a normal iris and pupillary ruff. The cup:disc ratio was 0.3 in both eyes. Gonioscopy showed an angle recess of approximately 15 degrees, with only the Schwalbe's line visible in primary position while using a 2-mm height of beam. On manipulation by asking the patient to look toward the mirror, the posterior trabecular meshwork (PTM) was visible in areas, but blotchy pigment clumps were seen over 3 o'clock (**Case 3-1**).

Points to consider

- Positive family history of PACG.
- Occludable angle.
- Past angle closure evidenced by the pigment clumping seen.

Diagnosis and Management

A diagnosis of PAC in both eyes was made and an iridotomy advised in both eyes. The lady had it done in the right eye, but for personal reasons did not return for the second eye. After 5 years she was found to have a cup:disc ratio of 0.3 in the right eye and 0.5 in the left eye, with IOPs of 12 and 24 mm Hg. Gonioscopy in the right eye showed mild inferior pigmentation of the trabecular meshwork, while the left eye showed goniosynechiae over 120 degrees. Perimetry was still within normal limits, so a diagnosis of PAC in the right eye and PAC with OHT in the left eye was made, an iridotomy done and timolol prescribed for the left eye.

Case 4

A 45-year-old lady was brought to casualty with severe pain in the right eye, and nausea for 1 day. On examination there was ciliary congestion, corneal edema, and a vertically oval, mid-dilated pupil. Her IOP was 54 mm Hg in the right eye and 12 mm Hg in the left eye. She was treated with IV mannitol 350 mL, oral acetazolamide 500 mg stat, timolol, brimonidine, and half an hour later pilocarpine 2% drops. A diagnosis of acute angle-closure in the right eye was made. After 2 hours the IOP was 32 mm Hg, topical medications were continued, and oral acetazolamide 250 mg was advised every 8 hours. The next day her IOP had reduced to 24 mm Hg, and the corneal edema and ciliary congestion reduced (**Case 4-1**).

Points to consider

- An acute attack for <24 hours may not lead to significant PAS formation or trabecular damage.
- Iridotomy should not be attempted in the presence of a congested eye.
- Ischemic optic nerve head damage may have occurred.

Diagnosis and Management

After 4 days the IOP had reduced to 16 mm Hg and an iridotomy was performed in both eyes. Medications were gradually tapered over 2 months. Regular review for 5 years showed sectoral areas of iris atrophy and glaucomflecken, but the IOP was controlled with a PG analog alone and her vision and perimetry were normal.

Case 5

A 52-year-old lady was brought with a history of loss of vision in the left eye with episodes of severe pain over the last 6 months. The patient gave a history of unilateral headaches over time. On examination the left eye had a vision of perception of light and projection of rays inaccurate in three quadrants, severe ciliary congestion, marked corneal edema, and a "stony hard eye" on palpation. The IOP was unrecordable by applanation tonometry. The other eye had a vision of 6/12, shallow anterior chamber, van Herick grade 1 with evidence of sphincter atrophy, IOP of 28 mm Hg, and cup:disc ratio of 0.7 with thinning and pallor of the neuroretinal rim inferiorly and temporally. A diagnosis of PACG in both eyes, with continuing acute episodes in the left eye, was made. Maximal medical therapy—acetazolamide, glycerol, pilocarpine, timolol, and brimonidine—reduced the IOP in the left eye to 32 mm Hg but the vision did not improve (**Case 5-1**).

Points to consider

- An acute angle closure attack of over 6 months duration.
- Very poor vision.
- Very high IOP.

Diagnosis and Management

A diagnosis of PACG in both eyes was made. The patient and relatives were counseled about the poor visual prognosis for the left eye, and the need for an iridotomy in the right eye and further lifelong medications, as required. A trabeculectomy with releasable sutures was done in the left eye after preoperative mannitol. After 6 months the

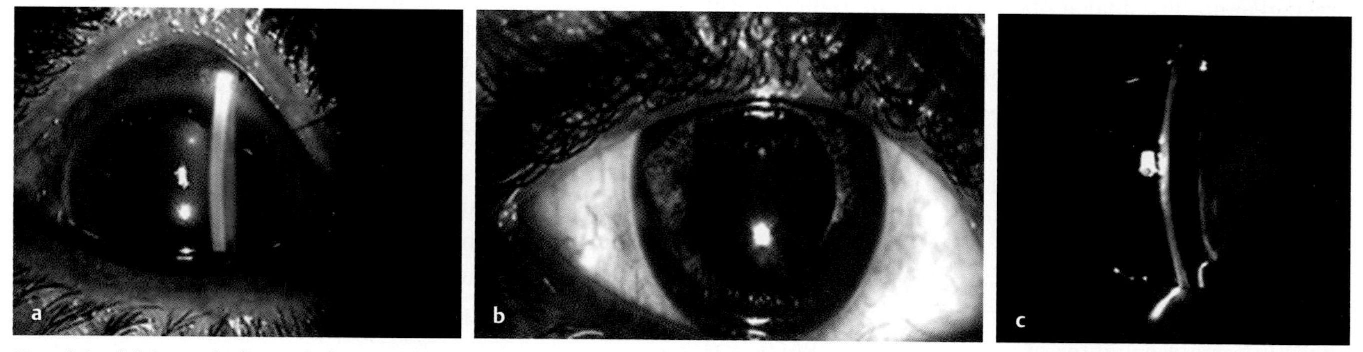

Case 4-1 **(a)** Corneal edema, shallow anterior chamber, and a vertically dilated pupil. **(b, c)** After 5 years, extensive iris atrophy can be seen with anterior subcapsular lenticular opacities—"glaucomflecken."

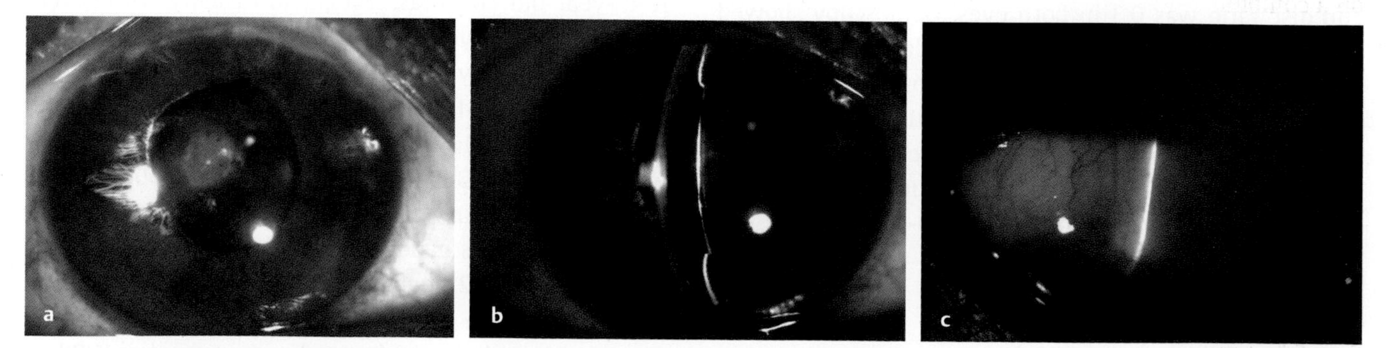

Case 5-1 **(a, b)** Vertically oval unreactive pupil and anterior subcapsular cataractous changes seen in a grade 2 anterior chamber. **(c)** Relatively avascular trabeculectomy bleb at 6 months.

IOP in the right eye was 12 to 14 mm Hg and 12 to 14 mm Hg in the left eye. The vision in the left eye only improved to 2/60. Perimetry in the right eye revealed a superior arcuate scotoma and the patient was advised to use a PG analog once a day, with a target IOP of 12 to 15 mm Hg in mind.

Case 6

A 60-year-old male had been diagnosed to have chronic simple glaucoma for 10 years, with a nasal step in both eyes. He was on regular treatment and follow-up, with IOPs recorded from 16 to 24 mm Hg, using an increasing number of glaucoma medications over time, but still continued to show visual field progression to a biarcuate scotoma in both eyes (**Case 6-1**). On gonioscopy, an angle recess of 15 degrees with PAS of >180 degrees was seen.

Points to consider

- Was the diagnosis correct? No earlier gonioscopic findings were recorded.
- Was the patient compliant?
- Target IOP for mild perimetric damage was not achieved.

Diagnosis and Management

The diagnosis was changed to PACG, and an iridotomy was done to prevent further angle closure and episodes of raised IOP. A target IOP of 10 to 12 mm Hg was set, and achieved using a PG analog, combination of timolol and pilocarpine, and a combination of brimonidine and brinzolamide. Both eyes have been stable for over 5 years. An iridotomy done at first diagnosis could have prevented angle-closure attacks, progression of PAS in a narrow angle, and progressively increasing IOP and glaucomatous neuropathy over time.

Case 7

A 49-year-old male had a baseline IOP was 18 mm Hg in the right eye and 46 mm Hg in the left eye. He was started on a combination of timolol and brimonidine drops in the left eye. On examination, best corrected visual acuity was 6/6 in the right eye and 6/18 in the left eye. IOPs were 16 and 28 mm Hg in in the right eye and left eye, respectively. A PG analog and dorzolamide were added to the left eye, but IOP remained high at 22 mm Hg.

On slit-lamp examination, anterior chamber of van Herick grade 2 was present with patchy pupillary ruff atrophy. A relative afferent pupillary defect was present in the left eye. On gonioscopy, occludable angles with visible goniosynechiae was seen in both eyes, left eye > right eye, with blotchy pigmentation in the left eye. Fundus examination of right eye showed a cup:disc ratio of 0.5:1 and cup:disc ratio of 0.9:1 in the left eye. Humphrey visual field examination showed right eye to be normal and in the left eye only a central island of vision remained (**Case 7-1**).

Points to consider

- Young male with angle closure bilaterally.
- Baseline IOP of >40 mm Hg is unlikely to be controlled on medication to achieve a target IOP of 12 mm Hg.
- Asymmetry of damage is more common in PACD than POAG.

Diagnosis and Management

A diagnosis of PAC in the right eye and chronic PACG in the left eye was made after ruling out microspherophakia or subluxated lenses. He underwent left eye trabeculectomy with 0.02% mitomycin C used for 1 minute subconjunctivally (**Case 7-2a**). The right eye underwent Nd:YAG peripheral iridotomy and was prescribed a PG analog (**Case 7-2b**). After 8 years he developed a visually significant cataract in the left eye and phacoemulsification was done. He was continued on topical drugs in the right eye and has had stable Humphrey visual fields.

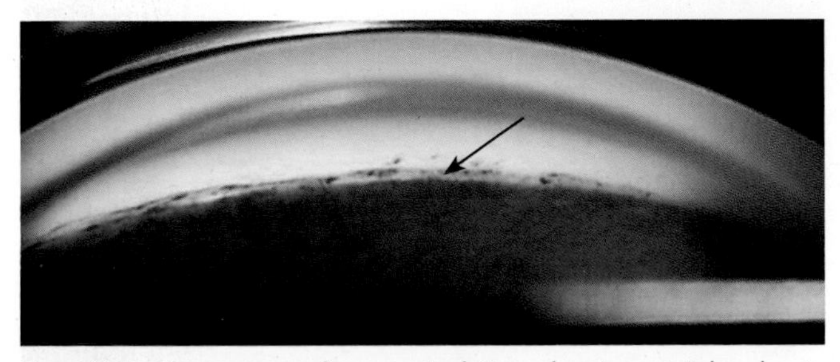

Case 6-1 Gonioscopy after manipulation showing peripheral anterior synechiae (*black arrow*) up to Schwalbe's line and pigmentation anterior to the Schwalbe's line.

Case 8

A 54-year-old man with a family history of glaucoma reported for a check-up. He was found to have a vision of 6/6 in both eyes, a shallow anterior chamber with a flat iris configuration, van Herick grade 2, pupillary ruff atrophy in both eyes, and sphincter atrophy in the left eye, with a sluggish pupillary reaction. Cup:disc ratio was 0.6 with a regular neuroretinal rim in the right eye and 0.8 with a very thin and pale neuroretinal rim at both poles in the left eye. IOPs were 20 and 32 mm Hg and his gonioscopy showed an angle recess of 15 degrees in the right eye with goniosynechiae of 90 degrees and pigmentation grade 2. In the left eye a completely closed angle was present. On perimetry there was a central island of vision in the left eye and the right eye was within normal limits (**Case 8-1**).

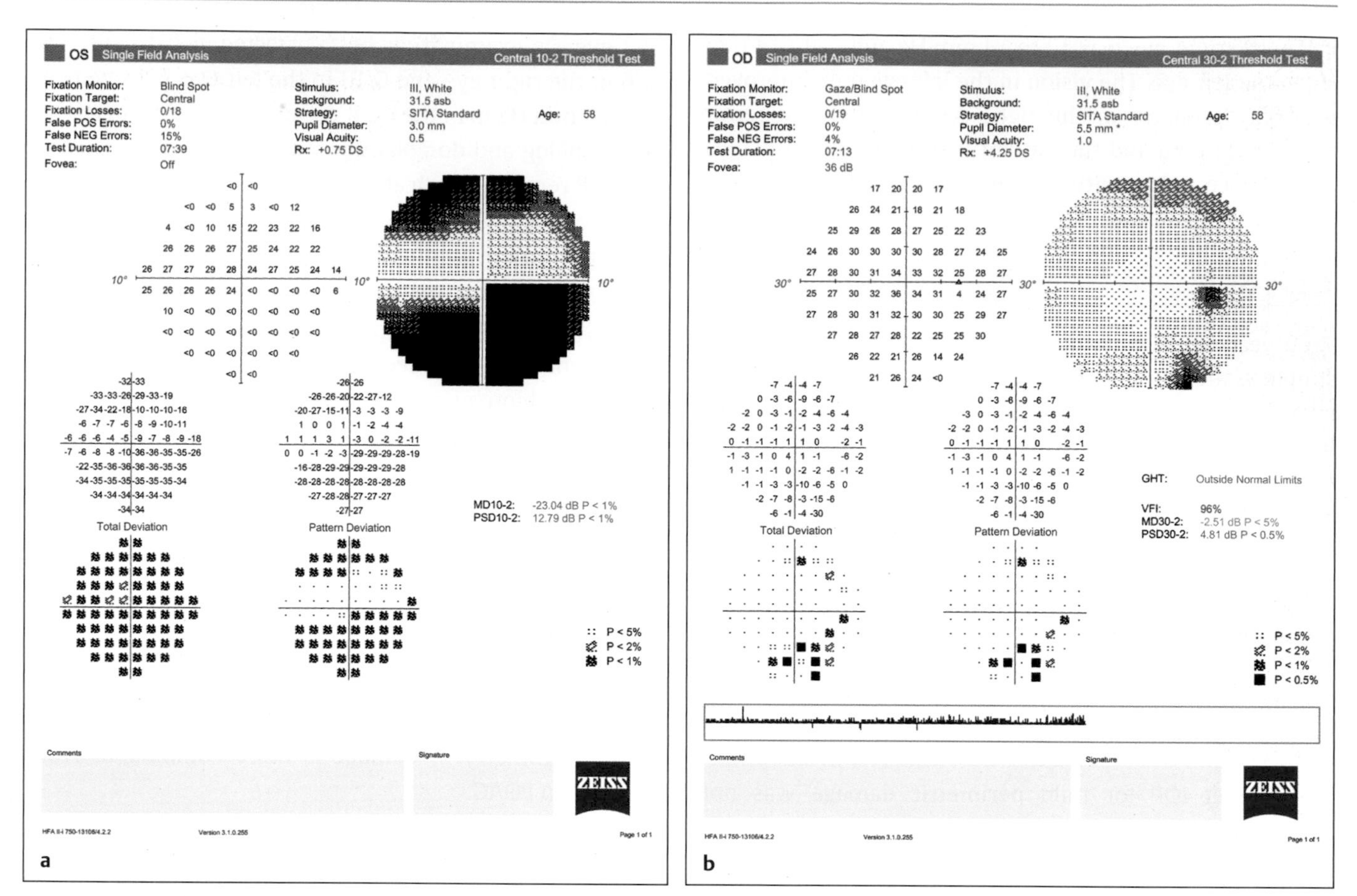

Case 7-1 Humphrey visual field examination showed no defect on 30-2 SITA Standard in right **(a)** and remaining central island of vision on 10-2 SITA Standard in left eye **(b)**.

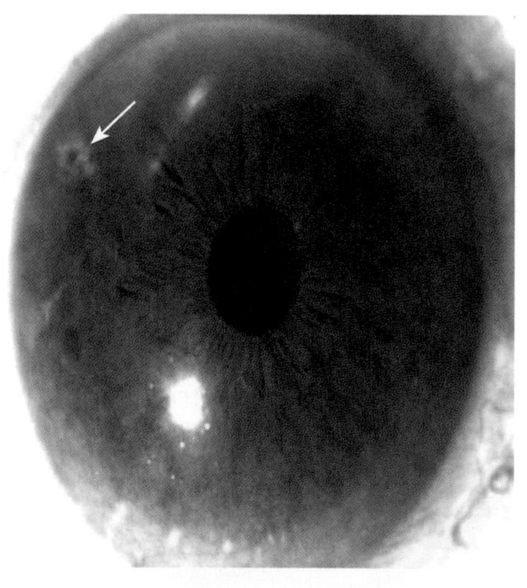

Case 7-2 **(a)** Clinical picture of the left eye showing a diffuse superonasal bleb which is mildly elevated, moderately vascular. **(b)** Clinical picture of the right eye showing a superotemporal patent peripheral iridotomy (*white arrow*).

Points to consider

- There was a flat iris configuration, not steep.
- Primary angle closure commonly presents asymmetrically.
- The target IOP for the left eye would be 10 to 12 mm Hg.

Diagnosis and Management

UBM before iridotomy showed ciliary processes pushing up the peripheral iris and a diagnosis of plateau iris syndrome was made. The patient was initially started on pilocarpine 2% every 8 hours, along with timolol and brimonidine. An iridotomy was done in both eyes to relieve any relative

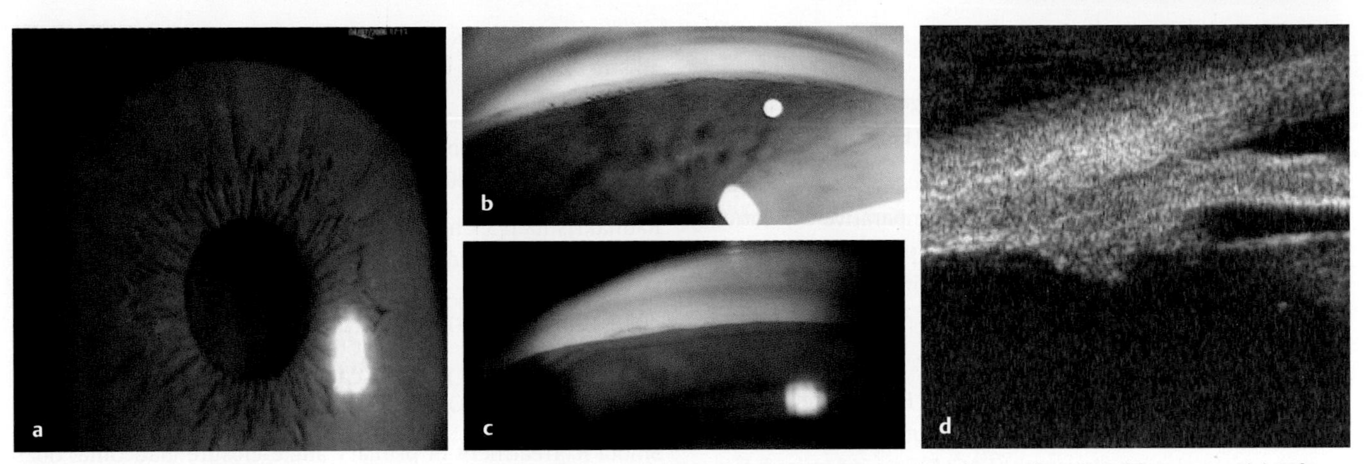

Case 8-1 **(a)** Pupillary ruff atrophy. **(b)** Right eye peripheral anterior synechiae with anterior trabecular meshwork visible in areas. **(c)** Left eye closed angle as only Schwalbe's line and cornea can be seen on manipulation. **(d)** Ultrasound biomicroscopy (UBM) showing ciliary processes pushing up the peripheral iris.

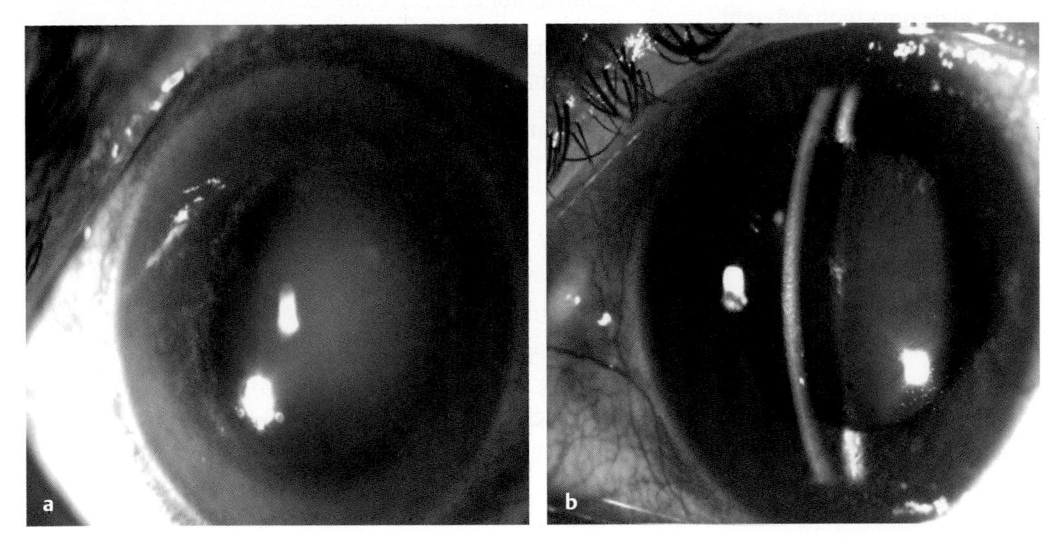

Case 9-1 **(a)** Corneal edema, vertically oval pupil, and a patchy sphincter atrophy. **(b)** After resolution of the corneal edema, pigment dispersion on the back of the cornea, and anterior subcapsular lenticular opacities, glaucomflecken were seen.

pupillary block that may be there additionally. Iridotomy in the left eye was done under cover of Diamox for 2 days to prevent loss of the remaining island of vision. Pilocarpine was then stopped in both eyes. A diurnal phasing on medications done after 4 weeks showed a peak IOP of 12 mm Hg in the right eye and 18 mm Hg in the left eye, and a PG analog was added to the left eye. Laser iridoplasty for thinning the peripheral iris was discussed with the patient, who was also counseled regarding the probable necessity for a filtering surgery in the left eye even after that to achieve target IOP. He chose to continue medications and review regularly.

Case 9

A 60-year-old female was diagnosed to have acute PACG in the left eye for 1 day, with an IOP of >60 mm Hg. Her IOP was lowered using IV mannitol, oral acetazolamide and glycerol, timolol, brimonidine, and later pilocarpine to 22 mm Hg. After an iridotomy her IOPs reduced to the range of 16 to 20 mm Hg in that eye on topical medications, cup:disc ratio was 0.5 with a concentric enlargement of the cup and mild neuroretinal rim pallor. On perimetry there were a few scattered loci of abnormal retinal sensitivity (**Case 9-1**).

Points to consider

- Duration of angle closure attack was only 1 day.
- Very high IOPs during the acute PACG may cause ischemic damage to the optic nerve head.
- Chronic medications may be required.

Management

The patient was counseled on the need to continue topical medications, and repeat a field after 2 to 3 months to look for field loss. Lifelong review was explained, with a possibility of decreasing or increasing target IOP as required. More than half the patients of acute PACG may have visual field loss and 10% may become blind, if the IOP is not reviewed in the long term.

Suggested Readings

Ahram DF, Alward WL, Kuehn MH. The genetic mechanisms of primary angle closure glaucoma. Eye (Lond) 2015;29(10): 1251–1259

Angmo D, Shakrawal J, Gupta B, et al. Comparative evaluation of phacoemulsification alone versus phacoemulsification combined with goniosynechiolysis in primary angle-closure glaucoma: a randomized controlled trial. Ophthalmol Glaucoma 2019;2(5):346–356

Azuara-Blanco A, Burr J, Ramsay C, et al; EAGLE study group. Effectiveness of early lens extraction for the treatment of primary angle-closure glaucoma (EAGLE): a randomised controlled trial. Lancet 2016;388(10052):1389–1397

Lau LI, Liu CJ, Chou JC, Hsu WM, Liu JH. Patterns of visual field defects in chronic angle-closure glaucoma with different disease severity. Ophthalmology 2003;110(10):1890–1894

Le JT, Rouse B, Gazzard G. Iridotomy to slow progression of angle-closure glaucoma. Cochrane Database Syst Rev 2016; 2016(6):12270

Mapstone R. Precipitation of angle closure. Br J Ophthalmol. 1974 Jan;58(1):46–54

Moghimi S, Torkashvand A, Mohammadi M, et al. Classification of primary angle closure spectrum with hierarchical cluster analysis. PLoS One 2018;13(7):e0199157

Nongpiur ME, Ku JY, Aung T. Angle closure glaucoma: a mechanistic review. Curr Opin Ophthalmol 2011;22(2):96–101

Nongpiur ME, Ku JY, Aung T. Angle closure glaucoma: a mechanistic review. Curr Opin Ophthalmol 2011;22(2):96–101

Quigley HA. Angle-closure glaucoma-simpler answers to complex mechanisms: LXVI Edward Jackson Memorial Lecture. Am J Ophthalmol. 2009 Nov;148(5):657–669

Radhakrishnan S, Chen PP, Junk AK, Nouri-Mahdavi K, Chen TC. Laser peripheral iridotomy in primary angle closure: a report by the American Academy of Ophthalmology. Ophthalmology 2018;125(7):1110–1120

Sihota R. An Indian perspective on primary angle closure and glaucoma. Indian J Ophthalmol 2011;59(Suppl):S76–S81

Sihota R. Treatment of primary angle-closure glaucoma: does early lens extraction help? Natl Med J India 2017;30(2):78–79

Sihota R. Classification of primary angle closure disease. Curr Opin Ophthalmol 2011;22(2):87–95

Sinha R, Kumar G, Bali SJ, et al. Changing concepts of angle closure glaucoma: a review. Indian J Ophthalmol 2011;59:75–78

Soh ZD, Thakur S, Majithia S, Nongpiur ME, Cheng CY. Iris and its relevance to angle closure disease: a review. Br J Ophthalmol 2021;105(1):3–8

Sun X, Dai Y, Chen Y, et al. Primary angle closure glaucoma: what we know and what we don't know. Prog Retin Eye Res 2017;57:26–45

Wang N, Jia SB. Phacoemulsification with or without goniosynechialysis for angle-closure glaucoma: a global meta-analysis based on randomized controlled trials. Int J Ophthalmol 2019;12(5):826–833

CHAPTER 12

Juvenile Open-Angle Glaucoma

Overview

- Inheritance and Genetics
- Pathophysiology
- Clinical Features
- Management
- Differential Diagnoses
- Prognosis
- Cases
- Suggested Readings

Introduction

Juvenile open-angle glaucoma (JOAG) is an idiopathic open-angle glaucoma that is detected between 3 and 40 years, or between 12 and 30 years, by different definitions. The *European Glaucoma Society uses the ages of 10 to 35 years as a cut-off.* The usual age at which it is seen is mid-teen to late teen, implying that patients have a long life expectancy, during which control has to be appropriate.

Inheritance and Genetics

JOAG may be familial or sporadic. *One-third of patients are likely to have familial JOAG with an autosomal-dominant transmission.* One-third of the patients have mutations seen in the trabecular meshwork-induced glucocorticoid response (TIGR) or MYOC, myocilin gene, chromosome 1-1q21-q23. In the presence of this mutation, abnormal proteins cause increased protein aggregates in the endoplasmic reticulum. This prevents normal protein production and cell death. Myocilin mutations can cause familial JOAG and also early onset adult open-angle glaucoma. Risk stratification has been suggested using the mutations seen: mild risk with the Gln368Stop mutation, intermediate risk with the Thr377Met and Gly252Arg mutations, and severe risk with the Pro370Leu mutation. Mutations in CYP1B1 (2p22.2) have also been reported.

Pathophysiology

There are trabecular abnormalities present in JOAG similar to those seen in developmental glaucomas. Compact and thickened trabecular beams, fewer spaces with extracellular material deposition, and an anterior insertion of the iris are seen.

Clinical Features

JOAG is predominantly seen in males and is often asymptomatic. Patients may complain of blurring of vision or pain only when glaucomatous neuropathy is severe, or with very high intraocular pressure (IOP). *Complaints of colored haloes in a "white" eye should indicate JOAG or steroid-induced glaucoma.* Patients generally present with vision loss when the glaucomatous neuropathy is advanced.

JOAG is *bilateral in about 80% of cases*, and if at presentation only one eye seems affected, close review of the fellow eye may detect glaucomatous changes later. JOAG patients are largely myopic, so that the optic nerve head should be looked at carefully in young myopes. Anterior segment examination is generally within normal limits with possibly a deep and quiet anterior chamber (**Fig. 12.1**).

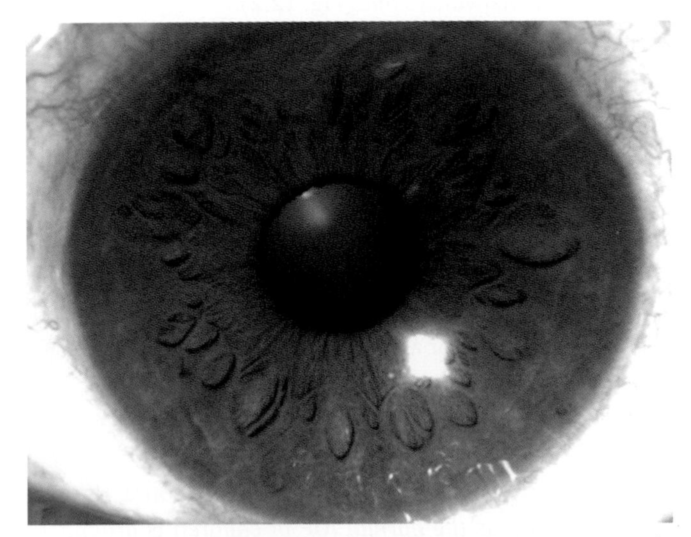

Fig. 12.1 Normal appearance of the anterior segment in juvenile open-angle glaucoma (JOAG).

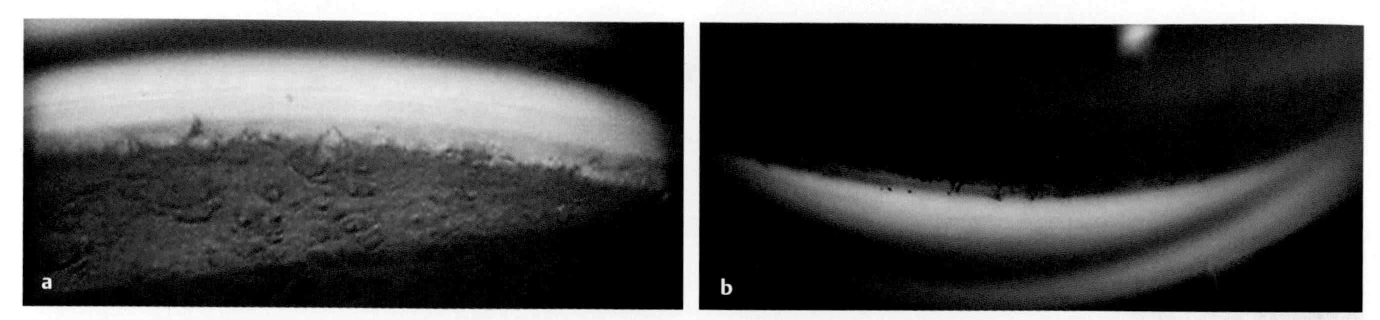

Fig. 12.2 (a, b) Juvenile open-angle glaucoma (JOAG). Multiple iris processes, following the contour of the angle, are seen.

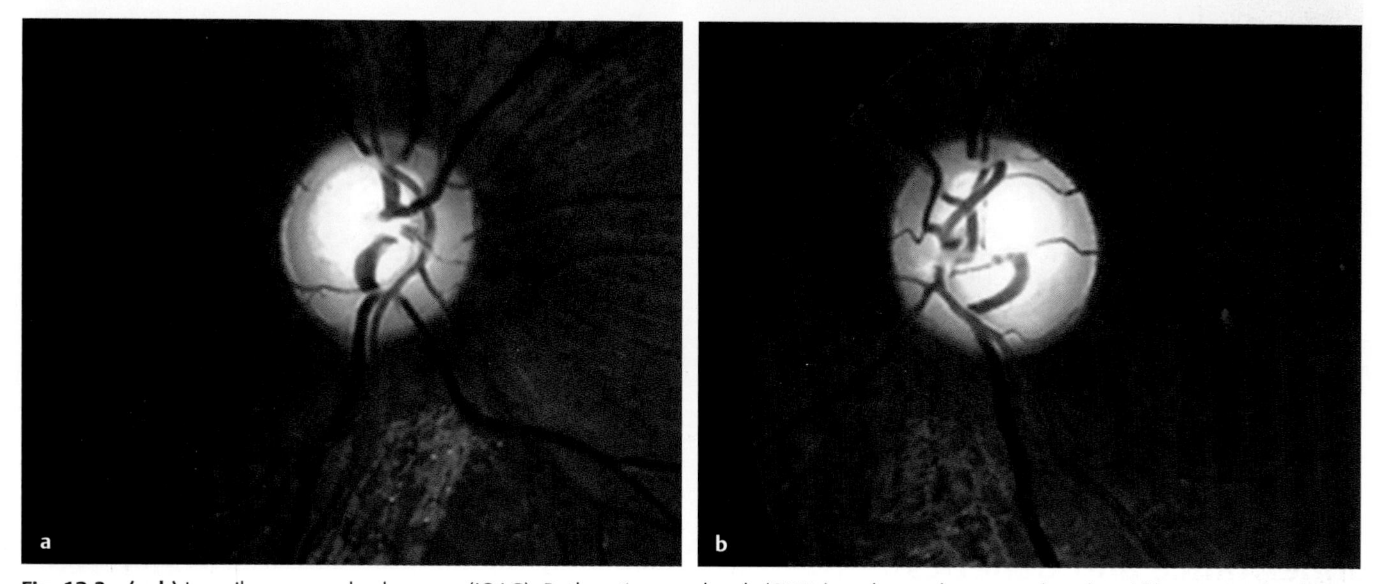

Fig. 12.3 (a, b) Juvenile open-angle glaucoma (JOAG). Both optic nerve heads (ONHs) are larger than normal, and could be expected to have a large cup. Asymmetry of the cup:disc ratio between the two eyes of >0.2 is a strong indicator of possible early JOAG. The left eye shows thinning and pallor of the inferior neuroretinal rim.

Gonioscopy shows a wide open angle with a featureless appearance. Some JOAG eyes show *developmental anomalies such as iris processes, an anterior insertion of the iris, or prominent Schwalbe's line* (**Fig. 12.2**).

On optic nerve head examination in JOAG, a large disc with a very deep cup, generalized thinning, and significant pallor of the neuroretinal rim is seen (**Figs. 12.3–12.6**).

The IOP in JOAG is extremely high, 40 to 50 mm Hg as compared to primary open-angle glaucoma (POAG), and also has large swings in diurnal and intervisit IOP. In some patients a high IOP alone is enough to make a diagnosis, even if the optic nerve head is within normal limits, if all secondary reasons for a raised IOP have been ruled out.

Management

Target IOP in JOAG needs to take into account the age of the patient, as *the normal IOP in children is around 12 to 15 mm Hg,* and also the degree of glaucomatous optic neuropathy. These patients are likely to live for 40 to 50 years. Therefore, an IOP of at least the mid-teens should be initially looked for, and can be reassessed and modified over time (**Flowchart 12.1**).

Response to medication is generally poor, and even if a reasonable response is seen, IOP fluctuations can occur between visits and the IOP may suddenly rise, so that a careful review is important. Prostaglandin (PG) analogs and β-blockers are most effective, and dorzolamide and brimonidine may be used additionally. Surgery is often required, and trabeculectomy is performed most commonly with over 80% achieving target IOP. *In JOAG, eyes care must be taken to avoid hypotony, as these eyes of young, myopic males are more prone to hypotony after trabeculectomy.* On the other hand, young patients have a stronger fibroblastic response. The use of low-dose, 0.01 mg/mL, short duration of mitomycin C (MMC), 1 minute subconjunctival is enough to lower the IOP in the long term. Other surgeries have been used such as drainage devices, but in children they are prone to tube migration and displacement due to low sclera rigidity and are also prone to corneal decompensation over time.

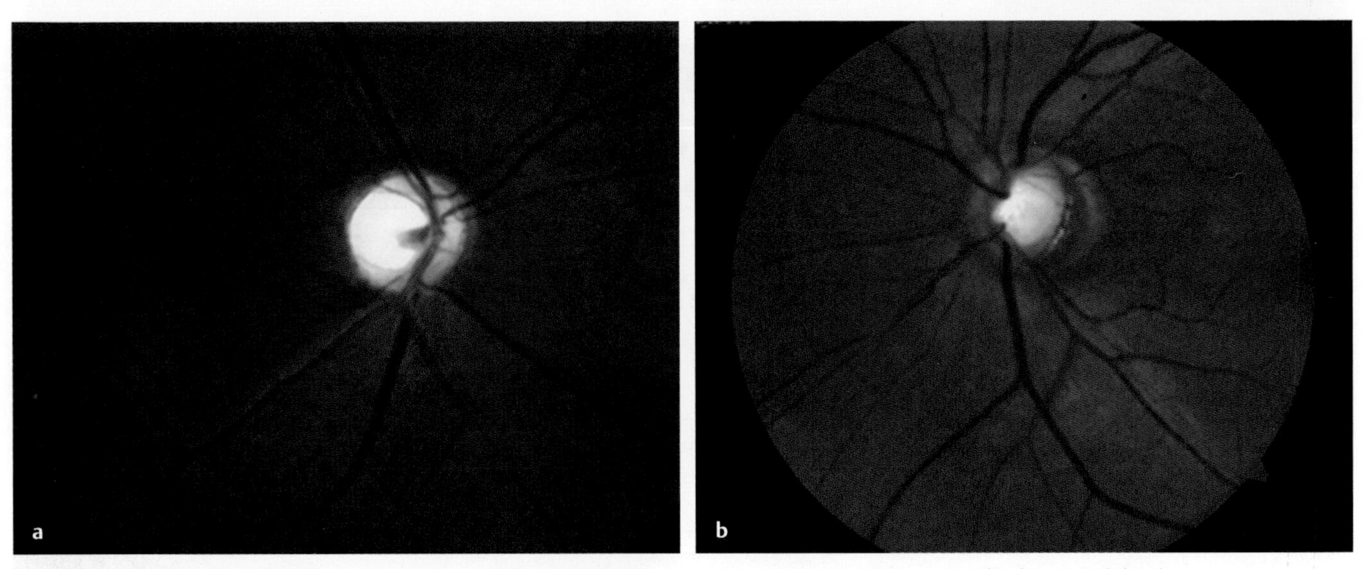

Fig. 12.4 **(a, b)** Asymmetry of the two eyes in size, shape, and cupping can be seen in juvenile open-angle glaucoma (JOAG).

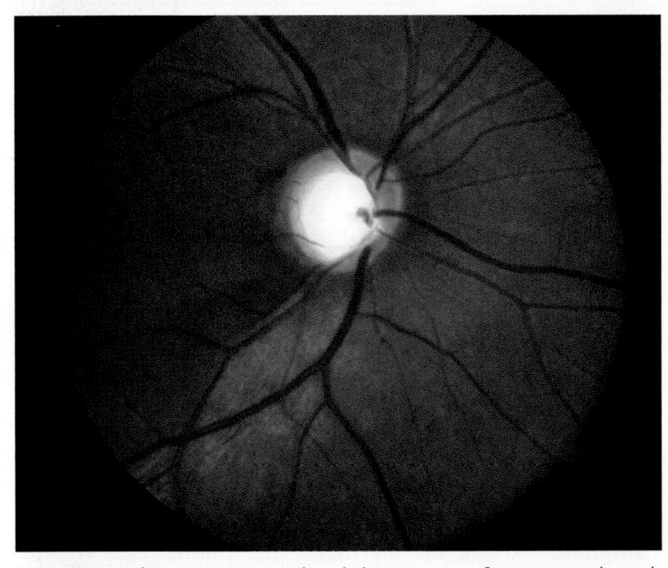

Fig. 12.5 A large optic nerve head showing an inferotemporal notch and retinal nerve fiber layer defect.

Keeping in mind the familial nature of the disease, it is important to screen both parents and siblings. In case a mutation has been identified, genetic testing may help identify family members at risk. However, not all individuals with a MYOC mutation develop glaucoma.

Differential Diagnoses

Differential diagnoses to be ruled out are steroid-induced glaucoma, angle recession, Posner-Schlossman syndrome, and pigment dispersion syndrome. Steroid use at this age could be dermatological, pulmonary, or muscle-enhancing supplements.

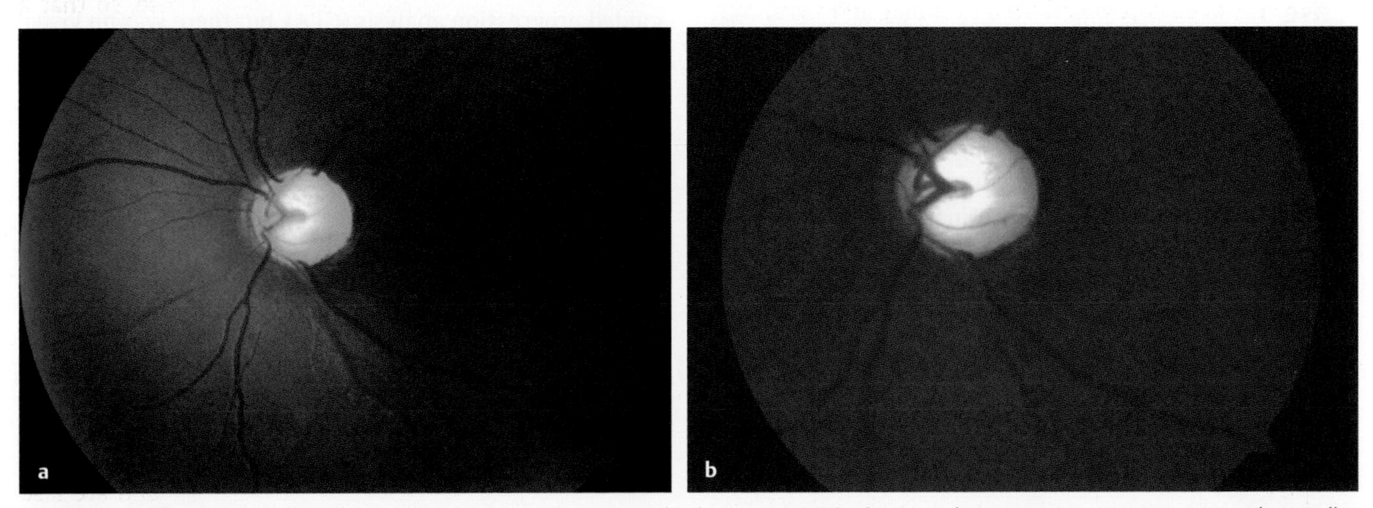

Fig. 12.6 **(a, b)** Optic nerve head in a patient with juvenile open-angle glaucoma (JOAG). There is a deep, extensive cupping seen, with 4+ pallor of the neuroretinal rim.

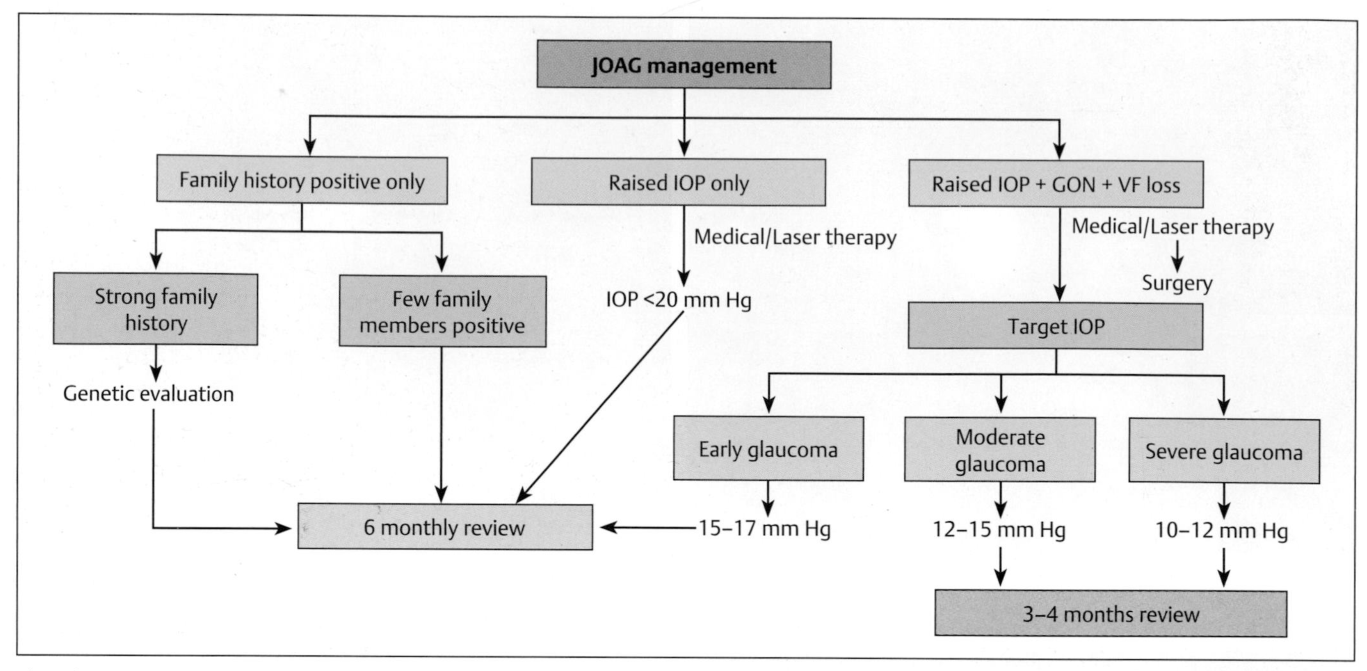

Flowchart 12.1 Algorithm for management of juvenile open angle glaucoma. GON, glaucomatous optic neuropathy; IOP, intraocular pressure; JOAG, juvenile open-angle glaucoma; VF, visual field.

Prognosis

JOAG patients present with severe glaucomatous neuropathy, and achieving a low-normal IOP quickly will stabilize this and in certain cases may even allow some reversal of the cupping. Counseling of parents and the patient about regular medications, regular review, and possibly further surgeries such as repeat filtration or bleb revisions is important.

Cases

Case 1

An 18-year-old male presented with recurrent, nonspecific headaches. Refraction was −2DS in both eyes. On examination, he was found to have a deep anterior chamber, van Herick (VH) grade 4, briskly reacting pupils, and a cup:disc ratio of 0.6:1, with mild neuroretinal rim pallor in both eyes. Gonioscopy revealed a wide open angle with the scleral spur visible. IOP was 36/38 mm Hg, with a central corneal thickness (CCT) of 520 µm in both eyes. He was started on a PG analog and a combination of timolol and brimonidine, and his IOP dropped to 16/18 mm Hg after 2 weeks. Perimetry was within normal limit (WNL) in both eyes (**Case 1-1**).

Points to consider

- Steroid-induced IOP rise should be ruled out.
- Prominent Schwalbe's line is often seen in JOAG.
- Significantly raised IOP is enough to make a diagnosis of early JOAG.

Diagnosis and Management

The patient had no history of steroid use; therefore, a diagnosis of JOAG suspect was made. Tapering of medications led to a rise in IOP again. Patient was advised good compliance using an alarm on his phone and regular review. Over a review for 8 years possible progression of the neuropathy was noted on optical coherence tomography guided progression analysis (GPA), but there was no visual field loss.

Case 2

A 19-year-old male, diagnosed as JOAG with baseline IOP of 42 mm Hg in the right eye and 44 mm Hg in the left eye, underwent a trabeculectomy in both eyes 10 years ago and IOPs were well controlled till 1 year ago without medications. He complained of recent gradual and painless diminution of vision in the right eye, with a best corrected visual acuity of 6/12 in the right eye and 6/6 in the left eye. The IOPs were 34 and 22 mm Hg in the right eye and left eye, respectively.

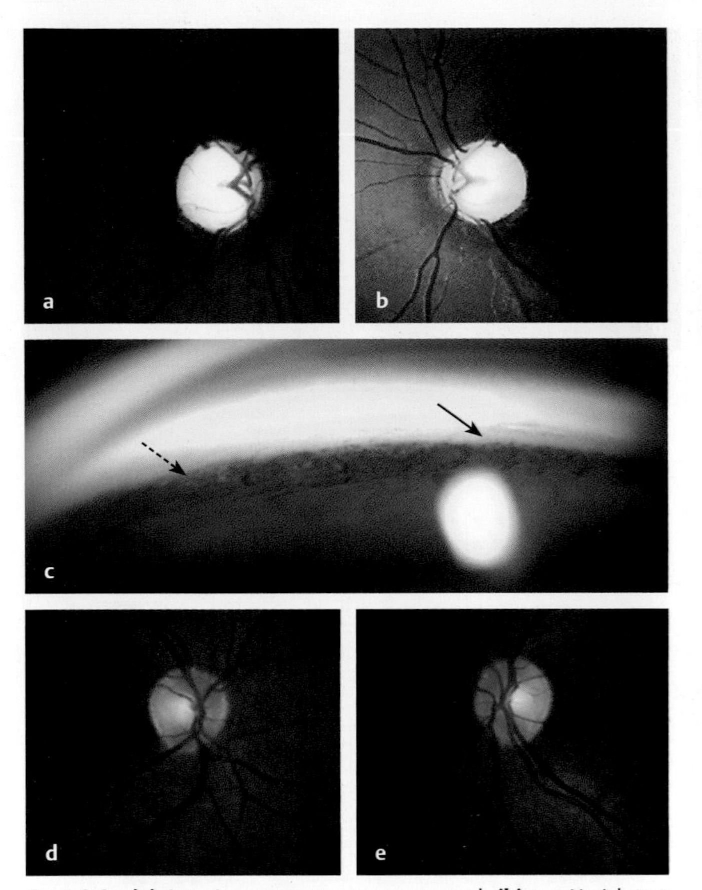

Case 1-1 **(a)** Anterior segment appears normal. **(b)** van Herick test reveals a deep anterior chamber. **(c)** Gonioscopy showing a wide open angle, prominent Schwalbe's line (*black arrow*), and scleral spur (*dashed arrow*). **(d, e)** Cup:disc ratio of 0.6:1, with mild neuroretinal rim pallor bilaterally.

On examination, anterior chamber of VH grade 3 was present with sluggish pupillary reaction in the right eye. Mildly elevated but vascular blebs were seen in both eyes (**Case 2-1**). Right eye showed a cup:disc ratio of 0.9:1 and left eye cup:disc ratio of 0.7:1. On gonioscopy, open angles with visible scleral spur were seen with a patent trabeculectomy ostium.

Points to consider

- Trabeculectomy ostium was patent.
- Trabeculectomy blebs may fail due to subconjunctival fibrosis.
- Steroid use of any kind should be looked for.

Diagnosis and Management

Target IOP should be 10 to 12 mm Hg in the right eye and <15 mm Hg in the left eye. Both eyes were started on a PG analog, with additional β-blocker in the right eye. IOP remained 24/14 mm Hg, after which 360 degrees selective laser trabeculoplasty (SLT) in the right eye was done. After 6 months, IOP was 12/14 mm Hg in both eyes.

Case 3

A 32-year-old male presented with gradual and painless diminution of vision in the right eye for the last 6 months. He was a known case of JOAG with a history of trabeculectomy in both eyes, which was done 1 year earlier. On examination, best corrected visual acuity was 6/6 in both the eyes. IOPs were 52 and 28 mm Hg in the right eye and left eye, respectively. A family history of glaucoma in father and brother was present. On examination, anterior chamber of VH grade 4 was present with iris hypoplasia. Relative afferent pupillary defect was present in the right eye. A mildly elevated, vascularized bleb over 2 o'clock hour was present superonasally in both the eyes. On gonioscopy, open angles with a completely blocked ostium in the right eye and partially blocked in the left eye were seen. Fundus examination of the right eye showed a cup:disc ratio of 0.9:1 and the left eye a cup:disc ratio of 0.7:1. Humphrey visual field (HVF) examination showed superior and inferior arcuate defect in the right eye and a normal visual field in the left eye.

Points to consider

- Failing blebs due to subconjunctival and scleral scarring within 1 year suggests an increased fibroblastic response.
- Surgeries to be considered are a repeat trabeculectomy or a drainage device.
- Postoperatively steroids may be required for a longer duration.
- Glaucoma medications may be necessary to reach target IOP.

Diagnosis and Management

The right eye underwent a retrabeculectomy with MMC of 0.2 mg/mL applied for a minute subscleral and a minute subconjunctivally. The left eye was started on topical travatan and timolol combination to attain target IOP of <18 mm Hg. The right eye developed a thin avascular bleb after 4 years of trabeculectomy, for which it underwent a bleb revision (**Case 3-1**). He was continued on topical drugs in the left eye only and had stable HVF after 10 years with IOP of 12/16 mm Hg in both eyes (**Case 3-2**).

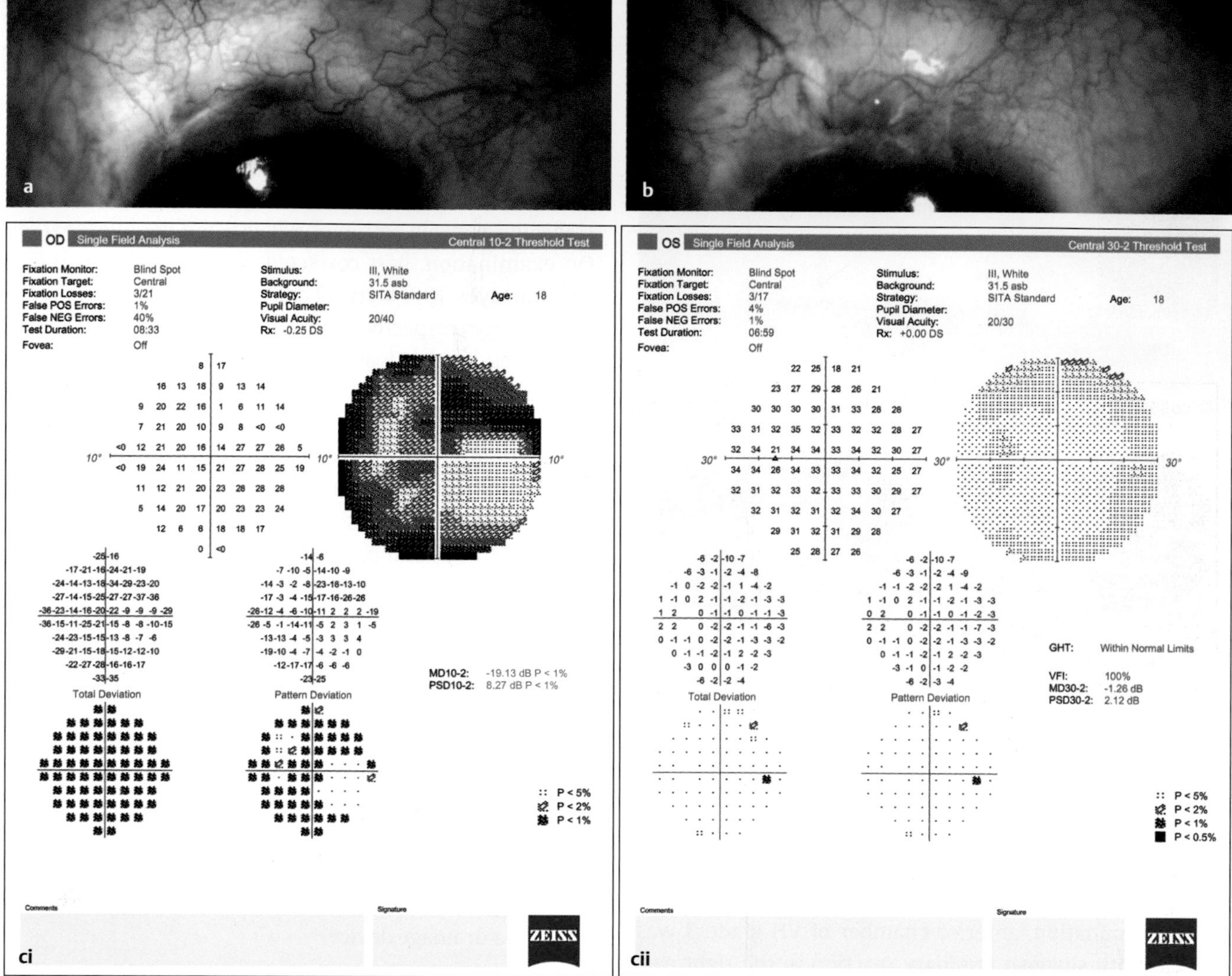

Case 2-1 **(a)** Clinical picture of the right eye showing a superonasal bleb which is mildly elevated, moderately vascular, with 2 o'clock hour extend. **(b)** Clinical picture of left eye showing a superonasal bleb which is moderately elevated, moderately vascular, with 2 to 3 o'clock hour extend. **(c)** Humphrey visual field examination showed biarcuate defect on 10-2 SITA standard program in right eye and no defect on 10-2 SITA standard in left eye.

Case 4

A 16-year-old girl noticed loss of vision in the left eye. On examination, her vision was 6/6 and 2/60, PR accurate. There was a normal anterior chamber and iris, with a cup:disc ratio of 0.7 with an inferior notch and retinal nerve fiber layer wedge defect of right eye, and 0.9 with neuroretinal rim thinning and pallor in the left eye. IOP was recorded as 22/40 mm Hg. Gonioscopy showed a prominent Schwalbe's line with multiple iris processes, more in the left eye. Perimetry in the right eye showed a superior arcuate scotoma, and in the left eye it could not be done due to poor vision (**Case 4-1**).

Points to consider

- Gonioscopic findings of a prominent Schwalbe's line and iris processes indicate JOAG.
- As the patient has significant visual loss in the left eye, it is important to maintain the right eye visual status for the patient's lifetime.
- Target IOP should be <15 mm Hg.

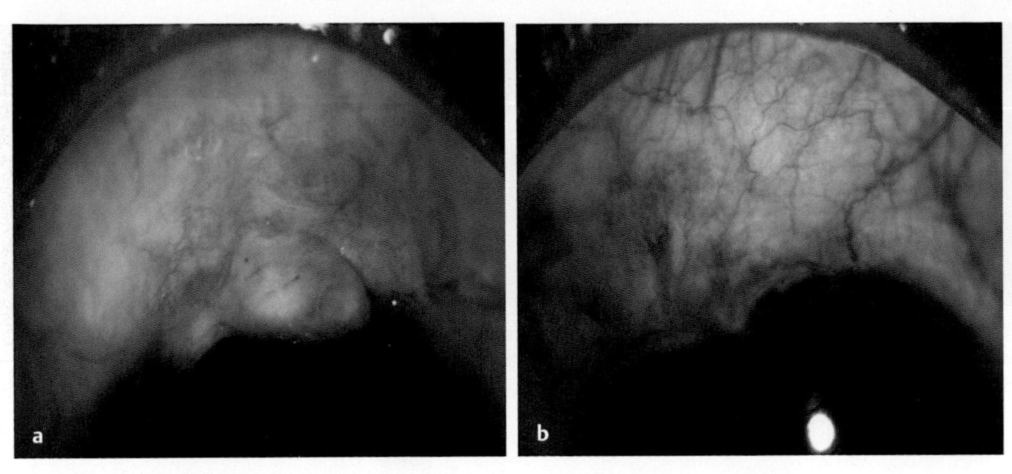

Case 3-1 **(a)** Clinical picture of the right eye after bleb revision showing a superior diffuse bleb which is moderately elevated, mildly vascular, and Seidel negative. **(b)** Clinical picture of left eye showing a superonasal bleb which is mildly elevated, moderately vascular, with 2 to 3 o'clock hour extent.

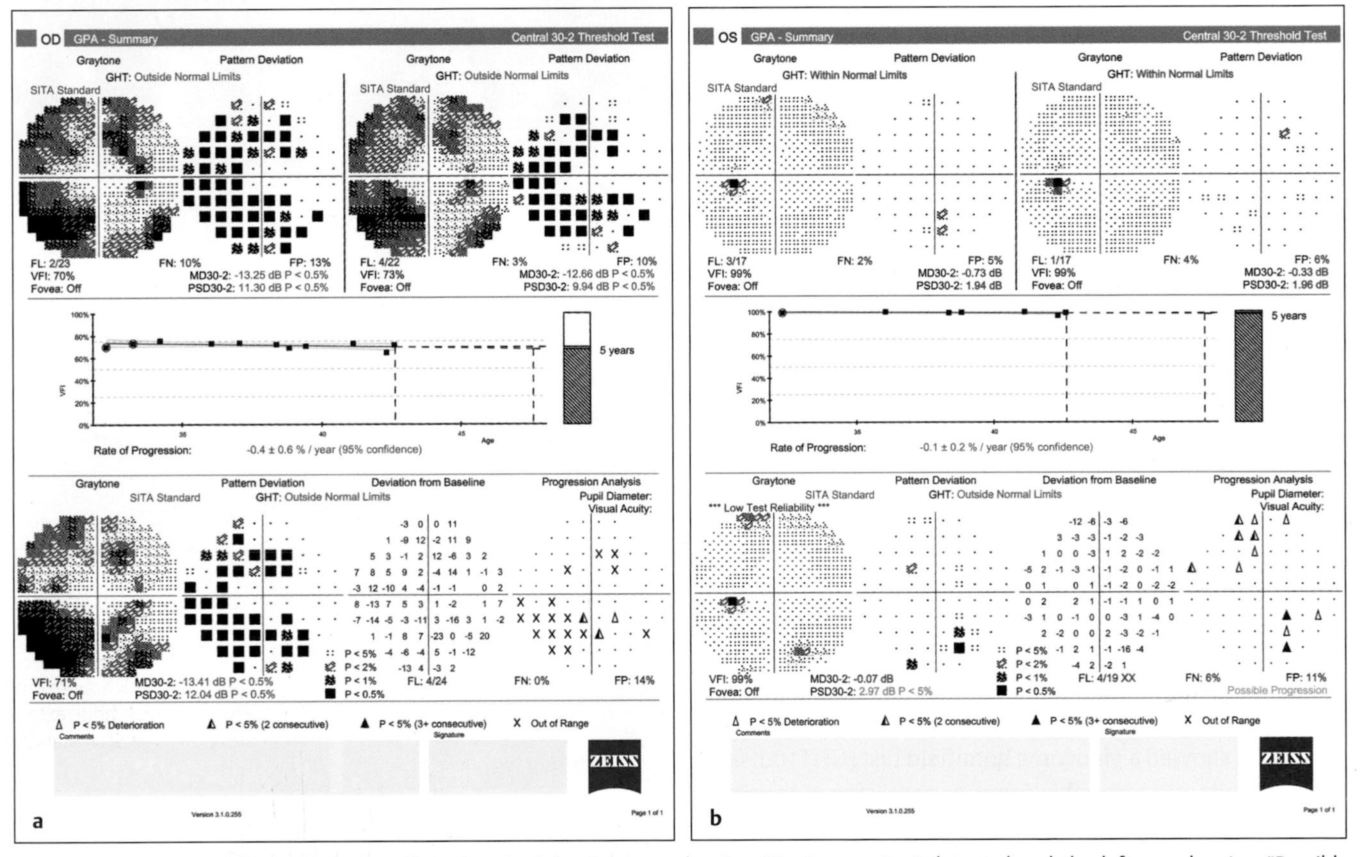

Case 3-2 (a, b) Guided progression analysis (GPA) of the right eye showing "No Progression" detected and the left eye showing "Possible Progression" compared to baseline in three or more tests. Rate of progression: right eye—0.6%/year; left eye—0.1%/year.

Diagnosis and Management

A diagnosis of JOAG was made and visual prognosis for the left eye explained. As the family could not afford lifelong medications, a trabeculectomy using 0.1 mg/mL MMC for 1 minute subconjunctivally was performed. The right eye was started on timolol drops. After 4 years, her IOP was 14/16 mm Hg and the right eye has not shown any progression of glaucoma on optical coherence tomography or perimetry.

Case 5

A 24-year-old myopic male presented for refractive surgery. On examination, best corrected visual acuity was 6/6 in both the eyes. IOPs were 12 and 14 mm Hg in the right eye and left eye, respectively.

On examination, a right-sided port wine stain was present on his face (**Case 5-1**). Ocular examination showed dilated and tortuous vessels in conjunctiva in all quadrants

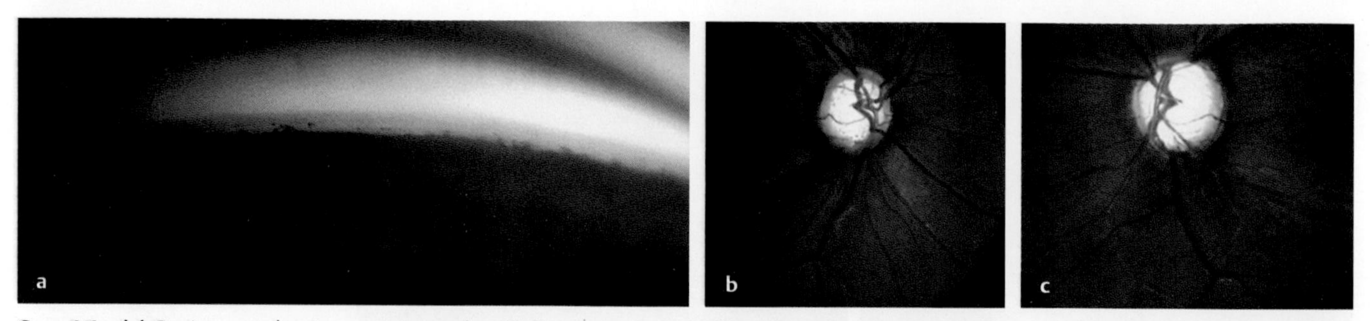

Case 4-1 **(a)** Gonioscopy showing an open angle with fine iris processes. **(b)** Right optic nerve head with a cup:disc ratio of 0.7 and an inferior notch associated with a retinal nerve fiber layer wedge defect. **(c)** Left eye cup:disc ratio of 0.9 with loss of inferior neuroretinal rim and a wide retinal nerve fiber layer defect from 5 to 7 o'clock.

of the right eye only (**Case 5-2**). There was a deep anterior chamber and the scleral spur was visible on gonioscopy in both eyes. Fundus examination of the right eye showed a cup:disc ratio of 0.8:1 with baring of circumlinear vessels (BCLV) and left eye cup:disc ratio of 0.7:1. A diagnosis of JOAG suspect with right Sturge-Weber syndrome was made.

Points to consider

- As the left eye had no evidence of abnormal episcleral vessels, but had a cup:disc ratio of 0.7, a developmental glaucoma in both eyes should be considered.
- Developmental glaucomas may also have deep ACs but this patient has corneal diameters within normal limits suggesting the IOP rose after 3 to 4 years of age.

Diagnosis and Management

A diagnosis of JOAG was made, with the additional effect of increased episcleral venous pressure in the right eye. Diurnal phasing of IOP showed a range of 18 to 24 mm Hg in the right eye and 14 to 18 mm Hg in the left eye. SITA fast perimetry showed a glaucoma hemifield test (GHT) outside normal limits and a possible superior nasal step in the right eye and scattered abnormal loci in the left eye (**Case 5-3**). The patient was advised topical timolol to reduce aqueous production in the right eye, and asked to repeat an SITA standard perimetry on Humphrey perimeter.

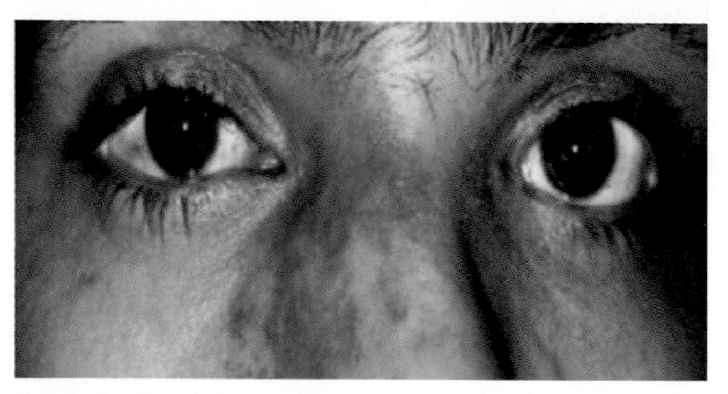

Case 5-1 Clinical picture of face showing right-side port wine stain involving right periocular area.

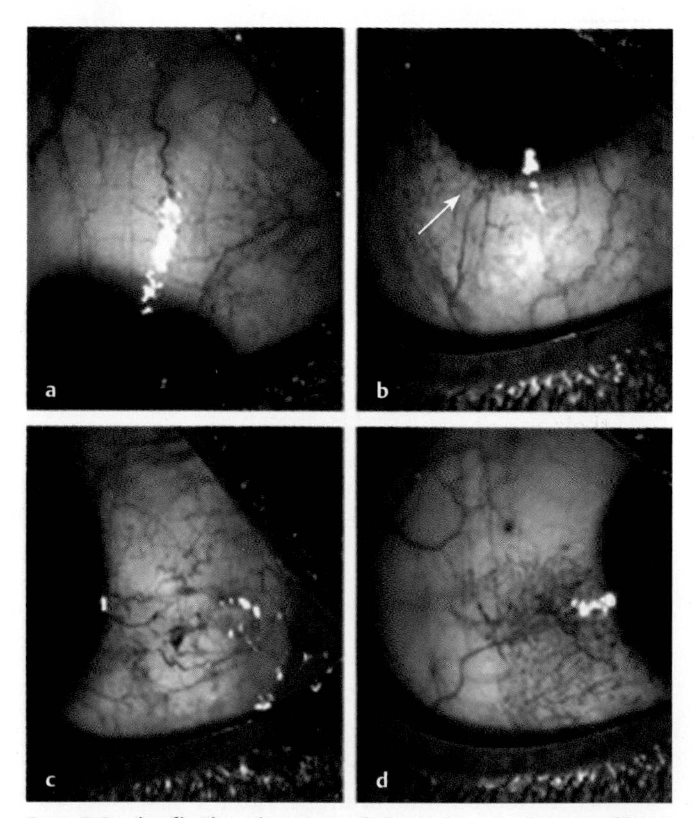

Case 5-2 **(a–d)** Clinical picture of the right eye showing dilated and tortuous vessels in conjunctiva in all quadrants with multiple hemorrhages near limbus inferiorly (*white arrow*).

Case 6

A 28-year-old lady was diagnosed as JOAG on the basis of a noncontact tonometry (NCT) reading of 22/20 mm Hg and some abnormal loci around the blind spot on automated perimetry (**Case 6-1**). She was advised a PG analog drop once at night.

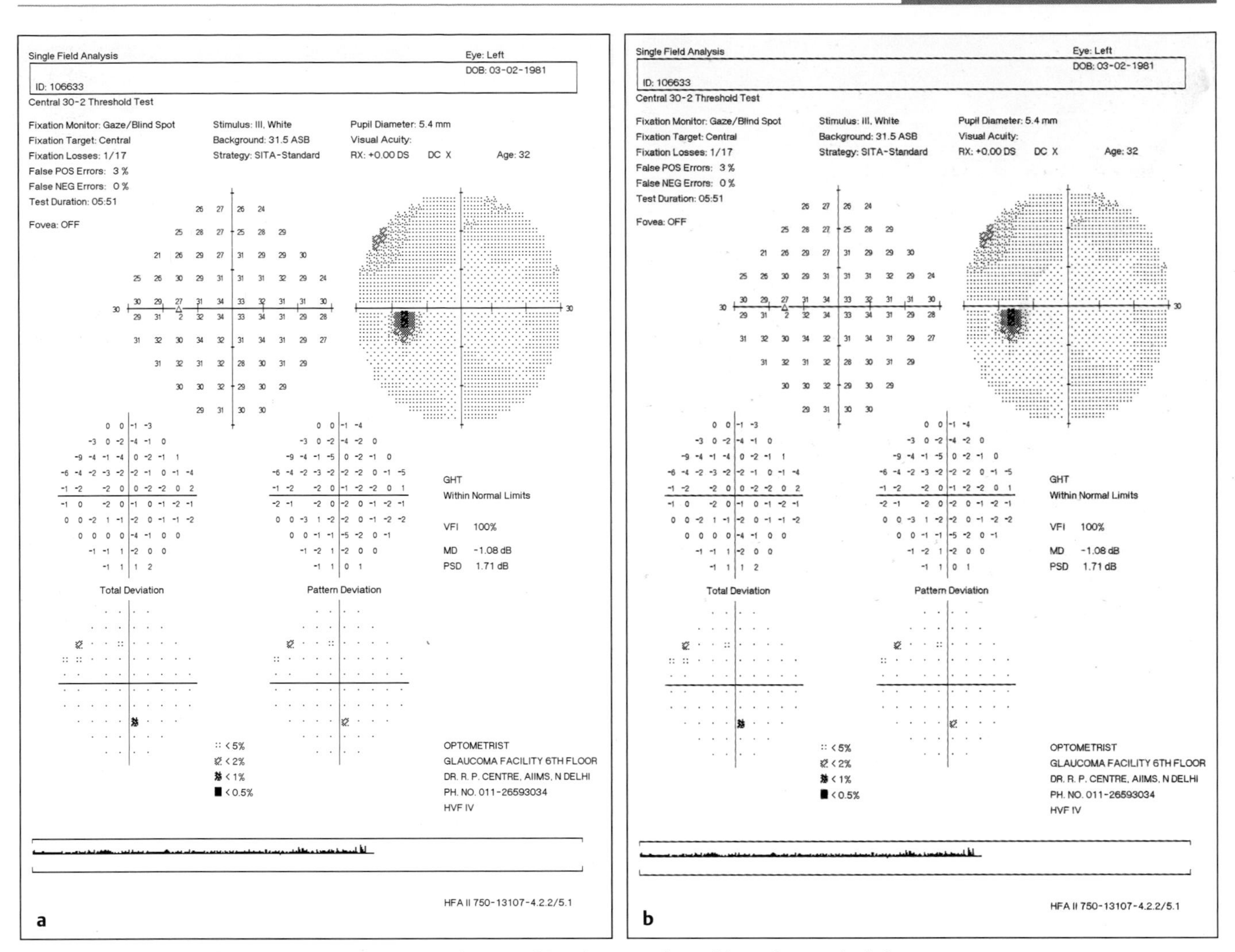

Case 5-3 **(a, b)** Humphrey visual field showing nasal step in the right eye and possible artifacts in the left eye.

Points to consider

- JOAG is more common in males.
- NCT readings may be erratic, especially when first performed, as patients are apprehensive and squeeze their eyelids.
- At least three IOP readings at different times of the day should be done before prescribing medications.

Diagnosis and Management

Applanation tonometry showed readings of 12/14 mm Hg. The right eye had a tilted disc with loss of the inferotemporal rim having adjacent loss of retinal layers, a possible coloboma of the optic nerve head with perimetry showing a superior arcuate scotoma. The left eye had a similarly tilted disc, and surrounding loss of retinal layers, but no field loss. PG analogs were continued, and she was explained about the possible congenital nature of the abnormality. Imaging and perimetry were repeated annually but have shown no change for over 10 years.

Case 7

A 24-year-old male complained of noticing a diminution of vision in the left eye. On examination, a deep anterior chamber, open angle with iris processes, and a left relative afferent pupillary defect (RAPD) was seen. The optic nerve head showed a cup:disc ratio of 0.9:1 with generalized pallor in the left eye and 0.7:1 with narrowing of the inferior rim in the right eye. Applanation tonometry showed 34 and 42 mm Hg in the right eye and left eye, respectively (**Case 7-1a–d**).

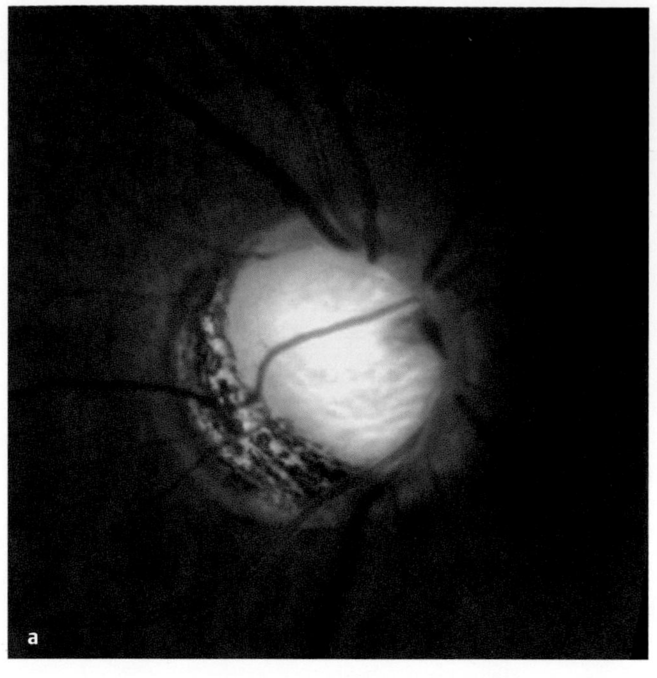

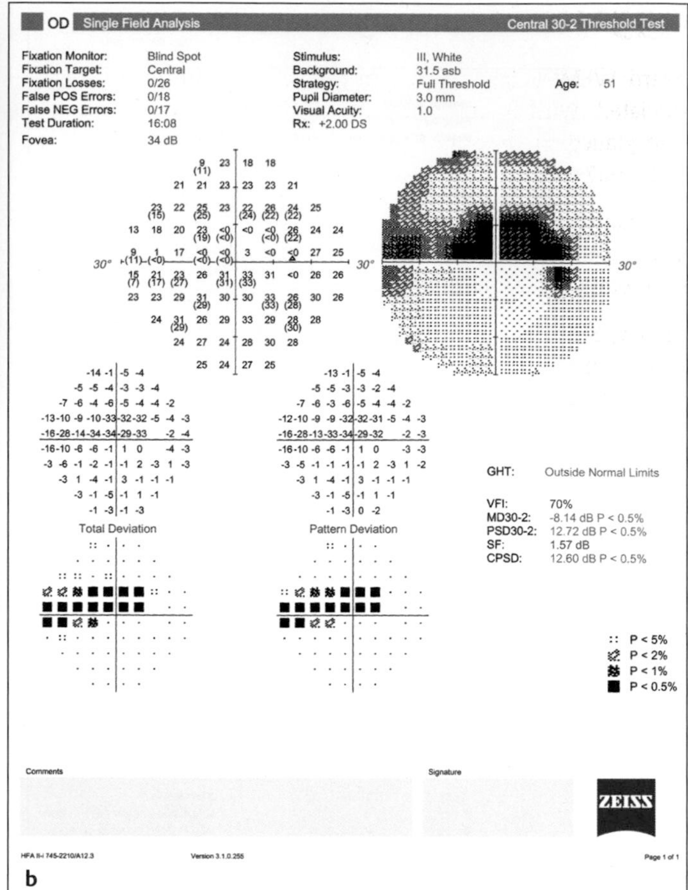

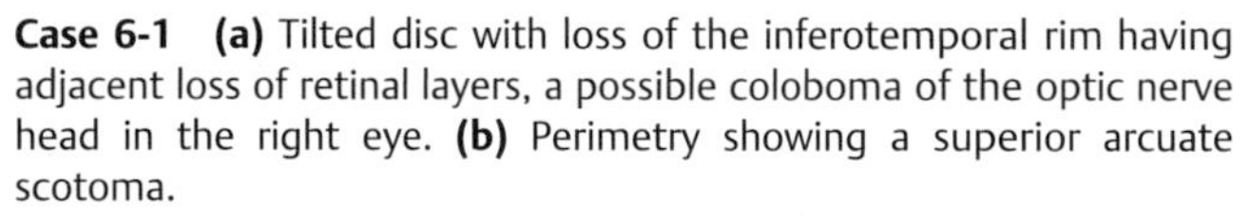

Case 6-1 **(a)** Tilted disc with loss of the inferotemporal rim having adjacent loss of retinal layers, a possible coloboma of the optic nerve head in the right eye. **(b)** Perimetry showing a superior arcuate scotoma.

Points to consider

- There was no history of steroid use; trauma or congestion of the eyes.
- The patient was started on latanoprost, timolol, and brimonidine topically and tablet acetazolamide 250 mg every 8 hours. After 3 days, the IOP recorded was 14 mm Hg in the right eye and 26 mm Hg in the left eye.

Diagnosis and Management

In view of IOP much in excess of "target" IOP of 10 to 12 mm Hg, the patient underwent a trabeculectomy with 0.02 mg/mL MMC applied for 1 minute subconjunctivally in the left eye and was controlled to an IOP of 10 to 12 mm Hg for the last 12 years. The right eye is on latanoprost and timolol and has maintained an IOP of 14 to 15 mm Hg over these years. The visual fields in both eyes are stable.

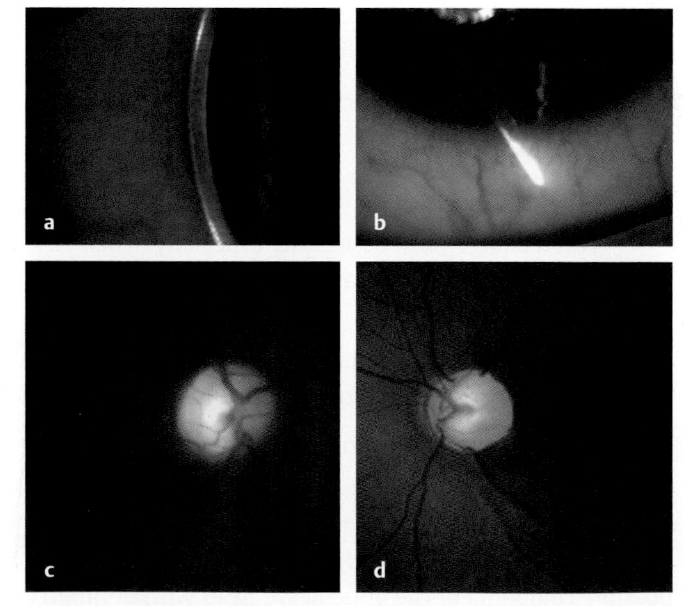

Case 7-1 **(a, b)** A deep anterior chamber with otherwise normal anterior segment. **(c, d)** Fundus photograph of left optic nerve head showing a cup:disc ratio of 0.9:1 with generalized pallor in the left eye and 0.7:1 with narrowing of the inferior rim in the right eye and some pallor of the neuroretinal rim.

Suggested Readings

Alward WLM, Fingert JH, Coote MA, et al. Clinical features associated with mutations in the chromosome 1 open-angle glaucoma gene (GLC1A). N Engl J Med 1998;338(15): 1022–1027

European Glaucoma Society Terminology and Guidelines for Glaucoma. 4th ed. Chapter 2 (2.2): Classification and terminology. Br J Ophthalmol; 2017:2017 ;101(5):73-127

Gupta V, Srivastava RM, Sihota R, Kaur J, Kumar S, Singh D. Determinants of severity at presentation among young patients with early onset glaucoma. Indian J Ophthalmol 2013; 61(10):546–551

Gupta V, Somarajan BI, Gupta S, et al. The inheritance of juvenile onset primary open angle glaucoma. Clin Genet 2017; 92(2):134–142

Hewitt AW, Bennett SL, Fingert JH, et al. The optic nerve head in myocilin glaucoma. Invest Ophthalmol Vis Sci 2007;48(1): 238–243

Menezes A, Panarelli J. How to manage juvenile open angle glaucoma. Rev Ophthalmol 2016

Turalba AV, Chen TC. Clinical and genetic characteristics of primary juvenile-onset open-angle glaucoma (JOAG). Semin Ophthalmol 2008;23(1):19–25

CHAPTER 13 Childhood Glaucomas

Overview

- Classification
- Pathogenesis
- Primary Congenital Glaucoma
  - Clinical Features
- Anterior Segment Dysgenesis Disorders
  - Axenfeld-Rieger Syndrome
  - Peters Anomaly
- Aniridia
  - Clinical Features
  - Management
- Sturge-Weber Syndrome
- Secondary Glaucomas in Childhood
- Examination of a Child with Glaucoma
- Management of Childhood Glaucomas
  - Surgeries
- Lifelong Review
- Prognosis
- Genetic Counseling
- Cases
- Suggested Readings

Introduction

Glaucomas occurring between birth and 12 to 15 years are not common, and may occur due to many causes, ranging from congenital/developmental anomalies to secondary glaucomas. There is an overlap in the age distribution mentioned in different texts, with glaucoma presenting within a month of birth being labeled neonatal glaucoma, from the age of 1 month to 2/3 years infantile glaucoma, and from then on developmental glaucoma. This was used to provide some idea about the severity of trabecular dysgenesis as well as prognosis; those presenting earlier such as neonatal glaucomas were thought to have greater trabecular abnormalities and a poorer prognosis.

Classification

A new classification of childhood glaucomas, Childhood Glaucoma Research Network classification, has included glaucoma and glaucoma suspects, with an emphasis on glaucoma following cataract surgery. The primary glaucomas include: primary congenital glaucoma (PCG) and juvenile open-angle glaucoma. The secondary glaucomas include: glaucoma following cataract surgery, glaucoma associated with nonacquired systemic diseases or syndromes, glaucoma associated with nonacquired ocular anomalies, and glaucoma associated with acquired conditions.

Commonly seen secondary glaucomas are: post-traumatic, steroid-induced, associated with uveitis or keratitis, or after congenital cataract surgery.

Hoskins, Shaffer, and Hetherington have proposed a prognostic classification using the extent of dysgenesis of angle structures as prognostic for control of intraocular pressure (IOP) (**Table 13.1**):

- Isolated trabecular dysgenesis alone having the best prognosis after surgery.
- Iridotrabecular dysgenesis having lower success.
- Corneotrabecular dysgenesis having the worst prognosis.

Pathogenesis

Congenital and developmental glaucomas show a rise in IOP due to dysgenesis of the trabecular meshwork, occurring due to abnormalities during fetal and neonatal life. The normal development of the trabecular meshwork starts at around the fourth month of gestation, while the Schlemm's canal and collector channels are seen around the limbus at the sixth month. Development of the trabecular meshwork is completed only a year or so after birth.

Many theories have been suggested for the occurrence of trabecular dysgenesis, seen as abnormal architecture of the trabecular meshwork—an anomalous membrane or abnormal tissue at the angle, absence of Schlemm's canal,

Table 13.1 Hoskins-Shaffer-Hetherington classification

Isolated trabecular dysgenesis	Iridotrabecular dysgenesis	Corneotrabecular dysgenesis
Flat iris insertion, at different levels, anterior or posterior	Iris stromal defects: hypoplasia or hyperplasia	Peripheral iridocorneal abnormalities, for example, Axenfeld anomaly
Wrap-around iris insertion	Anomalous iris vessels	Midperipheral, for example, Rieger anomaly
Any other	Structural anomalies: ▪ Holes ▪ Colobomata ▪ Aniridia	Central iridocorneal abnormalities, for example, Peters anomaly, anterior staphyloma

thickened beams, and few pleomorphic endothelial cells (**Fig. 13.1**):

- *Defective/arrested development of neural crest cells* is thought to lead to maldevelopment of the trabecular meshwork, a neurocristopathy.
- *Differential growth of the anterior segment* leading to an anteriorly retained iris and ciliary body.

Although 90% of cases are sporadic, congenital glaucomas are especially common in ethnicities where consanguinity is prevalent. Genetic mutations have been found to be responsible for some cases, with an overlap of phenotypes, and an autosomal recessive inheritance is common (**Fig. 13.2**). Penetrance varies from 40 to 70%. *The CYP1B1 gene is responsible for the formation of the CYP1B1 enzyme which is thought to help in the development of the anterior segment of the eye.* More than 140 mutations of this gene at short arm of chromosome 2 at position 22.2 have been found related to PCG. *Autosomal dominant inheritance is seen with mutations in angiopoietin receptor, TEK gene.* Identification of such biallelic mutations confirms the diagnosis, if clinical features are inconclusive. Angiopoietin receptor TEK mutations may cause a rise in IOP by affecting anterior chamber vascular formation, Schlemm's canal formation, or function.

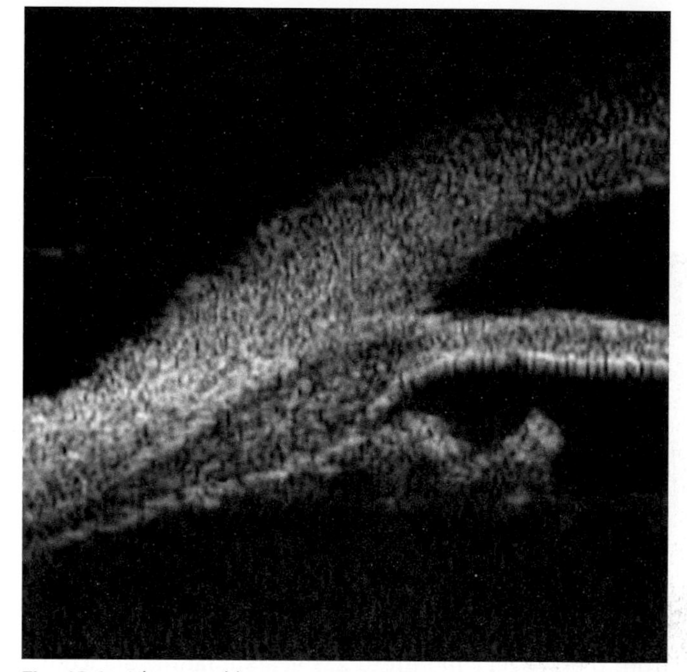

Fig. 13.1 Ultrasound biomicroscopy (UBM) of the anterior chamber angle in primary congenital glaucoma showing abnormal tissue over the trabecular meshwork, no Schlemm's canal visible, and a thinner ciliary body.

Primary Congenital Glaucoma

PCG is defined as having only an abnormal development of the trabecular meshwork and anterior chamber angle, thereby obstructing aqueous outflow. The cytochrome P450 1B1, CYP1B1, variant is seen in 44% of PCG in India, and 80 to 100% in Saudi Arabia. CYP1B1 can be seen in 20 to 100% of familial cases and in only about 10 to 15% of sporadic cases. Latent transforming growth factor 2, LTBP2, is seen in <40% of congenital glaucomas. Patients with a CYP1B1 variant are likely to have more corneal haze, and need more glaucoma medications. No genotype–phenotype correlations have been found with TEK.

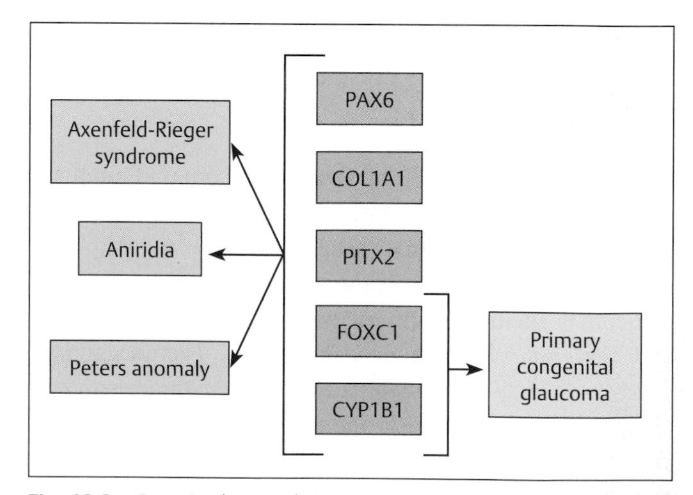

Fig. 13.2 Genetic abnormalities in anterior segment developmental anomalies with glaucoma.

Clinical Features

Males are more frequently affected than females, with both eyes being affected in over 80% of patients. A detailed family history should always be looked for.

The severity of symptoms and signs depends upon the age of onset, and the rate and degree of raised IOP. There is a triad of symptoms associated with PCG, caused by corneal epithelial edema present (**Fig. 13.3**):

- Photophobia: Babies with PCG show an increased sensitivity to light, often turning away from a light source.
- Epiphora: Tearing is a common complaint in such eyes, especially in bright light.
- Blepharospasm is a consequence of irritation and hypersensitivity to light.

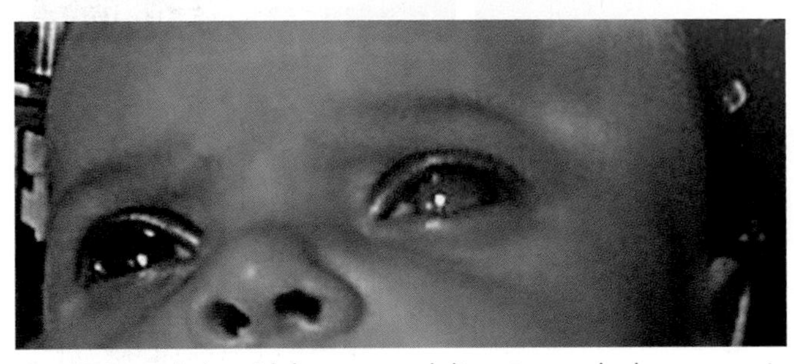

Fig. 13.3 A baby with large corneal diameters and edema, more in left than right eye, with tearing.

Common clinical features of PCG are due to the presence of chronically raised high IOPs, stretching and enlarging the eyeball in all directions, often asymmetrically. A large cornea in a large eye, together, giving the appearance of an ox's eye, is termed *buphthalmos*. Such an enlargement of the eye is seen generally up to the age of 3 years, while the collagen in the ocular coats is still immature.

There are no defined criteria for PCG, and common diagnostic features are as follows (**Flowchart 13.1**):

- High IOPs often over 30 mm Hg are seen. In a newborn, an IOP more than the normal of 10 to 12 mm Hg should be suspicious.
- Enlargement of the cornea: *An increase in corneal diameter of >11 mm in the first year and >12 mm thereafter is considered to be suggestive of PCG* (**Fig. 13.4**).
- A ground-glass appearance of the cornea, described by parents as a cloudy cornea, is due to corneal endothelial dysfunction caused by high IOPs, and resolves with lowering of IOP in most eyes.
- Haab's striae: Tears of the Descemet's membrane commonly appear as rail track–like lines in the peripheral cornea, concentric to the limbus. They may also be horizontal and cross the pupillary area, when they are likely to reduce visual acuity (**Fig. 13.5**).
- Optic nerve head cupping of >0.2:1, with a concentric loss of neuroretinal rim is seen, unlike loss at the superior and inferior poles in adults.

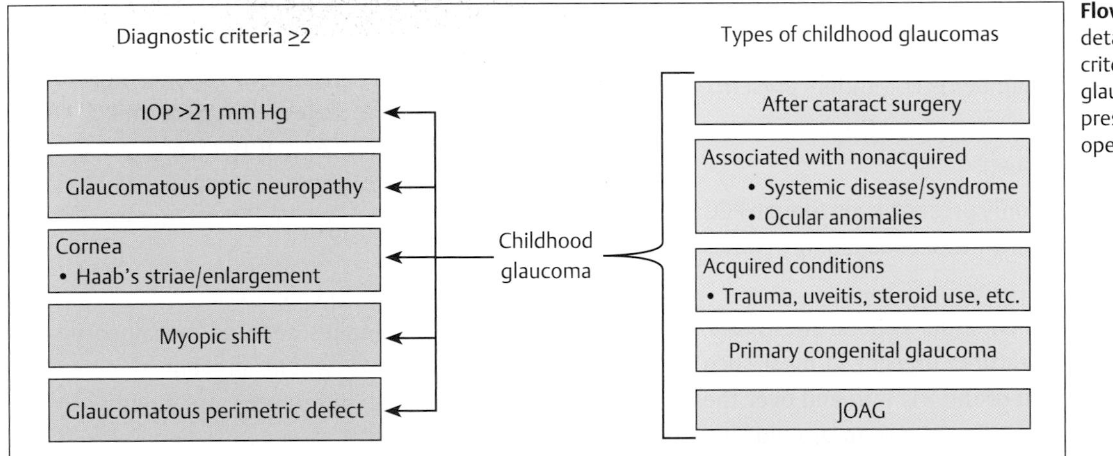

Flowchart 13.1 Algorithm detailing the diagnostic criteria of primary congenital glaucoma. IOP, intraocular pressure; JOAG, juvenile open-angle glaucoma.

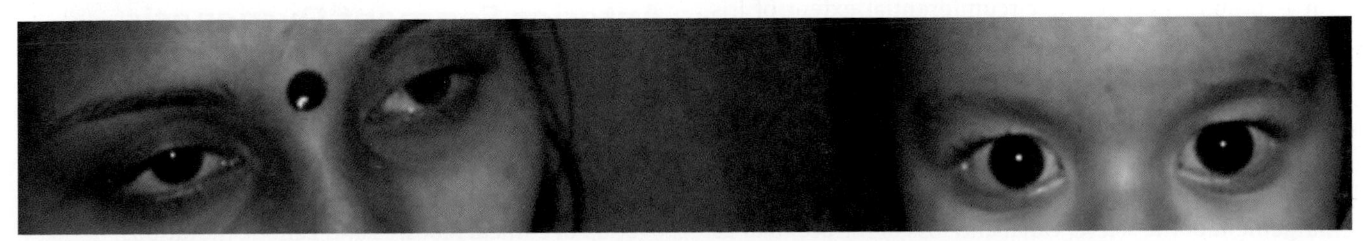

Fig. 13.4 A comparison of the corneal diameter of a baby with that of his mother allows an early diagnosis in some cases.

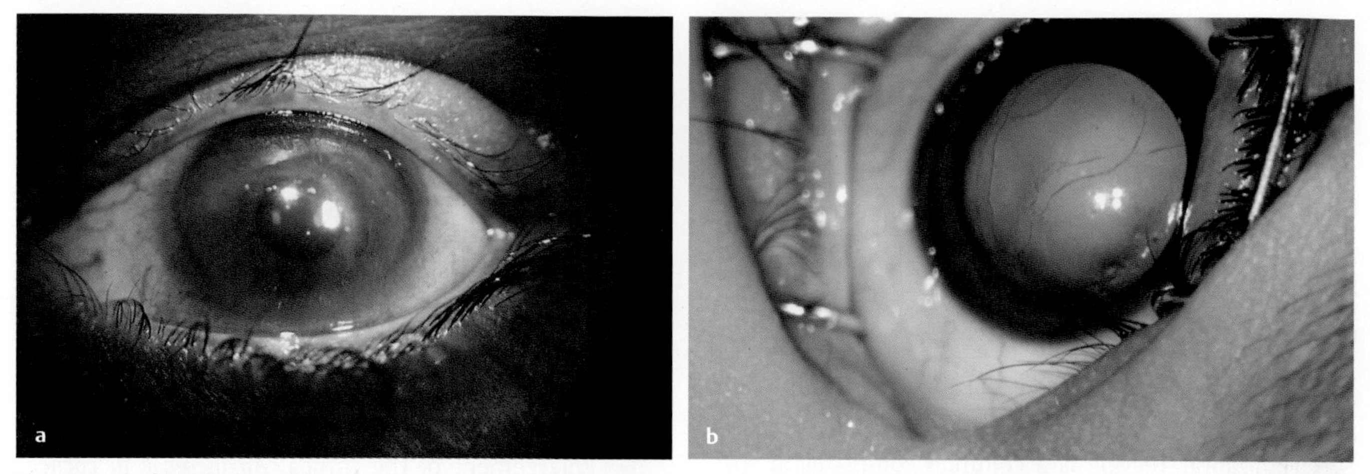

Fig. 13.5 (a, b) Multiple Haab's striae giving a train-track appearance across the visual axis and circumferentially.

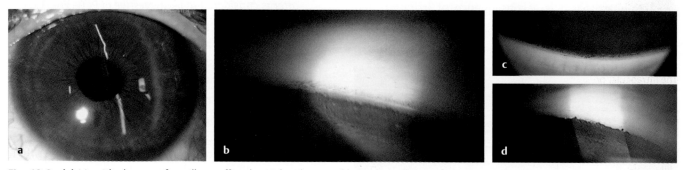

Fig. 13.6 (a) Iris with absence of pupillary ruff and peripheral areas of hypoplasia. **(b)** Anterior, "wrap-around" iris insertion, covering a large part of the trabecular meshwork, with a prominent Schwalbe's line. **(c)** Numerous iris processes and an anterior insertion of the iris covering the trabecular meshwork and almost reaching Schwalbe's line. **(d)** Peripheral iris hypoplasia seen as a darker area due to the loss of iris stroma and visibility of the pigment epithelium. Anterior insertion of the iris with no angle structures is seen.

- Elongation of the eye with an increased axial length leads to significant myopia.
- A very deep anterior chamber is commonly present.
- Stretching of the limbus, with an obliteration of the corneoscleral angle, is seen.
- Iris hypoplasia is commonly present, even though PCG is defined as having only trabecular abnormalities (**Fig. 13.6a**).

Gonioscopy of PCG is performed under general anesthesia, using a direct gonioscope. Features present in most such eyes are an anterior insertion of the iris into and over the trabecular meshwork, seen either as a "wrap-around" iris or as iris processes. Schwalbe's line can be identified easily, as it is prominent, and the circumferential extent of iris tissue approaching this provides some idea of trabecular dysfunction and baseline IOP (**Fig. 13.6b–d**).

In the early stages of congenital glaucoma, the rapid, concentric increase of cupping can be explained by distension of the optic nerve head and lamina cribrosa with enlargement of the scleral canal and loss of intracellular as well as intercellular fluid. In infants, there is an increased elasticity of the coats of the eyes, as there are fewer mature collagen fibers, so that there is stretching of the scleral canal leading to a larger disc area, and a larger cup:disc ratio, which can reverse if the IOP is adequately lowered. At a later stage, there is probable glial tissue changes with atrophy of neurons and therefore no reversal (**Fig. 13.7**).

Distinguishing congenital glaucoma from other anterior segment congenital anomalies such as megalocornea or anterior megalophthalmos would prevent unnecessary surgery. Some important differences are highlighted in **Table 13.2**.

Anterior Segment Dysgenesis Disorders

Anterior segment dysgenesis disorders are a spectrum of developmental disorders involving the iris, cornea, angle structures, and the lens in differing degrees, with an overlap of clinical features and genetic mutations.

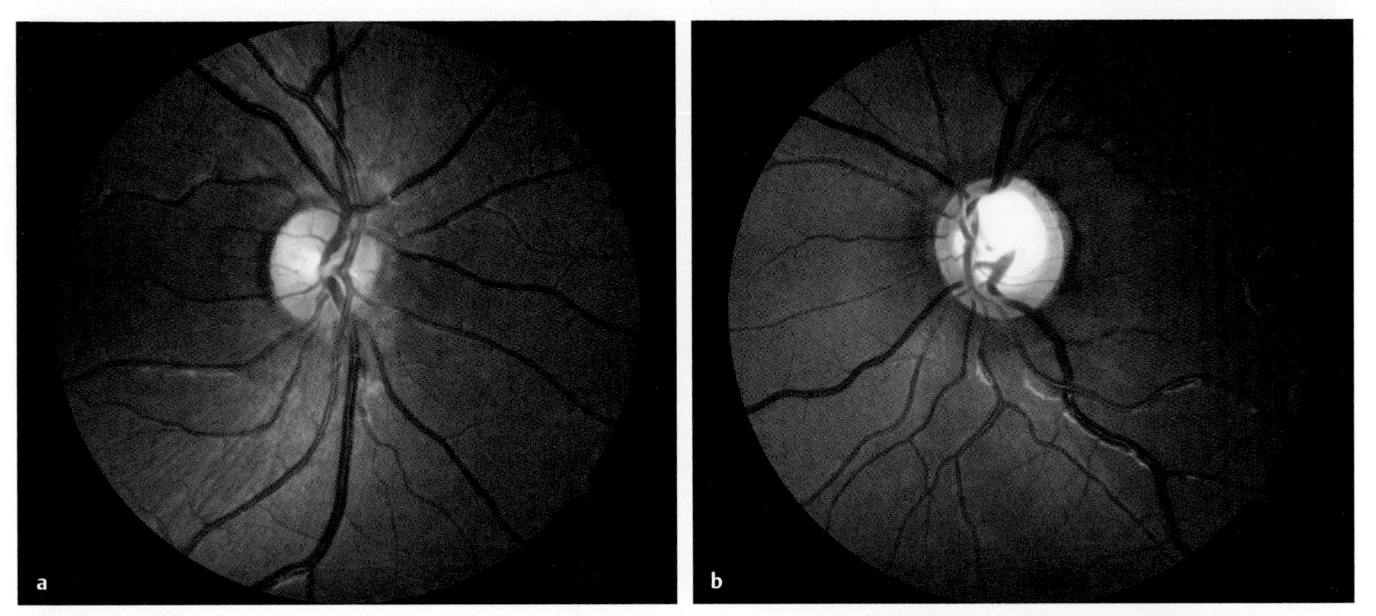

Fig. 13.7 (a, b) Unilateral primary congenital glaucoma (PCG). The right eye shows a normal optic nerve head with a cup:disc ratio of 0.2, and neuroretinal rim of good color, while the left has a larger optic nerve head, with a deep cup having concentric enlargement, cup:disc ratio of 0.8. The intraocular pressure (IOP) was maintained at 12 mm Hg after filtering surgery; therefore, the remaining neuroretinal rim color is good.

Table 13.2 Differentiating features of congenital glaucoma and megalocornea

	Congenital glaucoma	Megalocornea
Inheritance	Sporadic/autosomal recessive	Autosomal dominant
Gender	Males > females	Generally males
History	Progression over time	No change
Symptoms	Photophobia	Nil
Cornea	Edema, Haab's striae	Clear
Gonioscopy	Anterior insertion of iris/abnormal tissues	Normal or minimal iris processes
Axial length	Increased	Within normal limits
Refraction	Myopia, irregular astigmatism	With the rule, if present

This group of anomalies includes aniridia, Axenfeld anomaly, Rieger anomaly, Axenfeld-Rieger syndrome (**Fig. 13.8a**), iridogoniodysgenesis, Peters anomaly (**Fig. 13.8b**), and posterior embryotoxon.

Axenfeld-Rieger Syndrome

On clinical examination, a prominent, anteriorly displaced Schwalbe's line is present, and can be seen in the corneal periphery, when it is known as posterior embryotoxon. There are midperipheral iris strands adherent to the displaced Schwalbe's line. Iris abnormalities include extensive stromal hypoplasia, corectopia, and polycoria seen in different permutations and combinations.

On gonioscopy, iris strands can be seen attaching to Schwalbe's line, together with anterior insertion of the iris and often multiple iris processes. Approximately 50%

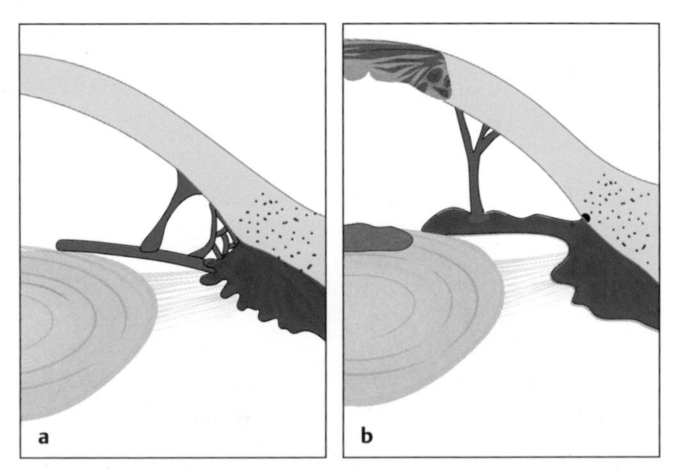

Fig. 13.8 (a) Axenfeld-Rieger spectrum: Prominent and anteriorly displaced Schwalbe's line, peripheral/midperipheral iridocorneal adhesions, and iris hypoplasia. **(b)** Peters anomaly: Prominent Schwalbe's line, iridocorneal adhesions to central corneal defect and leucoma, and iris hypoplasia.

of individuals with Axenfeld-Rieger syndrome develop glaucoma, generally in late childhood, but glaucoma may also occur in infancy if the trabecular dysgenesis is more severe.

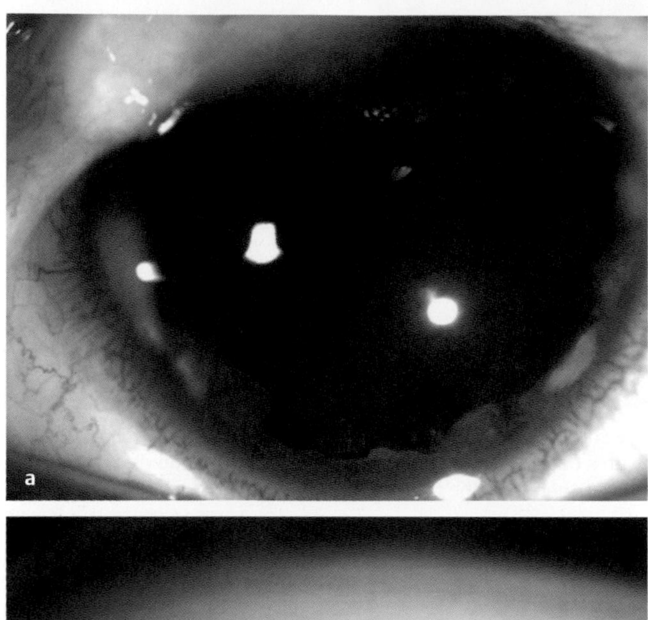

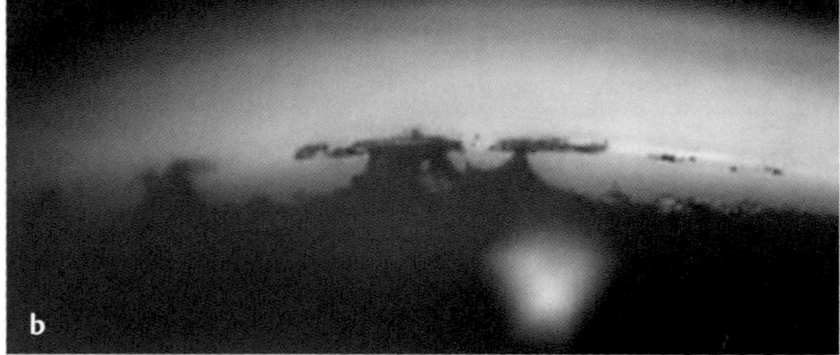

Fig. 13.9 **(a)** Extensive midperipheral iridocorneal adhesions seen with dark areas of iris hypoplasia. **(b)** Prominent and anteriorly displaced Schwalbe's line, posterior embryotoxon.

Systemic abnormalities are common; midfacial hypoplasia, telecanthus, dental anomalies such as microdontia, oligodontia, presence of redundant periumbilical skin, hypospadias, anal stenosis, and pituitary abnormalities causing growth retardation should be looked for (**Figs. 13.9** and **13.10**).

Axenfeld-Rieger spectrum can be divided into:

- *Axenfeld anomaly*: It has posterior embryotoxon to which fine or broad iris strands are attached.
- *Rieger anomaly*: It has the above plus significant iris stromal hypoplasia, polycoria, corectopia, and ectropion. The pupil in such eyes is distorted.
- *Axenfeld-Rieger syndrome (ARS)*: Combinations of the earlier features have been designated as ARS, if systemic features are seen.

ARS has an autosomal dominant inheritance with high penetrance. Mutations in PITX2, FOXC1, and occasionally in PAX6 have been found in such patients. Mutations in forkhead box C1, FOXC1, are associated with ocular anomalies and less so with systemic features, while those with mutations in pair, like homeodomain transcription factor 2, PITX2, commonly have systemic abnormalities in the cardiovascular, skeletal, and craniofacial tissues.

Peters Anomaly

Patients with Peters anomaly have a developmental defect of central corneal endothelium, Descemet's membrane, and stroma, with a variety of associated ocular and systemic abnormalities. The anomaly occurs due to an abnormal migration of neural crest cells causing maldevelopment of

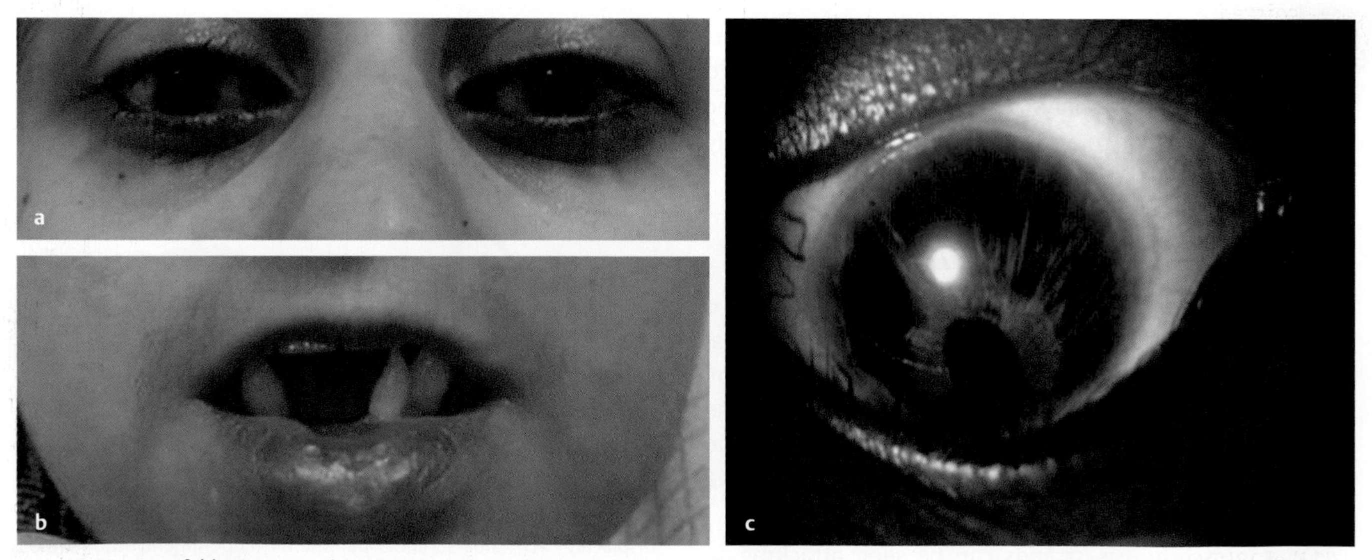

Fig. 13.10 Axenfeld-Rieger syndrome. **(a)** Asymmetrical presentation. **(b)** Malar hypoplasia with dental anomalies. **(c)** Left eye posterior embryotoxon, iris adhesions, extensive iris hypoplasia, and corectopia.

anterior chamber and angle, and faulty separation of lens vesicle from surface ectoderm. It is bilateral in 80% of cases, but not necessarily symmetric. The inheritance is usually sporadic or autosomal recessive, with mutations in paired box gene-6, PAX6, and also PITX2 and FOXC1 seen.

Clinical Features

Peters anomaly presents in various forms (**Fig. 13.11**):

- *Peters anomaly type I*: This type has a varying size and depth of the posterior corneal defect associated with iris strands extending from the collarette to the edges of the defect and overlying stromal edema. The lens is not involved and is clear.
- *Peters anomaly type II*: This type has additional lens abnormalities, for example, lens adherence to the posterior corneal defect, central cataract, or even an absent anterior chamber. This is often associated with microphthalmos and aniridia.
- *Peters Plus*: Peters anomaly with associated systemic abnormalities such as short stature, cleft lip and palate, cardiac, genital abnormalities, and general developmental delay.

Glaucoma is seen in around 50 to 80% of such eyes, reportedly more prevalent in eyes with involvement of the lens—cataract and corneolenticular adherence.

Aniridia

Aniridia is a rare congenital anomaly characterized by varying levels of iris hypoplasia, from partial absence to only a stump of iris tissue. Approximately two-thirds are familial, commonly autosomal dominant, and the rest sporadic.

Isolated aniridia is caused by heterozygous mutations in the paired box gene-6, PAX6, on chromosome 11p13 or deletion of a regulatory region controlling its expression. Other genes where mutations cause aniridia are FOXC1, PITX2, and PITX3. The pathogenesis of glaucoma in aniridia is thought to be due to trabecular developmental abnormalities, especially when the presentation is early. Progressive angle closure by the stump of the iris has also been described.

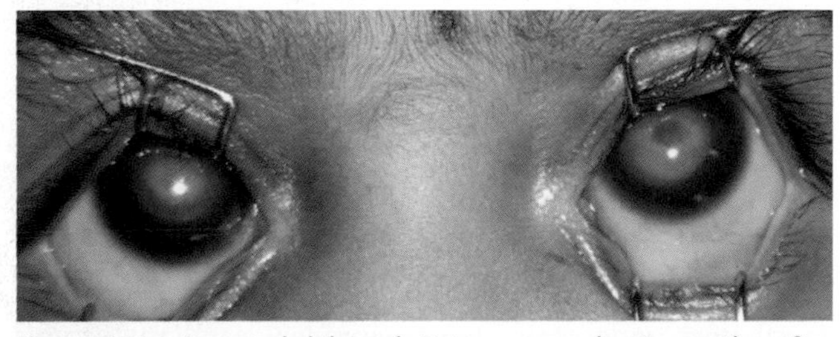

Fig. 13.11 Operated bilateral Peters anomaly 6 months after trabeculectomy cum trabeculotomy having an intraocular pressure (IOP) of 12/10 mm Hg. Peripheral corneal edema has cleared but the central corneal opacity will need a keratoplasty.

Clinical Features

Aniridia patients commonly have other developmental anomalies involving the cornea, angle, lens, fovea, and optic nerve. *Glaucoma in aniridia occurs in nearly 50 to 75% of cases, with ocular hypertension and glaucoma occurring in the second decade.* Systemic associations seen are WAGR (Wilm tumor, ataxia, genitourinary abnormalities, and mental retardation) or Miller syndrome. About 60% of children with WAGR syndrome and 25 to 33% of patients with sporadic aniridia may develop nephroblastoma.

Clinically, aniridia has been described with some differing features (**Fig. 13.12**):

- Partial or complete absence of the iris.
- Limbal stem cell deficiency, leading to pannus and aniridic keratopathy of some degree in 90% of eyes.
- Congenital cataract with lenticular subluxation in about 50 to 80%.
- Foveal hypoplasia in about 50%.
- Optic nerve hypoplasia in 10%.
- Associated intellectual disability.
- Pendular nystagmus in about 90%.

All patients with aniridia complain of photophobia and glare. Many have poor vision and pendular nystagmus due to foveal hypoplasia. There is often a complaint of chronic irritation as well.

On examination, there is 360-degree pannus due to limbal stem cell deficiency with irregular thickening and conjunctivalization, and a significant dry eye, in almost all eyes. A congenital corneal opacity may also be present. The iris shows varying degrees and locations of iris hypoplasia, from coloboma like iris loss, ectropion, eccentric pupil, to a rudimentary stump. On gonioscopy, the trabecular meshwork is visible in infants, but is thought to get covered by rotation of the iris stump over time. More than 50% of aniridic patients develop cataract and often have a subluxated lens. Fundus examination shows a vascularized fovea with poor foveolar reflex and macular hypopigmentation. There may also be associated optic nerve hypoplasia.

IOP measurements need to take into account the presence of a thicker central cornea and other changes in the central cornea. The IOP may increase over years as the iris stump changes are seen.

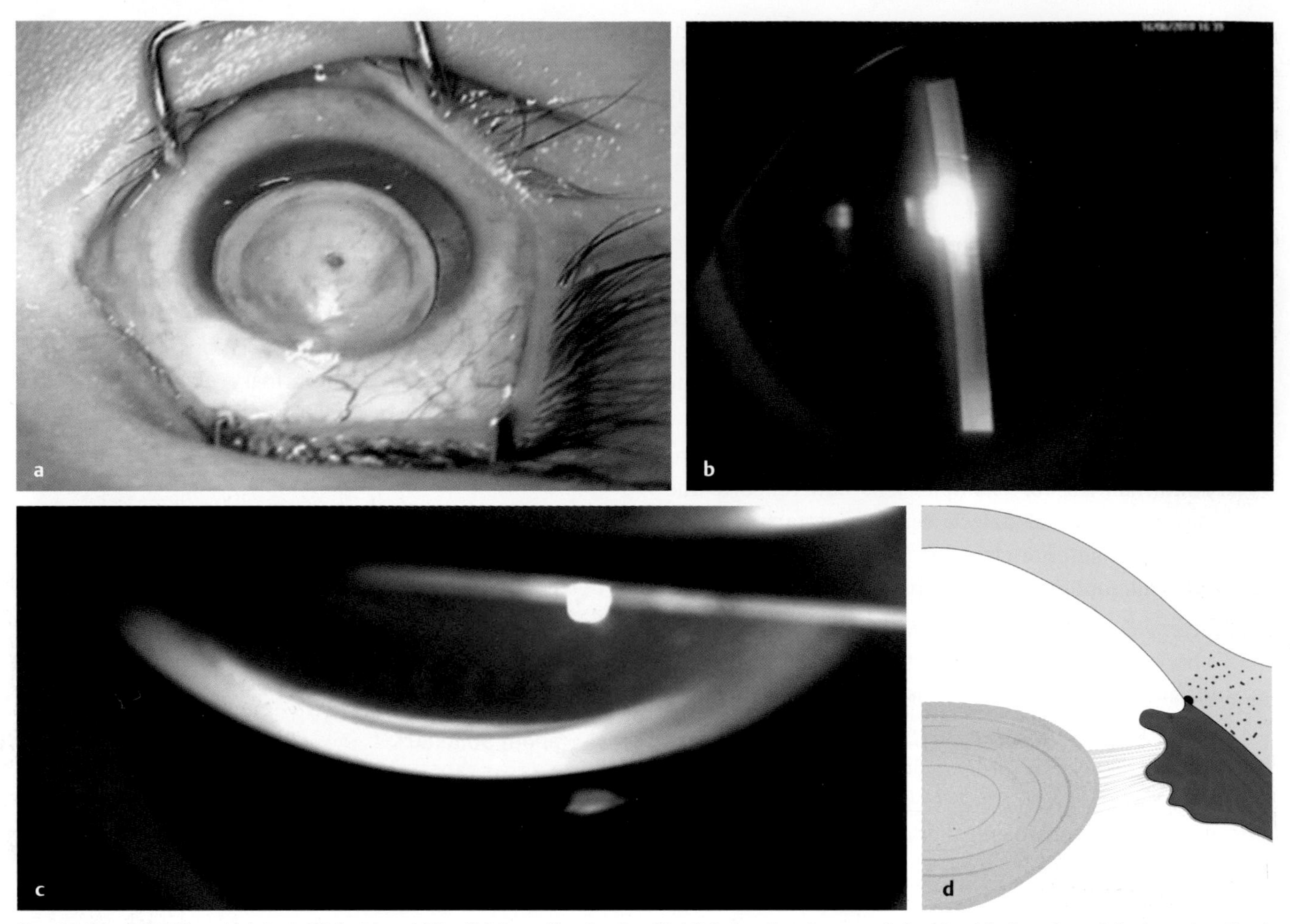

Fig. 13.12 **(a)** Diffuse bleb in a child with aniridia. **(b)** Retroillumination highlighting the absence of the iris with the edge of the lens visualized. **(c)** Gonioscopy of an aniridic eye with visibility of ciliary processes. **(d)** Diagrammatic representation of aniridia.

Management

The medical treatment suggested is the use of miotics to pull the iris away from the trabecular meshwork and drugs that decrease aqueous production, such as β-blockers, alpha agonists, and carbonic anhydrase inhibitors.

Currently, no single surgery has been uniformly accepted as the first choice for aniridic glaucoma. Prophylactic goniotomy was shown to be effective in preventing or delaying the onset of glaucoma in aniridic eyes, but therapeutic goniotomy for glaucoma was associated with poor success of around 20%, while trabeculotomy was more successful. Trabeculectomy with mitomycin C (MMC) and releasable sutures has shown a much greater success over time. Glaucoma drainage devices such as Baerveldt, Molteno, and Ahmed glaucoma valves have shown good success rates; however, they cannot be considered as first line in view of the high risk of complications. Common complications with surgery are vitreous loss, flat anterior chamber, choroidal effusions, suprachoroidal hemorrhage, etc. An increased incidence of retinal detachment has been described after surgeries for cataract and glaucoma.

Aniridic glaucoma is frequently resistant to conventional medical and surgical management, and therefore considered intractable. It is also associated with other ocular anomalies causing visual dysfunction and therefore has a poor visual prognosis overall.

Sturge-Weber Syndrome

This is a phakomatosis with hamartomas in the skin, meninges, and the eye due to a somatic mutation in the GNAQ gene. This affects blood vessel development, leading to abnormal and excessive formation of blood vessels in certain tissues. The classical triad consists of a facial port wine stain, leptomeningeal capillary venous malformations, and ocular vascular abnormalities.

The cutaneous port wine stain or facial venous dilation occurs in the distribution of the trigeminal nerve—ophthalmic and maxillary, generally unilateral, but may be seen bilaterally as well. These lesions can also be seen on the extremities. In a newborn these are flat, but become more raised and nodular with hypertrophy of underlying tissues with age (**Fig. 13.13**).

In the eye, vascular malformations are seen in the eyelid, conjunctiva, episclera, retina, and all the uvea. *Honey comb appearance of dilated vessels is common in the episclera, and the circumferential extent of this malformation at the limbus is thought to correlate with the occurrence of a rise in IOP, as it raises episcleral venous pressure.* Choroidal hemangiomas occur in 50% of cases, presenting as a deeper red orange-colored mass, sometimes with pigmented edges or subretinal fluid (**Fig. 13.14**). The characteristic ultrasonography sign of high internal reflectivity and no attenuation can be seen, and on optical coherence tomography a smooth lesion with expansion of both medium and large choroidal vessels is visualized.

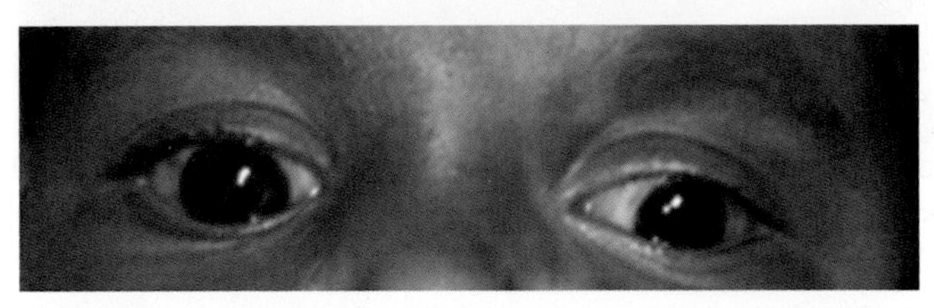

Fig. 13.13 Port wine stain of the face may be unilateral or bilateral, over the distribution of the trigeminal nerve, with glaucoma presenting in infancy or in the teens.

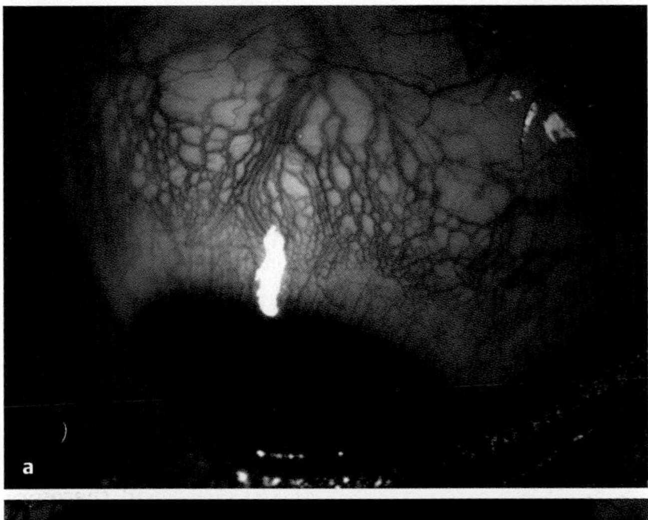

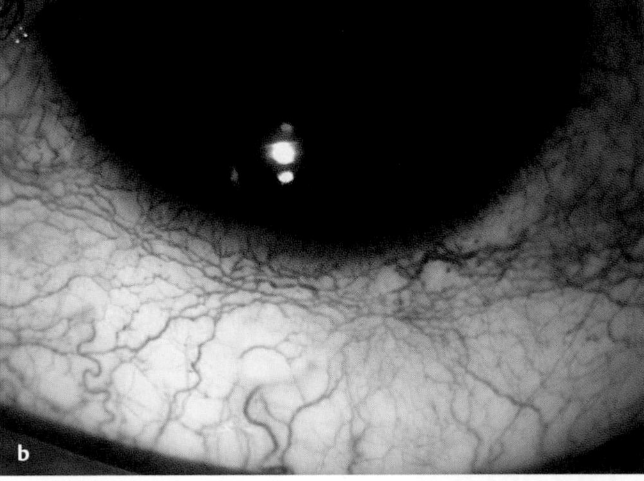

Fig. 13.14 **(a)** Extensive "honey comb" appearance of episcleral hemangioma. **(b)** A narrow band of limbal hemangiomatous changes can also be responsible for the rise in intraocular pressure (IOP).

Glaucoma occurs in 50 to 70% of cases, especially when the eyelid is involved and extensive episcleral malformations are present. Additional dysgenesis of the trabecular meshwork often leads to early and severe glaucoma (**Fig. 13.15**).

Leptomeningeal vascular malformations are present ipsilaterally in 10% of patients, involving the parietal and occipital areas. They are more often associated with larger and bilateral hamartomata. Underlying venous stasis causes ischemic damage and later calcification leads to the characteristic "rail track" double lines. Epileptic seizures occur in more than 75% of such patients.

Management of the glaucoma is initially with medications, but often requires surgery. Trabeculectomy alone or combined with trabeculotomy is commonly done. The most common complication seen after lowering of IOP is choroidal effusion. The use of MMC, releasable/adjustable sutures, and viscoelastics has decreased the chances of complications, and improved prognosis. Early control of IOP appropriate for the glaucomatous neuropathy present leads to best visual function. Lifelong review has to be explained to all patients.

Differential diagnosis of congenital corneal opacification is sometimes confused with the corneal edema seen in childhood glaucomas, and the causes are easily remembered by the mnemonic—STUMPED:

- S—Sclerocornea.
- T—Tears in Descemet's membrane; birth trauma/ glaucoma.

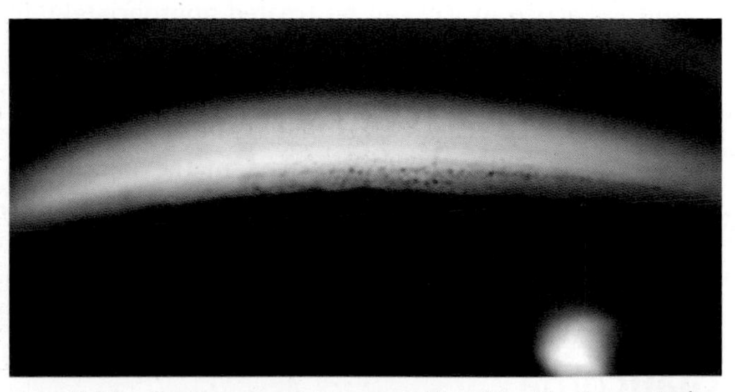

Fig. 13.15 Gonioscopy of a 4-year-old child with Sturge-Weber syndrome showing congenital anomalies such as an anterior insertion of the iris.

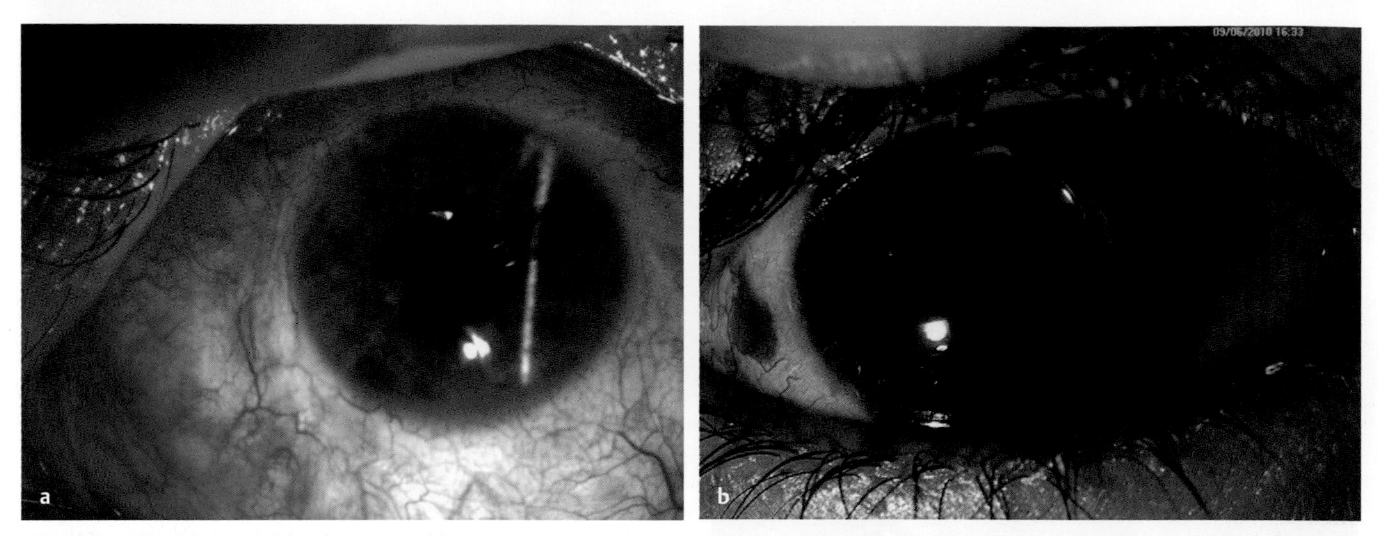

Fig. 13.16 **(a)** A 14-year-old male, operated for congenital cataract, with sclera-fixated lens, failed **Ahmed glaucoma valve** (AGV) placed through pars plana, and a functioning trabeculectomy. **(b)** Pseudophakic glaucoma in a 3-year-old. There is an updrawn pupil with evidence of healed uveitis.

- U—Ulcers; congenital rubella.
- M—Mucopolysaccharidosis.
- P—Peters anomaly.
- E—Endothelial dystrophy; CHED, posterior polymorphous.
- D—Dermoid.

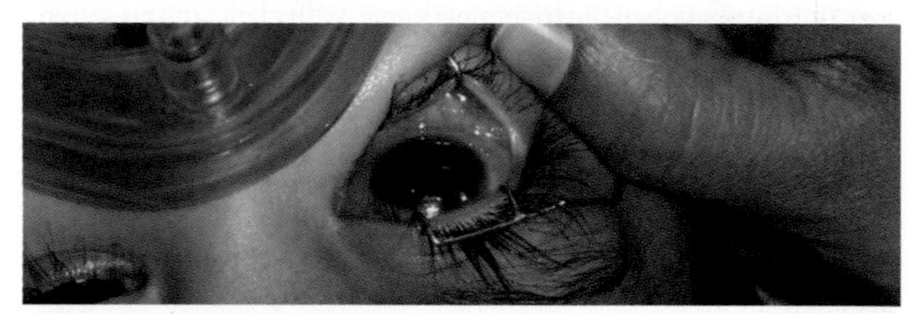

Fig. 13.17 Examination under anesthesia.

Secondary Glaucomas in Childhood

Common causes of secondary childhood glaucoma in India are trauma, steroid induced, uveitis, corneal ulcers, pseudophakia, and aphakia.

As ophthalmologists treat the primary pathology, the possibility of ensuing or attendant glaucoma is often overlooked. A high degree of suspicion in the pathologies named above would identify the rise in IOP before glaucomatous neuropathy develops. Secondary glaucomas need to have the cause identified first, followed by a gonioscopy to look for open or closed angles, so that the reason for a rise in IOP can be treated appropriately. In the presence of a normal optic nerve or mild neuropathy, reducing the IOP to a range of 18 to 20 mm Hg may be acceptable for a week or so, as there is no inherent optic nerve susceptibility to IOP. However, in the long term, reducing the IOP to the teens would give best results (**Fig. 13.16**).

Examination of a Child with Glaucoma

Examination of a child is fraught with difficulty, and the most physiological way is to *keep the child fasting for a while, so that he or she sleeps when he or she has milk at the hospital.* Most children of up to 2 years can then have an anterior segment evaluation, Perkins applanation tonometry, and a dilated fundus examination. They may be sedated if uncooperative, for example, chloral hydrate 25 to 50 mg/kg orally 30 minutes prior, but an anesthesia or pediatric backup is required in case of any untoward respiratory or central nervous system (CNS) side effects.

Examination under anesthesia is necessary to allow a detailed evaluation of the eye, IOP, and any other associated ocular anomalies (**Fig. 13.17**). This can be performed using a standardized protocol of inhalational sevoflurane and laryngeal mask airway, without muscle relaxants to have as minimal an effect as possible on IOP and further examinations on review are comparable. The important parameters to be recorded on a standard proforma are: corneal diameters, corneal clarity, cup:disc ratio, applanation tonometry, axial length, and refraction under cycloplegia.

Management of Childhood Glaucomas

Optic nerve head cupping in children is reversible due to the elasticity of optic nerve head tissues initially with a significant lowering of IOP. Early diagnosis and treatment can restore near-normal vision.

Target IOP in children is not the same as in adults, as the normal IOP in children has been recorded under anesthesia to be much lower, and related to age. A normal infant has an IOP ranging from 8 to 12 mm Hg, and children up to 14 years from 10 to 14 mm Hg. The treated IOP in a child's eye with glaucomatous optic neuropathy (GON) should therefore be brought down to such levels as well.

After pediatric review, betaxolol 0.25%, pilocarpine 2%, dorzolamide, or brinzolamide, and systemic acetazolamide are prescribed and can be evaluated.

There are few studies on the response to glaucoma medications in children, with variable results. There is lower efficacy of medications as compared to adults, and the number of nonresponders is much higher. The best efficacy is seen with oral acetazolamide 10 to 30 mg/kg/24 hours divided over every 8 hours to a maximum of 1,000 mg/24 hours, topical carbonic anhydrase inhibitors (CAIs), and β-blockers. However, even a combination of these is often not enough to lower the IOP to <15 mm Hg, and acetazolamide cannot be used for long periods (**Table 13.3**). Therefore, surgery is the treatment of choice, and medical therapy is used as a temporizing measure while awaiting surgery.

Surgeries

As the cause of the raised IOP in congenital glaucomas is a maldevelopment of the trabecular outflow pathways, specific surgeries have been aimed at relieving the obstruction to aqueous outflow present internal to Schlemm's canal—goniotomy and trabeculotomy (**Fig. 13.18**).

Goniotomy is performed ab interno from the temporal limbus. After the anterior chamber is filled with viscoelastic, a knife/blade is passed across the anterior chamber to disinsert any abnormal tissue from Schwalbe's line across 120 degrees. A success rate of 50 to 70% in infantile glaucoma has been reported with one to two procedures over 4 to 5 years. However, in neonatal or developmental glaucomas, eyes with severe glaucomatous neuropathy, or eyes with severe trabecular dysgenesis, this is not successful. It cannot be performed in the presence of a hazy cornea.

Trabeculotomy also aims to open a path through abnormal trabecular tissues to the Schlemm's canal, but ab externo. After making a radial incision at the junction of the posterior limbus and sclera, the Schlemm's canal is identified by a gush of aqueous and visibility of the canal floor. A trabeculotome is introduced into the canal to the right and the left without any force, and rotated into the anterior chamber keeping the arms parallel to the iris and away from the cornea. This opens up 90 to 180 degrees of the angle, and has been reported to have similar success rates as with goniotomy (**Fig. 13.19**). A 360-degree trabeculotomy can be performed using a 6–0 polypropylene suture or an illuminated cannula passed through the canal and pulled into the anterior chamber, with better success, again in mild glaucomas.

Both goniotomy and trabeculotomy can cause a hyphema while cutting through tissue, and hypotony or cataract if there is entry into the supraciliary space or iris trauma.

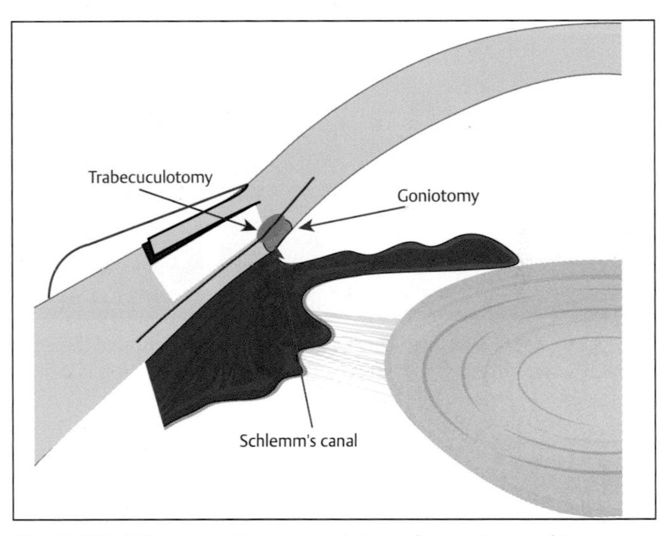

Fig. 13.18 Diagrammatic representation of surgeries used to increase access of aqueous to the Schlemm's canal in congenital glaucoma—goniotomy ab interno (*blue arrow*) and trabeculotomy ab-externo (*red arrow*).

Table 13.3 A summary of medications and their reported efficacy

Drug	Systemic side effects	Approximate IOP lowering	Nonresponse
Dorzolamide/brinzolamide	Nil	4–5 mm Hg	
β-blockers	Bronchial spasm	2–4 mm Hg	50%
Prostaglandin analogs	Nil	2–4 mm Hg	60%
Brimonidine	Central nervous system (CNS) toxicity		
Oral acetazolamide	Poor weight gain, acidosis	6–10 mm Hg	

Abbreviation: IOP, intraocular pressure.

A *combined trabeculotomy with trabeculectomy* with or without MMC has been shown to result in lower IOPs with better control even in severe glaucomas, or patients with reduced corneal clarity, of 70 to 90%. A 6- to 8-mm high, limbus-based conjunctival flap is made and a 4 × 4 mm superficial sclera flap dissected. In infants, 0.04%/0.02% MMC is applied for 2 minutes subscleral and 1 minute subconjunctival, followed by a copious wash with saline. After making a radial incision at the junction of the posterior limbus and sclera, Schlemm's canal is identified by a gush of aqueous and visibility of its floor. A trabeculotome is introduced to the right and the left without any force, and rotated into the anterior chamber, keeping the arms parallel to the iris and away from the cornea, over 120 degrees (**Fig. 13.20**). A full-thickness sclera ostum of 1 × 3 mm is excised, and an iridectomy performed. The corners of the superficial sclera flap are sutured with 10/0 monofilament and the conjunctiva with continuous 8/0 Vicryl.

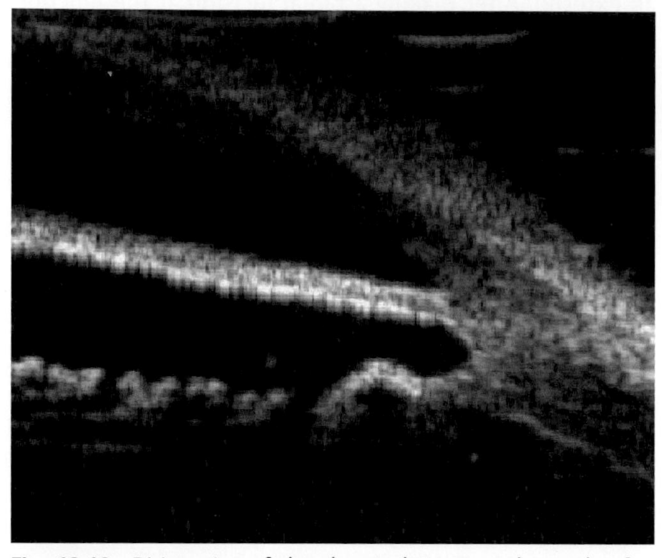

Fig. 13.19 Disinsertion of the abnormal tissue at the angle after trabeculotomy.

A *trabeculectomy with MMC* alone has also been reported to have a success of 60 to 65% (**Figs. 13.21** and **13.22**). However, over time bleb changes may occur, either as fibrosis and failure, or thinning of the epithelium over the bleb. About 4 to 6 years after combined surgery or trabeculectomy alone, thin or avascular blebs may predispose children to blebitis or traumatic rupture, and a *bleb revision* is required. An epithelial exchange without disturbing the bleb architecture preserves function over

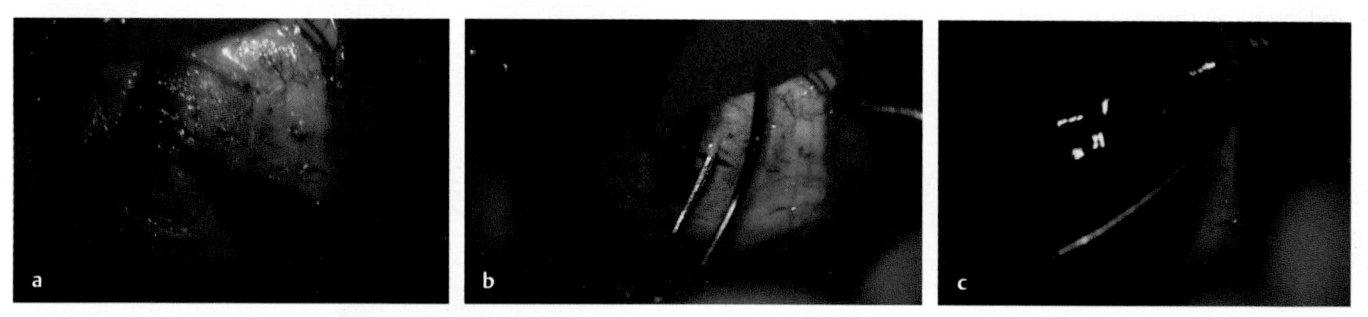

Fig. 13.20 **(a)** Identifying Schlemm's canal at the junction of the white sclera with the blue gray limbus. **(b)** Passing one arm of the trabeculotome through Schlemm's canal parallel to the limbus. **(c)** Rotating it into the anterior chamber, keeping the arm away from the cornea and parallel to the iris.

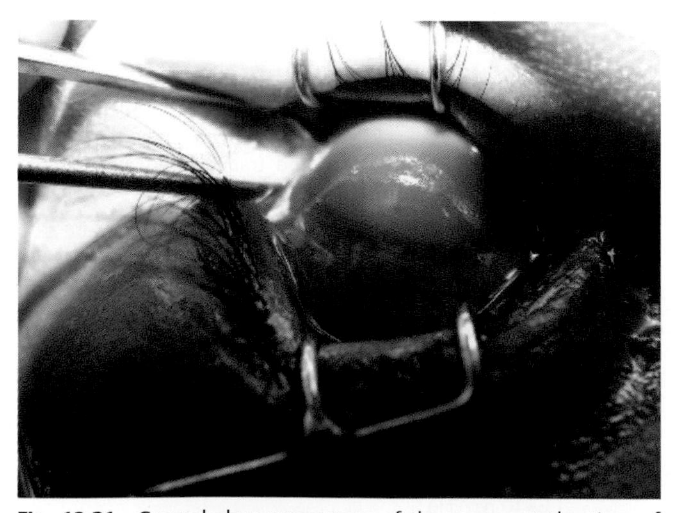

Fig. 13.21 Ground-glass appearance of the cornea at the time of surgery.

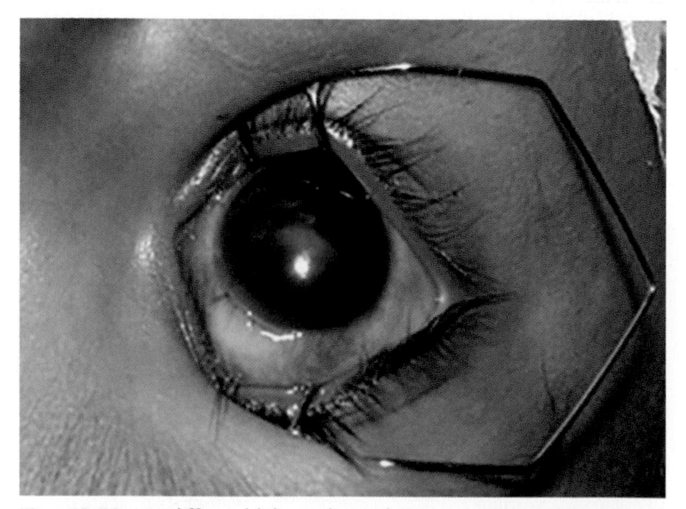

Fig. 13.22 A diffuse bleb and resolving central corneal edema 3 months after surgery.

the years (**Fig. 13.23**). Further filtering surgery may be required in eyes with a failing bleb (**Fig. 13.24**).

Glaucoma drainage devices have also been used, with a reported success similar or slightly better than trabeculectomy with MMC. However, rates of tube and plate erosion and extrusion are much higher in children over time due to thinner sclera, as is failure requiring a resurgery (**Flowchart 13.2**).

Lifelong Review

Patients need regular review examinations under anesthesia, 1 month after surgery, every 3 months for a year, and thereafter every 6 months. Anterior segment examination is performed using an operating microscope, for corneal changes, iris pattern, lens status, and bleb appearance. Corneal diameters, white to white, horizontal, and vertical, are recorded by Castroviejo calipers. The fundus should be examined by a direct ophthalmoscope to record cup:disc ratio and neuroretinal rim status, as well as any associated retinal anomalies. Any change in cup:disc ratio recorded should be seen in at least a subsequent examination and should persists till the last review. IOP with Perkins tonometer and ultrasonic corneal pachymetry should be done. Cycloplegic refraction under tropicamide provides best corrected visual acuity for patients.

As childhood glaucoma is frequently asymmetrical, and corneal irregularities are common, refractive errors need to be adequately corrected periodically. Amblyopia therapy and correction of any strabismus seen are very important for final visual acuity. Corneal opacities as in Peters anomaly need keratoplasty and careful control of IOP after that.

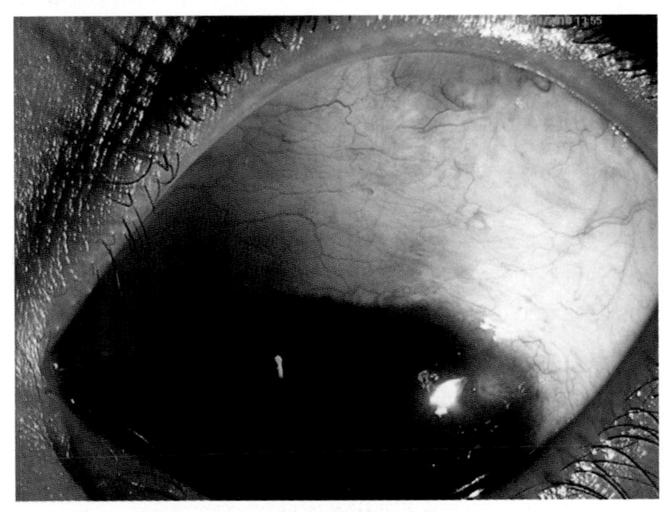

Fig. 13.23 Diffuse bleb following bleb revision necessitated by avascularity and sweating in a primary congenital glaucoma bleb.

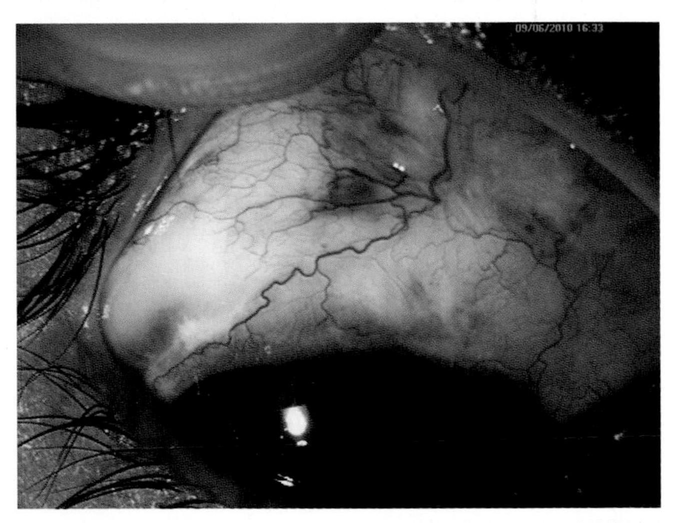

Fig. 13.24 Multiple surgeries are required in some childhood glaucomas to control intraocular pressure (IOP).

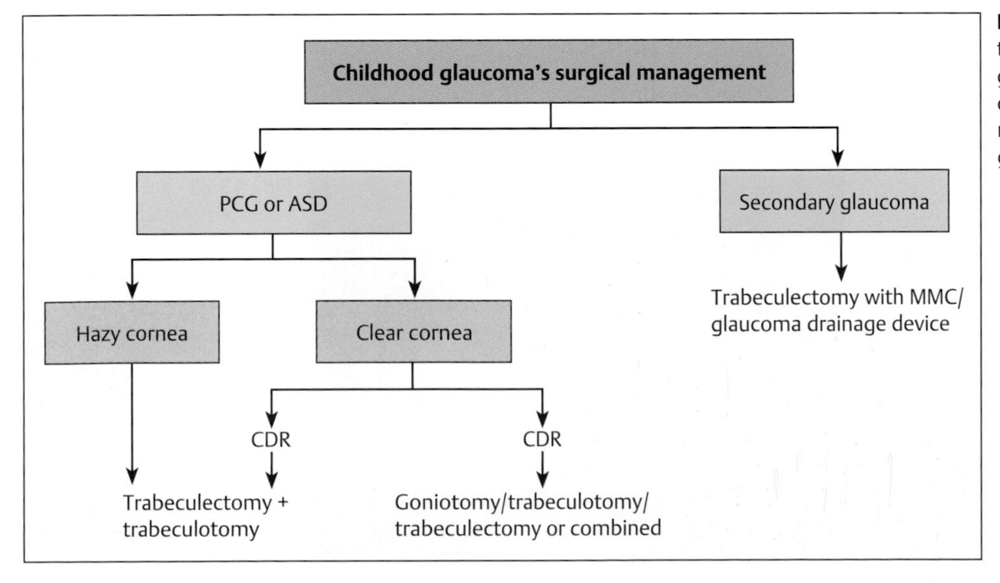

Flowchart 13.2 Algorithm explaining the surgical management of childhood glaucoma. ASD, anterior segment dysgenesis; CDR, cup:disc ratio; MMC, mitomycin C; PCG, primary congenital glaucoma.

In a few years the filtering bleb epithelium becomes thin and transparent, or is seen to be avascular with the use of MMC. These are prone to traumatic rupture, leaks, or sweating, and need a bleb revision. Bleb-related endophthalmitis is more common in children, 7 to 14%, with an increase over time. Bleb-sparing epithelial exchange has been shown to maintain IOP control in the long term.

Prognosis

Prognosis in childhood glaucomas for control of IOP has improved dramatically over the past decade. However, prognosis for vision is still lagging due to ensuing amblyopia or concomitant anterior and posterior segment anomalies, or any associated neurologic impairment.

Final visual outcome is dependent on baseline optic nerve head damage, corneal opacification, associated ocular abnormalities, amblyopia, strabismus, and IOP control in the long term. Children with PCG presenting between 1 month and 2 years of birth have the best success rates for control of IOP and good vision (**Fig. 13.25**).

Genetic Counseling

In the presence of a positive mutation of known genes, counseling becomes more specific. The autosomal recessive inheritance of CYP1B1 and LTGB mutations means that parents of affected children are heterozygotes or carriers. Congenital glaucoma is expected in 25% of siblings, 50% would be carriers, and 25% normal. Siblings of the parents have a 50% risk of being carriers. Prenatal testing for a mutation is now possible.

The morbidity from childhood glaucoma is often very severe as it is diagnosed late and not treated adequately. In treating and reviewing children, it has to be remembered that the normal IOP is in the low teens, and glaucomatous eyes should achieve such pressures to stabilize/reverse the glaucomatous neuropathy present. The lifelong review has to be emphasized as further medications or surgery may often be required.

Cases

Case 1

A 12-year-old girl with a family history of glaucoma and a cup:disc ratio of 0.5 both eyes in large optic nerve heads, underwent perimetry. Her fields showed a few central abnormal loci.

Points to consider

- Abnormal loci are not in Bjerrum's area.
- There is no normative data for children in the Humphrey machine.
- Their attention spans are short, so short programs should be used.
- Goldmann kinetic perimetry should be recorded.

Diagnosis and Management

A diagnosis of developmental glaucoma was made. There were large areas of "white-out" in the visual field suggesting a very high retinal sensitivity, or that the child was randomly pressing the buzzer (**Case 1-1**). The field was repeated on kinetic perimetry and was within normal limits.

Case 2

A newborn child is noticed to have tearing and photophobia by the pediatrician. On examination, large corneas having a ground-glass appearance were seen with a sleeping IOP of 32/36 mm Hg by Perkins tonometer. After pediatric consultation, betaxolol 0.25% twice a day and pilocarpine 2% 8 hourly with acetazolamide at 15 mg/kg 8 hourly was started, but IOP was 24/26 mm Hg.

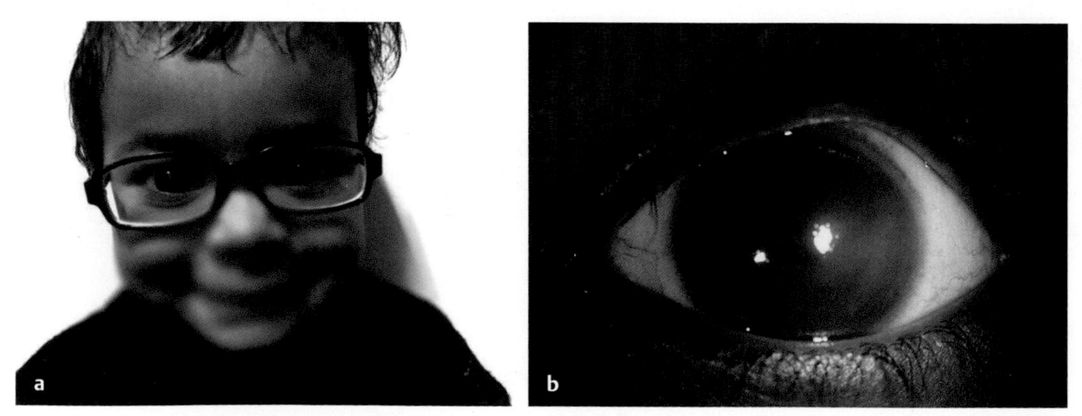

Fig. 13.25 (a, b) Bilateral operated primary congenital glaucoma with clear corneas and appropriate refractive correction.

Points to consider

- The response to glaucoma medications in children is significantly less than in adults.
- Around 25 to 30% may be nonresponders.
- Normal IOP in children is 10 to 14 mm Hg.

Diagnosis and Management

A diagnosis of congenital glaucoma was made and the patient underwent bilateral trabeculectomy plus trabeculotomy augmented by MMC 0.2 mg/mL. Topical antibiotic steroids and tropicamide drops were continued for 2 months. An examination under anesthesia at 6 weeks showed a significant clearing of both corneas with a normal anterior segment, and at 6 months clear corneas in both eyes with Haab's striae in the left eye (**Case 2-1**). At 9 years of age, the cup:disc ratio was 0.4 in both eyes, and refractions −2.5DS −0.75 DCYL at 180 degrees.

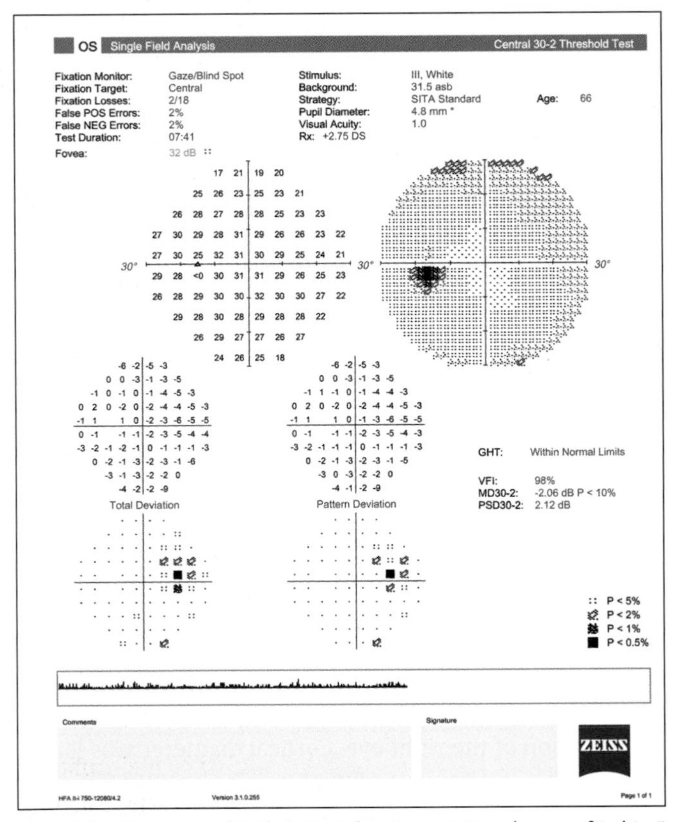

Case 1-1 Humphrey field printout showing scattered areas of "white" in the grayscale, which show up as a pattern defect; the algorithm highlights it as a significant change from normal, even if it is a higher sensitivity not lower.

Case 3

In a 3-month-old child with photophobia, asymmetric cloudy corneas, sleeping IOP of 40/30 was seen. On examination under anesthesia (EUA), corneal diameters of 14/12 mm, with Haab's striae, cup:disc ratio of 0.9/0.8, and IOP 40/28 mm Hg were noted. The patient was prescribed betaxolol 0.5% twice a day, dorzolamide and pilocarpine 2% every 8 hours, and systemic acetazolamide 8 to 30 mg/kg/24 hour doses were given every 8 hours.

Points to consider

- Large corneal diameters are a marker for severe glaucomatous neuropathy.
- Baseline severe GON may not reverse.
- Parents should be counseled that the eyes will remain large.

Diagnosis and Management

Bilateral trabeculectomy with trabeculotomy was done with MMC 0.2 mg/mL applied both subscleral and subconjunctival. A year later the IOPs were 10/12 mm Hg, corneal edema had resolved leaving a linear macular opacity over Haab's striae, and cup:disc ratio was 0.8/0.5 (**Case 3-1**). The patient was advised registration for endothelial keratoplasty, in case required.

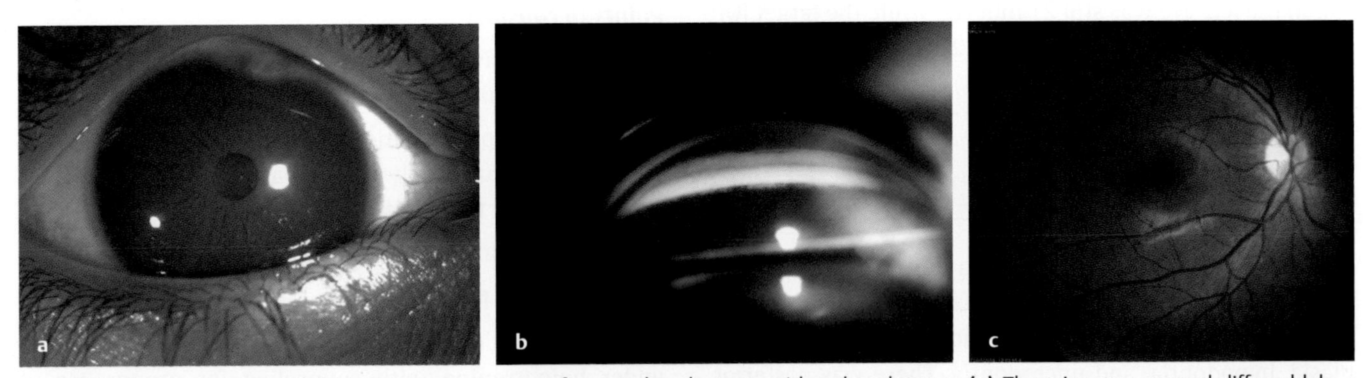

Case 2-1 A primary congenital glaucoma eye 5 years after a trabeculectomy with trabeculotomy. **(a)** There is a superonasal diffuse bleb, a clear cornea with a loss of normal pattern of the iris. **(b)** An anterior insertion of the iris can be appreciated. **(c)** Cup:disc ratio of 0.4 with regular neuroretinal rim of good color.

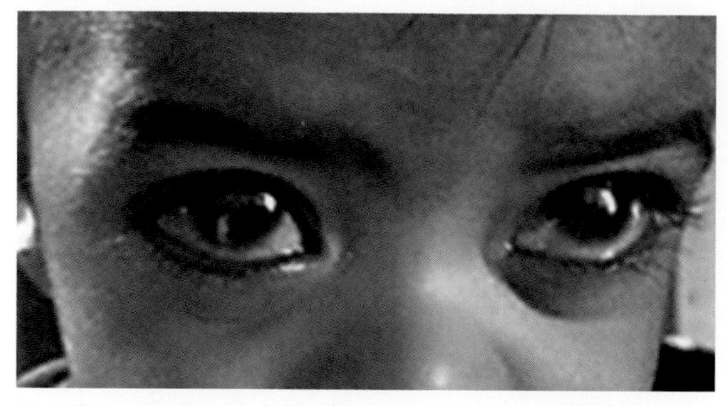

Case 3-1 Large corneal diameters, right > left, with linear corneal opacities in both eyes. The patient is no longer photophobic.

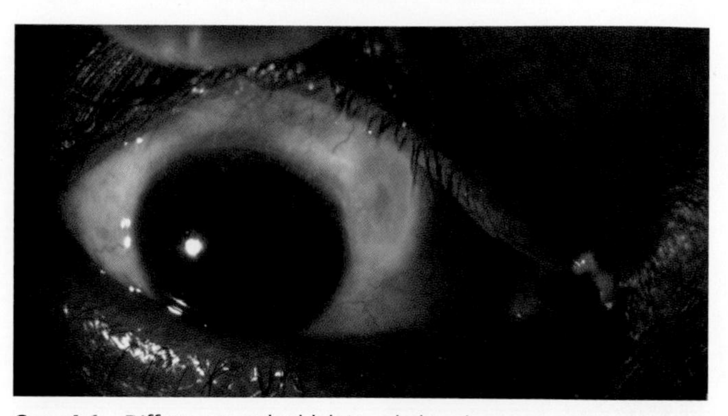

Case 4-1 Diffuse avascular bleb in aphakic glaucoma.

Case 4

A 2-year-old child complained of pain in the left eye. He had been operated for congenital cataract at the age of 3 months, lens aspiration with anterior vitrectomy was done, and the patient was left aphakic. On examination there was corneal edema, a deep anterior chamber with vitreous present, a cup:disc ratio of 0.8 with pallor, and concentric thinning of the neuroretinal rim. Sleeping IOP by Perkins tonometer was 16/36 mm Hg. The patient was advised a prostaglandin (PG) analog at bedtime and timolol twice a day. An EUA after 2 weeks showed a central cornea thickness (CCT) of 580/650 µm, a decrease in corneal edema, and an IOP of 14/28 mm Hg.

Points to consider

- Glaucoma is common after congenital cataract surgery.
- Aphakic eyes in children have thicker corneas; therefore, corrected IOPs should be documented.

Diagnosis and Management

The patient was advised a trabeculectomy as corrected IOP in the left eye was still 21 mm Hg, while the target IOP should be 12 to 14 mm Hg. After 2 years, his IOP in the left eye was 12 mm Hg (**Case 4-1**). Lifelong review was advised.

Case 5

A 10-year-old girl presented with a diminution of distant vision in the left eye noted since childhood and banging into objects recently. She was found to have malar hypoplasia, hypodontia, and microdontia. There was posterior embryotoxon, iris stromal hypoplasia, and ectopic pupils in both eyes (**Fig. 13.10**). IOP was 36/40 mm Hg. Perimetry of right eye showed only a central island of vision.

Points to consider

- Response to glaucoma medications is very poor in eyes having anterior segment dysgenesis.
- Target IOP would be 10 to 12 mm Hg, as the glaucoma is severe.

Diagnosis and Management

A diagnosis of Axenfeld-Rieger syndrome was made and a trabeculectomy augmented by MMC, 0.2 mg/mL, for 1 minute subconjunctival was done for both eyes. After 2 years, IOPs were 10/14 mm Hg with stable 10-2 Humphrey field analyzer (HFA) perimetry.

Case 6

A 6-year-old girl, diagnosed and operated for PCG in both eyes at 6 months of age, with left congenital partial ptosis, c/o deviation of the right eye. Corneal diameter was larger in the right eye with central Haab's striae, and the cup:disc ratio was 0.7/0.3. Diurnal IOP showed the highest IOP to be 24/14 mm Hg. Refractive error was −4.5D/−3D cyl, and −0.5D/−2D cyl with best corrected visual acuity of 6/60 and 6/6 (**Case 6-1**).

Points to consider

- Lower vision in the right eye can be attributed to central Haab's striae and strabismus.
- Larger cup:disc ratio in the right eye may be due to a comparatively higher baseline IOP in the right compared to the left eye.
- The normal for children this age is in the low teens.

Diagnosis and Management

Timolol, twice a day, was advised for both eyes. Refraction under homatropine with counseling for proper use of spectacles, and conventional occlusion 1:6 was done. After 6 months, the visual acuity was 6/24 and 6/6. Conventional occlusion and glaucoma medications were continued.

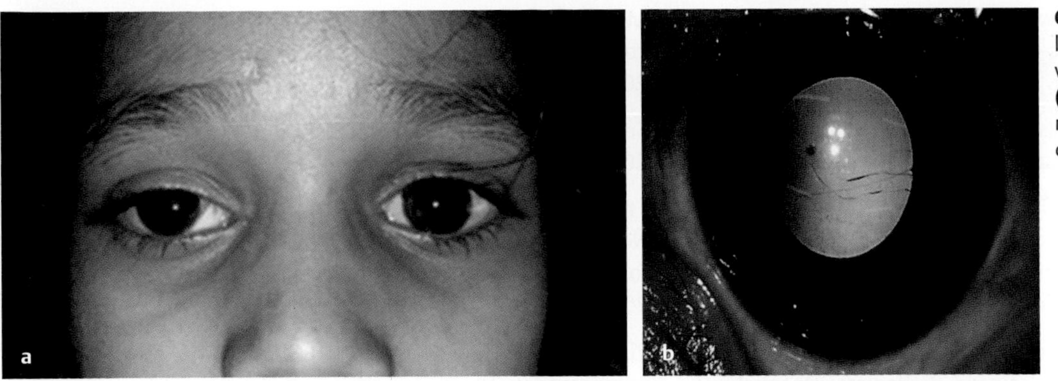

Case 6-1 **(a)** Right cornea is larger, both corneas are clear, with a right divergent squint. **(b)** Haab's striae can be seen running across the central cornea.

Case 7

A 2-week-old baby with white corneas in both eyes underwent an EUA. There was a central leucomatous opacity in both eyes with stromal edema extending to the limbus, corneal diameters were 12 mm Hg both eyes, and IOP was 34/36 mm Hg by Perkins tonometer (**Case 7-1**).

Points to consider

- Bilateral central leucomatous opacity.
- High IOP.
- Large corneal diameters.

Diagnosis and Management

A diagnosis of Peters anomaly was made and the parents counseled about other possible abnormalities such as cataract, iris hypoplasia, etc., and the need for keratoplasty after IOP control. Bilateral trabeculotomy + trabeculectomy was done, and after 6 months a clearing of the peripheral cornea was seen, IOP was 12 mm Hg in both eyes with a diffuse bleb. The patient was referred for a penetrating keratoplasty.

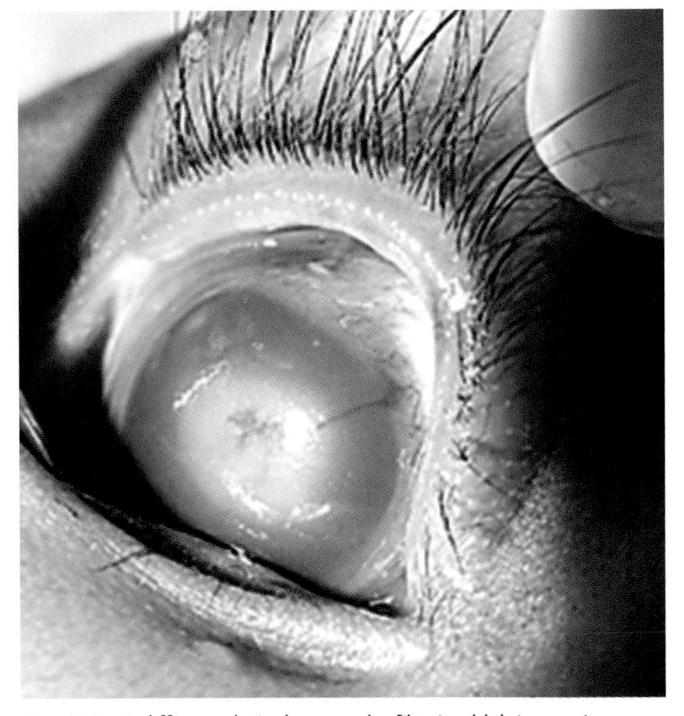

Case 7-1 A diffuse, relatively avascular filtering bleb is seen in an eye with a central leucomatous corneal opacity, that is, Peters anomaly.

Suggested Readings

Al-Hazmi A, Awad A, Zwaan J, Al-Mesfer SA, Al-Jadaan I, Al-Mohammed A. Correlation between surgical success rate and severity of congenital glaucoma. Br J Ophthalmol 2005; 89(4):449–453

Badawi AH, Al-Muhaylib AA, Al Owaifeer AM, Al-Essa RS, Al-Shahwan SA. Primary congenital glaucoma: an updated review. Saudi J Ophthalmol 2019;33(4):382–388

Chang JW, Kim JH, Kim S-J, Yu YS. Congenital aniridia: long-term clinical course, visual outcome, and prognostic factors. Korean J Ophthalmol 2014;28(6):479–485

Ghate D, Wang X. Surgical interventions for primary congenital glaucoma. Cochrane Database Syst Rev 2015;1:CD008213

Giangiacomo A, Beck A. Pediatric glaucoma: review of recent literature. Curr Opin Ophthalmol 2017;28(2):199–203

Gramer E, Reiter C, Gramer G. Glaucoma and frequency of ocular and general diseases in 30 patients with aniridia: a clinical study. Eur J Ophthalmol 2012;22(1):104–110

Hoskins HD Jr, Shaffer RN, Hetherington J. Anatomical classification of the developmental glaucomas. Arch Ophthalmol. 1984 Sep;102(9):1331–6

Idrees F, Vaideanu D, Fraser SG, Sowden JC, Khaw PT. A review of anterior segment dysgeneses. Surv Ophthalmol 2006;51(3): 213–231

Ito YA, Walter MA. Genomics and anterior segment dysgenesis: a review. Clin Exp Ophthalmol 2014;42(1):13–24

Lewis CJ, Hedberg-Buenz A, DeLuca AP, Stone EM, Alward WLM, Fingert JH. Primary congenital and developmental glaucomas. Hum Mol Genet 2017;26(R1):R28–R36

Malik R, AlDarrab A, Edward DP. Contemporary management of refractory pediatric glaucoma. Curr Opin Ophthalmol 2020;31(2):123–131

Mantelli F, Bruscolini A, La Cava M, Abdolrahimzadeh S, Lambiase A. Ocular manifestations of Sturge-Weber syndrome: pathogenesis, diagnosis, and management. Clin Ophthalmol 2016;10:871–878

Silverstein M, Salvin J. Ocular manifestations of Sturge-Weber syndrome. Curr Opin Ophthalmol 2019;30(5):301–305

Midha N, Sidhu T, Chaturvedi N, et al. Systemic associations of childhood glaucoma: a review. J Pediatr Ophthalmol Strabismus 2018;55(6):397–402

Moore DB, Tomkins O, Ben-Zion I. A review of primary congenital glaucoma in the developing world. Surv Ophthalmol 2013;58:287–285

Seifi M, Walter MA. Axenfeld-Rieger syndrome. Clin Genet 2017

Thau A, Lloyd M, Freedman S, Beck A, Grajewski A, Levin AV. New classification system for pediatric glaucoma: implications for clinical care and a research registry. Curr Opin Ophthalmol 2018;29(5):385–394

Yu Chan JY, Choy BNK, Ng AL, Shum JW. Review on the management of primary congenital glaucoma. J Curr Glaucoma Pract 2015;9(3):92–99

CHAPTER 14

Secondary Glaucomas I: Pseudoexfoliation and Pigment Dispersion

Overview

- Pseudoexfoliation Syndrome with Glaucoma
  - Pathogenesis
  - Clinical Features
  - Ocular Examination
  - Management
- Pigment Dispersion Syndrome and Pigmentary Glaucoma
  - Pathomechanism
  - Clinical Features
  - Ocular Examination
  - Differential Diagnosis
  - Management
  - Prognosis
- Cases
- Suggested Readings

Introduction

Secondary glaucomas are those that have an identifiable, acquired cause for the rise in intraocular pressure (IOP) and are associated with ocular or systemic pathology or therapy. Ophthalmologists concentrate on managing the initial pathology—trauma, infections, etc., and by the time glaucoma is diagnosed, it is usually advanced. Most secondary glaucoma patients have poor vision, partly due to the primary pathology and partly to the glaucomatous damage before the diagnosis of glaucoma is made.

Secondary glaucomas can be broadly divided by pathogenesis into open-angle and closed-angle secondary glaucomas based upon the trabecular status. *Commonly more than one mechanism may contribute to the rise in IOP and the optic neuropathy, that is, a mixed mechanism causes the raised IOP* (**Table 14.1**).

Secondary angle closure is caused by many mechanisms, grossly divided into pupillary block, pathology pulling the iris anteriorly, or abnormalities behind the iris pushing it forward (**Table 14.2**).

In this chapter, some common secondary glaucomas are discussed.

Table 14.1 Common secondary glaucomas

Angle	Ocular pathology
Open	▪ Pigmentary glaucoma ▪ Pseudoexfoliation glaucoma ▪ Blunt ocular trauma ▪ Steroid-induced ▪ Phacolytic ▪ Increased episcleral venous pressure (e.g., dysthyroid orbitopathy, Sturge-Weber syndrome) ▪ Posner-Schlossman syndrome ▪ Uveitis with trabeculitis ▪ Ghost cell glaucoma
Closed	▪ Pseudophakic/aphakic ▪ Chronic uveitis ▪ Neovascular glaucoma ▪ Iridocorneal endothelial syndrome ▪ Uveal effusion ▪ Aqueous misdirection syndrome ▪ Microspherophakia
Mixed mechanism	Almost all of the above

Table 14.2 Causative mechanisms of secondary angle closure

Pupil block	Posterior pushing mechanisms	Anterior pulling mechanisms
Seclusio/occlusion pupillae	Malignant glaucoma	Neovascular membranes
Phacomorphic	Choroidal effusions	Epithelial ingrowth
	Ciliary body cysts and tumors	ICE syndrome
	Ciliary effusions—sulfonamides, tamoxifen	
	Retinopathy of prematurity	
	Choroidal hemorrhage	

Abbreviation: ICE, iridocorneal endothelial syndrome.

Pseudoexfoliation Syndrome with Glaucoma

Pseudoexfoliation syndrome is an *age-related generalized fibrillopathy* characterized by the deposition of white, powdery, or fluffy material within the anterior segment of the eye, including lens, angle, pupil, and cornea. The deposits are most visible on the anterior lens capsule. Pseudoexfoliation can cause secondary open-angle glaucoma which is more aggressive in its clinical course with a high IOP at onset, progresses at a faster rate, and responds poorly to medical therapy, compared to primary open-angle glaucoma (POAG). *Pseudoexfoliation glaucoma (PXG) is seen in up to 50% of eyes with pseudoexfoliation, and can be associated with angle closure as well.*

Pseudoexfoliation is seen worldwide with a higher prevalence in Scandinavian countries. Its incidence varies between 1.5 and 27%, increasing with age. It is also known to be present in tissues such as lung, liver, kidney, gall bladder, and cerebral meninges.

Pathogenesis

It has been seen to be associated with single-nucleotide polymorphisms (SNPs) of lysyl oxidase-like 1 (LOXL1) gene on chromosome 15q24.1. The deposits are composed of amyloid, laminin, collagen, elastic fibers, and basement membrane. They block trabecular spaces, together with pigment released from the iris, preventing aqueous outflow.

Clinical Features

The patient may present with pain and redness, usually unilateral, with gradually diminishing vision for distance. Patients with an anatomically narrow angle may present with headaches or blurring of vision during angle-closure attacks. Those with an open angle may be completely asymptomatic.

Ocular Examination

The corneal endothelium may have small, whitish powdery flakes or pigment deposition on it, and early corneal endothelial decompensation is common. The anterior chamber may be shallow in pseudoexfoliation syndrome due to zonular laxity or an inherently small eye. Pigment dispersion, with particles floating in the anterior chamber can be seen.

A common feature is the dandruff-like whitish deposits at the pupillary margin and on the iris. A loss of pupillary ruff is seen. Due to contact between the iris and anterior lens surface, there is pigment release from the pigment epithelium, leading to peripupillary transillumination defects in light-colored irides. These are rare in brown irises and can be appreciated as a moth-eaten pattern of iris. Sphincter atrophy causes an asymmetric pupil and poor dilation. Posterior synechiae may also be seen.

Similar whitish deposits on the anterior lens capsule form three distinct zones, better visible after dilation. A homogenous central disc of the size of the pupil is surrounded by a clear zone, and further peripherally a ring of powdery deposits can be seen, forming a *target sign* (**Fig. 14.1**). Phacodonesis may be present with a subluxated or dislocated lens due to weakness of the zonules.

The mean IOP in pseudoexfoliation syndrome patients is higher than that of POAG as greater fluctuations are seen and it progresses faster than POAG. The optic nerve head often has asymmetrical or unilateral glaucomatous neuropathy with diffuse neuroretinal rim damage corresponding to the quantity of pseudoexfoliative material present (**Fig. 14.2**).

Gonioscopy shows the presence of white flakes, moderate-to-severe pigmentation of the trabecular meshwork, and a dark, dense, uneven, and wavy deposition above the Schwalbe's line, which is known as Sampaolesi's line (**Fig. 14.3**). In 9 to 18% of patients the angle may be occludable in pseudoexfoliation syndrome.

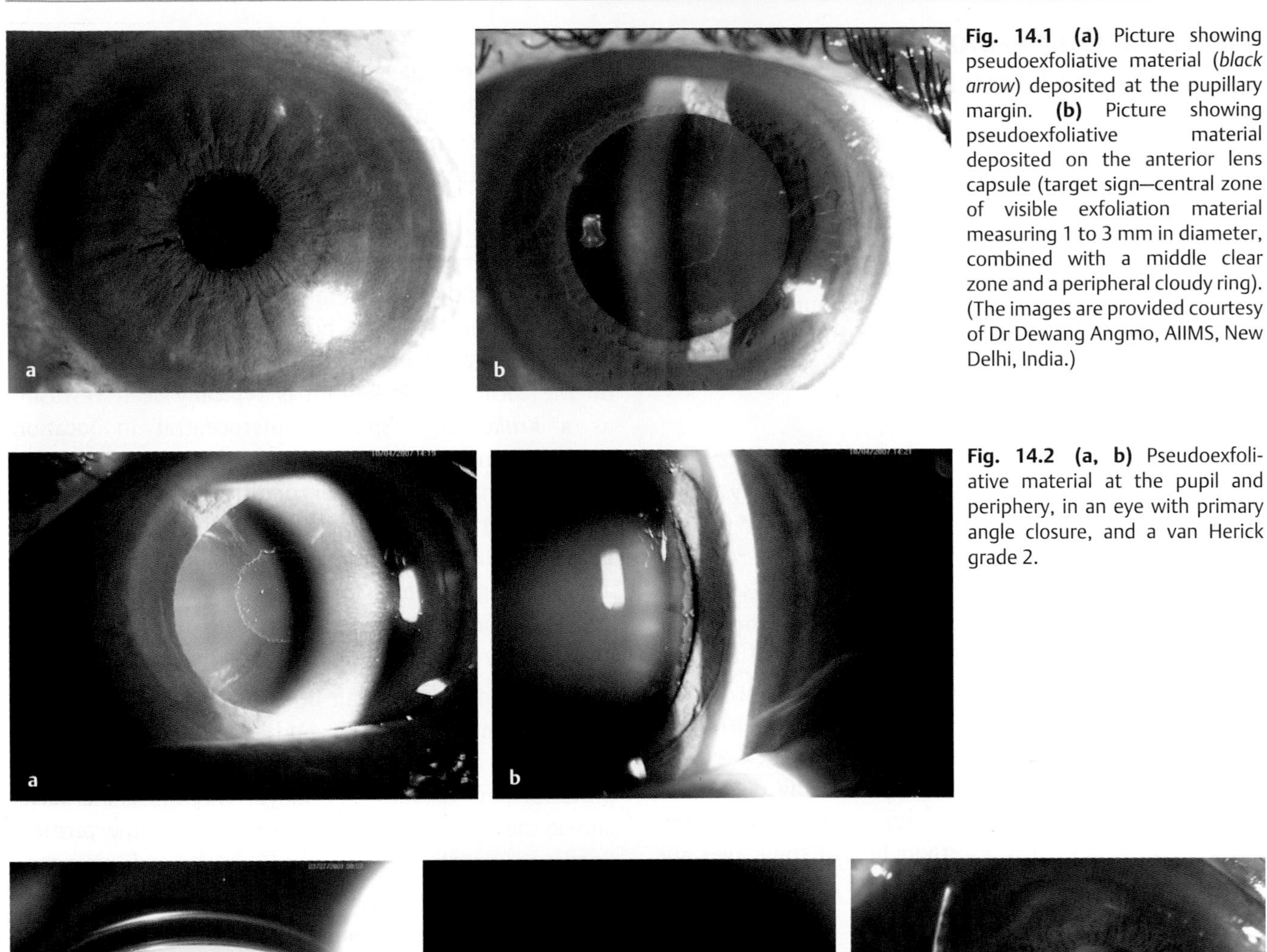

Fig. 14.1 (a) Picture showing pseudoexfoliative material (*black arrow*) deposited at the pupillary margin. **(b)** Picture showing pseudoexfoliative material deposited on the anterior lens capsule (target sign—central zone of visible exfoliation material measuring 1 to 3 mm in diameter, combined with a middle clear zone and a peripheral cloudy ring). (The images are provided courtesy of Dr Dewang Angmo, AIIMS, New Delhi, India.)

Fig. 14.2 (a, b) Pseudoexfoliative material at the pupil and periphery, in an eye with primary angle closure, and a van Herick grade 2.

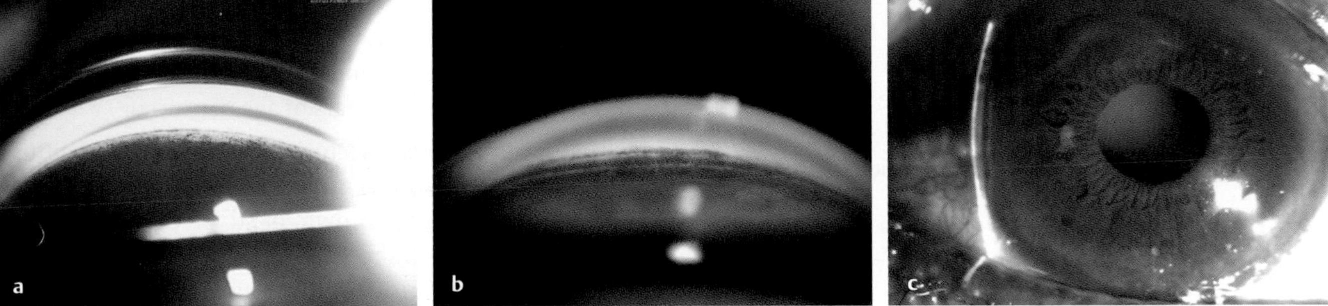

Fig. 14.3 (a, b) Gonioscopy of an open angle with pseudoexfoliation syndrome, heavy pigmentation of the trabecular meshwork, and Sampaolesi' line. **(c)** van Herick test showing a shallow anterior chamber in a patient with pseudoexfoliation.

Management

Medical treatment is similar to that of POAG, first-line drugs being prostaglandin (PG) analogs, β-blockers, and alpha-adrenergic agonists. Combination therapy is generally necessary, but may still not achieve target IOP.

Laser trabeculoplasty is successful and well tolerated for reducing IOP in PXG associated with open angles. Selective laser is the modality of choice at present.

Filtering surgery such as trabeculectomy is indicated when medical or laser therapy has failed to obtain target IOP or when there is progression of the glaucomatous neuropathy. A higher incidence of postoperative inflammation and choroidal effusion is seen.

Combined trabeculectomy and cataract surgery is indicated in PXG when there is intractable glaucoma with cataract. A heparin-coated posterior chamber intraocular lens (PCIOL) reduces the risk of postoperative inflammation. Common complications anticipated during combined or cataract surgery in PXG are poor dilation of pupil, zonular dialysis and vitreous loss, dislocation or decentration intraocular lens (IOL), and increased postoperative ocular inflammation.

Pigment Dispersion Syndrome and Pigmentary Glaucoma

Pigment dispersion syndrome (PDS) occurs due to pigment release from the iris into the aqueous. This is seen bilaterally in young, myopic males, 20 to 40 years of age. This can lead to pigmentary glaucoma (PG), a secondary open-angle glaucoma, if the pigment release is excessive enough to significantly hamper aqueous outflow, causing glaucomatous optic neuropathy. *The risk of developing PG from PDS is 10 to 50%* in different studies.

Pathomechanism

Posterior bowing of the iris with "reverse pupillary block" is thought to result from the posterior surface of the iris rubbing on anterior lens zonules, leading to pigment release from the iris pigmented epithelium. This is seen with blinking, pupillary movements, on dilation, and during strenuous exercise such as jogging and cycling. Aqueous currents deposit the pigment vertically on the central corneal endothelium. Trabecular meshwork cells phagocytize the released pigment, but pigment overload leads to their dysfunction and death causing disruption of trabecular meshwork architecture and cellular debris blocking the spaces. It is also thought that some eyes are predisposed to pigment release, with associated genes identified in some patients.

In asymmetric presentations, the eye with more posterior iris bowing, greater trabecular pigmentation, or higher IOP was more likely to show glaucomatous neuropathy.

Clinical Features

Most patients are asymptomatic. Patients may experience transient visual blurring or halos during episodes of IOP rise, particularly after exercise or pupillary dilation. Uncommonly, this may be associated with mild-to-moderate pain.

A history of trauma should be ruled out.

The disease can have varied clinical presentations:

- *PDS* with bilateral dispersion of iris pigment.
- *Pigmentary ocular hypertension* (POH), PDS with elevated IOP but without glaucomatous optic neuropathy. This is more likely to progress to glaucoma.
- *PG*, where there is glaucomatous optic neuropathy with PDS.
- *Regressed phase.* In older patients, decreased pigmentation of the trabecular meshwork is seen with IOP in the normal range, while optic nerve head and visual field changes do not reverse. This then mimics normal tension glaucoma.

A family history may be present in PDS, but is seen in 25 to 50% of patients with PG.

Ocular Examination

PDS may be either unilateral or bilateral. A deep anterior chamber with backward bowing of the peripheral iris, *concave iris configuration*, is seen. Pigment deposition on the corneal endothelium is typically seen vertically as a *Krukenberg's spindle*, inferocentral in location, corresponding to aqueous convection currents. A similar deposition may occur in other conditions such as exfoliation syndrome. Free-floating pigment granules may be present in the aqueous. Midperipheral iris transillumination defects are seen in light-colored irises in a radial spoke-like pattern due to pigment loss, best visible with retroillumination. This is rarely seen in pigmented races such as Indians.

Pigment deposition can be seen all over the anterior segment, on the anterior and posterior lens capsule, iris surface, at the level of insertion of zonules into the posterior lens capsule (Zentmayer ring or Scheie strip), and on the anterior hyaloidocapsular ligament, where it is known as Egger line.

IOP is typically elevated, with large fluctuations and spikes seen on dilation and strenuous exercise. A gradual decrease of IOP after 60 years of age may occur.

Gonioscopy shows a posterior iris insertion and diffuse, uniformly dense trabecular meshwork pigmentation: A homogeneous dark brown band of pigmentation in the superior angle more than inferior with concave iris configuration is definitive. Schwalbe's line also has pigment deposition (**Figs. 14.4** and **14.5**).

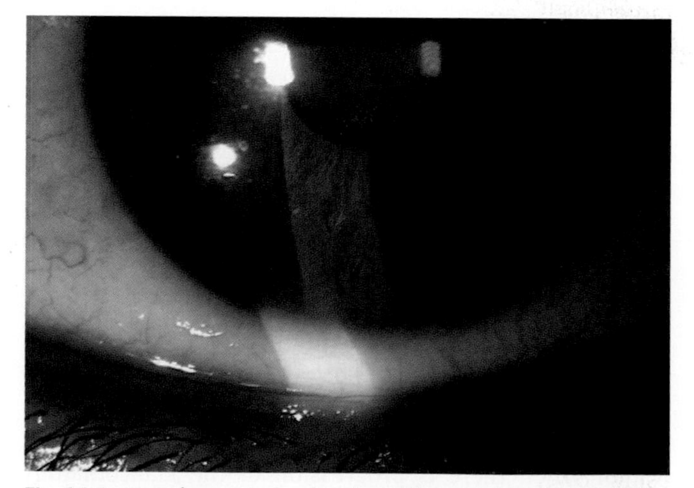

Fig. 14.4 Very deep anterior chamber with a peripheral iris concavity.

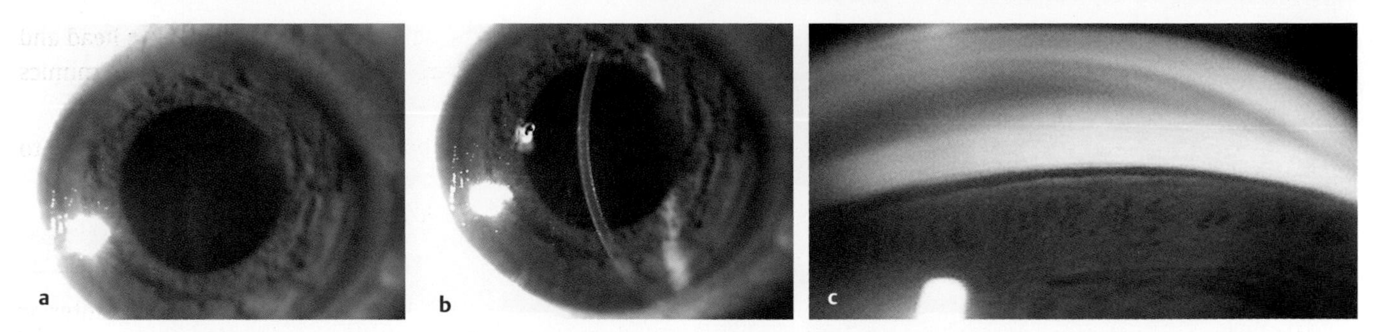

Fig. 14.5 **(a, b)** Krukenberg's spindle seen as linear pigment deposition on the central corneal endothelium, inferocentral in location corresponding to the convection currents of aqueous. **(c)** Densely pigmented trabecular meshwork seen as a uniform band.

Patients with PDS have an *increased frequency of peripheral retinal degenerations* such as lattice degeneration and retinal breaks. A rhegmatogenous retinal detachment is seen in 6 to 7% cases of PDS, irrespective of the amount of myopia. A dilated peripheral retinal screening is therefore essential.

Ultrasound biomicroscopy (UBM) can image the concave configuration of the iris and its proximity to the anterior zonules, and can be helpful to confirm reverse pupillary block, and be an indicator for laser iridotomy (**Fig. 14.6**).

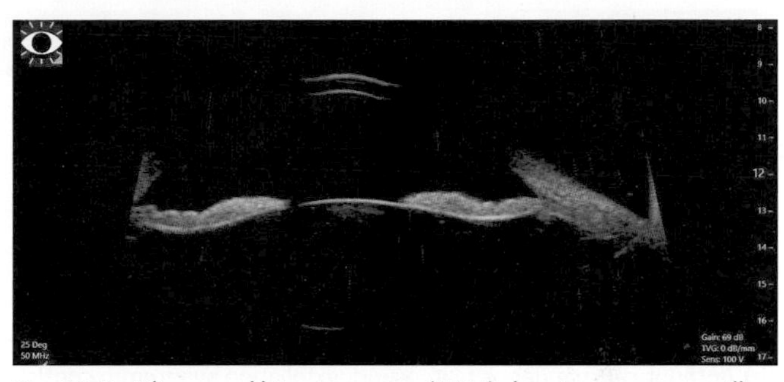

Fig. 14.6 Ultrasound biomicroscopy (UBM) showing reverse pupillary block. (The image is provided courtesy of Dr Dewang Angmo, AIIMS, New Delhi, India.)

Differential Diagnosis

All conditions that cause liberation of pigments and deposition in various structures of the anterior segment form a differential diagnosis for PDS, for example,

- Pseudoexfoliation syndrome.
- Blunt trauma.

Management

As patients are young, it is imperative that they understand the need for *appropriate lowering of IOP lifelong.*

Medical treatment is the first line to reduce IOP to target levels depending upon the severity of glaucomatous neuropathy and visual field defects, as for POAG. Pilocarpine was used to prevent the backward bowing of the iris, but is no longer a preferred drug.

Nd:YAG (neodymium:yttrium aluminum garnet) laser peripheral iridotomy (LPI) has been proposed as a means for eliminating reverse pupillary block. The iridotomy prevents pressure differentials across the anterior and posterior chamber, decreasing contact between the iris and zonular fibers and has been shown to lower IOP over the long term. Iridotomy alone may not prevent progression of PDS to PG, and additional medications are required.

Laser trabeculoplasty has been shown to be effective, using lower power settings on the heavily pigmented trabecular meshwork, and a post-laser IOP spike should be expected in such eyes and treated. There is an initial lowering of IOP, but this may be lost over time. Repeat selective laser trabeculoplasty (SLT) can be done and may be successful.

Filtering procedures are usually as successful as in POAG; however, the patients being young and myopic they are at increased risk of hypotony maculopathy.

Prognosis

With lifestyle modifications such as avoiding jogging and martial arts, fluctuations in IOP may be reduced. Appropriate therapy maintaining target IOP and regular review can stabilize glaucomatous damage.

Cases

Case 1

A 24-year-old myopic male was referred to the glaucoma clinic. His IOP was OD: 22 mm Hg, OS: 24 mm Hg. On gonioscopy, angles were open with increased pigmentation. Also, a concave iris configuration was noted. Humphrey visual field (HVF) showed no defect. Fundus examination showed large optic discs with a large cup. Central corneal thickness (CCT) was 540 and 546 µm (**Case 1-1**). Diurnal variation showed IOP ranging from 22 to 28 mm Hg. UBM confirmed reverse pupillary block.

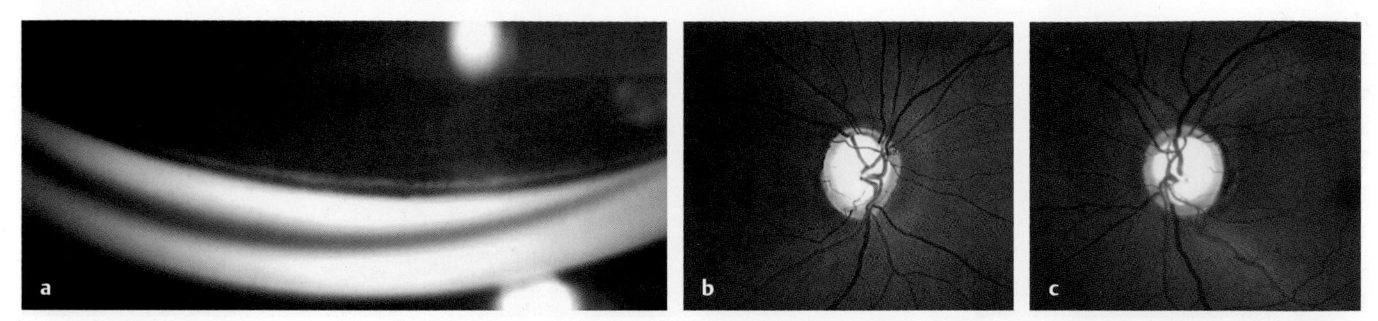

Case 1-1 **(a)** Gonioscopy of an open angle, with a heavily pigmented trabecular meshwork. **(b, c)** Fundus photographs of bilateral symmetrical large optic nerve heads with cup:disc ratio of 0.7. (The images are provided courtesy of Dr Dewang Angmo, AIIMS, New Delhi, India.)

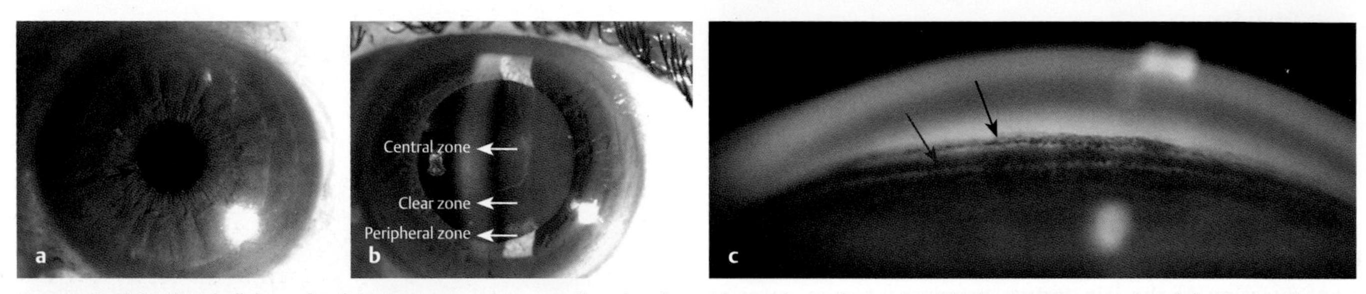

Case 2-1 **(a)** Whitish flakes of exfoliative material on pupillary border with patchy ruff atrophy (*black arrow*) in pseudoexfoliation syndrome. **(b)** Anterior capsule deposits in pseudoexfoliation syndrome, consisting of three distinct zones. A central zone known as disc, a clear zone, and a peripheral zone with striations; all together forms a classic "target sign." **(c)** Gonioscopy picture of pseudoexfoliation syndrome showing open angles with an uneven pigmentation of the trabecular meshwork (*red arrow*) and pigmentation anterior to the Schwalbe's line, also known as Sampaolesi's line (*black arrow*). (The images are provided courtesy of Dr Dewang Angmo, AIIMS, New Delhi, India.)

Points to consider

- Young patients do not normally have a pigmented trabecular meshwork.
- Look for a Krikenberg spindle or pseudoexfoliation.
- Trabeculoplasty works well in PDS.

Diagnosis and Management

A Krukenberg's spindle was seen on the corneal endothelium. A diagnosis of PG suspect was made and SLT was done. The IOP reduced to 14 to 16 mm Hg at 3 and 6 months follow-up. Lifelong review has been recommended.

Case 2

A 61-year-old male presented with complaints of gradual and painless diminution of vision in both eyes for the last 3 months. On examination, best corrected visual acuity was 6/9 in right eye and 6/12 in left eye. IOPs were 22 and 26 mm Hg in the right eye and left eye, respectively. No history of any systemic disease was present.

On slit-lamp examination, anterior chamber of van Herick grade 3 was present with normal iris pattern. Pupillary reaction was sluggish in both the eyes. White flakes of exfoliative material were present on the pupillary margin with patchy ruff atrophy (**Case 2-1a**). "Target sign" was visible (**Case 2-1b**). On gonioscopy, open angles with increased, irregular pigmentation of the trabecular meshwork were present in both eyes. Pigmentation anterior to the Schwalbe's line, also known as Sampaolesi's line, was present in the inferior angle (**Case 2-1c**). Fundus examination of right eye showed a cup:disc ratio of 0.5:1 and left eye cup:disc ratio of 0.7:1.

Points to consider

- Pseudoexfoliative glaucoma is more aggressive than POAG.
- Pseudoexfoliation may cause episodes of raised IOP.
- Perimetry should be done.

Diagnosis and Management

Pseudoexfoliative glaucoma with immature senile cataract was diagnosed in both eyes. Perimetry showed superior nasal step in the left eye. He was started on topical latanoprost in both eyes, and diurnal phasing after 2 weeks showed IOPs of 14 to 16 mm Hg. Review every 6 months was advised.

Case 3

A 65-year-old female complained of gradual diminution of vision in both eyes. On examination a shallow anterior chamber, van Herick grade 1 was seen, with pupillary ruff atrophy and a sluggish pupillary reaction. There was dandruff-like material deposited on the pupil and anterior surface of the lens. The lens had nuclear sclerosis grade 3 with a posterior subcapsular cataract (PSC). The fundus was hazily visible; a cup:disc ratio of about 0.8 was noted in both eyes. The IOP was 32/30 mm Hg. Gonioscopy of both eyes showed an occludable angle, posterior trabecular meshwork was not visible over >180 degrees, which opened on asking the patient to look toward the mirror up to the posterior trabecular meshwork, with iridotrabecular synechiae seen over >180 degrees (**Case 3-1**).

Points to consider

- Pseudoexfoliation may be seen in eyes with a narrow angle.
- Zonular weakness may lead to secondary narrowing of the angle.
- Primary angle-closure glaucoma (PACG) may be more severe in the presence of pseudoexfoliation.

Diagnosis and Management

A diagnosis of PACG with pseudoexfoliation was made, and the patient was immediately started on dorzolamide/timolol combination drops twice a day and 3 days later underwent an Nd:YAG iridotomy in both eyes. After 2 weeks, patency of the iridotomy was confirmed by direct visualization of the lens capsule; the IOP was 22/20 mm Hg. Perimetry showed a biarcuate scotoma in the right eye and a superior arcuate defect in the left. As the target IOP was in the low teens a PG analog was added.

Case 4

A 50-year-old male was diagnosed with early POAG, having a superior nasal step in the right eye, and a baseline IOP of 26/22 mm Hg, recorded thrice at different occasions. The patient was advised the use of PG analog at bedtime, and reviewed in 2 weeks, when the IOPs were 15/16 mm Hg. However, the field defect in the right eye was seen to progress over the year, with fluctuating IOPs of the late-teens/early 20s and he was referred to a tertiary center (**Case 4-1**).

Points to consider

- Was the patient compliant?
- Was he using the prescribed drug?
- Was there some other additional factor such as steroid use or pseudoexfoliation?

Diagnosis and Management

The patient claimed to be very compliant and could afford the medications. On repeating gonioscopy a few white flakes were seen on the trabecular meshwork which was heavily pigmented. On dilation of the pupil a "target" sign was seen. A diurnal phasing showed a range of IOP of 14 to 22 mm Hg, and a β-blocker twice a day was added to dampen this. On subsequent review at 5 years, the IOPs and perimetry were stable.

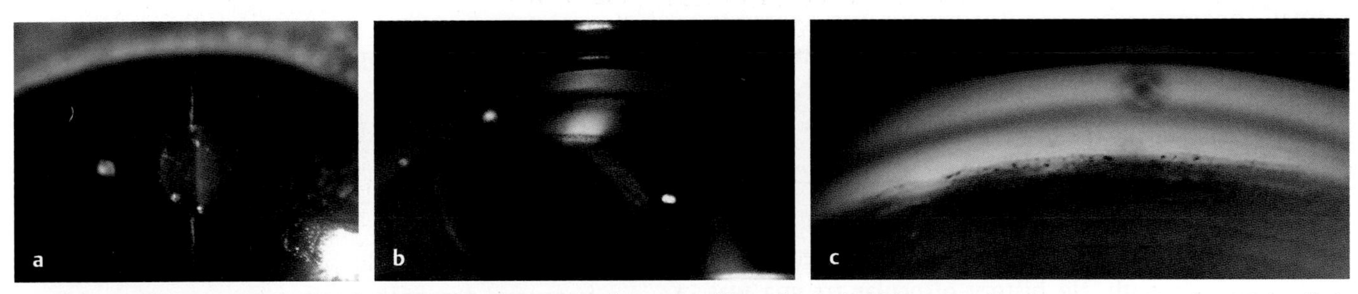

Case 3-1 **(a)** Shallow anterior chamber with white deposits on the pupil and lens. **(b)** Occludable angle with pigment seen anterior to Schwalbe's line. **(c)** After manipulation, peripheral anterior synechiae and irregular pigmentation can be seen.

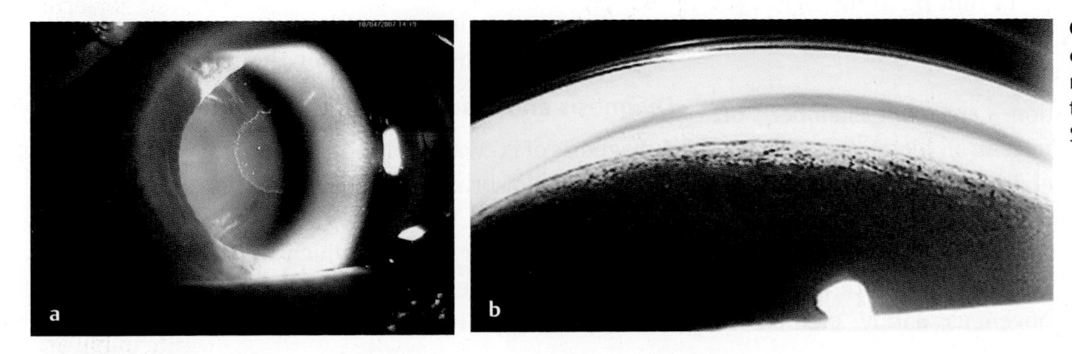

Case 4-1 **(a)** Central circular deposit of pseudoexfoliative material. **(b)** Pigmented trabecular meshwork and a Sampaolesi's line seen.

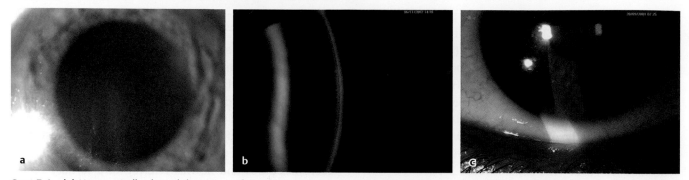

Case 5-1 **(a)** Linear spindle-shaped deposition of pigment on the cornea. **(b)** "S"-shaped iris concavity. **(c)** Uniform, dense band of trabecular meshwork pigmentation 3+.

Case 5

A 20-year-old fitness instructor complained of episodes of blurring during exercise for which his blood pressure, etc., had been evaluated. On examination, Krukenberg's spindle was visible in both eyes, with a concave, relatively featureless iris. The cup:disc ratios were 0.4 and 0.3, with IOPs of 20/22 mm Hg (**Case 5-1**).

Points to consider

- The IOPs were borderline high.
- IOP could be much higher during certain exercises.
- Both optic nerve heads are within normal limits.

Diagnosis and Management

A diagnosis of pigment dispersion syndrome was made. On UBM significant iridozonular contact was seen and an Nd:YAG iridotomy was done. The patient was advised to avoid strenuous exercise and review for IOP, etc., twice a year.

Case 6

A 29-year-old male presented with complaints of gradual and painless diminution of vision in the right eye, noticed for the last 1 month. No history of ocular trauma was present. On examination, best corrected visual acuity was hand movement close to face in the right eye and 6/6 in the left eye. IOPs were 20 and 14 mm Hg in the right eye and left eye, respectively. No history of any other systemic illness or drug use was present.

On slit-lamp examination, anterior chamber of van Herick grade 4 was present in both eyes. Heavy pigmentation on the central corneal endothelium, also known as "Krukenberg's spindles," was seen in the right eye (**Case 6-1**). Relative afferent pupillary defect was present in the right eye. On gonioscopy, open angles with a concave iris configuration and homogenous darkly pigmented trabecular meshwork grade 4 in the right eye and grade 2 in the left eye were present. Fundus examination of the right eye showed a cup:disc ratio of 0.9:1 and left eye cup:disc ratio of 0.4:1.

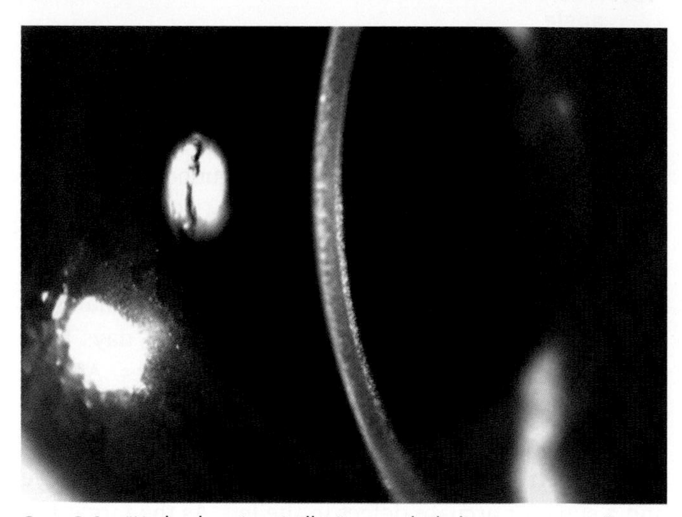

Case 6-1 "Krukenberg's spindles" on endothelium—pigment deposition on corneal endothelium in a triangle shape due to aqueous currents.

Points to consider

- Krukenberg's spindle present in both eyes, right larger and denser than left.
- Trabecular pigmentation was much more in the right eye.
- Asymmetric optic nerve damage commensurate with extent of pigment dispersion.

Diagnosis and Management

A diagnosis of PG was made and the patient was prescribed topical timolol-brimonidine combination in both eyes and a PG analog in the right eye. He underwent a diurnal phasing of IOP after 4 weeks, which showed an IOP of 10 to 12 mm Hg in both eyes through the day. He was advised 3 monthly review to recheck efficacy and compliance.

Suggested Readings

Ayala M. Long-term outcomes of selective laser trabeculoplasty (SLT) treatment in pigmentary glaucoma patients. J Glaucoma 2014;23(9):616–619

Buffault J, Leray B, Bouillot A, Baudouin C, Labbé A. Role of laser peripheral iridotomy in pigmentary glaucoma and pigment dispersion syndrome: a review of the literature. J Fr Ophthalmol 2017;40(9):e315–e321

Jensen PK, Nissen O, Kessing SV. Exercise and reversed pupillary block in pigmentary glaucoma. Am J Ophthalmol 1995;120(1):110–112

Liu L, Ong EL, Crowston J. The concave iris in pigment dispersion syndrome. Ophthalmology 2011;118(1):66–70

Michelessi M, Lindsley K. Peripheral iridotomy for pigmentary glaucoma. Cochrane Database Syst Rev 2016;2(2):CD005655

Plateroti P, Plateroti AM, Abdolrahimzadeh S, Scuderi G. Pseudoexfoliation syndrome and pseudoexfoliation glaucoma: a review of the literature with updates on surgical management. J Ophthalmol 2015;2015:370371

Schlötzer-Schrehardt U, Naumann GO. Ocular and systemic pseudoexfoliation syndrome. Am J Ophthalmol 2006;141(5): 921–937

Scuderi G, Contestabile MT, Scuderi L, Librando A, Fenicia V, Rahimi S. Pigment dispersion syndrome and pigmentary glaucoma: a review and update. [Published correction appears in Int Ophthalmol. 2019 Jun 6;] Int Ophthalmol 2019;39(7): 1651–1662

Sugar HS. Pigmentary glaucoma: a 25-year review. Am J Ophthalmol 1966;62(3):499–507

Wang W, He M, Zhou M, Zhang X. Ocular pseudoexfoliation syndrome and vascular disease: a systematic review and meta-analysis. PLoS One 2014;9(3):e92767

CHAPTER 15

Secondary Glaucomas II: Pseudophakic, Aphakic, Malignant, and Post-Uveitic Glaucomas

Overview

- Pseudophakic and Aphakic Glaucomas
  - Etiology
  - Clinical Features
  - Management
  - Complications
  - Prognosis
- Aqueous Misdirection Syndrome or Malignant Glaucoma
  - Pathophysiology
  - Clinical Features
  - Management
  - Prognosis
- Uveitic Glaucoma
  - Pathophysiology
  - Clinical Features
  - Management
  - Prognosis
- Cases
- Suggested Readings

Introduction

Secondary glaucomas are defined as those that have an identifiable, acquired cause for the rise in intraocular pressure (IOP) and are associated with ocular or systemic pathology or therapy. Some secondary glaucomas may be caused by inflammatory or other changes following ocular surgery or other ocular pathology, and commonly have both open angle and closed angle trabecular damage. Some secondary glaucomas are discussed below:

- Pseudophakic and aphakic glaucomas.
- Aqueous misdirection syndrome.
- Uveitic glaucoma.

Pseudophakic and Aphakic Glaucomas

Glaucoma secondary to changes in or pathology of the crystalline lens is called lens induced glaucoma, while a rise in IOP caused due to cataract surgery is termed pseudophakic or aphakic glaucoma.

A rise of IOP may be seen in up to 40% of eyes 6 to 12 hours after an uncomplicated cataract surgery, which returns to baseline in a day.

Pseudophakic or aphakic glaucoma is defined as a raised IOP caused as a consequence of cataract surgery or its aftereffects, and is generally seen in eyes which had some complication during surgery. There are many reasons for such a rise in IOP after cataract surgery, and these have to be identified, so that appropriate therapy is instituted to reduce the raised IOP and prevent glaucomatous neuropathy.

The Chennai Glaucoma Study found a prevalence of 1.38% of pseudophakic or aphakic glaucomas among all glaucomas identified. *Glaucoma was found in 18.59% of aphakes and 5.99% of pseudophakes.* As a result of glaucoma, 18.52% of people with glaucoma in aphakia/pseudophakia were blind in one eye and 3.70% in both eyes.

Etiology

Multifactorial glaucomas are due to many factors that cause trabecular outflow dysfunction, and the rise in IOP can occur in the presence of an open angle or with evidence of angle closure or often with both.

Intraoperative complications leading to secondary rise in IOP include posterior capsular rupture, vitreous loss, or lens drop. Postoperatively the occurrence of a shallow anterior chamber can lead to peripheral anterior synechiae (PAS) or significant postoperative inflammation may cause trabeculitis and synechiae. *Commonly identified reasons for pseudophakic or aphakic glaucoma are postoperative inflammation, posterior and peripheral synechiae, residual lens material, and intraocular lens (IOL) related problems such as haptic malposition* (**Table 15.1**).

Clinical Features

Pseudophakic or aphakic glaucomas tend to occur in eyes with a history of preoperatively complicated or displaced cataracts, or eyes in which intraoperative and postoperative problems have occurred. *Such eyes therefore have many associated features, such as uveitis, corneal endothelial cell loss, fibrous endothelial metaplasia, PAS, and pigment dispersion, which have to be identified.* Examination should be aimed at detecting the abnormalities affecting trabecular outflow, any associated intraocular damage, and the effects of raised IOP.

Aphakic glaucoma is more common in patients below the age of 15 years, with about three-fourths being seen after congenital cataract surgeries and most others after ocular trauma.

Pseudophakic glaucoma on the other hand is more frequent in adults, with 90% of eyes having a history of complications during cataract surgery. *Anterior chamber IOLs are more likely to cause a secondary glaucoma, which is seen in 5 to 6%,* often due to a posterior chamber IOL placed wrongly in the anterior chamber, or pupillary capture of the IOL (**Fig. 15.1**). *Iris fixated IOLs can result in pseudophakic glaucoma in around 4% of eyes while posterior chamber IOLs cause the least glaucoma, in 2 to 3% of eyes.*

Viscosurgical device use during cataract surgery is ubiquitous, and increased IOP is recorded commonly 4 to 8 hours after surgery due to high molecular weight material blocking trabecular spaces. IOP generally returns to normal in 1–7 days or so, but may reach levels of 30 mm Hg, which should be looked for. *Sodium hyaluronate causes a higher IOP rise than methylcellulose.* This is also used to keep the anterior chamber formed after posterior capsular rupture, and may enter the vitreous, from where absorption or removal is extremely slow therefore leading to chronically high IOPs (**Fig. 15.2**).

Chronic uveitis is an integral part of the ocular response to complications such as excessive manipulations in the eye, retained lens matter, and the use of anterior chamber IOLs. It is accompanied by trabeculitis which can cause trabecular edema decreasing trabecular spaces, an inflammatory membrane, or ultimately heal with fibrosis causing a chronically decreased aqueous outflow. Pupillary block can be caused by iris adhesions to an anterior chamber or posterior chamber IOL, a large air bubble, or the vitreous face. The occurrence of an occlusio/seclusio pupillae can

Table 15.1 Multiple factors alone and together that contribute to pseudophakic/aphakic glaucoma

Open angle factors	Angle closure factors
Viscoelastics that are incompletely removed/or enter the vitreous	IOL malposition
Vitreous in anterior chamber	Pupillary block by IOL or vitreous face
Pigment dispersion	Uveitis causing seclusio or occlusio pupillae
Trabeculitis with uveitis	Prolonged shallow anterior chamber after surgery
Steroid-induced glaucoma	Iris prolapse
Epithelial ingrowth	Malignant glaucoma
Residual lens matter	

Abbreviation: IOL, intraocular lens.

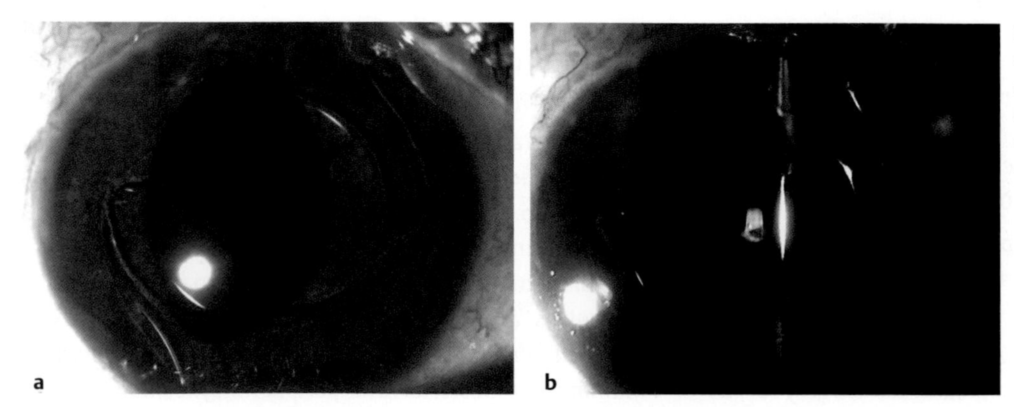

Fig. 15.1 **(a)** Pseudophakic glaucoma after anterior chamber intraocular lens (IOL) and vitreous in the anterior chamber. **(b)** Pseudophakic glaucoma, secondary angle closure after an anterior chamber IOL.

lead to chronic angle closure. Therapy with long-term steroids is an additional reason for a rise of IOP in such eyes. The uveitis-glaucoma-hyphema (UGH) syndrome was more prevalent earlier, with the frequent use of anterior chamber IOLs, but can occasionally occur with sulcus and posterior chamber IOL placement also, due to ongoing iris microtrauma (**Fig. 15.3**). This presents commonly with repeated episodes of uveitis, cystoid macular edema, and microhyphemas.

Congenital cataract surgery leads to a secondary glaucoma in 10 to 40% of eyes, being more common after aphakia than pseudophakia, and in eyes operated in infancy, less than 2 to 3 months of age, rather than later (**Fig. 15.4**). Congenital anterior segment or trabecular anomalies may preexist in eyes with congenital cataract, increasing the possibility of a rise in IOP after surgery. The incidence of glaucoma continues to increase with time after congenital cataract surgery, and repeated lifelong tonometry and optic nerve head examination in such eyes is important.

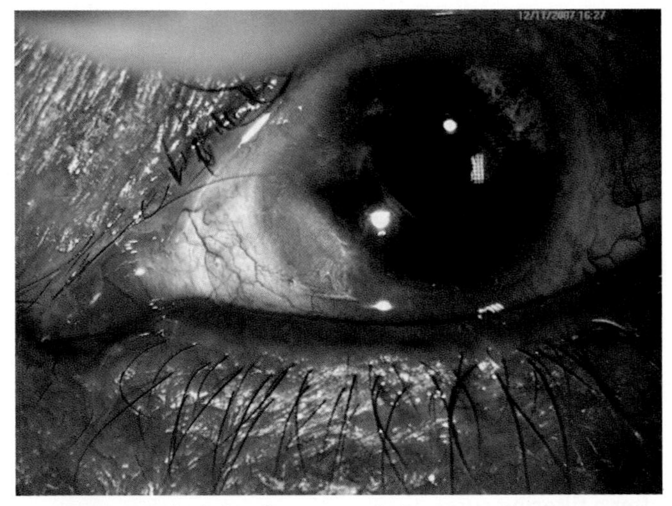

Fig. 15.2 Pseudophakic glaucoma with chronic uveitis after posterior capsular rupture.

Management

Prevention is as always the best policy. For example, the necessity for an iridectomy in aphakic eyes, especially children, and doing a thorough vitrectomy in case of intraoperative problems during cataract surgery. The use of perioperative steroids in eyes expected to have significant inflammation would also reduce the later occurrence of glaucoma.

IOP control in the early postoperative period should be aimed at reducing IOP to the early 20s, as the optic nerve would be normal. In the presence of chronically raised IOP, a target range based upon the extent of glaucomatous damage will need to be set. The first line of therapy for pseudophakic or aphakic glaucoma is medical control, avoiding latanoprost and pilocarpine while inflammation is present. These may be added once inflammation subsides. *Open angle pseudophakic or aphakic glaucomas generally respond to medical therapy, or a laser trabeculoplasty may help to reach the target IOP.*

Pupillary block due to any cause—inflammatory membrane, IOL, or vitreous—is initially treated conservatively with mydriatics and steroids to break any synechiae and lift the iris off. If this is not effective, an Nd:YAG laser iridotomy performed over a pocket of aqueous will allow the iris to fall back relieving iridotrabecular contact. This may require a number of attempts, with a gap of a few days

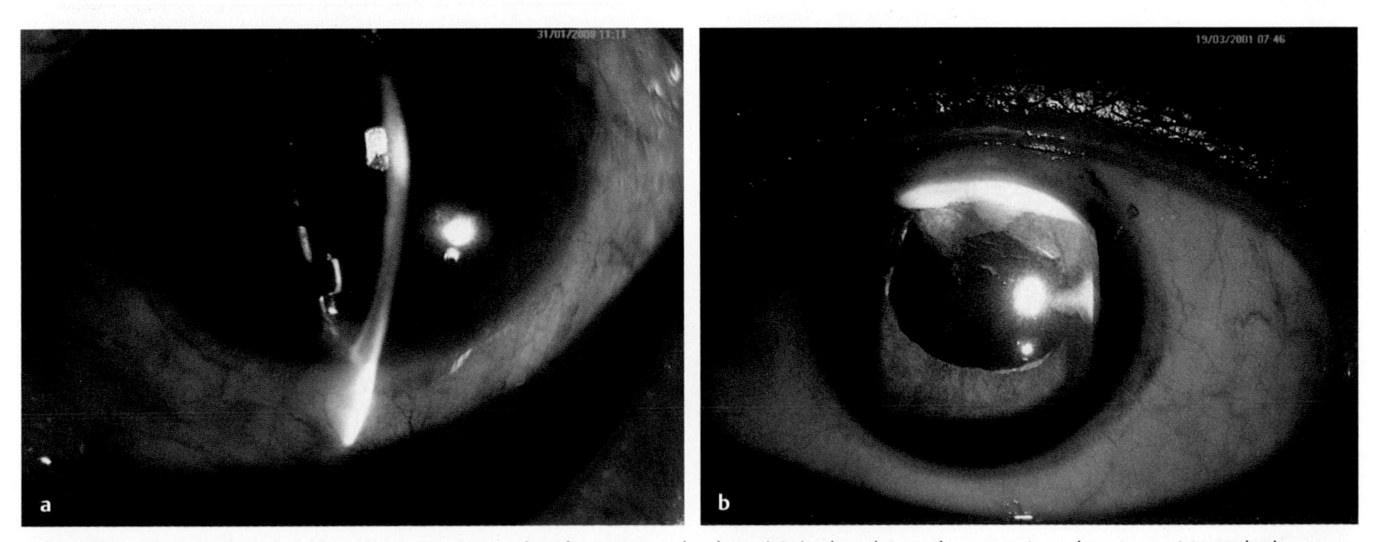

Fig. 15.3 **(a)** Pseudophakic glaucoma. Posterior chamber intraocular lens (IOL) placed in sulcus causing chronic uveitis and glaucoma. **(b)** Pseudophakic glaucoma having vitreous in the wound, with stromal and epithelial ingrowth.

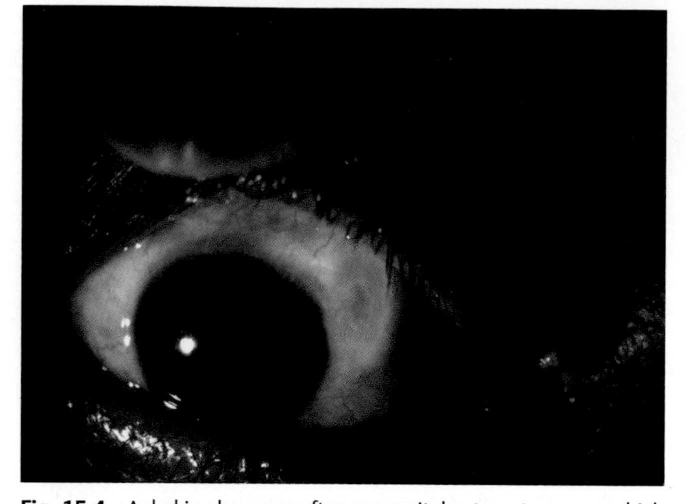

Fig. 15.4 Aphakic glaucoma after congenital cataract surgery which required a trabeculectomy.

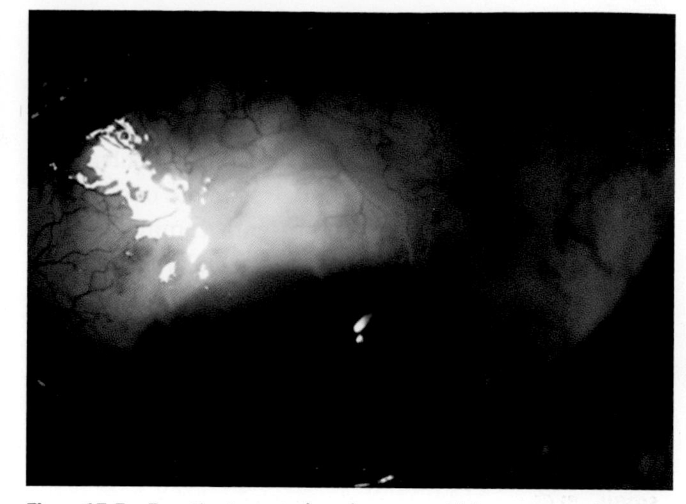

Fig. 15.5 Functioning trabeculectomy bleb in pseudophakic glaucoma.

to allow inflammation to settle between laser applications. A small iridotomy may close over time, and therefore it needs to be large and preferably multiple.

IOL explantation or exchange may be required in UGH syndrome and malpositioned lenses, once inflammation and IOP have been controlled medically.

Surgery in the early postoperative period is only required if there is residual lens matter in the anterior chamber or vitreous, causing severe inflammation. The lens matter in such cases needs to be removed early and as much as possible. Eyes that have chronically raised IOP need filtering surgery, which has to overcome existing inflammation, fibrosis, and the presence of free vitreous. Any such surgery should be attempted in as quiet an eye as possible.

Trabeculectomy augmented by mitomycin C (MMC) has improved the success rate in such eyes, and may need the application of MMC 0.2 mg/mL for 1 minute, subconjunctival and/or subscleral depending upon the fibrosis encountered during dissection. Long-term efficacy of trabeculectomy can be improved by:

- Waiting for a quiet eye.
- Use of releasable scleral sutures with early removal to maintain the anterior chamber and prevent endothelial cell loss.
- Postoperative globe massage/MMC application over the conjunctiva at the first signs of scarring.
- Longer postoperative use of topical steroids for up to 2 months.

Glaucoma drainage devices have been used, but are plagued with problems of vitreous plugging the tube and fibrosis. Placement in the ciliary sulcus decreases corneal complications and has improved success.

Complications

Complications after filtering surgery are seen more often in aphakic eyes especially in children. A flat or shallow anterior chamber, choroidal effusions, suprachoroidal hemorrhage, and bleb failure due to fibrosis are common (**Fig. 15.5**). In aphakic glaucomas, it has been suggested that putting an anterior chamber/posterior chamber IOL at the time of trabeculectomy or a drainage device may prevent or decrease effusions and suprachoroidal hemorrhages after a filtering surgery.

Prognosis

The prognosis for IOP control in pseudophakic glaucomas is better than for aphakic glaucomas, while visual prognosis depends on the amount of glaucomatous neuropathy present at diagnosis and accompanying ocular pathology such as pseudophakic bullous keratopathy. In children, management of amblyopia after IOP control is exceedingly important.

Aqueous Misdirection Syndrome or Malignant Glaucoma

Malignant glaucoma is a recalcitrant glaucoma with very shallow anterior chambers, and often very high IOPs, in the presence of a patent iridotomy. It is variously known as aqueous misdirection or ciliary block glaucoma, reflecting its pathophysiology. *This is difficult to treat and more importantly needs chronic therapy to prevent recurrences.*

Pathophysiology

Shaffer and Hoskins have suggested that aqueous may be misdirected into the vitreous, pushing the lens iris diaphragm forward, so that the anterior chamber becomes very shallow or flat and the IOP becomes extremely high. The vitreous face appears to prevent the movement of this aqueous anteriorly. Quigley et al suggest choroidal thickening and supraciliary effusion as the cause for recalcitrant shallowing of the anterior chamber.

Clinical Features

Malignant glaucoma occurs in anatomically predisposed, small eyes, especially in eyes with chronic primary angle closure with high IOP, after laser, surgery, or even spontaneously. It tends to occur in both eyes of a patient due to an inherent predisposition.

As aqueous misdirection tends to occur after a trabeculectomy or iridotomy in primary angle-closure glaucoma (PACG) eyes, the first sign to look for is a shallowing of the anterior chamber, with a tense eyeball, sometimes even while the surgery is in progress. Aqueous misdirection is accompanied by pain and severe diminution of vision. On examination there is ciliary congestion, an absent or very shallow anterior chamber, corneal stromal and epithelial edema, and a stony hard eye (**Fig. 15.6**).

It is important to rule out the more common cause of a shallow anterior chamber and pupillary block by doing or checking for a prior iridotomy. A suprachoroidal hemorrhage may also cause shallowing of the anterior chamber with a raised IOP, and an ultrasound would help distinguish it.

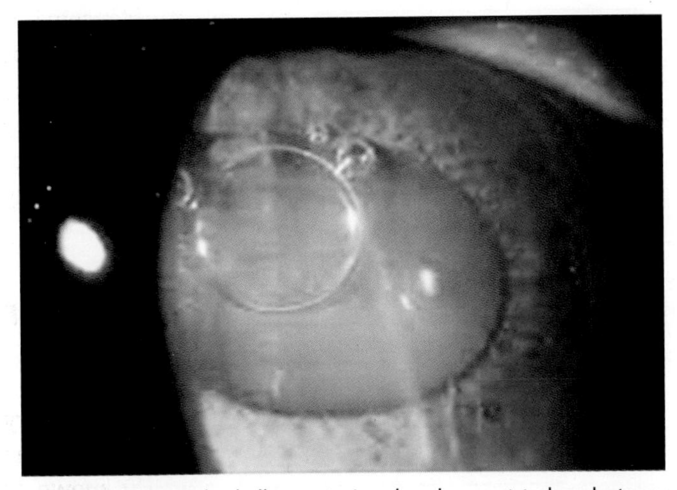

Fig. 15.6 Extremely shallow anterior chamber post trabeculectomy on first postoperative day, immobile air bubble, corneal edema, and an intraocular pressure (IOP) of 42 mm Hg.

On ultrasound biomicroscopy (UBM), the lens iris diaphragm is seen to have rotated forward, and iris and ciliary body are seen plastered to the cornea and sclera, with ciliary effusion present (**Fig. 15.7**). The ciliary processes are rotated anteriorly and seen to be in contact with the lens equator in some eyes.

Management

Aqueous misdirection does not respond to routine glaucoma medicines, and a decrease in aqueous formation with cycloplegia is the mainstay of initial medical therapy. Full doses of acetazolamide, timolol, and brimonidine should be immediately started to reduce aqueous production so that further fluid build-up in the posterior segment is halted. Intravenous (IV) mannitol adds to the effect of these medications by decreasing vitreous volume. *Cycloplegia pulls on the zonules, moving the lens back.* Cycloplegia and mydriasis are important, and higher doses of phenylephrine and atropine 1 to 2% are advocated. *Topical steroids help reduce inflammation and the ciliary effusion present.* The anterior chamber forms and IOP falls with medication in 3 to 5 days in some patients, but the medication needs to be continued for months with a gradual taper. It is suggested that atropinization should continue for up to a year or even lifelong.

If the IOP does not fall with medical therapy as detailed above, and the anterior chamber remains shallow, *the anterior hyaloid face has to be disrupted to allow fluid from the vitreous to flow into the anterior chamber, and reform the anterior chamber. An Nd:YAG laser capsulotomy and hyaloidotomy* may be tried in pseudophakic eyes or if a large iridotomy is present, and this may be effective. A *laser cyclophotocoagulation over 180 degrees may shrink the ciliary processes, pulling them away from the lens in some eyes, breaking ciliolenticular block.*

Often, all these measures are either not possible, or fail, and surgery is required. The first reported method was central vitreous aspiration using an 18-gauge needle. However, currently, a more controlled pars plana vitrectomy with or without lensectomy is undertaken. In phakic eyes a stepwise surgical approach is safer, with a core vitrectomy providing adequate space for subsequent phacoemulsification and IOL implantation, following this up with a posterior capsulectomy and anterior complete vitrectomy. The final vitrectomy should not be only a core vitrectomy, but a thorough and complete one, to prevent a recurrence. Even if the anterior chamber reforms, in the long term a further glaucoma surgery may still be required to control IOP (**Flowchart 15.1**).

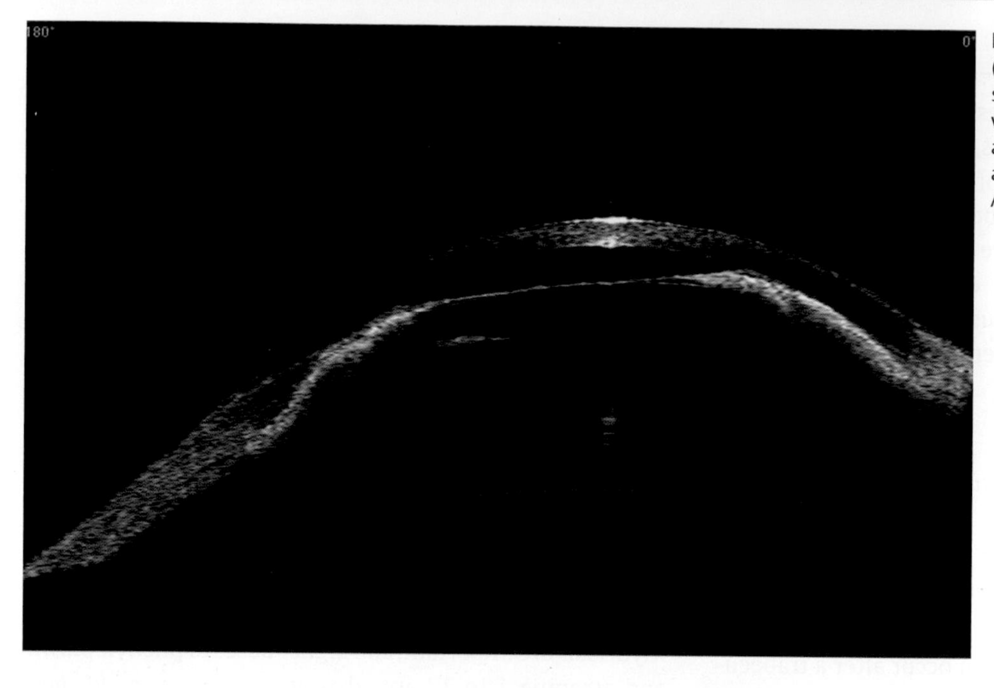

Fig. 15.7 Ultrasound biomicroscopy (UBM) picture of malignant glaucoma showing a very shallow anterior chamber with forward displacement of the lens, and the iris and ciliary body flattened and plastered to the cornea and sclera. A mild ciliary effusion is seen to the left.

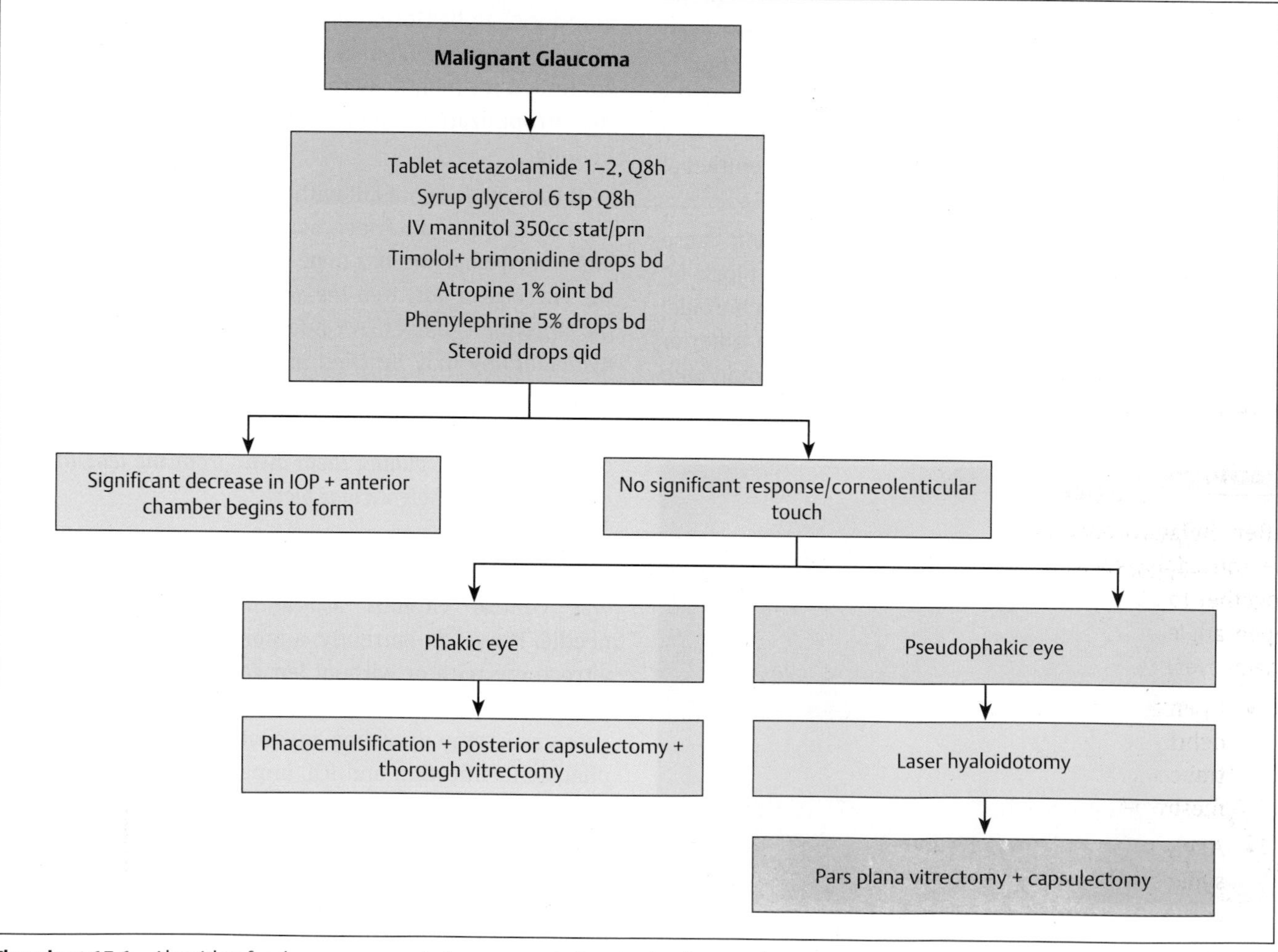

Flowchart 15.1 Algorithm for the management of aqueous misdirection/malignant glaucoma.

The fellow eye has the same predisposition for malignant glaucoma, and prophylactic steps need to be taken to avoid this whenever laser or any ocular surgery is required. These include a preoperative laser iridotomy in PACG eyes prior to trabeculectomy, use of atropine postoperatively, and stopping any miotics that may be in use, prior to surgery.

Prognosis

The long-term prognosis of malignant glaucoma has improved significantly, but care needs to be taken to diagnose aqueous misdirection early, use maximal glaucoma therapy initially, and use the stepwise approach suggested.

Uveitic Glaucoma

Uveitis and glaucoma are commonly seen together. *In approximately 10% of eyes with uveitis a preexisting glaucoma may be exacerbated or a secondary glaucoma caused.* Uveitis can cause glaucoma in a number of ways, and trabecular dysfunction can occur with an open angle, angle closure, or with a mixture of both. *In children, glaucoma is seen in about half of those with juvenile rheumatoid arthritis.*

Glaucoma in the presence of acute uveitis, with a duration of <3 months, is rare, as iridocyclitis is associated with some degree of ciliary effusion which lowers the IOP. An acute rise in IOP with uveitis is only common with herpes, with an IOP rise seen in about half the eyes with herpes zoster or simplex. Episodes of high IOP in the presence of very mild iridocyclitis may be seen in Posner-Schlossman syndrome, a forme fruste of herpetic uveitis, or Fuchs' heterochromic iridocyclitis.

Pathophysiology

After inflammation subsides, uveitic glaucomas may be caused by many concomitant mechanisms working together to cause trabecular meshwork dysfunction, with open angle and angle closure mechanisms both seen in many eyes:

- Open angle mechanisms: Trabeculitis, inflammatory debris, healing with scarring/membrane over the trabecular meshwork, pigment in the trabecular meshwork, a steroid-induced IOP rise.
- Angle closure mechanisms: Extensive posterior synechiae forming occlusio pupillae that prevents aqueous flow from the posterior to anterior chamber, and leads to iris bombe formation, iridotrabecular contact, trabecular damage, and a raised IOP.

Clinical Features

The patient may complain of pain, photophobia, and diminution of vision. A systemic history should be carefully taken.

On examination, features of the type, cause, and the effect of the uveitis have to be identified. In active anterior uveitis, ciliary congestion with keratic precipitates, aqueous flare and cells, miosis, and sometimes iris nodules are seen (**Figs. 15.8** and **15.9**). In healed anterior uveitis, posterior synechiae, old crenated and pigmented keratic precipitates, pigment dispersion, and a complicated cataract may be present. *A secondary pupillary block is seen with occlusio or seclusio pupillae*, synechiae to the lens, or inflammatory membrane, causing an iris bombe with variable PAS (**Fig. 15.8**). *Another kind of pupillary block may sometimes be seen in which the iris is plastered to the anterior lens surface and the anterior chamber appears deep, but aqueous cannot reach or pass through the pupil.* Pupillary block is more frequent in patients with HLA B27 or sarcoidosis.

Gonioscopy in all cases must be done to look for the presence of pigmentation or synechiae (**Fig. 15.10**). *PAS in uveitis are most common inferiorly and are broad based, in the shape of a table top.*

In intermediate uveitis, in addition to some of the features outlined above, the vitreous shows condensations, snow banking, and the appearance of snow balls. The peripheral retina also shows signs of inflammation. Posterior uveitis as in Vogt-Koyanagi-Harada disease or scleritis may cause ciliary effusion and secondary angle closure. Glaucoma is less common in intermediate or

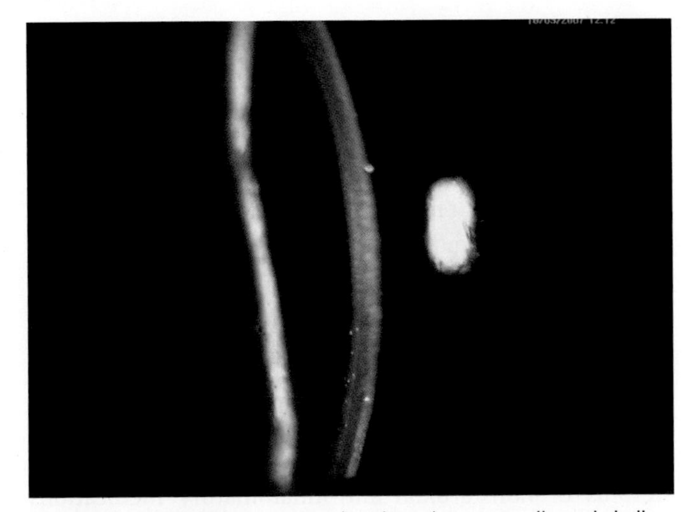

Fig. 15.8 An irregular anterior chamber, deep centrally and shallow peripherally, keratic precipitates at the back of the cornea, and a miosed, bound down pupil are seen.

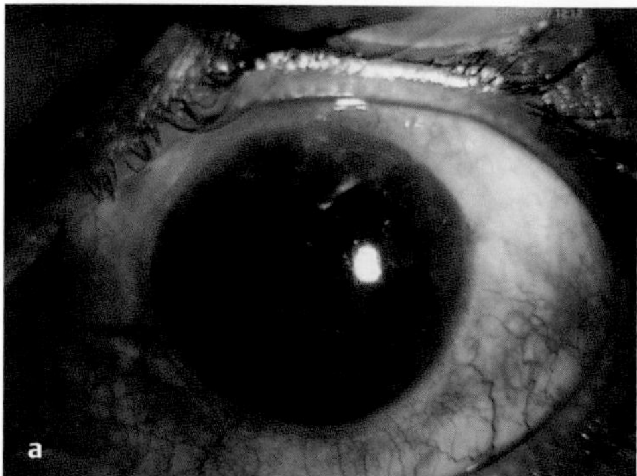

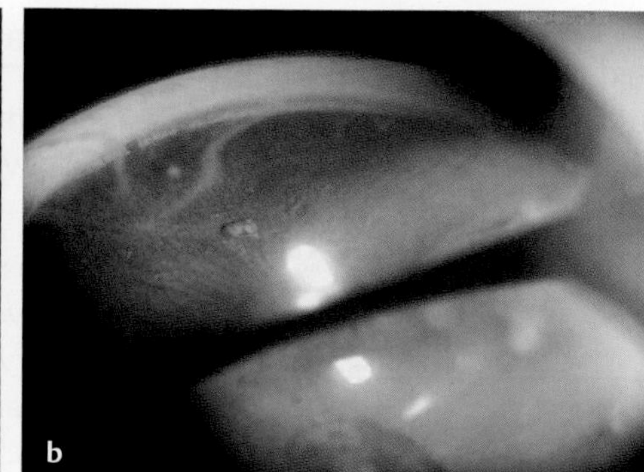

Fig. 15.9 **(a)** Extensive midperipheral anterior synechiae (PAS), occlusio pupillae, and iris bombe. **(b)** Gonioscopy showing iris nodules and PAS in an eye with active uveitis.

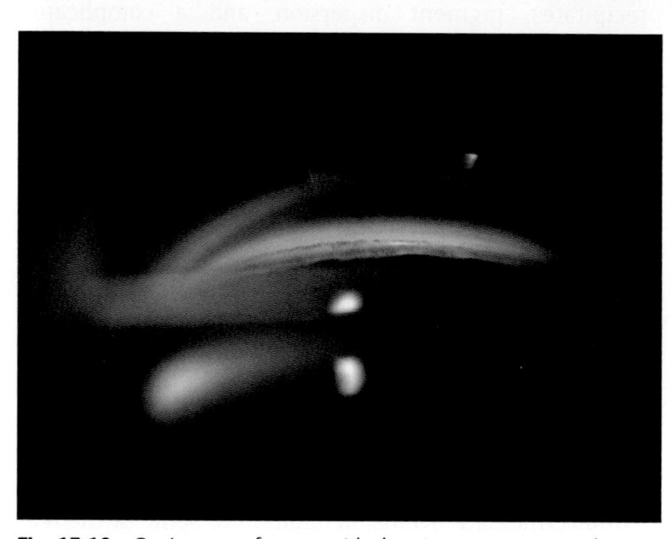

Fig. 15.10 Gonioscopy of an eye with chronic anterior uveitis showing broad synechiae inferiorly in an otherwise open angle, together with pigment dispersion.

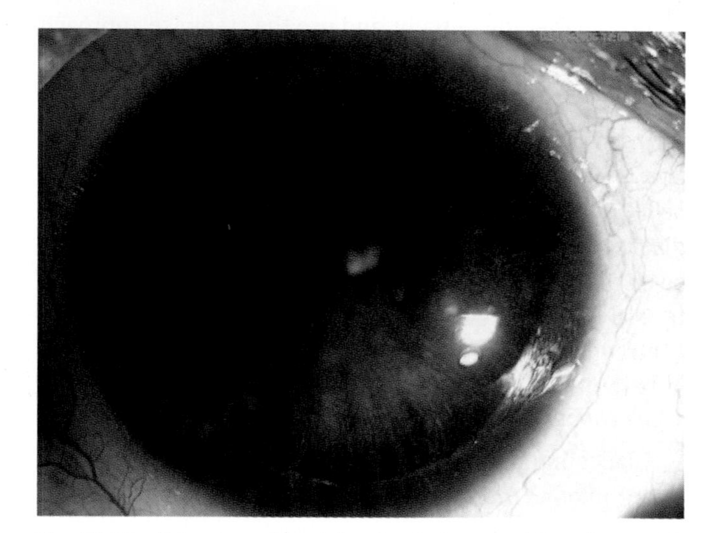

Fig. 15.11 Extensive midperipheral anterior synechiae after uveitis for which a more central and large iridotomy was done.

posterior uveitis per se, but IOP may rise due to steroid depots or implants used for the treatment of chronic inflammation.

Management

It is important to assess the severity of inflammation, so that adequate steps to control this are taken first. In the presence of a raised IOP, the use of lower potency steroids and cycloplegics is recommended. Difluprednate has been seen to cause steroid-induced glaucoma more frequently than any other steroid, and should be discontinued in an eye with uveitic glaucoma.

The initial management of the patient is aimed at controlling IOP medically and finding a possible cause of the uveitis. Treating the cause will reduce inflammation and further attacks. Ocular therapy using minimal, low-dose steroids or nonsteroidal anti-inflammatory medications to control the inflammation is essential. Additionally, glaucoma medications, β-blocker, alpha agonists, and carbonic anhydrase inhibitors (CAI) can be added one at a time to assess response and control IOP. Target IOP in uveitic glaucoma would depend on the degree of glaucomatous neuropathy seen. If diagnosed early before the onset of optic nerve damage, an IOP below 20 mm Hg may be low enough.

If there is an occlusio pupillae with iris bombe and peripheral iridocorneal touch, an iridotomy should be done as soon as possible to relieve the pupillary block and open up any parts of the trabecular meshwork still functioning. Even if extensive PAS have formed, an iridotomy may open some part of the trabecular meshwork still functioning, and decrease the need for medications. *These iridotomies may be difficult to place in the midperipheral area because of extensive PAS, and should be done more centrally, in areas away from the cornea. Multiple large iridotomies are required as further attacks of uveitis may close a small iridotomy* (**Fig. 15.11**).

Viral keratouveitis, especially herpes zoster or simplex, is often found to have a high IOP due to associated trabeculitis, and may not be controlled on Acyclovir and glaucoma medications. It frequently needs a trabeculectomy or implant.

In recalcitrant uveitis, topical or systemic immunosuppression may help control inflammation, decrease the use of steroids, and help control IOP.

If medical therapy is unable to control IOP, surgery, either a trabeculectomy or drainage device, may be done, always in a quiet eye (**Fig. 15.12**). Depending on the chances of recurrence of the uveitis and any subconjunctival scarring present, anitifibroblastic agents such as MMC may need to be applied subconjunctivally or subsclerally, intraoperatively. Prolonged use of postoperative steroids is recommended, 2 to 3 months in eyes with chronic uveitis. Recurrent attacks of uveitis may lead to failure of filtering surgery over time.

Prognosis

Uveitic glaucoma has a very good prognosis if detected early, before glaucomatous optic neuropathy has occurred, and if a cause of the uveitis can be found and treated. Recurrent or chronic uveitis causing glaucoma has a poorer response to glaucoma medications, and often needs surgery to control the IOP so that steroids can be continued to control inflammation.

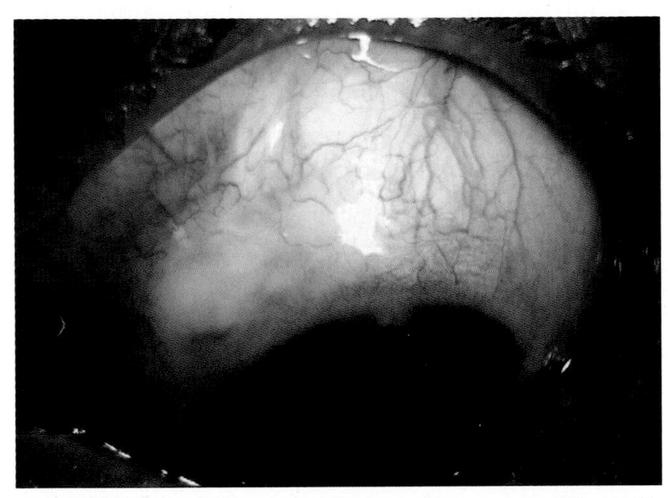

Fig. 15.12 Functioning trabeculectomy in an eye with uveitic glaucoma after >5 years.

Cases

Case 1

A 60-year-old female diagnosed to have chronic PACG in both eyes, uncontrolled on maximal tolerated medical therapy after iridotomy, underwent a trabeculectomy under local anesthesia, followed by a sudden diminution of vision and pain. On the first postoperative day, she was found to have peripheral iridocorneal touch and a centrally shallow anterior chamber, with an IOP of 50 mm Hg (**Case 1-1a**).

Points to consider

- Preoperative uncontrolled IOP in chronic PACG.
- Patent iridotomy was present.
- Very shallow anterior chamber and high IOP on first postoperative day.

Diagnosis and Management

Ultrasonography (USG) showed no suprachoroidal hemorrhage. A diagnosis of aqueous misdirection was made and the patient was started on acetazolamide 500 mg tablet and syrup glycerol 1 oz 8 hourly with topical brimonidine, timolol, and IV mannitol. Atropine ointment 1% and phenylephrine 5% thrice a day were given. The IOP fluctuated between 34 and 40 mm Hg. On the third day, a phacoemulsification with posterior capsulotomy and anterior vitrectomy was done, and the IOP reduced to 22 mm Hg on topical glaucoma medications and atropine. The anterior chamber reformed, but corneal edema persisted for 3 weeks. On follow-up at 6 months, the IOP was 16 mm Hg on timolol, brimonidine, and atropine (**Case 1-1b**).

Case 2

A 65-year-old lady complained of gradual diminution of vision in both eyes for 1 year and was diagnosed to have PACG for which a laser was performed. Since then there was acute pain in the left eye with a gross loss of vision. On

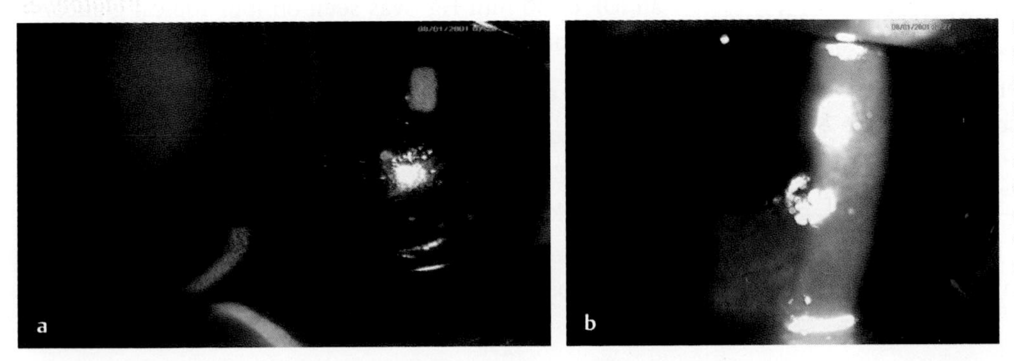

Case 1-1 **(a)** Extensive iridocorneal touch with an intraocular pressure (IOP) on maximal glaucoma medications of 32 mm Hg. **(b)** After phacoemulsification with posterior capsulotomy and anterior vitrectomy the anterior chamber is formed, and corneal edema can be seen. IOP was 22 mm Hg on topical glaucoma medications and atropine.

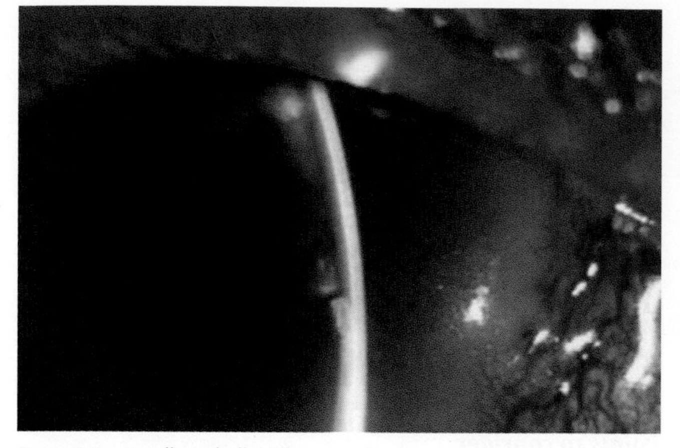

Case 2-1 Small eyeball with corneal edema and conjunctival congestion and a very shallow anterior chamber. (The image is a provided courtesy of Dr Digvijay Singh, Noble Eye Center, Gurugram, Haryana, India.)

examination, ciliary congestion, corneal stromal edema, very shallow anterior chamber, and an IOP of 64 mm Hg were observed. The other eye had a shallow anterior chamber, pupillary ruff atrophy, a cup:disc ratio of 0.7, and an IOP of 26 mm Hg. Gonioscopy of right eye showed an occludable angle with synechiae over more than 180 degrees.

Points to consider

- Post-iridotomy high IOP in PACG eye.
- Patent iridotomy rules out a pupillary block.
- USG showed no suprachoroidal hemorrhage.

Diagnosis and Management

The patient was diagnosed to have bilateral PACG with possible malignant glaucoma and was put on maximal glaucoma medications which did not reduce the IOP. After IV mannitol, a left phacoemulsification with posterior capsulotomy and vitrectomy was done. The IOP was 14 mm Hg for 2 weeks, but rose again to 44 mm Hg with corneal edema and a very shallow anterior chamber. The patient was advised systemic acetazolamide, timolol–brimonidine combination, atropine 1% ointment three times a day and phenylephrine drops. Over 3 months the IOP remained at 18/20 mm Hg. The patient was asked to taper acetazolamide but continue cycloplegia for at least a year. She was advised to be cautious about any surgery in the other eye, as this too could result in aqueous misdirection (**Case 2-1**).

Case 3

A 70-year-old lady has a high IOP of 34 mm Hg on first postoperative day after uneventful cataract surgery, with blurring of vision and pain. On examination, there was a deep anterior chamber and a mild flare (**Case 3-1**).

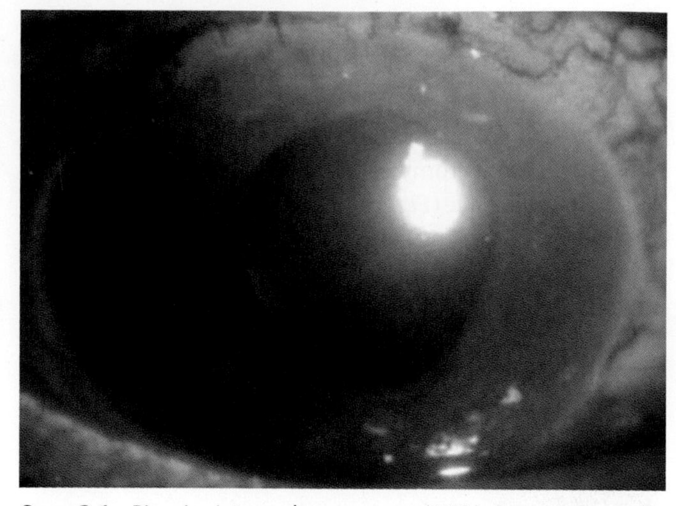

Case 3-1 Rise in intraocular pressure (IOP) after extracapsular cataract surgery, maintained anterior chamber with corneal edema.

Points to consider

- No prior history of glaucoma.
- No lens matter or free vitreous present.
- IOP rise after cataract surgery reduces within 2 to 7 days if due to viscoelastics.

Diagnosis and Management

A diagnosis of possible viscoelastic-induced IOP rise was made. Medical therapy to control IOP with timolol, brimonidine, and acetazolamide was started. The patient was reviewed in 24 hours when IOP was 24 mm Hg. The medications were tapered gradually, by asking the patient to stop Diamox after 4 days, then drops one at a time on weekly review till normal IOP was restored in 4 weeks.

Case 4

A 50-year-old lady underwent cataract surgery in a camp 3 months earlier, following which there was very little gain in vision. On examination, pupillary capture of the IOL, with extensive iris atrophy and corneal decompensation with an IOP of 30 mm Hg, was seen on four topical glaucoma medications (**Case 4-1**).

Points to consider

- Chronically raised IOP for months after cataract surgery.
- No known preexisting glaucoma.
- No evidence of retained lens matter, UGH syndrome, pupillary block, or a steroid response.

Diagnosis and Management

A diagnosis of pseudophakic glaucoma with healed uveitis was made. The patient was advised the use of timolol and brimonidine combination with tablets of long acting acetazolamide at bedtime. The patient refused further surgery when visual prognosis was explained. Therefore, a 180-degree diode laser cyclophotocoagulation (DLCP) was done and the IOP reduced to 16 mm Hg. The patient was advised a review every 3 months as further DLCP may be required.

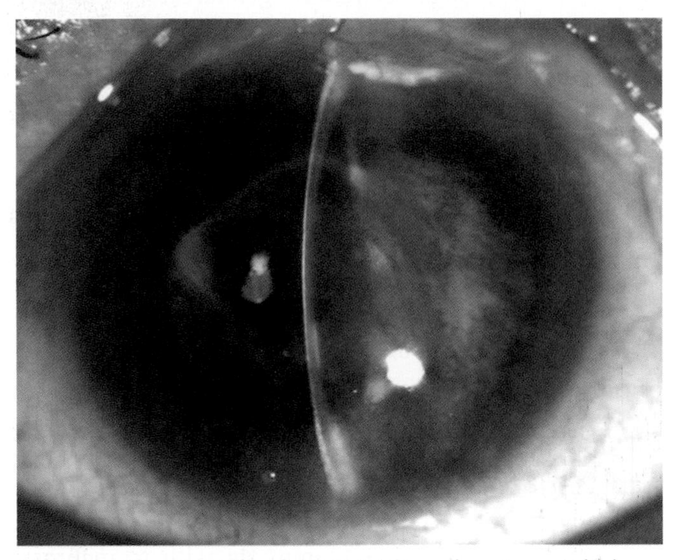

Case 4-1 After 3 months of cataract surgery there is corneal edema, sectors of iris atrophy, extensive peripheral anterior synechiae (PAS), and pupillary capture of intraocular lens (IOL).

Case 5

A 42-year-old female presented with complaints of gradual and painless diminution of vision in both eyes for the last 8 months. She had a history of cataract surgery in both eyes 2 years back. On examination, best corrected visual acuity was 2/60 in the right eye and 1/60 in the left eye. Baseline IOPs were 20 and 38 mm Hg in the right eye and left eye, respectively.

On slit-lamp examination, both eyes showed few pigments on endothelium with a three-piece posterior chamber IOL in anterior chamber. Pupillary reaction was sluggish in both eyes (**Case 5-1a**). On gonioscopy, closed angles with multiple PAS and IOL haptic abutting the trabecular meshwork were seen in both the eyes. Fundus examination showed a cup:disc ratio of 0.9:1 in both the eyes.

Points to consider

- Bilateral glaucoma in pseudophakia could be preexisting.
- PAS were seen to be caused by IOLs placed wrongly.
- Severe glaucomatous neuropathy.

Diagnosis and Management

A diagnosis of pseudophakia in both eyes with posterior chamber IOL in anterior chamber, with glaucoma was made. Left eye underwent trabeculectomy with 0.04% MMC with two releasable sutures to prevent corneal decompensation. Right eye was started on topical

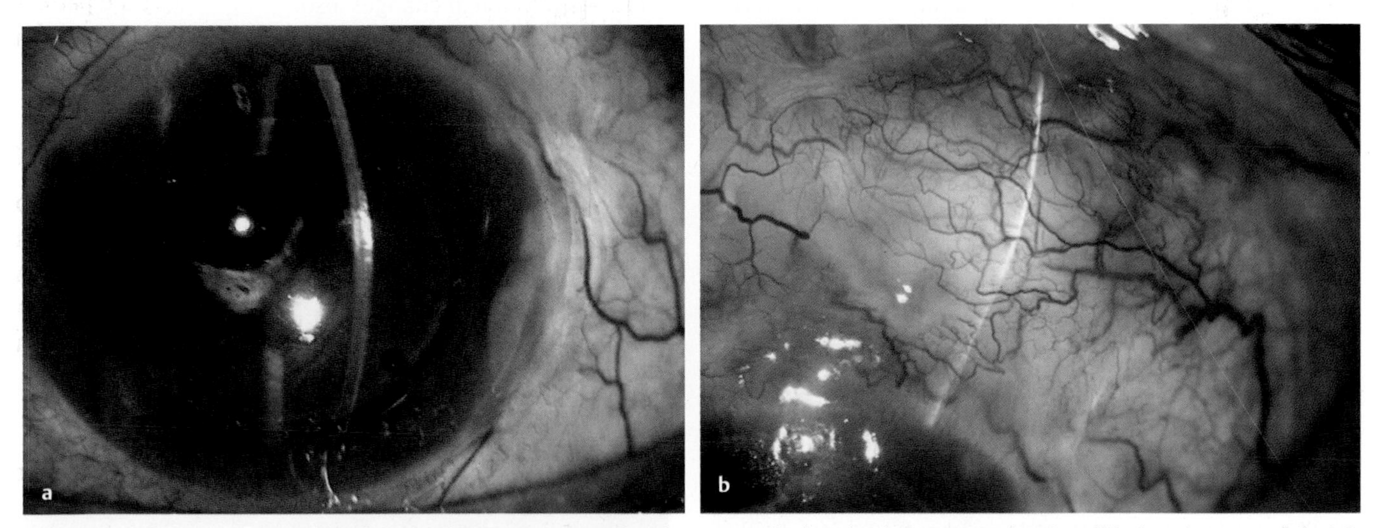

Case 5-1 **(a)** Clinical picture of the left eye showing posterior chamber intraocular lens (IOL) in anterior chamber. **(b)** Clinical picture of the left eye showing diffuse, mildly elevated and moderately vascular bleb.

travatan and pilocarpine. After 2 months of the surgery, IOPs were 12 and 10 mm Hg in the right eye and left eye, respectively, with a diffuse, mildly elevated and slightly vascular bleb in the left eye (**Case 5-1b**).

Case 6

A 53-year-old male presented with complaints of gradual and painless diminution of vision in the right eye for the last 5 months. He had a history of right eye cataract surgery 1 year earlier. On examination, best corrected visual acuity was 6/36 in the right eye and 6/9 in the left eye. IOPs were 46 and 18 mm Hg in the right eye and left eye, respectively.

On slit-lamp examination, the right eye had a shallow anterior chamber with anterior chamber IOL and a posterior capsular rent, suggestive of complicated cataract surgery. Irregular, nonreacting pupil, iris atrophy, and vitreous in anterior chamber were seen (**Case 6-1**). On gonioscopy, closed angles due to the IOL haptic pushing up the iris were present. Fundus examination showed a cup:disc ratio of 0.8:1 in the right eye and 0.3:1 in the left eye.

Points to consider

- Evidence of complicated cataract surgery.
- Angle closure due to IOL haptics.
- Severe glaucomatous neuropathy.

Diagnosis and Management

A diagnosis of right eye pseudophakic glaucoma due to secondary angle closure was made. Right eye was started on maximal topical medication. IOP was 22 mm Hg after 1 week. With a high baseline IOP and a target of <12 mm Hg, trabeculectomy with MMC was the first option. Drainage device may be blocked by vitreous and cause endothelial cell loss. Right eye underwent trabeculectomy with 0.04% MMC with two releasable sutures to prevent the anterior chamber IOL contact with the endothelium. Postoperatively IOP was 10 mm Hg in the right eye till 7 months, after which it became 18 mm Hg, for which topical timolol was started. IOP was 12 mm Hg after 3 years of surgery.

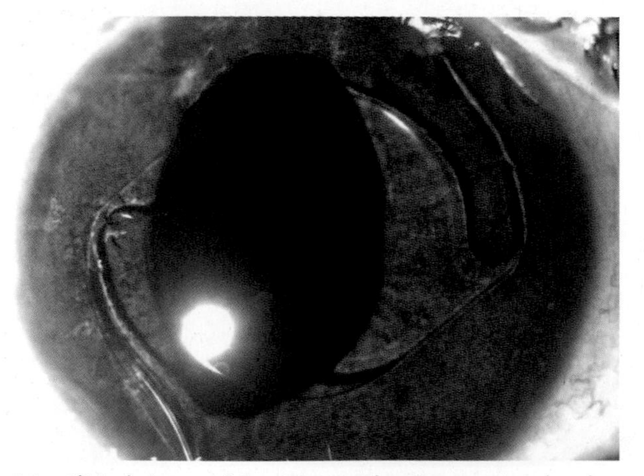

Case 6-1 Clinical picture of the right eye showing anterior chamber intraocular lens (IOL) with irregular and nonreacting pupil and iris pushed into the angle inferiorly.

Case 7

An 18-year-old man underwent congenital cataract surgery both eyes at the age of 3 months and was left aphakic. A raised IOP of 28/30 mm Hg was recorded only at the age of 12 years when a cup:disc ratio of 0.9 was noticed. Ocular examination revealed an open angle, with central corneal thickness (CCT) of 650/630 µm (**Case 7-1**). Perimetry showed a central island of vision in both eyes.

Points to consider

- IOP should be corrected for CCT.
- Cup:disc ratio of 0.9 needs an IOP in the low teens.
- Long life expectancy.

Diagnosis and Management

A diagnosis of childhood glaucoma after congenital cataract surgery was made. The corrected IOP was 21/23 mm Hg, and was controlled to 12/14 mm Hg with latanoprost, dorzolamide, and timolol, keeping in mind the CCT corrections of approximately minus 7 mm Hg due to the thicker corneas. Regular specular microscopy is required to monitor endothelial changes also.

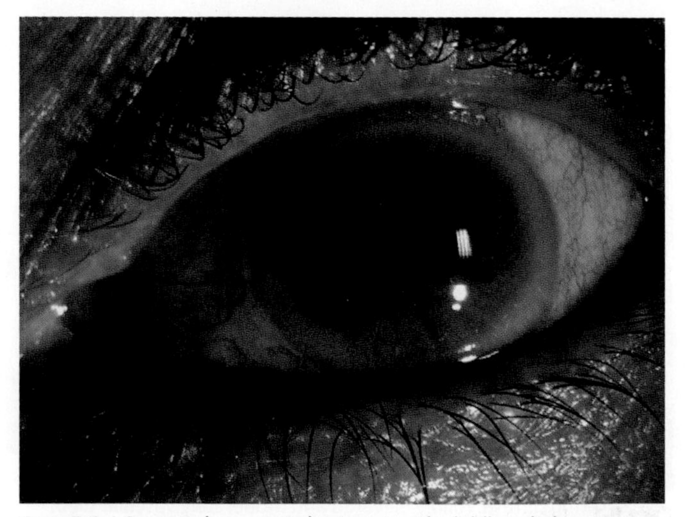

Case 7-1 Operated congenital cataract with childhood glaucoma.

Case 8

A 24-year-old lady had recurrent uveitis in both eyes. On examination there were posterior synechiae, with a complicated cataract. This was operated upon uneventfully, and perioperative steroids were prescribed. After 6 weeks there was an anterior chamber flare of 1+, a cup:disc ratio of 0.5 with regular neururetinal rim, and an IOP of 32/30 mm Hg (**Case 8-1**).

Points to consider

- IOP prior to cataract surgery was within normal limits.
- No residual lens matter, vitreous, etc., were present.
- Bilateral IOP rise after 6 weeks could be a possible steroid response.

Diagnosis and Management

A diagnosis of a steroid-induced response in both eyes was made. The IOP was managed medically with a combination of dorzolamide–timolol and brimonidine twice a day and long-acting acetazolamide twice a day. The patient was reviewed every 2 weeks to record IOP and taper medications. The long-acting acetazolamide was first reduced to once a day, then brimonidine and later dorzolamide was stopped. The patient was reviewed for IOP before every reduction in medications. The patient was on only timolol twice a day 3 months after cataract surgery and the IOPs recorded early morning and late in the evening were 14 to 18 mm Hg. Further follow-up would be required to try stopping timolol, as repeated episodes of uveitis continued.

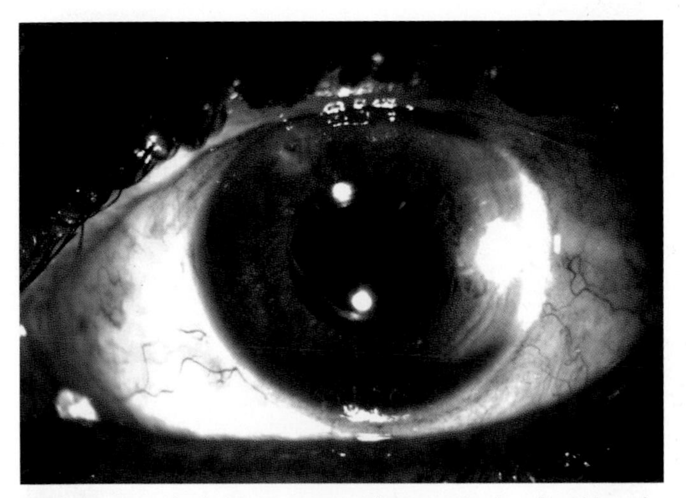

Case 8-1 Pseudophakia in an eye with past episodes of uveitis and a steroid-induced rise in intraocular pressure (IOP).

Suggested Readings

Ahmad SS. Acute lens-induced glaucomas: a review. J Acute Dis 2017;6(2):47–52

Bitrian E, Caprioli J. Pars plana anterior vitrectomy, hyaloido-zonulectomy, and iridectomy for aqueous humor misdirection. Am J Ophthalmol 2010;150(1):82–87.e1

Byrnes GA, Leen MM, Wong TP, Benson WE. Vitrectomy for ciliary block (malignant) glaucoma. Ophthalmology 1995; 102(9):1308–1311

Debrouwere V, Stalmans P, Van Calster J, Spileers W, Zeyen T, Stalmans I. Outcomes of different management options for malignant glaucoma: a retrospective study. Graefes Arch Clin Exp Ophthalmol 2012;250(1):131–141

Ellant JP, Obstbaum SA. Lens-induced glaucoma. Doc Ophthalmol 1992;81(3):317–338

Shaffer RN, Hoskins HD Jr. Ciliary block (malignant) laucoma. Ophthalmology. 1978 Mar;85(3):215-21

Kaplowitz K, Yung E, Flynn R, Tsai JC. Current concepts in the treatment of vitreous block, also known as aqueous misdirection. Surv Ophthalmol 2015;60(3):229–241

Kok H, Barton K. Uveitic glaucoma. Ophthalmol Clin North Am 2002;15(3):375–387, viii

Layden WE. Pseudophakia and glaucoma. Ophthalmology 1982;89(8):875–879

Little BC. Treatment of aphakic malignant glaucoma using Nd:YAG laser posterior capsulotomy. Br J Ophthalmol 1994; 78(6):499–501

Nche EN, Amer R. Lens-induced uveitis: an update. Graefes Arch Clin Exp Ophthalmol 2020;258(7):1359–1365

Papaconstantinou D, Georgalas I, Kourtis N, et al. Lens-induced glaucoma in the elderly. Clin Interv Aging 2009;4:331–336

Quigley HA, Friedman DS, Congdon NG. Possible mechanisms of primary angle-closure and malignant glaucoma. J Glaucoma. 2003 Apr;12(2):167–80

Shaffer RN. The role of vitreous detachment in aphakic and malignant glaucoma. Trans Am Acad Ophthalmol Otolaryngol 1954;58(2):217–231

Shahid H, Salmon JF. Malignant glaucoma: a review of the modern literature. J Ophthalmol 2012;2012:852659

Tsai JC, Barton KA, Miller MH, Khaw PT, Hitchings RA. Surgical results in malignant glaucoma refractory to medical or laser therapy. Eye (Lond) 1997;11(Pt 5):677–681

van Oye R, Gelisken O. Pseudophakic glaucoma. Int Ophthalmol 1985;8(3):183–186

CHAPTER 16

Traumatic Glaucoma

Overview

- Etiology
- Closed Globe Injury
  - Clinical Features
  - Management
  - Ghost Cell Glaucoma
- Open Globe Injuries
- Chemical Injuries
- Cases
- Suggested Readings

Introduction

Ocular trauma is very common, especially in the younger age group, where it may occur during work or while playing a sport. As ophthalmologists concentrate on treating the acute symptoms and signs, a raised intraocular pressure (IOP) is often missed, leading to a delay in therapy and unnecessary visual loss. Further, the socioeconomic consequences are very significant, ranging from expenses for prolonged therapy, visual disability, a loss of employment opportunities, and disfigurement.

The term "traumatic glaucoma" represents the state of an eye, which, due to an injury per se, or the subsequent reparative processes, has a chronically elevated IOP incompatible with the normal functioning of the optic nerve.

Etiology

Traumatic glaucoma is not a single entity, but a basket diagnosis of many causes resulting from trauma, which lead to a rise in IOP. The eye is well protected by the orbital bones on its superior, nasal, and inferior aspects, but is prone to damage by objects coming from the anterior or temporal aspects. The inferotemporal area is most often involved in closed and open globe injuries. In India this is commonly caused by cricket ball, fire crackers, or stone-related injuries.

A rise in IOP can occur soon after an injury or even years later due to many, often coexisting, pathologies:

- Causes of glaucoma in closed globe/concussional injuries:
  - *Early onset:*
    - Hyphema.
    - Trabecular tears/trabeculitis.
    - Phacotopic changes: Lens dislocation/subluxation.
    - Free vitreous in anterior chamber.
  - *Late onset:*
    - Healing of angle recessioncausing trabecular fibrosis.
    - Ghost cell glaucoma.
    - Glass membrane formation.
- Causes of glaucoma in open globe/penetrating injuries:
  - *Early onset:*
    - Inflammatory membranes and synechiae.
    - Lens particles.
    - Hyphema.
    - Phacoanaphylactic glaucoma.
  - *Late onset:*
    - Secondary angle closure.
    - Epithelial/fibrous ingrowth.

Closed Globe Injury

Around the world, sports-related injuries in young males are the commonest reason for traumatic glaucoma, especially injuries with smaller balls, cricket, golf, etc., or with a shuttle cock. Unsupervised use of firecrackers is the second-most common cause in India.

Clinical Features

All patients suspected to have traumatic glaucoma should undergo a detailed history and careful comprehensive evaluation, as early and appropriate therapy can significantly improve visual prognosis and is necessary for medicolegal purposes.

A detailed history of the mode of injury, the direction from which the injury occurred, time since injury, extent of vision loss, and any treatment already administered is important. Prior ocular complaints and any significant family history of glaucoma are also important.

An assessment of visual acuity with a record of projection of rays is essential. A comprehensive examination of the eye to identify all tissues that have been damaged would provide information about the probability of the occurrence of a significant IOP rise and its cause. The optic nerve head status on presentation is important for determining further management.

Concussive forces on the eye lead to an anteroposterior compression, forcing intraocular contents backward and centrifugally, leading to *shearing forces that damage circumferential structures* (**Fig. 16.1**). Damage is caused by many mechanisms once concussion occurs (**Flowchart 16.1**), for example:

- Anteroposterior compression.
- Equatorial expansion and return.
- Coup—injury at the point of contact.
- Contrecoup—injury opposite to contact.

When the force generated exceeds the elasticity of tissues it impinges upon, it disrupts any weak attachments or areas in the eye. This is seen generally in *one or more of seven locations or rings:*

1. Pupil: Tears in the sphincter muscle at the pupil lead to an irregular pupillary margin and traumatic mydriasis (**Figs. 16.2** and **16.3**).
2. Iridodialysis: The root of the iris is torn from its attachment to the ciliary body leading to a D-shaped pupil with a visible peripheral iris edge (**Fig. 16.4**).
3. Angle recession: Splitting of the ciliary body face between its central circular and peripheral

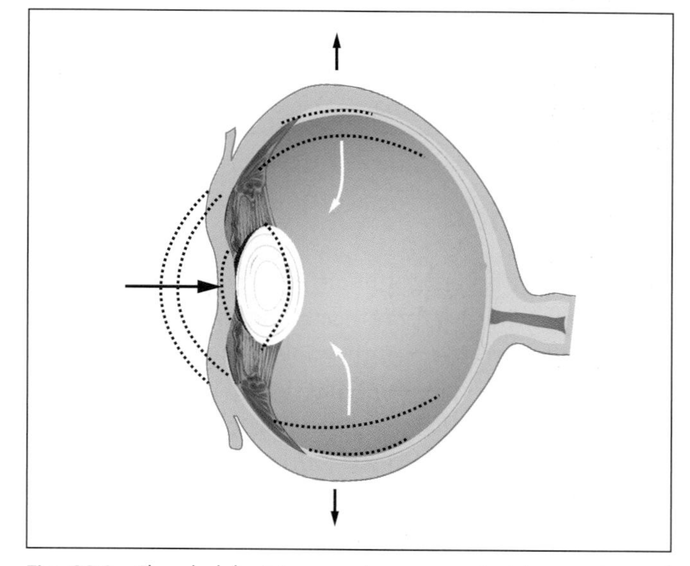

Fig. 16.1 Closed globe injury causing an equatorial expansion and return of the globe and shearing forces within the eye.

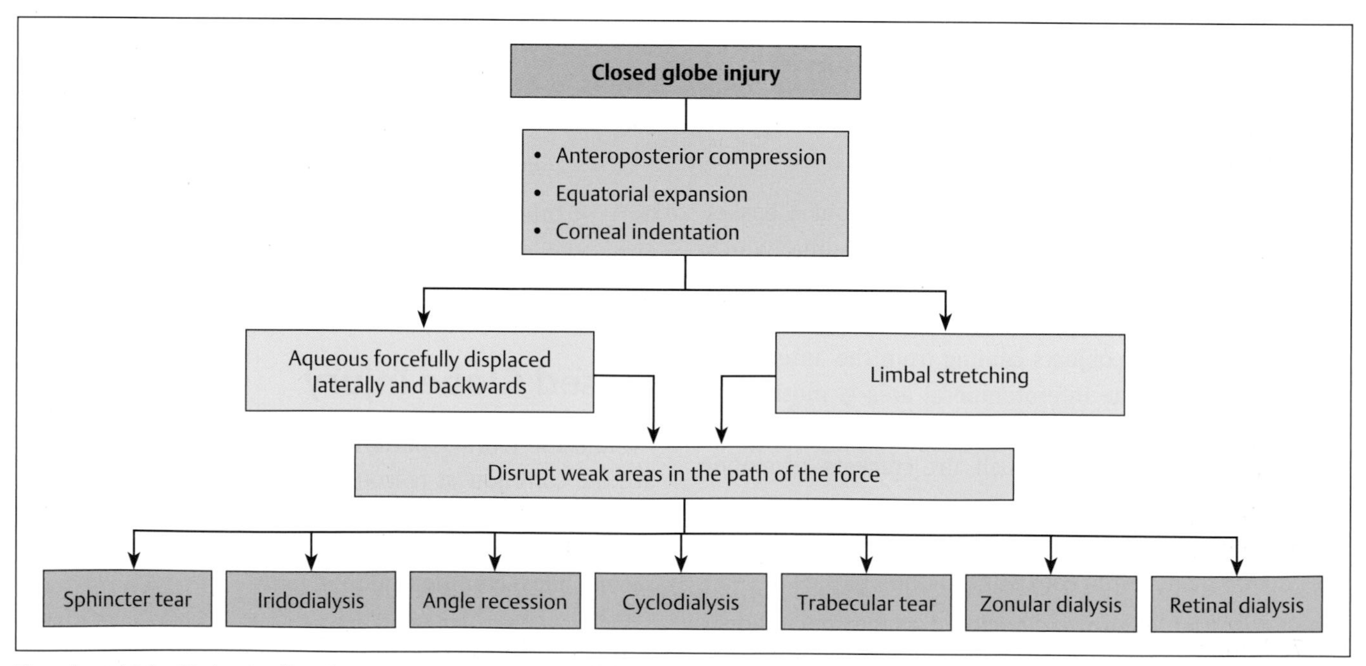

Flowchart 16.1 Understanding the common consequences of closed globe injury.

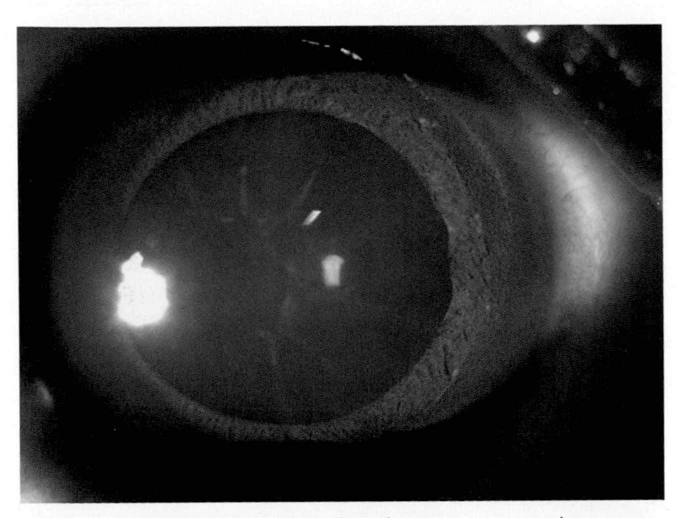

Fig. 16.2 Mid-dilated pupil with sphincter tears, and a rosette cataract after closed globe injury.

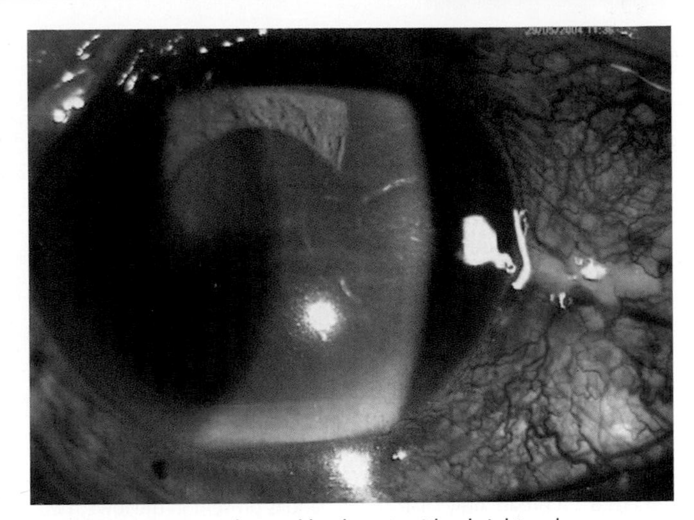

Fig. 16.3 Traumatic layered hyphema, with a bright red appearance of a rebleed. There is an irregular pupil, pigmentation/clots on the corneal endothelium, and ciliary and conjunctival congestion.

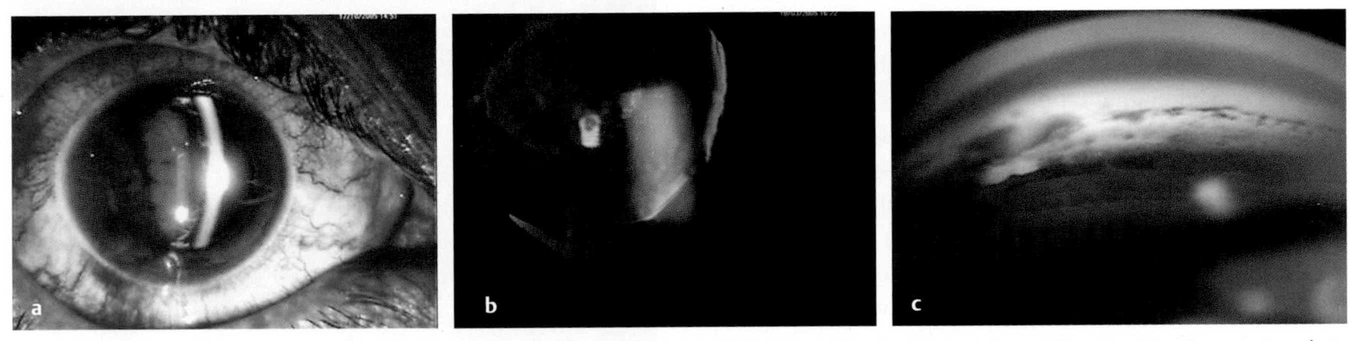

Fig. 16.4 **(a)** Anterior segment photograph showing large temporal iridodialysis associated with post-traumatic cataract, vitreous strands in the anterior chamber, and streaks of hyphema. **(b)** Posterior rosette cataract in a subluxated lens after blunt trauma. **(c)** Goniophotograph of the inferior angle following resolution of hyphema, where extensive pigment dispersion and peripheral anterior synechiae are visible.

longitudinal muscle fibers leads to a widening of the ciliary body band on gonioscopy and an irregular posterior displacement of the iris and lens (**Figs. 16.4c, 16.5,** and **16.6**).

4. Cyclodialysis: A disinsertion of the ciliary body from its attachment to the scleral spur allows the scleral wall to be seen as a white strip posterior to the ciliary body band. This provides an alternative path for drainage of IOP, and if large can prevent a significant IOP rise (**Figs. 16.6** and **16.7**).
5. Tears in the trabecular meshwork: Damage may be seen at the intracameral face of the trabecular meshwork.
6. Zonular dialysis: Stress on the zonules leads to stretching and breaking, causing instability or subluxation of the lens (**Fig. 16.4b**).
7. Retinal dialysis: A pull on the vitreous base can cause disinsertion of the retina at the ora serrata.

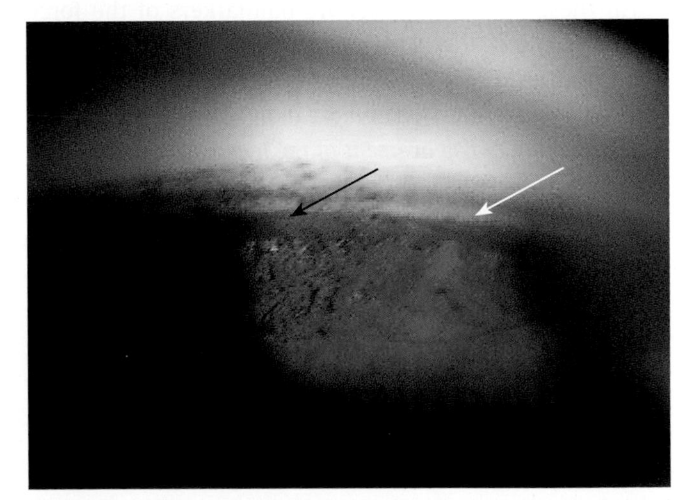

Fig. 16.5 Angle recession seen as a broad gray ciliary body band (*black arrow*). The white glistening scleral spur is clearly visible (*white arrow*), with some peripheral anterior synechiae and significant pigment dispersion, 1 week after closed globe injury.

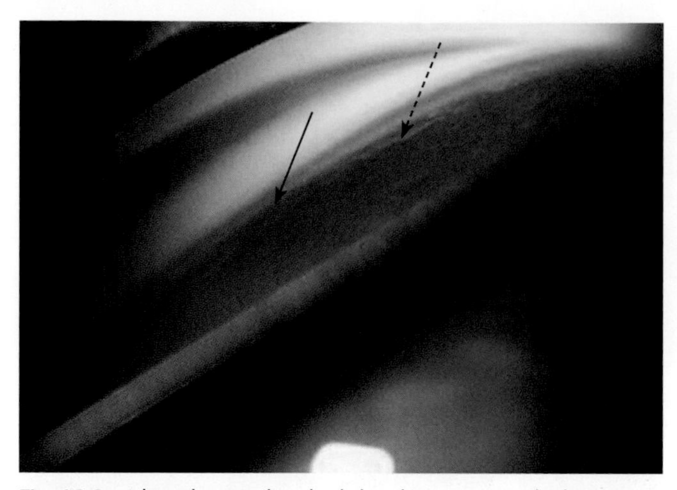

Fig. 16.6 A broad, gray ciliary body band is present in the lower two-thirds of the angle seen (*black arrow*), with a cyclodialysis; the white of the sclera seen posterior to the ciliary body (*dashed arrow*), years after closed globe injury.

On gonioscopy it is common to see an irregular, widened, gray ciliary body band, with a clearly visible white scleral spur, increased pigmentation of the trabecular meshwork, and often peripheral anterior synechiae at the edge of the recession. Subtle signs of trauma on gonioscopy are *areas of broken iris processes*, and a difference in ciliary body width on comparing the two eyes. *Gonioscopy of the involved eye must always be compared with the fellow normal eye* in case of doubt, as myopic eyes may also show a wide ciliary band, which would be regular and symmetric in the two eyes.

Fundus examination shows Berlin edema initially and evidence of choroidal ruptures concentric to the disc. Later extensive scarring of the retina can be seen (**Fig. 16.8**).

All these clinical findings are biomarkers of the force magnitude and therefore of prognostic significance in blunt injuries. *There is a common association of traumatic cataracts, angle recession of more than 180 degrees, injuries to the iris, and a displacement of the lens with concussional glaucoma.* An association of at least two of these clinical features is commonly present in all patients having traumatic glaucoma. Glaucoma may develop in 9% of patients with an angle recession over 10 years. *Other early factors suggestive of possible chronic glaucoma are a moderate-to-large hyphema, older age, and poor visual acuity* (**Figs. 16.9** and **16.10**).

Common biomarkers for chronic traumatic glaucoma in closed globe injuries are:

- Hyphema.
- Traumatic cataract.
- Angle recession of more than 180 degrees.
- Iris injuries.
- Displacement of lens.

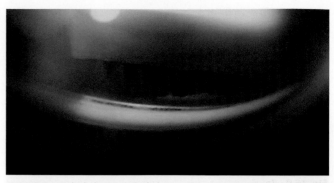

Fig. 16.7 Iridodialysis, cyclodialysis, and pigmentation of the trabecular meshwork after closed globe injury.

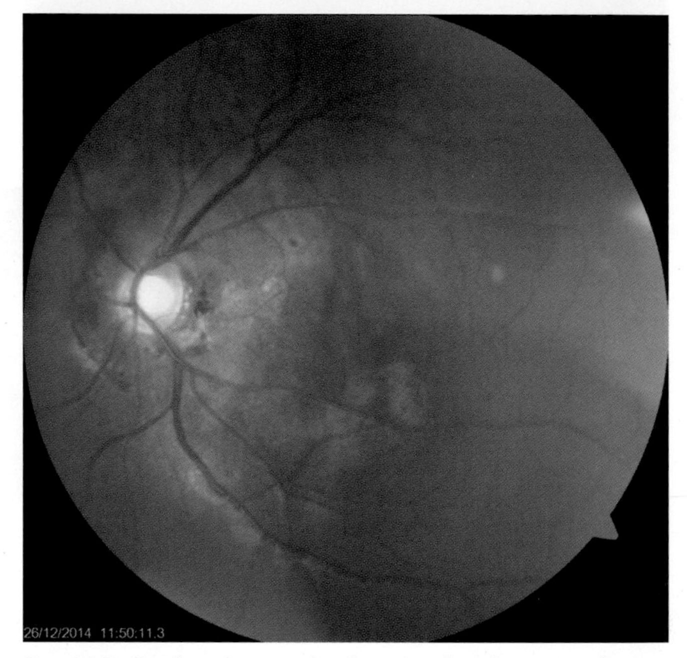

Fig. 16.8 Fundus photograph after closed globe injury showing multiple peripapillary healed choroidal ruptures and hypo- and hyperpigmented scars at the posterior pole. A cup:disc ratio of 0.7 and inferior thinning of the neuroretinal rim are indicators of traumatic glaucomatous neuropathy.

In the presence of media opacification or hyphema, ultrasound biomicroscopy (UBM) can help pick up anterior segment pathology such as angle recession or a cyclodialysis cleft (**Fig. 16.11**). Angle recession shows up as a rupture of the ciliary body that is still attached to the scleral spur. Cyclodialysis on the other hand can be seen as a disinsertion of the ciliary body from the scleral spur with a clear space between ciliary body and sclera, and posterior displacement of iris and ciliary body.

The rise in IOP after closed globe injury has been attributed to trabecular meshwork injury, inflammation, debris, scarring, red blood cells (RBCs) from hyphema, or ghost cells from a longstanding vitreous hemorrhage. Histopathology of trabecular samples has shown extensive pigment dispersion and in a few late cases a hyaline-like

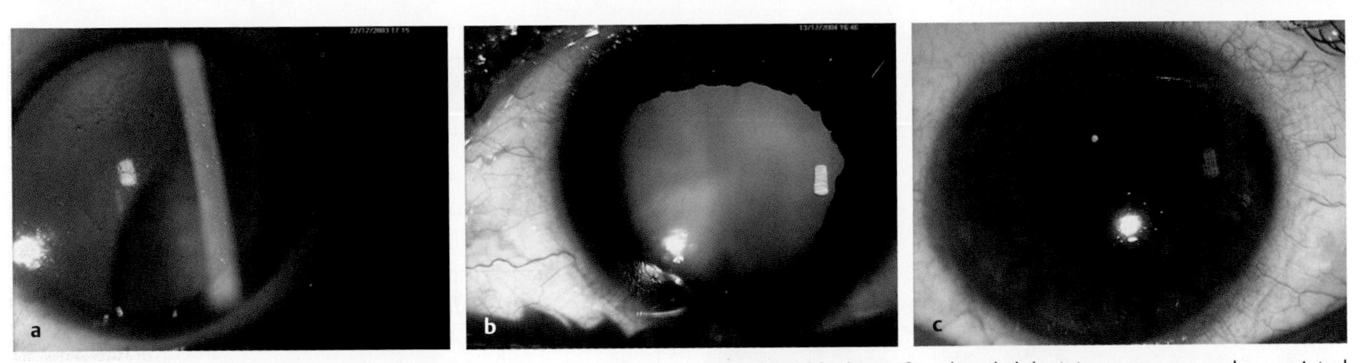

Fig. 16.9 **(a–c)** Cataractous or subluxated lens and iridodialysis are seen. These clinical findings after closed globe injury are commonly associated with chronic traumatic glaucoma.

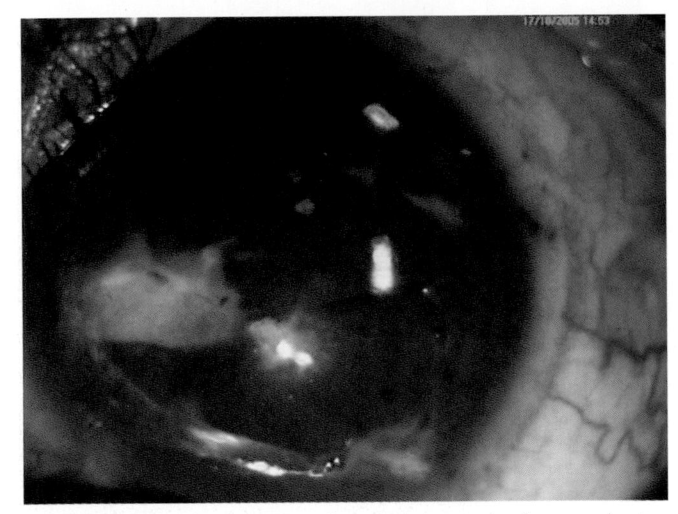

Fig. 16.10 Anterior segment clinical photograph of an eye having chronic glaucoma after firecracker injury. Multiple superficial corneal foreign bodies, post-traumatic cataract with healed uveitis, and posterior synechiae are visible.

glass membrane, similar to Descemet's membrane, over the intracameral surface of the trabecular meshwork. There also appears to be proliferation of corneal endothelial-type cells over the trabecular meshwork after concussive injury (**Fig. 16.12**).

The rise in IOP is therefore secondary to reduced aqueous outflow through the trabecular outflow. However, in the presence of a cyclodialysis cleft, an unrestricted flow of aqueous to the supraciliary space may lead to normal or low IOPs. Cyclodialysis can be seen on gonioscopy; however, in the presence of hypotony or iris obscuring the area, UBM may allow better visualization. In some eyes, iris tissue may block a cyclodialysis preventing the onset of hypotony and raising IOP.

Management

All patients have to be managed appropriately for any concomitant uveitis, with cycloplegics and steroids, as well as for any immediate raised IOP with β-blockers,

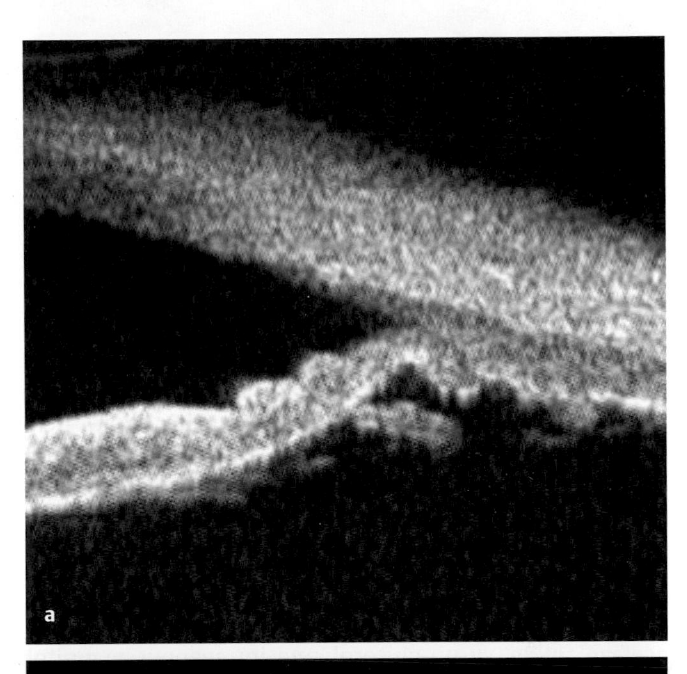

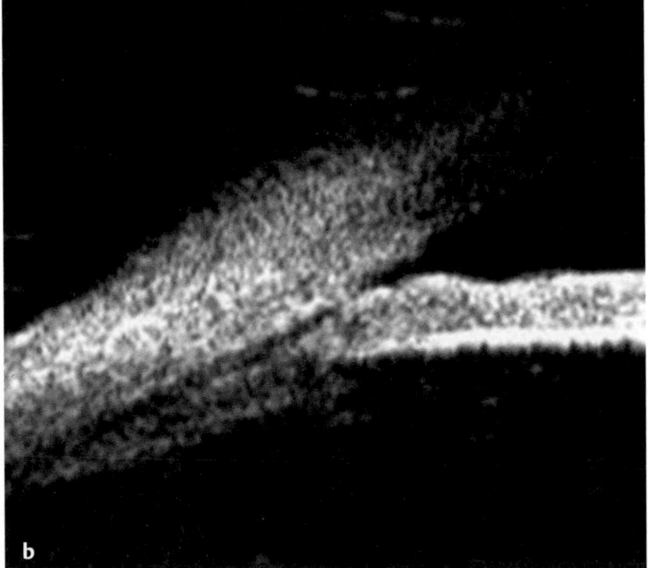

Fig. 16.11 Ultrasound biomicroscopy (UBM) after closed globe injury. **(a)** Showing rupture of the ciliary body that is still attached to the scleral spur, angle recession. **(b)** Disinsertion of the ciliary body from the scleral spur with an echolucent space between ciliary body and sclera, cyclodialysis.

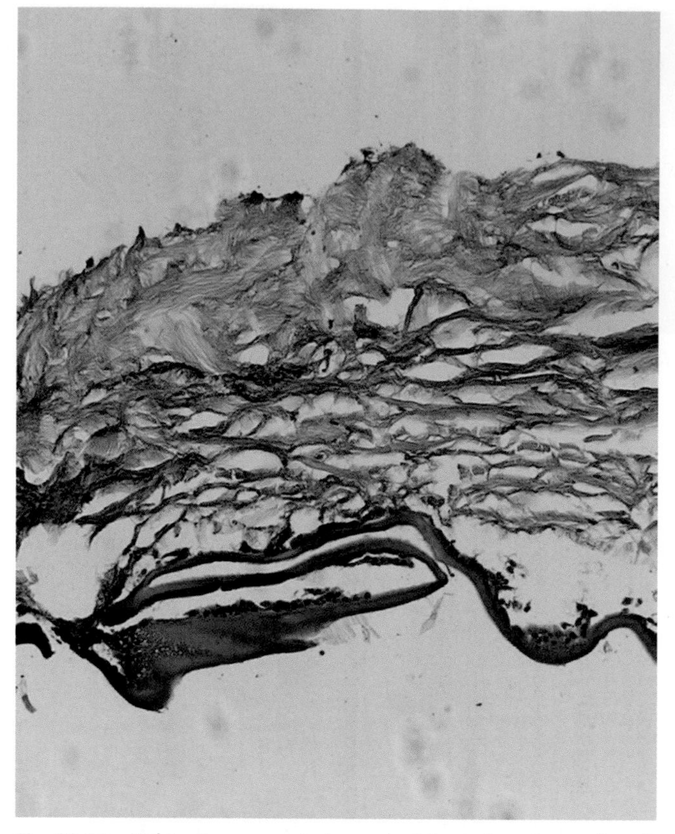

Fig. 16.12 Light microscopy photograph of the trabecular meshwork (hematoxylin and eosin preparation) in late traumatic glaucoma showing distortion of trabecular meshwork architecture and a glass membrane.

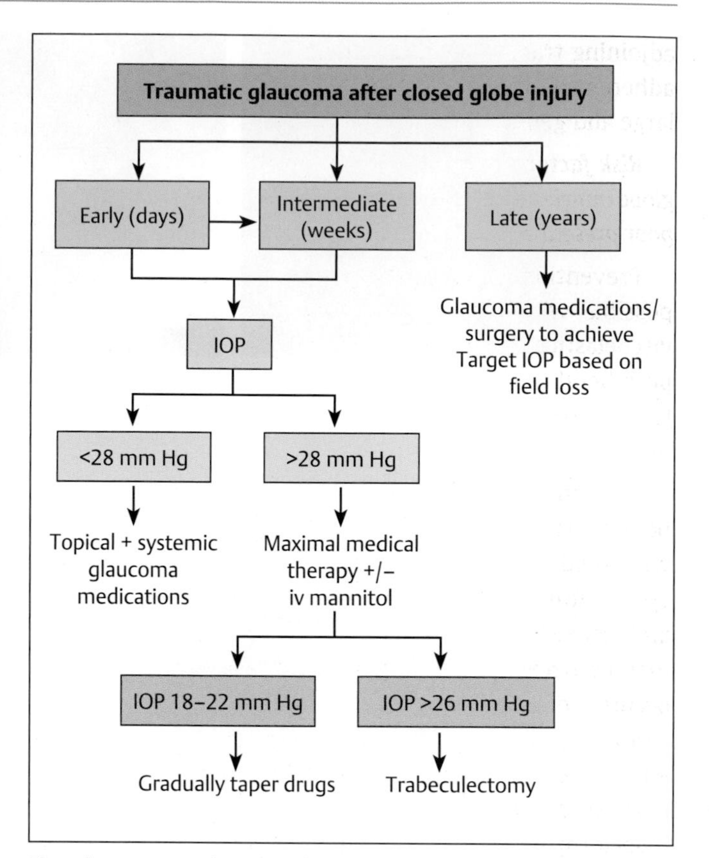

Flowchart 16.2 Algorithm depicting the management of traumatic glaucoma after closed globe injury. IOP, intraocular pressure.

brimonidine, Rho kinase inhibitors and carbonic anhydrase inhibitors topically. Systemic glaucoma medications, acetazolamide, syrup glycerol, and intravenous mannitol may be added as required to achieve an IOP of <21 mm Hg. In a large percentage of such eyes, medications can be gradually tapered off, over weeks or months. *Trabeculectomy would be considered if the IOP remains above 26 to 28 mm Hg on maximal medical therapy* (**Flowchart 16.2**).

Patients should be re-evaluated at 2 and 4 weeks and 3 and 12 months after trauma, even if the IOP appears to have reached normal levels.

In the presence of a hyphema, patients should be evaluated more frequently to monitor the IOP and look for earliest signs of corneal blood staining. *Surgery for a large hyphema is indicated if (i) IOP cannot be controlled to at least 20 to 24 mm Hg on maximal medical therapy, or (ii) a total hyphema lasts beyond a couple of days, or (iii) if corneal blood staining is seen.* Draining of the hyphema carries a risk of iris/lens injury, or a rebleed. Therefore, a trabeculectomy with spontaneous, partial drainage of hyphema results in a good control of IOP, relief to injured corneal endothelium, and a smaller residual hyphema that resolves with time.

Ghost Cell Glaucoma

After concessional injury with a resolving vitreous hemorrhage, *RBCs over 2 to 3 weeks old become spherical, rigid, and of a khaki color.* If there is an associated break in the zonules, these rigid RBCs come into the anterior chamber forming a pseudohypopyon and blocking trabecular outflow. Therapy is prolonged medical control of IOP in most cases, but in recalcitrant cases a vitrectomy and anterior chamber wash may be required to lower IOP.

Open Globe Injuries

In open globe injuries, the IOP generally rises once a repair has been done or there is spontaneous closure. Therefore, it is commonly seen late, associated with healed uveitis, secondary angle closure, and epithelial or fibrous downgrowth. This has been seen to occur in 5 to 20% of cases. Eyes having traumatic glaucoma after open globe injury were frequently found to have an adherent leukoma and evidence of lenticular damage or displacement. This evidence of injury to the lens–iris diaphragm possibly indicates the degree of damage and dysfunction of the adjoining trabecular meshwork, leading to glaucoma. The adherent leukomas causing glaucoma are not necessarily large and generally tend to involve the limbus.

Risk factors for the development of glaucoma after open globe injuries have been reported to be older age, lens injuries, poor presenting visual acuity, and early cataract surgery.

Prevention of glaucoma after open globe injuries is possible with care taken during primary repair to use viscoelastics to reform the anterior chamber and prevent peripheral anterior synechiae. The use of systemic and topical steroids to dampen inflammation is also effective in preventing later rise in IOP.

It is imperative that eyes be followed closely for a possible rise in IOP, which can be managed appropriately with medications in most cases. Measuring IOP in such eyes is fraught with difficulty due to corneal irregularity and coexistent inflammation and a digital assessment may be necessary. As inflammation subsides and healing occurs, medications can be tapered gradually. For secondary angle closure, early and large laser iridotomies will reopen the angle. Surgery may be required in some cases, and a trabeculectomy with mitomycin C gives good long-term results. Drainage devices have been used but need to be placed away from an already damaged cornea. Cyclophotocoagulation has not been found to be effective in the long term, and multiple applications are required. A review should be maintained to prevent glaucomatous morbidity (**Fig. 16.13**).

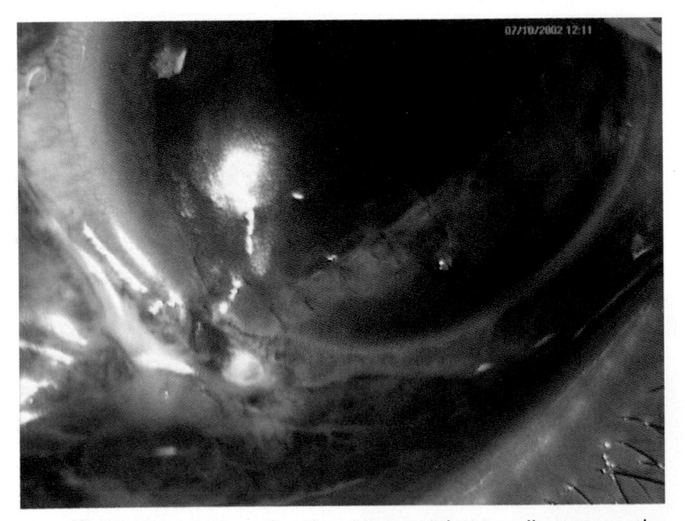

Fig. 16.13 Repaired perforating injury with iris adherent to the wound. This eye is likely to develop a chronic glaucoma and needs review.

Chemical Injuries

Chemical injuries, especially after alkali burns, lead to marked inflammation and ischemia of the limbus and intraocular structures, including the trabecular meshwork. A rise of IOP can be seen in 25 to 75% of chemical injuries. Glaucoma may be seen early, or as a late complication, with a phase of low pressure in between, due to suggested ciliary body shutdown. An early rise in IOP has been attributed to collagen shrinkage shortening the angle and increasing uveal blood flow, while the later rise may be multifactorial—trabecular meshwork scarring, angle closure, and steroid therapy.

Clinically, *a rise in IOP is seen most often in grade 3 and 4 chemical injuries*, where there is a total loss of corneal epithelium, stromal opacification, and limbal ischemia of more than one-third of the circumference. IOP measurement is difficult and digital assessment needs to be done regularly.

Chemicals commonly involved are ammonium hydroxide and ammonia in fertilizers, calcium hydroxide in whitewash and cement, magnesium hydroxide in firecrackers, and sodium and potassium hydroxides in soaps.

Management

Immediate therapy should be a copious wash with any clean fluid available, to normalize pH to between 7 and 7.2. Any particles of lime, etc., in the fornices should be looked for and removed. For grade 2 or worse injuries, hourly steroid drops, and a cycloplegic and topical antibiotic for 7 to 10 days will reduce inflammation. Thereafter, the steroids should be tapered. To lower IOP, aqueous suppressants such as timolol and brimonidine may be used. However, in the presence of severe inflammation, oral acetazolamide may be given initially and then tapered. Chronically raised IOP may require surgical intervention, trabeculectomy, or drainage devices, with a guarded prognosis as the conjunctiva is also involved in the chemical injury. Laser cyclophotocoagulation may be considered, but should be done in a graded manner, 180 degrees at a time.

Glaucoma after ocular trauma should be prevented as far as possible by taking due precautions in hazardous industries and sports. However, if an ocular injury occurs, a comprehensive ocular examination including evaluation of the anterior chamber and IOP would help detect glaucoma early and prevent any neuropathy. In view of associated ocular damage, prognosis in most eyes is guarded.

Cases

Case 1

A 14-year-old male presented with complaints of sudden, painful diminution of vision in right eye for the last 3 days following a firecracker injury. Best corrected visual acuity was hand movements close to face in the right eye and 6/6 in the left eye. IOPs were 44 and 16 mm Hg in the right eye and left eye, respectively. On slit-lamp examination, right eye anterior chamber was deep with multiple sphincter tear, traumatic mydriasis, and a rosette cataract (**Case 1-1**). On gonioscopy of right eye, angle recession was present, extending for more than 300 degrees with increased pigmentation in the inferior angle (**Case 1-2**). Fundus examination of right eye showed a cup:disc ratio of 0.3:1 and left eye cup:disc ratio of 0.2:1.

Points to consider

- A raised IOP of 44 mm Hg with no significant glaucomatous optic neuropathy.
- Due to the raised IOP, a diagnosis of right eye post-traumatic ocular hypertension was made.

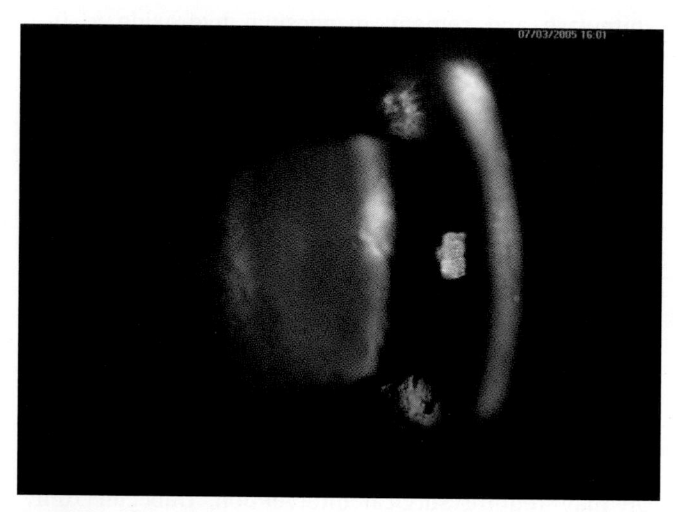

Case 1-1 Clinical picture of the right eye showing traumatic mydriasis and rosette-shaped cataract.

Diagnosis and Management

He was started on maximum oral and topical medications in the right eye for immediate control of IOP. After 1 week, IOP was 16 mm Hg and vision improved to 6/18 in the right eye. Topical medications were continued in the right eye. Keeping in mind the extent of angle recession, lifelong follow-up was advised.

Case 2

A 45-year-old male presented with complaints of gradual and painless diminution of vision in the left eye for the last 30 days, after injury with a cricket ball. On examination, best corrected visual acuity was 6/24p in the left eye and 6/9 in the right eye. IOPs were 14 and 24 mm Hg in the right eye and left eye, respectively. On slit-lamp examination, the anterior chamber in the left eye was irregularly deep, and there was an irregular, oval, dilated pupil with sluggish pupillary reaction. A cataractous lens subluxated from 12 o'clock to 5 o'clock was also present (**Case 2-1**). On gonioscopy, small areas of angle recession, increased trabecular pigmentation, and possible resolving blot clots were seen in the left eye (**Case 2-2**). Fundus examination of right eye showed a cup:disc ratio of 0.3:1 and left eye cup:disc ratio of 0.7:1. Hence, a diagnosis of left eye post-traumatic glaucoma with a subluxated cataractous lens was made.

Points to consider

- Target IOP of <15 mm Hg to be achieved.
- Followed by lifelong follow-up.

Diagnosis and Management

He was advised Humphrey visual field examination and refraction. A diurnal variation of IOP is required to be noted to determine what medications are required.

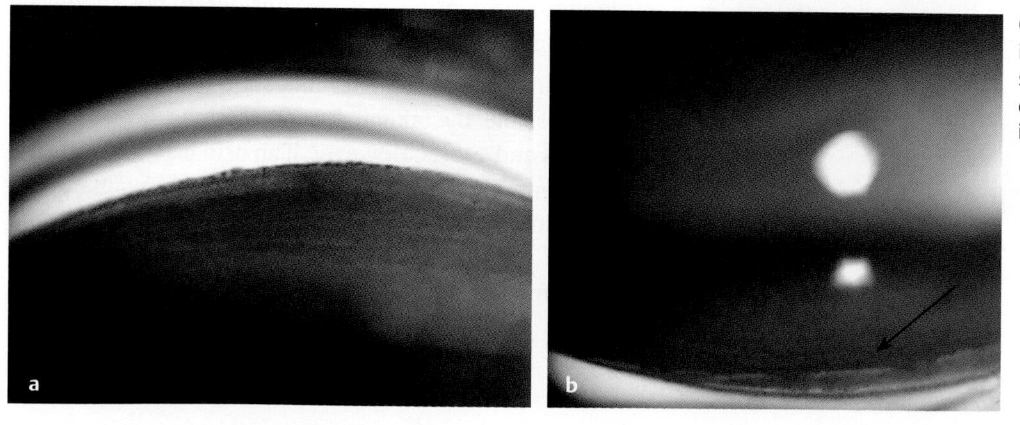

Case 1-2 Gonioscopy picture: **(a)** inferior angle and **(b)** superior angle showing angle recession (*black arrow*) with increased pigmentation in the inferior angle.

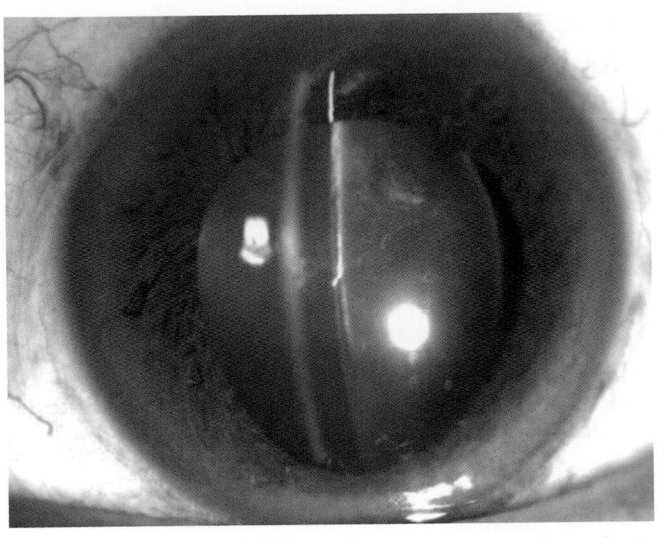

Case 2-1 Clinical picture of the left eye showing irregular mydriatic pupil and nasally subluxated cataractous lens.

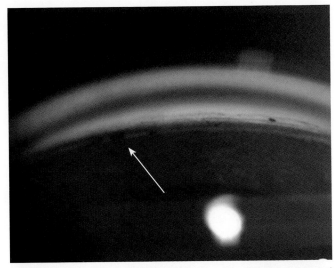

Case 2-2 Gonioscopy picture of inferior angle showing increased pigmentation with resolved hyphema clots (*white arrow*).

Case 3

A 16-year-old male complained of diminution of vision and pain in the right eye after being hit by a cricket ball 2 hours earlier. His vision was perception of light (PL) with an accurate projection of rays (PR), and there was corneal edema, ciliary congestion, hyphema filling two-thirds of the anterior chamber, and no view of the pupil or fundus. The IOP was 46 mm Hg.

Points to consider

- An IOP over 28/30 mm Hg over a number of days can cause retinal venous occlusions, and corneal blood staining if a hyphema is present.
- Although there was traumatic inflammation, the use of cycloplegia is debatable and could be avoided as it may cause a rebleed.

Diagnosis and Management

The patient was put on maximal tolerable glaucoma medications, timolol, brimonidine, Rho kinase inhibitors acetazolamide tablets, and syrup glycerol. IV mannitol 350 mL was given stat. The IOP reduced to 28/30 mm Hg in 2 hours, and remained so over the next 2 days on maximal therapy. To reduce IOP further, a trabeculectomy was done. IV mannitol was given preoperatively, intracameral wash was not done as iris damage could not be evaluated, but blood that spontaneously came out of the trabecular ostium on air injection was cleared. After 24 hours the IOP was 14 mm Hg and the hyphema had reduced considerably. A month later, the hyphema had resolved. The patient had a vision of 6/12, resolving Berlin edema and choroidal rupture, cup:disc ratio of 0.4, and a well-controlled IOP of 12 mm Hg (**Case 3-1**).

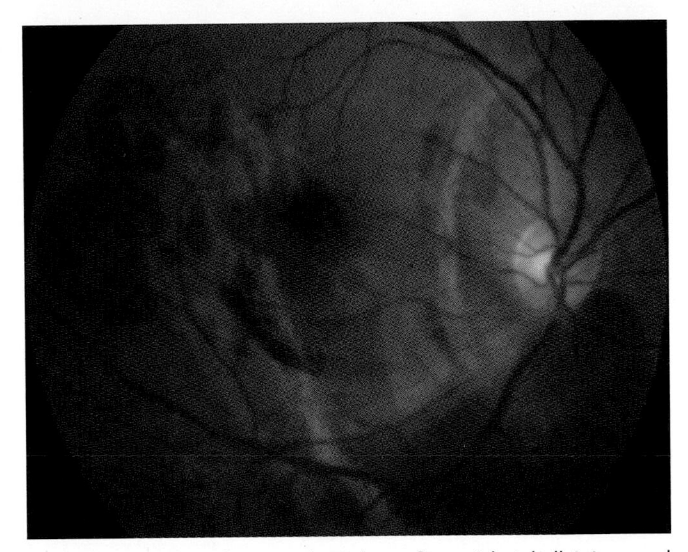

Case 3-1 Fundus photograph 2 days after cricket ball injury and control of intraocular pressure (IOP) with trabeculectomy. There were crescentic choroidal ruptures with subretinal hemorrhage involving the macula.

Case 4

A 14-year-old female gave a history of firecracker injury 5 years earlier with pain, redness, and diminution of vision A lens aspiration with posterior chamber intraocular lenses was done 3 days after trauma with some gain in vision. The patient noted sudden onset of pain, redness with an IOP of 46 mm Hg, and vision of 6/24. IV mannitol and all topical glaucoma medications were given, but IOP remained at 30 mm Hg. Fundus examination revealed extensive chorioretinal scarring and a cup:disc ratio of 0.8 with significant neuroretinal rim pallor (**Case 4-1**).

Points to consider

- High IOP can occur years after trauma.
- The visual field appears to show defects due to retinal pathology as well as glaucoma.
- Target IOP should be <15 mm Hg.

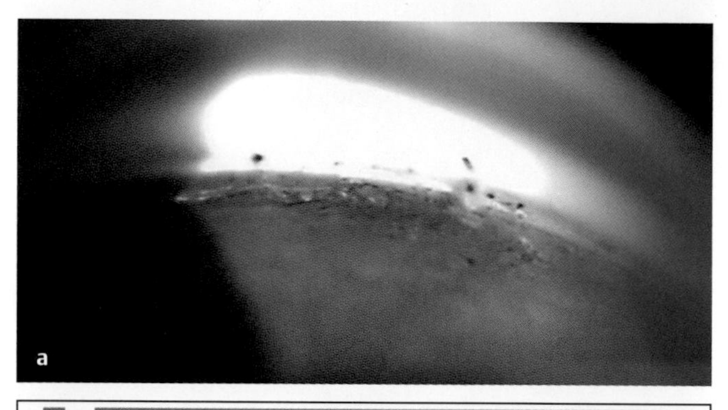

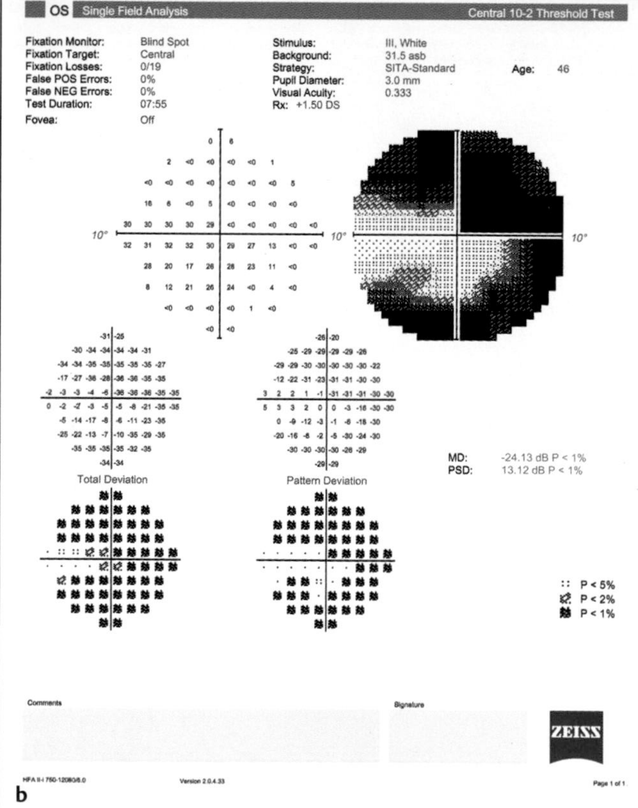

Case 4-1 **(a)** Gonioscopy shows an extensive angle recession with areas of cyclodialysis. **(b)** Visual field has extensive generalized loss of sensitivity with scotomas seen within and outside Bjerrum's area.

Diagnosis and Management

Visual prognosis was explained and a trabeculectomy performed. After 5 years her vision is 6/12, IOP is 12 to 15 mm Hg, and visual field is stable.

Case 5

A 4-year-old child presented with a history of a fall, and repair of an ocular perforation 3 months earlier, with significant DV. On examination, a superior leucomatous corneal opacity, with iris adhesions and remnants of the lens capsule, was seen. The IOP was 30 mm Hg and the cup:disc ratio was 0.7 with some inferior neuroretinal rim pallor (**Case 5-1**).

Points to consider

- There is evidence of glaucomatous neuropathy and corneal damage.
- Carbonic anhydrase inhibitors and alpha agonists should be avoided.

Diagnosis and Management

Timolol drops were prescribed, which reduced the IOP to 23 mm Hg. Thereafter a combination of timolol and a prostaglandin (PG) analog was prescribed at bedtime, and the IOP was 16 mm Hg. The parents were advised the need for long-term review for glaucoma and corneal evaluation.

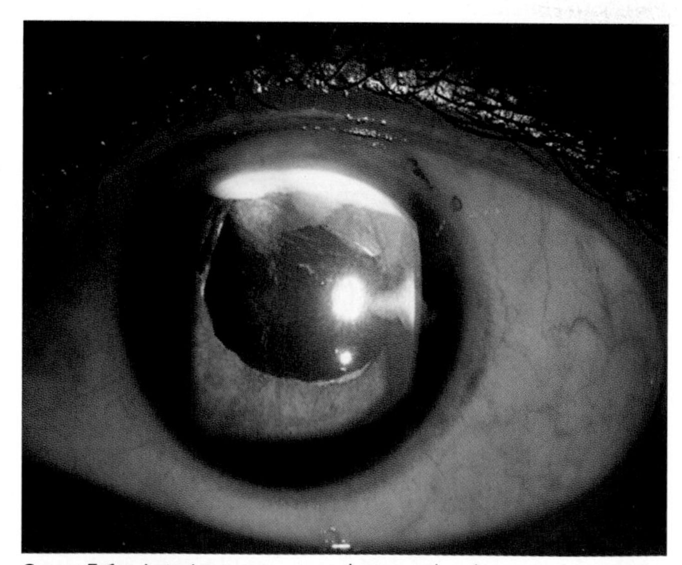

Case 5-1 Anterior segment photograph showing a superior leucomatous corneal opacity with iris adhesions including remnants of the lens capsule.

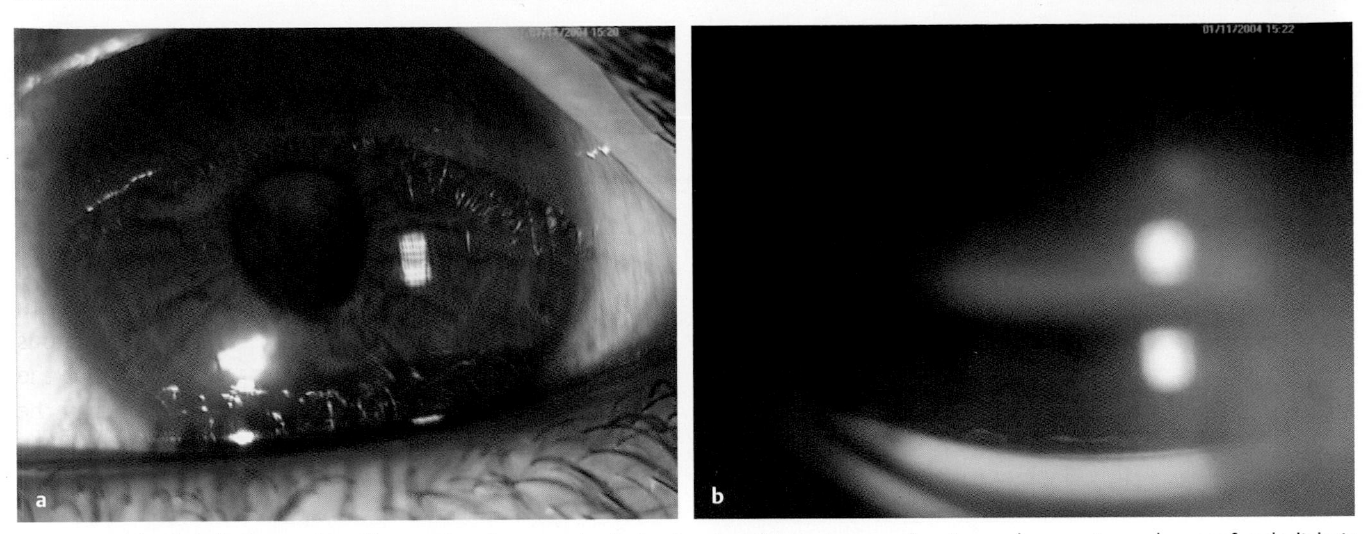

Case 6-1 **(a)** Inferiorly distorted pupil in an otherwise normal anterior chamber. **(b)** Gonioscopy showing angle recession and areas of cyclodialysis with significant pigmentation and peripheral anterior synechiae.

Case 6

A 50-year-old gentleman complained of noticing a loss of peripheral vision in his right eye. He had been diagnosed as POAG and was on latanoprost drops. On examination, vision in the right eye was 6/24 and in the left eye was 6/6, with an inferiorly distorted pupil in the right eye, a cup:disc ratio of 0.9 in the right eye and 0.3 in left eye, and IOP of 32/16 mm Hg. Gonioscopy revealed angle recession and areas of cyclodialysis with significant pigmentation and peripheral anterior synechiae (**Case 6-1**).

Points to consider

- POAG is generally bilateral with little asymmetry.
- Always look for a secondary cause of raised IOP, with gonioscopy, if asymmetrical glaucomatous neuropathy is seen in the presence of an open angle.

Diagnosis and Management

A target IOP of around 12 mm Hg was explained, which was achieved using a combination of PG analog and timolol with another combination of brinzolamide and brimonidine.

Suggested Readings

Bai HQ, Yao L, Wang DB, Jin R, Wang YX. Causes and treatments of traumatic secondary glaucoma. Eur J Ophthalmol 2009; 19(2):201–206

Gharaibeh A, Savage HI, Scherer RW, Goldberg MF, Lindsley K. Medical interventions for traumatic hyphema. Cochrane Database Syst Rev 2019;1:CD005431

Razeghinejad R, Lin MM, Lee D, Katz LJ, Myers JS. Pathophysiology and management of glaucoma and ocular hypertension related to trauma. Surv Ophthalmol 2020; 65(5):530–547

Sihota R, Sood NN, Agarwal HC. Traumatic glaucoma. Acta Ophthalmol Scand 1995;73(3):252–254

Tumbocon JAJ, Latina MA. Angle recession glaucoma. Int Ophthalmol Clin 2002;42(3):69–78

Turalba AV, Shah AS, Andreoli MT, Andreoli CM, Rhee DJ. Predictors and outcomes of ocular hypertension after open-globe injury. J Glaucoma 2014;23(1):5–10

CHAPTER 17

Steroid-Induced Glaucoma

Overview

- Risk Factors
- Steroid Potency
- Route of Administration
- Pathophysiology
- Clinical Features
- Management
  - Therapy
- Prognosis
- Cases
- Suggested Readings

Introduction

Steroid-induced glaucoma is a secondary glaucoma occurring as a response to corticosteroids, exogenous or endogenous. Steroids are ubiquitously used in medicine and ophthalmology, making this a common cause of iatrogenic glaucoma. It is usually associated with topical steroid use, but it may develop with oral, intravenous, inhaled, intravitreal, or periocular steroid administration. The rise in intraocular pressure (IOP) can occur at all ages, with children younger than 10 years reported to have more frequent and severe IOP elevations. No gender or racial predilection has been reported, and it is more frequently seen in patients with trabecular outflow abnormalities such as primary open-angle glaucoma (POAG) and other glaucomas.

Steroid-induced ocular hypertension is a term used when there is a chronic rise in IOP, but no glaucomatous neuropathy, while ***steroid-induced glaucoma*** has both raised IOP and glaucomatous neuropathy.

Two seminal studies by Armaly and Becker found that approximately one-third of normal individuals experience a moderate increase in IOP, 6 to 15 mm Hg, after topical steroid use for 4 to 6 weeks, with 5 to 6% developing a marked increase in IOP, >31 mm Hg. Thus, around 35% of the general population are "steroid responders," that is, have a tendency to develop steroid-induced glaucoma when steroids are administered. It was also seen that patients with POAG and their relatives were more likely to be high steroid responders (**Table 17.1**).

Risk Factors

Following are the conditions which are associated with an increased risk of steroid-induced glaucoma:

- Patients with POAG.
- First-degree relatives of POAG patients.
- Children below 10 years.
- High myopia.
- Connective tissue disorders (especially rheumatoid arthritis).
- Eyes with traumatic angle recession and their fellow eyes.
- Endogenous hypercortisolism.
- Diabetes mellitus.

Table 17.1 IOP response to topical corticosteroid administration in two seminal studies

	Becker (Absolute IOP)	Armaly (Rise in IOP)
Steroid eye drops / *Grade of response*	Betamethasone QID (6 weeks)	Dexamethasone TDS (4 weeks)
Low	<20 mm Hg (58%)	<6 mm Hg (66%)
Intermediate	20–31 mm Hg (36%)	6–15 mm Hg (29%)
High	>31 mm Hg (6%)	>15 mm Hg (5%)

Abbreviations: IOP, intraocular pressure; QID, four times daily; TDS, three times daily.

Individuals with pre-existing POAG have a much greater tendency to develop an elevated IOP from topical corticosteroids. Corticosteroids were used earlier as a test to unmask or diagnose early POAG. Conversely, normal individuals with a high steroid response are more likely to develop POAG. Patients with primary angle-closure glaucoma (PACG) and patients with secondary glaucoma are thought to behave in the same manner as normal eyes with regard to steroid response.

Steroid Potency

The risk of developing a steroid-induced rise in IOP is also related to the *anti-inflammatory potency of the steroid used*, with betamethasone, dexamethasone, and difluprednate being most likely to cause a significant rise in IOP and loteprednol, rimexolone, and hydrocortisone the least (**Table 17.2**). Difluprednate has been introduced as having a highly potent anti-inflammatory effect with raised IOP reported in 3 to 4% of individuals; however, when it occurs the rise in IOP can be substantial, especially in children.

Table 17.2 Anti-inflammatory effect of different steroids, which is generally directly correlated with the rise of intraocular pressure caused

Anti-inflammatory potency	Steroid
Highly potent	▪ Betamethasone ▪ Dexamethasone ▪ Difluprednate ▪ Clobetasol propionate ▪ Flucinonide ▪ Fluticasone
Moderately potent	▪ Prednisolone ▪ Triamcinolone acetonide ▪ Loteprednol etabonate ▪ Fluorometholone
Less potent	▪ Hydrocortisone ▪ Medrysone

The concentration or frequency of dosing of a steroid also influences the likelihood of producing an IOP elevation.

Route of Administration

Most cases of steroid-induced glaucoma occur due to exogenous steroids which may be administered topically, periocularly, or systemically (**Table 17.3**). A few examples of exogenous steroids are:

- Ocular:
  - Drops, ointments, intravitreal injections, etc.
  - Periocular: Subtenon injections.
- Systemic:
  - Asthma: Inhalational, oral.
  - Dermatological: Creams, IV.

However, endogenous steroids can also cause this condition, for example:

- Pituitary adenomas.
- Cushing's syndrome.

Steroid response varies with the route of administration: Topical steroids produce an elevated IOP in a larger number of people in 2 to 6 weeks, and systemic steroids have to be used over months to years for an elevated IOP to be seen in fewer.

Most people have a steroid response from topically applied eye drops that are commonly used for uveitis or allergic conjunctivitis. Periocular steroid injections, subtenon, orbital floor, or retrobulbar, are used to treat inflammation such as uveitis or macular edema. The depot forms have a prolonged duration of action, and are more likely to lead to a steroid response. *There is no way to predict a steroid response with intraocular or periocular steroid use, as IOP changes after topical use do not correlate*

Table 17.3 Route, duration, and suggested doses related to steroid-induced glaucoma

Route	Average dose	Approximate time taken for IOP rise
Oral	25 mg hydrocortisone/day 50 mg prednisolone	1 year 2–15 months
Inhalational	1,500 µg flunisolide or >1,600 µg of beclomethasone, budesonide, or triamcinolone 200 µg fluticasone	3 months 1 year
Pulse steroids (repeated)	140 mg repeated 4 weeks	6 months
Dermatological	Betamethasone cream (0.1%)	3 months
Topical (eye)	More than QID dose of a potent steroid (dexamethasone)	2–6 weeks

Abbreviations: IOP, intraocular pressure; QID, four times daily.

with IOP seen following intra- or periocular steroid use. After posterior subtenon injection of triamcinolone, a rise in IOP has been shown in 21 to 44% cases at 5 to 9 weeks, with a chronic rise in IOP in 9% cases.

Intravitreal injections of steroids are commonly used to treat diabetic macular edema, and other causes of macular edema. IOP may show a sustained rise after intravitreal injections of steroid in 5 to 15% of eyes, but generally returns to baseline within days. A sustained rise is especially seen if access to the anterior segment is facilitated by pseudophakia or vitrectomy (**Fig. 17.1**). Any persistent rise subsides over 5 to 6 months. However, with repeat injections, more eyes show an IOP of >30 mm Hg. Risk factors for IOP elevation after intravitreal triamcinolone acetonide (IVTA) include younger age, high myopia, and multiple injections. Intravitreal implants of 0.2 µg/day fluocinolone caused a rise in IOP of >25 mm Hg in about 25% of eyes, while dexamethasone intravitreal implants caused a rise in IOP of >25 mm Hg in about 10% of South Asian eyes. It is therefore necessary to check IOP in the first week after intravitreal steroid injections and 2 weeks after implants, as the IOP rise does not tend to reduce, and may require filtering surgery.

Systemic administration of corticosteroids is least likely to induce glaucoma; however, the IOP elevation may occur as long as weeks later. Chronic use over months to years can lead to a cataract and glaucoma. The incidence of steroid-induced IOP elevation in patients on systemic corticosteroids has not been well studied. In studies after renal transplant, increased IOP has been recorded in 5 to 12.5%. In a population-based study, a strong association was found between inhaled corticosteroid use and presence of either glaucoma or elevated IOP; the risk increased with more than four puffs per day.

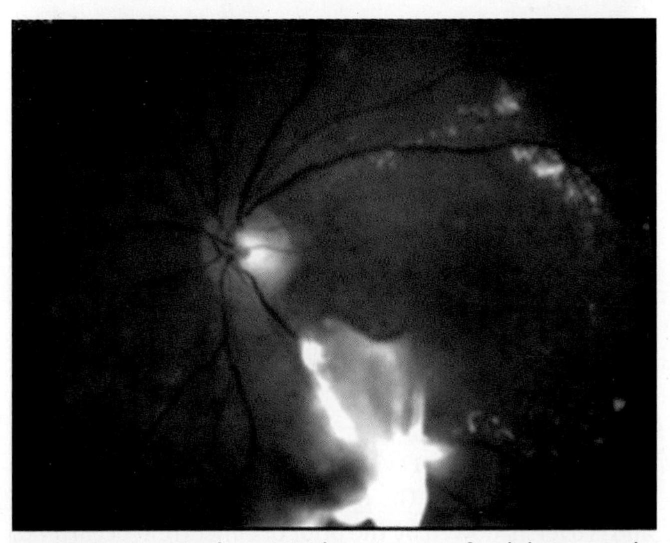

Fig. 17.1 Intravitreal triamcinolone injection for diabetic macular edema; intraocular pressure (IOP) should be rechecked after 1 week, and on every review.

Elevated IOP may also be caused by increased endogenous corticosteroids as seen in Cushing disease, and with pituitary adenomas.

Pathophysiology

Steroids lead to a rise in IOP by reducing the spaces present in the trabecular meshwork in a number of ways.

The main mechanism by which steroids cause a rise in IOP is their membrane-stabilizing action. Hyaluronidase-sensitive glycosaminoglycans and mucopolysaccharides are normally present in the aqueous outflow system. Lysosomes in the trabecular meshwork endothelial cells keep this depolymerized, as the polymerized form may undergo hydration, and decrease aqueous outflow. Steroids stabilize lysosomal membranes and lead to an accumulation of polymerized glycosaminoglycans in the trabecular meshwork, reducing spaces and increasing outflow resistance. An increased expression of collagen, elastin, fibronectin, and sialoglycoprotein is also seen. Fibrillar material and collagen have also been seen deposited around Schlemm's canal and the trabecular meshwork.

Mutations in the myocilin gene lead to misfolding and aggregation of myocilin protein within the trabecular meshwork cells, causing endoplasmic reticulum stress leading to apoptosis. This was earlier known as the trabecular meshwork-inducible glucocorticoid response gene (TIGR gene), as it was seen to cause a rise in IOP after the use of dexamethasone (**Table 17.4**).

Clinical Features

As the effect of steroid use takes time to set in and the IOP rise is gradual, most patients have no symptoms till a very high IOP occurs. *The occurrence of such high IOPs in young adults can cause colored haloes and blurring of vision, distinguished from angle-closure glaucoma by the fact that the eye remains "white."*

The use of systemic steroids over a long duration typically leads to a posterior subcapsular cataract (PSC) and glaucoma. *A history of systemic or ocular diseases requiring chronic corticosteroid use, for example, uveitis, collagen vascular disease, asthma, dermatitis, etc., should be elicited in patients having open-angle glaucoma with a high IOP, as IOPs in POAG generally do not rise above 30 mm Hg.*

The age of the affected patient may determine clinical features seen: infants may present with photophobia and cloudy corneas, juveniles with colored haloes, and adults with an open-angle glaucoma.

Table 17.4 Effect of steroids on the trabecular outflow channel

Trabecular meshwork component	Effect of steroids
Trabecular endothelium function	Inhibition of phagocytosis, proliferation, and migration Inhibition of proteases
Extracellular matrix	Increased deposition of ECM Thickened trabecular beams MYOC-induced increase in expression of fibronectin, elastins, glycosaminoglycans
Cytoskeleton	Cross-linking of actin fibers Microtubule tangles
Gene expression	Increased expression of MYOC (TIGR) Decreased expression of matrix metalloproteinases

Abbreviations: ECM, extracellular matrix; MYOC; myocilin gene; TIGR, trabecular meshwork-inducible glucocorticoid response gene.

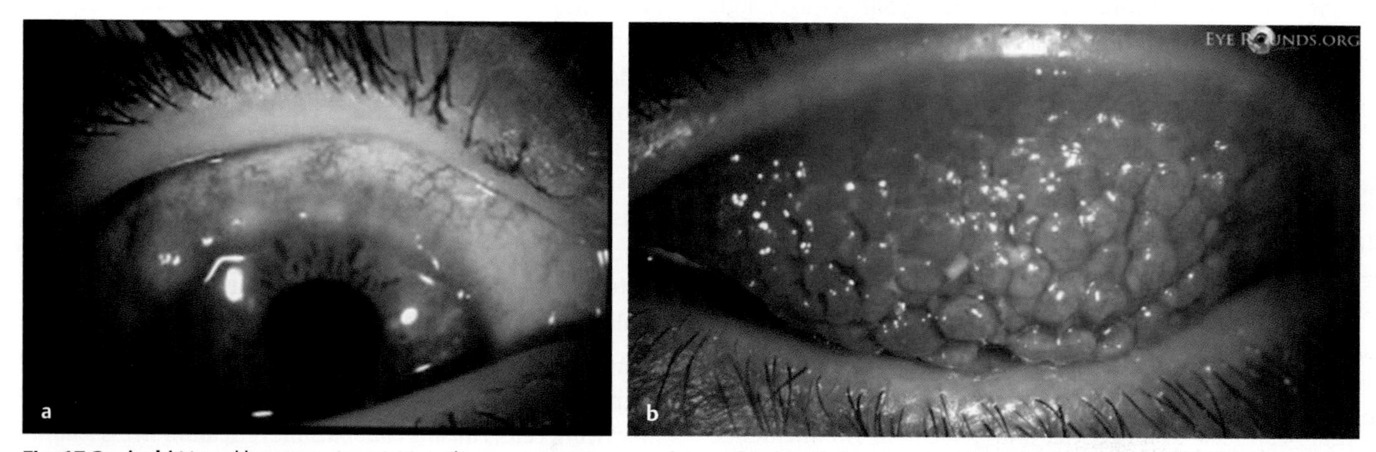

Fig. 17.2 (a, b) Vernal keratoconjunctivitis is the commonest cause of steroid-induced glaucoma in children. Tonometry and fundus examination should be done for diagnosis.

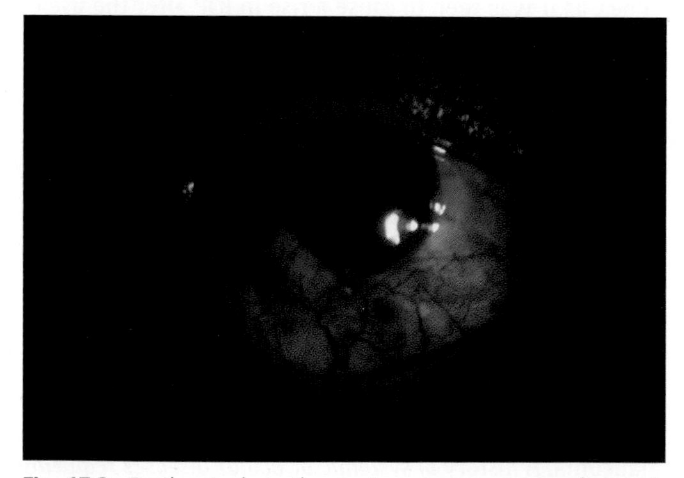

Fig. 17.3 Postkeratoplasty therapy is a common cause of steroid-induced glaucoma.

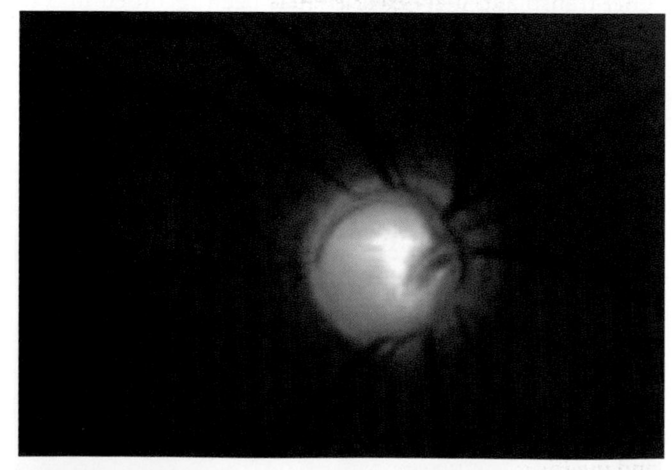

Fig. 17.4 High intraocular pressures (IOPs) after topical use of steroids loften leads to a cup:disc ratio of 0.9 with generalized thinning and pallor of the neuroretinal rim.

The chronic use of topical steroids also causes mydriasis, increased corneal thickness, PSCs, ptosis, and atrophy of the eyelid skin (**Figs. 17.2–17.5**). These may help diagnose past steroid use, if patients are unaware of the medication used.

Cumulative dose of systemic steroids appears to cause a rise in IOP over time. The rise in IOP is generally moderate, and is overshadowed by the prior or concurrent occurrence of a PSC. The drop in vision because of a cataract brings such patients to an ophthalmologist early, with early to

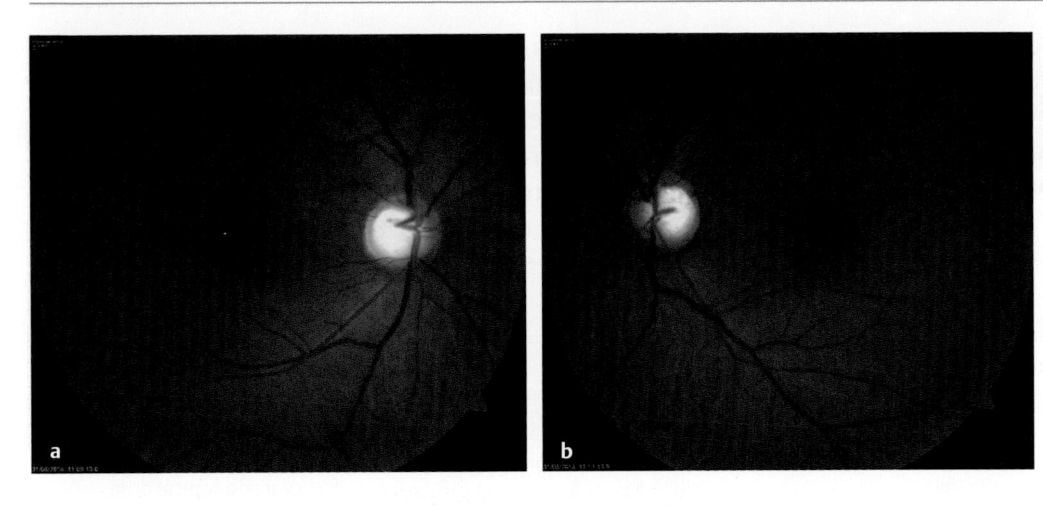

Fig. 17.5 (a, b) Steroid-induced glaucoma due to a dermatological cream used for eczema, lead to a cup:disc ratio of 0.7 and 0.8 with focal inferotemporal neuroretinal rim loss in right eye.

moderate glaucomatous optic neuropathy. IOP rise after systemic use of steroids over months is generally lower, and also shows a gradual decrease in IOP over months once the steroids are stopped.

In the majority of cases where topical steroids have been used for a limited time, around 3 months, IOP reduces gradually to baseline within weeks to months upon stopping the steroid. In such patients, an initial medical control of IOP with a slow taper of glaucoma medications over time is required. However, a quarter to third of patients with prolonged use of steroids will show chronically raised IOPs, generally in the thirties or even up to 50 mm Hg. In such cases, patients present only when the glaucomatous optic neuropathy is advanced, as subcapsular cataracts occur later. The optic nerve head shows a generalized cupping with thinning and pallor of the neuroretinal rim. A prolonged rise in IOP in infants can present as a congenital glaucoma with photophobia and an enlarged eyeball, while in older children this leads to a deep cup and severe glaucomatous optic neuropathy.

The steroid-related IOP response wanes with time, leaving behind past evidence of glaucomatous neuropathy. This "burnt-out" glaucoma can be mistaken as normal tension glaucoma later.

The differential diagnosis of steroid-induced glaucoma includes juvenile open-angle glaucoma (JOAG), POAG, and other secondary open-angle glaucomas such as a traumatic and uveitic glaucomas.

Management

Prevention is best, and in eyes with conditions commonly associated with steroid-induced glaucoma, as in vernal keratoconjunctivitis (VKC), parents need to be educated to avoid steroids and use decongestants, mast cell–stabilizing agents, and lubricants instead.

Steroids are a Schedule H drug, and prescribing physicians and dispensing pharmacists should advise caution in their use, with monitoring of IOP in those with a family history of glaucoma. When prescribed, regular drug holidays should be explained, as in VKC, where steroids may be advised for 7 to 10 days, with a break for a similar period to prevent glaucoma.

Monitoring of patients on whom periocular or intravitreal steroids are used is especially important, and an IOP rise may be prevented by using glaucoma medications such as a brimonidine–timolol combination prior to and for a few days after the procedure.

Therapy

The first and most effective management is the discontinuation of the steroid and controlling IOP to "target" depending upon the optic nerve head damage with glaucoma medications. A lower potency steroid such as prednisolone phosphate, loteprednol etabonate, fluorometholone, rimexolone, or medrysone may be substituted if absolutely required. Nonsteroidal anti-inflammatory drops such as nepafenac or diclofenac may be tried, but their anti-inflammatory efficacy is much less than that of steroids.

The presence of a steroid depot subtenon, visible intravitreal steroid, or an intravitreal implant in an eye with medically uncontrolled IOP would require removal at the earliest. This would need to be followed by maximal tolerated medical therapy of the glaucoma, and a gradual taper as the effect of the steroid on the trabecular meshwork wears off.

Patients who used systemic steroids can be expected to have more moderate rises in IOP and a mild-to-moderate glaucoma. After discontinuation or reduction in the use of the offending steroid, glaucoma medications will usually control IOP to <18 or <15 mm Hg for a mild/moderate glaucoma. After 3 to 4 weeks these medications can be tapered gradually to maintain such a target IOP. There are patients having renal transplant, nephrotic syndrome, etc., in whom steroids will be continued, so that they will need appropriate, long-term glaucoma medications (**Table 17.5**).

A treatment algorithm for steroid-induced glaucoma is suggested in **Flowchart 17.1**.

Glaucoma occurring due to the use of topical steroids needs maximal medical therapy—topical and oral to reduce IOP to a level apposite to their glaucoma severity. When medical therapy is ineffective, laser trabeculoplasty can be added. Argon laser and selective laser trabeculoplasty (SLT) have been shown to be effective in several cases. *In some eyes, the IOP remains elevated despite maximal*

Table 17.5 Management guidelines for steroid-induced glaucoma

Route of steroid administration	Topical and systemic	Subtenon	Intravitreal
Initial treatment	▪ Discontinue steroid in all forms if possible ▪ Medical control of IOP with oral and topical drugs for the washout period of steroid	▪ Excise steroid depot ▪ Medical control of IOP with oral and topical drugs	▪ Medical control of IOP with oral and topical drugs
Intermediate treatment (week)	▪ Substitute with other nonsteroidal/low potency drugs if necessary ▪ Taper oral glaucoma medications	▪ Glaucoma medications during washout period	▪ Medications/laser trabeculoplasty ▪ Vitrectomy with or without trabeculectomy
Long-term treatment (month)	▪ Medical, laser trabeculoplasty, or surgery till target IOP is achieved	▪ Medications, laser trabeculoplasty, or surgery till target IOP is achieved	▪ Medications, laser trabeculoplasty, or surgery till target IOP is achieved
Review (year)	▪ To adjust medications as steroids continue to wash out and lower IOP as age-related trabecular changes raise IOP further		

Abbreviation: IOP, intraocular pressure.

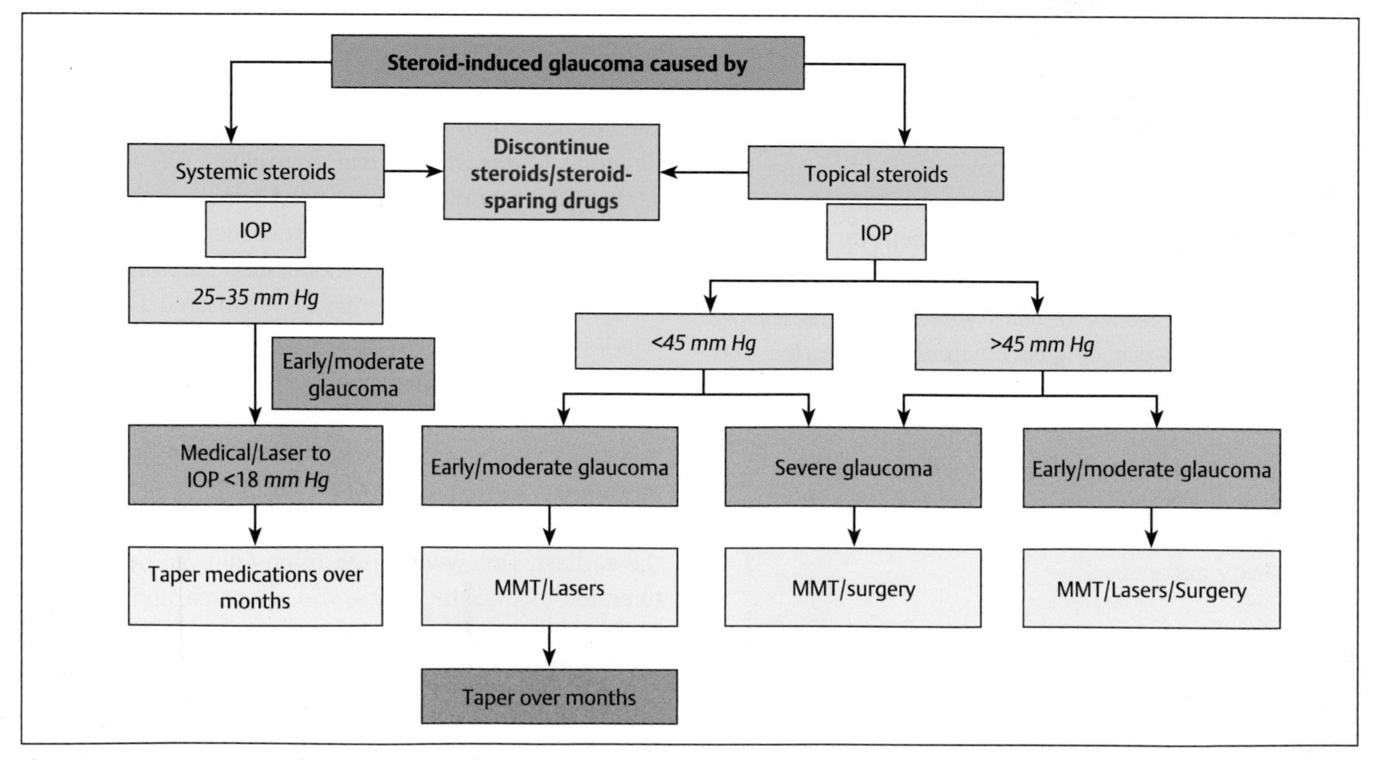

Flowchart 17.1 Treatment algorithm for steroid-induced glaucoma. IOP, intraocular pressure; MMT, maximal medical therapy.

glaucoma medications at levels likely to cause further optic nerve head damage. This is seen in younger patients who have used topical steroids for about a year, had baseline IOPs of around 50 mm Hg, and baseline evidence of glaucomatous optic neuropathy. These eyes need surgery to control their IOP, with trabeculectomy being the first choice.

Glaucoma following intravitreal triamcinolone is managed medically, till the intravitreal steroid crystals resolve, commonly about 6 months after the injection. Intractable secondary glaucoma persists in some cases which requires removal of the corticosteroid by pars plana vitrectomy, and if necessary combined with trabeculectomy. Glaucoma following an intravitreal steroid implant would need to be controlled medically or by laser trabeculoplasty, and if not controlled, by a filtering surgery.

A subtenon injection of anecortave acetate has been used as a means of reducing IOP in steroid-induced glaucoma.

Prognosis

Steroid-induced glaucoma can be stabilized with appropriate steps to reduce IOP, commensurate to the extent of glaucomatous damage. As the steroid washes out of the trabecular meshwork, the IOP appears to reduce over months in most patients who used systemic steroids and in those on topical steroids with no glaucomatous optic neuropathy at baseline. Those with baseline optic nerve damage need chronic glaucoma therapy and review.

Steroid-induced glaucoma is iatrogenic, and if a steroid response occurs, it should be diagnosed early by the ophthalmologist or physician who advised steroid therapy. Control of IOP and stabilization of glaucomatous neuropathy is possible in all cases, keeping in mind the appropriate target IOP for each individual.

Cases

Case 1

An 8-year-old child presented with severe pain, redness, and itching in both eyes for 2 years. The parents noticed a diminution of vision a month ago. On examination there was generalized conjunctival congestion with large papillae on the palpebral conjunctiva and limbus. There was a normal anterior chamber, van Herick grade 3, corneal epithelial edema, PSCs, and cup:disc ratio of 0.9 in both eyes (**Case 1-1**). The IOP was 34/42 mm Hg. A history of topical steroid use intermittently over 2 years was elicited. A diagnosis of VKC with steroid-induced glaucoma was made.

Points to consider

- Target IOP in this child would be 10/12 mm Hg both for the advanced glaucomatous neuropathy and his life expectancy.
- Congestion at the limbus decreases success of filtering surgery.

Diagnosis and Management

Maximal medical therapy resulted in IOPs of only 24/28 mm Hg; therefore, the patient underwent a trabeculectomy using mitomycin C (MMC) 0.2 mg/mL for 1 minute subconjunctival. The IOP after 6 months was 12/14 mm Hg and the Humphrey field analyzer (HFA) showed a central island of vision in both eyes. Due to continued recurrences of VKC, the bleb became more vascularized and the IOP rose to 20/24 mm Hg after 2 years. Topical timolol and dorzolamide combination was given to reach target IOP. As VKC is a chronic disease, parents were counseled to avoid steroids and use olopatadine 0.1%, and 0.03% tacrolimus ointment twice a day.

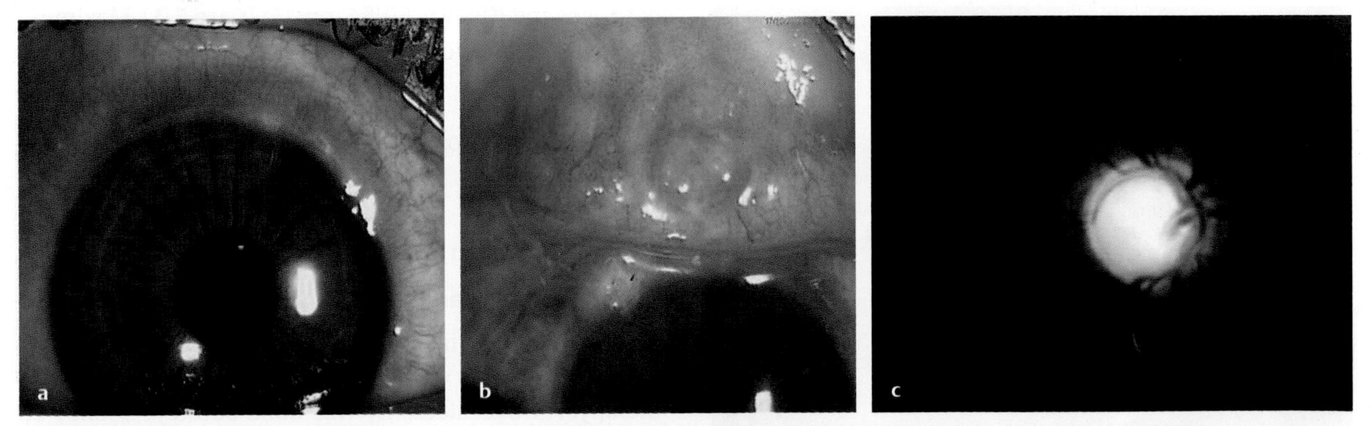

Case 1-1 **(a)** Limbal nodules. **(b)** Palpebral large papillae. **(c)** Cup:disc ratio of 0.9 with generalized pallor of the neuroretinal rim.

Case 2

A 35-year-old lady was diagnosed to have clinically significant diabetic macular edema for which 2 mg/0.05 mL intravitreal triamcinolone acetonide was given. After 3 weeks her IOP had risen to 24 mm Hg and at 6 weeks to 28 mm Hg. Her fundus examination showed a resolution of the macular edema, a cup:disc ratio of 0.6, and neuroretinal rim within normal limits (**Case 2-1**).

Points to consider

- Moderate steroid response seen in 10 to 20% of such eyes, and chronic IOP rise in <5%.
- Avoid prostaglandins (PGs) in the control of IOP.

Diagnosis and Management

The patient was prescribed a combination of timolol and brimonidine for 6 weeks and was then tapered to only timolol, keeping the IOP at <20 mm Hg at all times.

Case 3

A 50-year-old male diagnosed to have chronic PACG was adequately controlled on two glaucoma medications for 2 years, and then presented with high IOPs of 28 mm Hg OD and 26 mm Hg OS. He was noticed to have an acromegalic habitus (**Case 3-1**).

Points to consider

- Sudden increase in IOP could be due to a pituitary adenoma.
- The right eye visual field had a possibly quadrantic defect.

Diagnosis and Management

Magnetic resonance imaging (MRI) was done and showed a macroadenoma. The patient had elevated serum cortisol, prolactin, and growth hormone. One month after resection of the adenoma, the IOP reduced to 14/16 mm Hg on his earlier glaucoma medications.

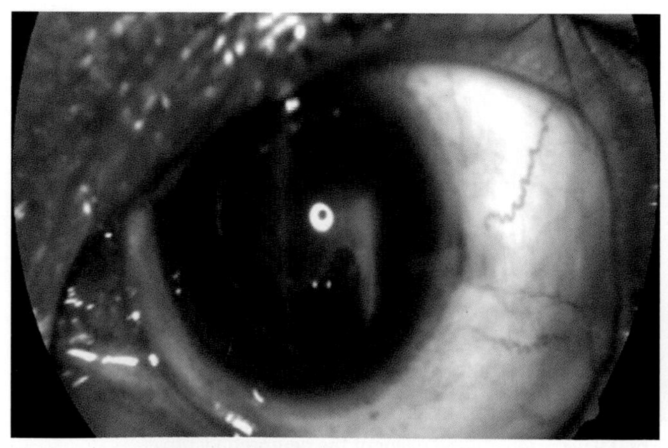

Case 2-1 Intravitreal triamcinolone injected for diabetic macular edema, seen in the midvitreous.

Case 4

A 19-year-old male presented with complaints of redness and itching in both eyes for the last 5 to 6 years. He was using an unknown topical medication on and off for 5 years. On examination, best corrected visual acuity was 6/9 and 6/6, and IOPs were 24 and 26 mm Hg in in the right eye and left eye, respectively.

On slit-lamp examination, conjunctival papillae, anterior chamber van Herick grade 3 was present with normal iris pattern. Mild PSC was present in both eyes (**Case 4-1**). On gonioscopy, open angles with visible scleral spur were present in both eyes (**Case 4-2**). Fundus examination of right eye showed a cup:disc ratio of 0.7:1 and left eye cup:disc ratio of 0.8:1 (**Case 4-3**). Hence, steroid-induced glaucoma with PSC was diagnosed in both eyes.

Points to consider

- Topical steroids used on and off.
- Moderate rise in IOP.
- Mmoderate glaucoma.

Diagnosis and Management

Steroids were stopped in both eyes, and the patient was started on timolol twice a day and advised close follow-up. Diurnal control after 4 weeks showed IOPs of 16 to 20 mm Hg. He was advised regular review for IOP and possible cataract surgery.

Case 5

A 21-year-old male presented with vernal keratoconjunctivitis and having used topical steroids for 6 years. His cup:disc ratio was 0.9 in both eyes with generalized and severe pallor of the neuroretinal rim. There were PSCs in both eyes and IOP was 50/54 mm Hg (**Case 5-1**). Maximum glaucoma medications were started.

Points to consider

- Severe glaucoma in a young patient needs an IOP of <12 mm Hg.
- PGs should be avoided as they may increase inflammation.

Diagnosis and Management

As medicines did not reduce IOP, an SLT was done, but after 1 week, IOPs were again 26/28 mm Hg on maximal therapy. A trabeculectomy was done both eyes, followed by phacoemulsification 3 months later. After 5 years, his IOPs were 10/12 mm Hg.

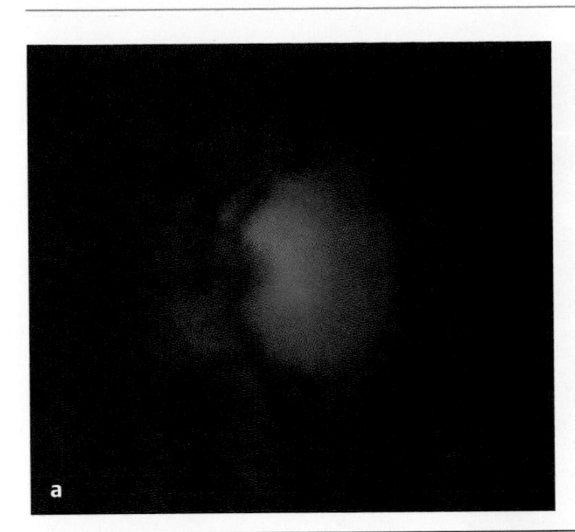

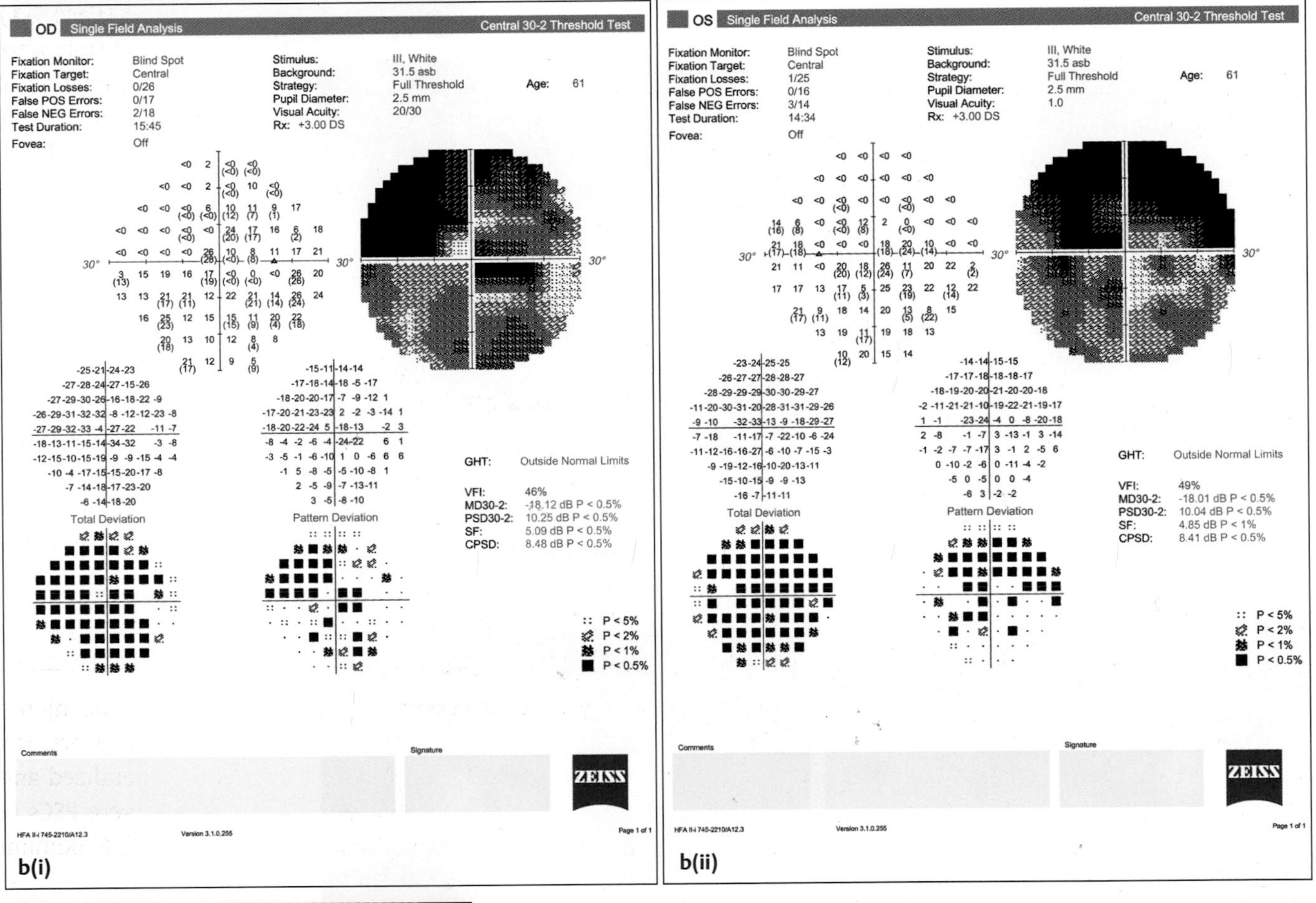

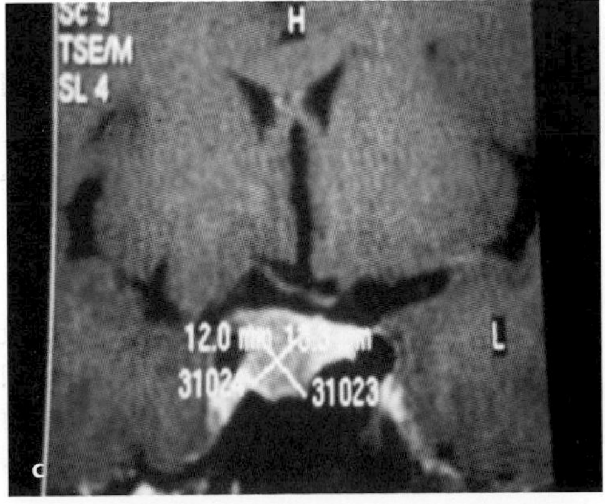

Case 3-1 **(a)** Optic nerve head showing cup:disc ratio of 0.7 and 0.8. **(b)** Perimetry shows a possible superior quadrantic loss in the right eye. **(c)** Magnetic resonance imaging (MRI) showing a pituitary macroadenoma.

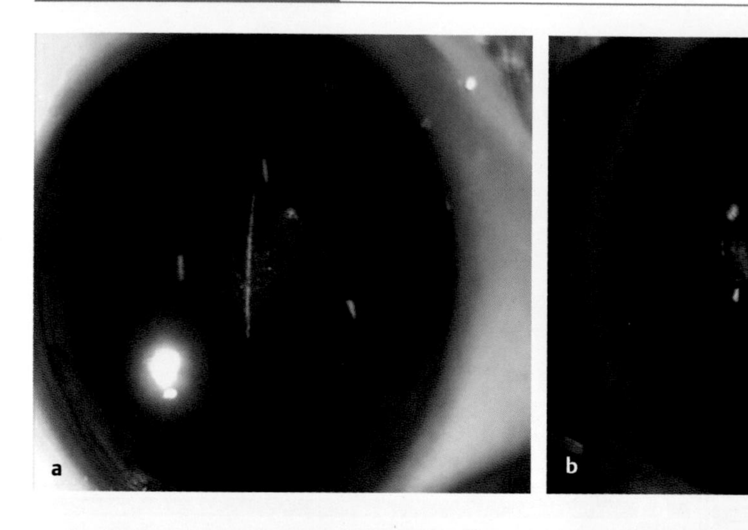

Case 4-1 (a, b) Clinical picture showing posterior subcapsular cataract.

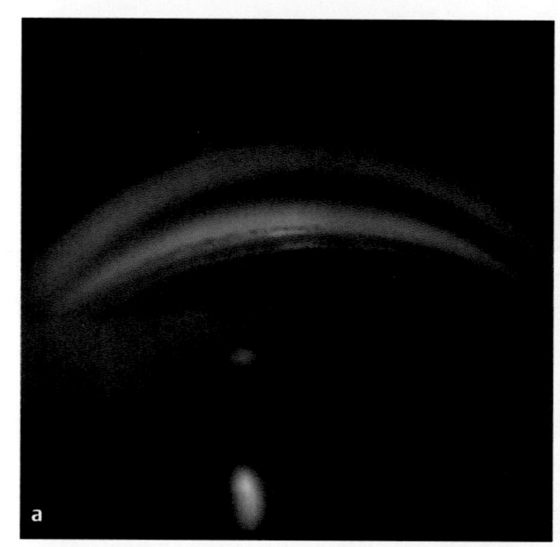

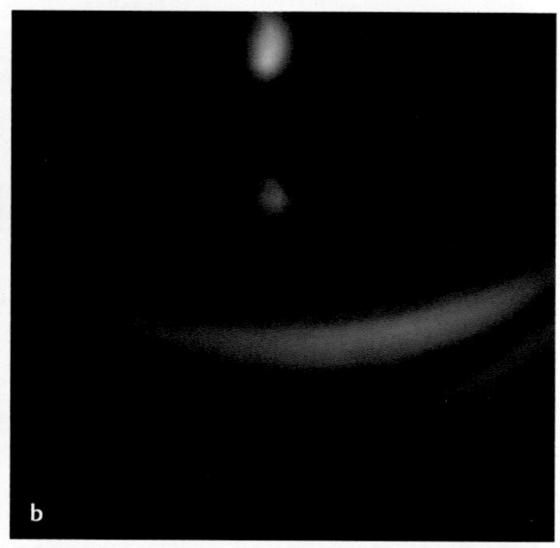

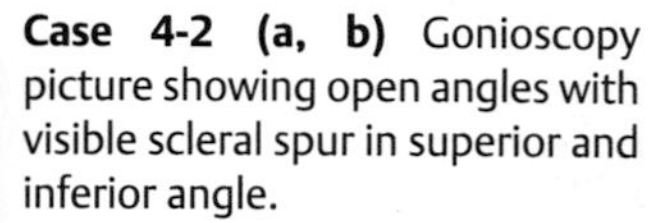

Case 4-2 (a, b) Gonioscopy picture showing open angles with visible scleral spur in superior and inferior angle.

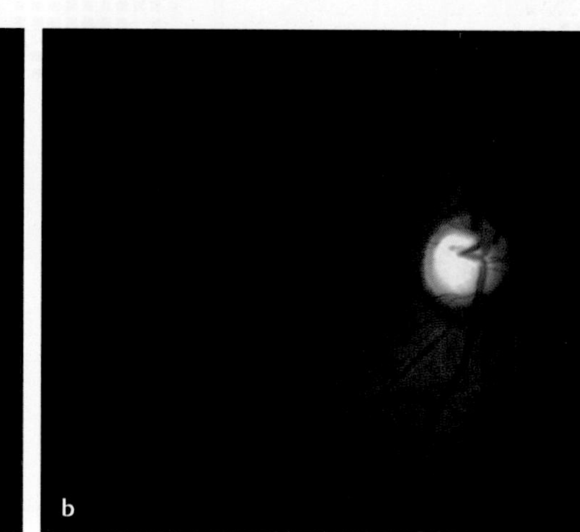

Case 4-3 (a, b) Fundus photograph of right eye showing a cup:disc ratio of 0.7:1 and left eye showing a cup:disc ratio of 0.8:1.

Case 6

A 28-year-old patient with lamellar ichthyosis was treated with betnovate skin cream for 2 years. The patient had additionally been on topical steroids for 6 months in the right eye for allergic conjunctivitis. His cup:disc ratios were 0.9 and 0.4 in the right eye and left eye, respectively, with IOPs at presentation of 36 mm Hg in the right eye and 28 mm Hg in the left eye. Topical steroids were stopped. The patient was started on 0.5% timolol twice a day and 0.2% brimonidine twice a day (**Case 6-1**).

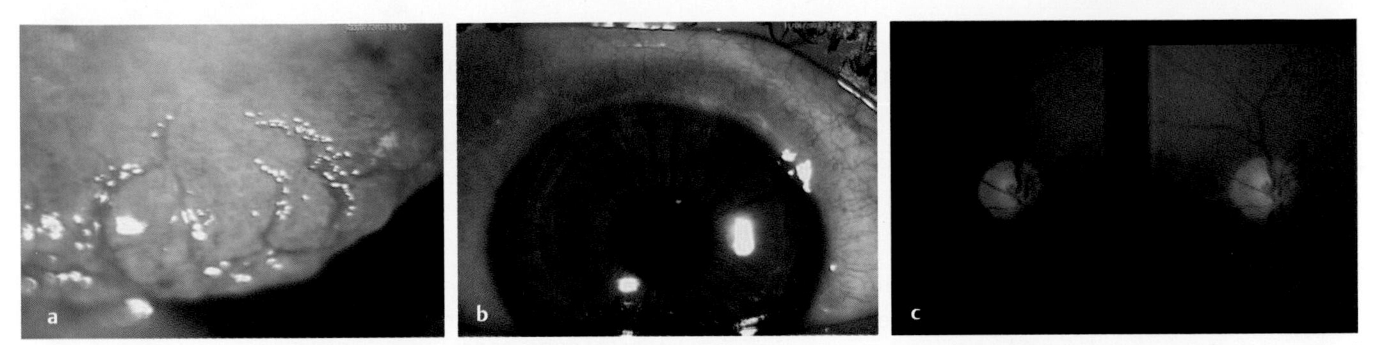

Case 5-1 **(a)** Large palpebral papillae. **(b)** Limbal nodules. **(c)** Optic nerve head showing a cup:disc ratio of 0.6 with a very significant neuroretinal rim pallor.

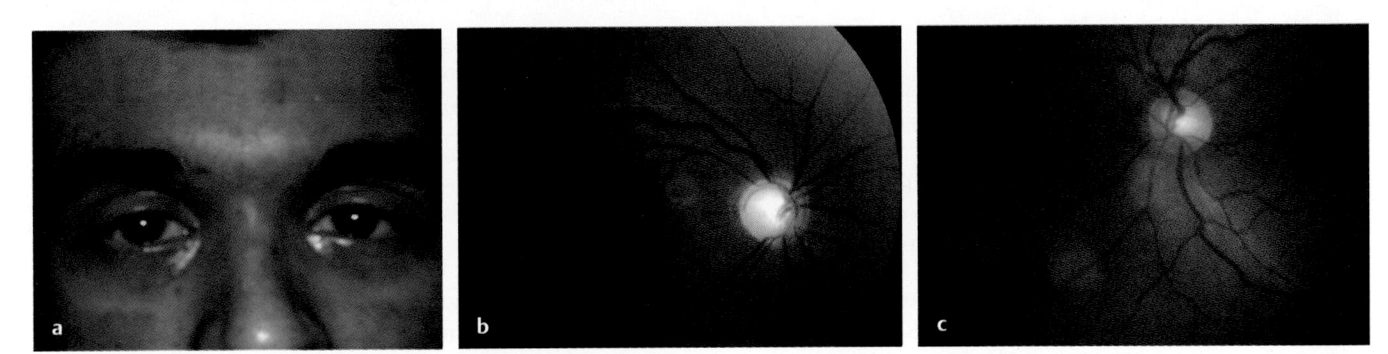

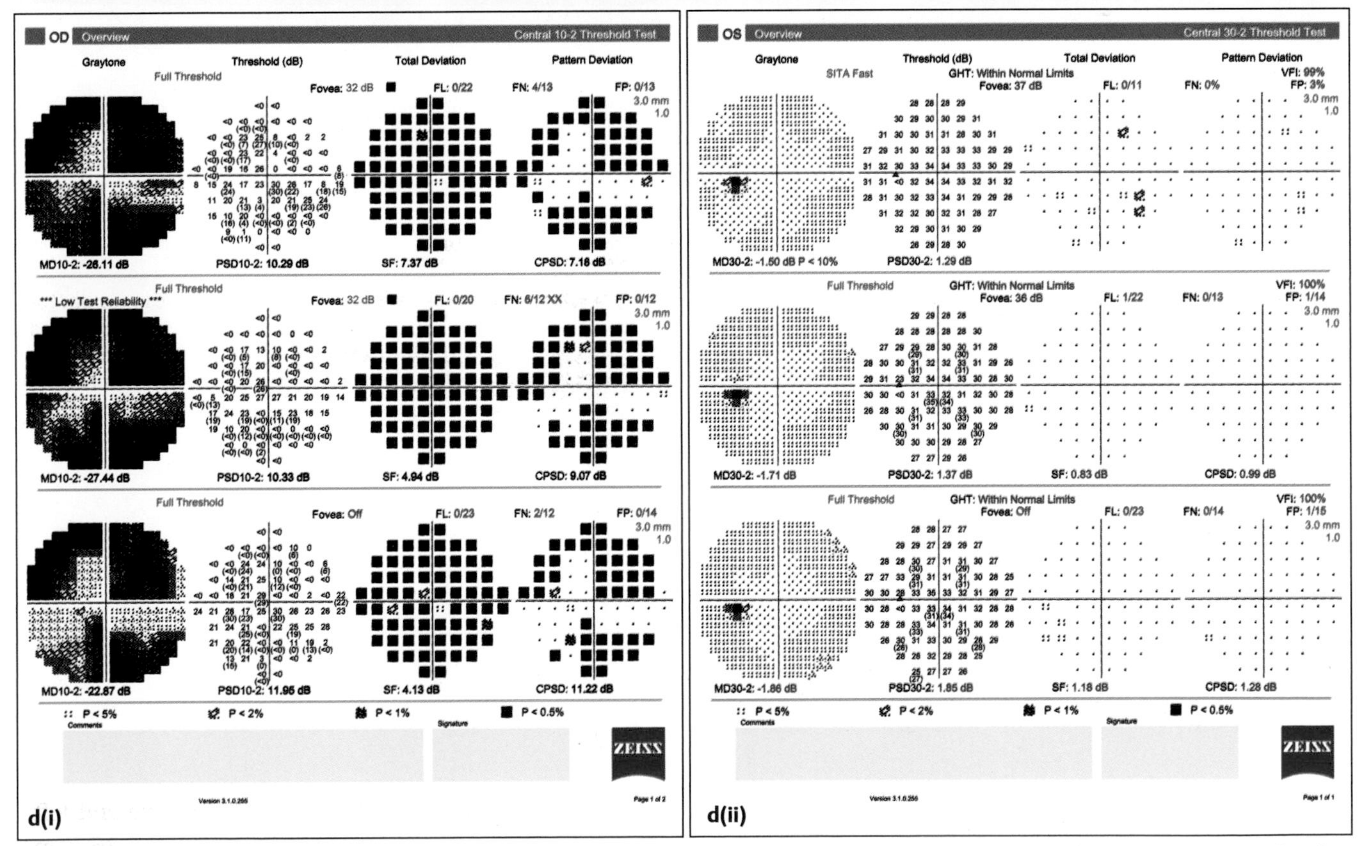

Case 6-1 **(a)** Erythema of the eyelids and face. **(b)** Right eye optic nerve head had a cup:disc ratio of 0.9 with generalized pallor. **(c)** Left eye optic nerve head with a cup:disc ratio 0.5 with normal neuroretinal rim. **(d)** Right eye has small central island of vision and left eye has normal field.

Points to consider

- Chronic dermatological problems may need non-steroidal therapy.
- Asymmetrical glaucoma was seen probably because of topical steroid use in one eye only.

Diagnosis and Management

On discussion with the dermatologist, the patient was weaned off topical betnovate. After 1 year, on timolol maleate alone, his IOP was 16 mm Hg in the right eye and 14 mm Hg in the left eye, with stable perimetry.

Suggested Readings

Armaly MF. Inheritance of dexamethasone hypertension and glaucoma. Arch Ophthalmol 1967;77(6):747–751

Armaly MF. Statistical attributes of the steroid hypertensive response in the clinically normal eye. 1: The demonstration of three levels of response. Invest Ophthalmol 1965;4:187–197

Becker B. Intraocular pressure response to topical corticosteroids. Invest Ophthalmol 1965;4:198–205

Bui Quoc E, Bodaghi B, Adam R, et al. Intraocular pressure elevation after subtenon injection of triamcinolone acetonide during uveitis. J Fr Ophthalmol 2002;25(10):1048–1056

Mindel JS, Tavitian HO, Smith H Jr, Walker EC. Comparative ocular pressure elevation by medrysone, fluorometholone, and dexamethasone phosphate. Arch Ophthalmol 1980; 98(9):1577–1578

Mitchell P, Cumming RG, Mackey DA. Inhaled corticosteroids, family history, and risk of glaucoma. Ophthalmology 1999; 106(12):2301–2306

Nuyen B, Weinreb RN, Robbins SL. Steroid-induced glaucoma in the pediatric population. J AAPOS 2017;21(1):1–6

Roberti G, Oddone F, Agnifili L, et al. Steroid-induced glaucoma: epidemiology, pathophysiology, and clinical management. Surv Ophthalmol 2020;65(4):458–472

Sihota R, Konkal VL, Dada T, Agarwal HC, Singh R. Prospective, long-term evaluation of steroid-induced glaucoma. Eye (Lond) 2008;22(1):26–30

Yuksel-Elgin C, Elgin C. Intraocular pressure elevation after intravitreal triamcinolone acetonide injection: a meta-analysis. Int J Ophthalmol 2016;9(1):139–144

CHAPTER 18

Neovascular Glaucoma

Overview

- Pathogenesis
- Clinical Features
- Management
- Prevention and Prognosis
- Cases
- Suggested Readings

Introduction

Neovascular glaucoma (NVG) is a recalcitrant glaucoma caused by ischemia to the retina, which presents with very high intraocular pressures (IOPs) and can cause blindness in a short time. The common associated retinal vascular diseases are *proliferative diabetic retinopathy (PDR), central retinal vein occlusion (CRVO), Eales' disease, and carotid insufficiency*. Other less common causes are central retinal artery occlusion, tumors, and retinal vasculitis.

Pathogenesis

In the presence of retinal hypoxia vascular endothelial growth factors (VEGFs) are released, that cause formation of new vessels at the retina. These factors also pass into the anterior segment where similar new vessel formation can be seen.

In diabetics, there is a 5% chance of neovascularization of the iris (NVI) in nonproliferative diabetic retinopathy (NPDR), but almost half of untreated PDR patients can develop NVI and NVG. Among eyes with ischemic CRVO, especially if the patient is elderly, hypertensive, or having hyperlipedemia, 50% may develop NVI and NVG.

Clinical Features

Patients present with severe pain, diminution of vision, and redness. They also commonly have systemic diseases such as hypertension, diabetes, ischemic heart disease, and nephropathy.

Normal iris vessels lie in the stroma, run radially without branching, and are not normally visible in eyes with dark irises. However, visible vessels with an irregular course and branching over the iris are new vessels. As new vessels of iris do not have a normal vascular wall, there is a leak of proteins into the anterior chamber, causing aqueous flare, which can be mistaken as inflammation. With time, a fibrovascular membrane forms over the iris and angle, which contracts causing ectropion uveae, and closure of the angle. At this stage the IOP rises significantly leading to corneal edema, and a rapid fall in vision occurs if not treated. Fundus examination when possible shows optic nerve damage depending on the extent and duration of the rise in IOP.

In patients with PDR or ischemic CRVO early NVI may be picked up on careful pupillary examination, iris angiography or Retcam angiography (**Figs. 18.1** and **18.2**).

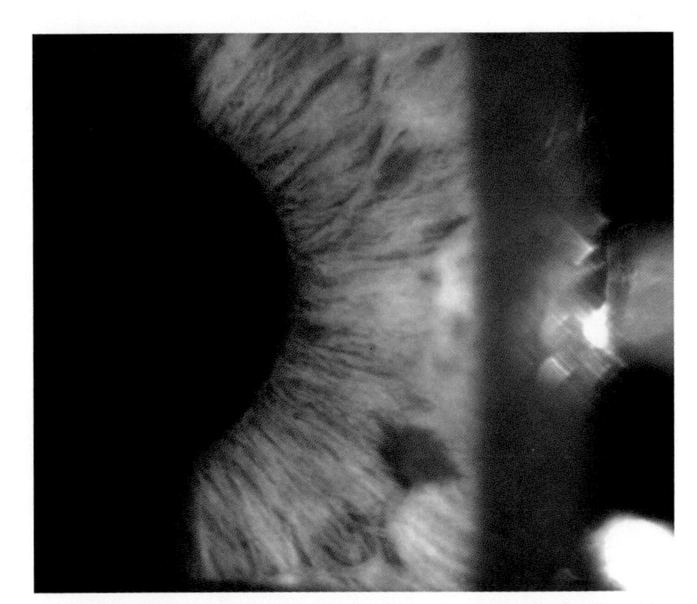

Fig. 18.1 The ophthalmologist should look specifically for knuckles of red at the pupil or fine vessels in the angle in patients with proliferative diabetic retinopathy or central retinal vein occlusion.

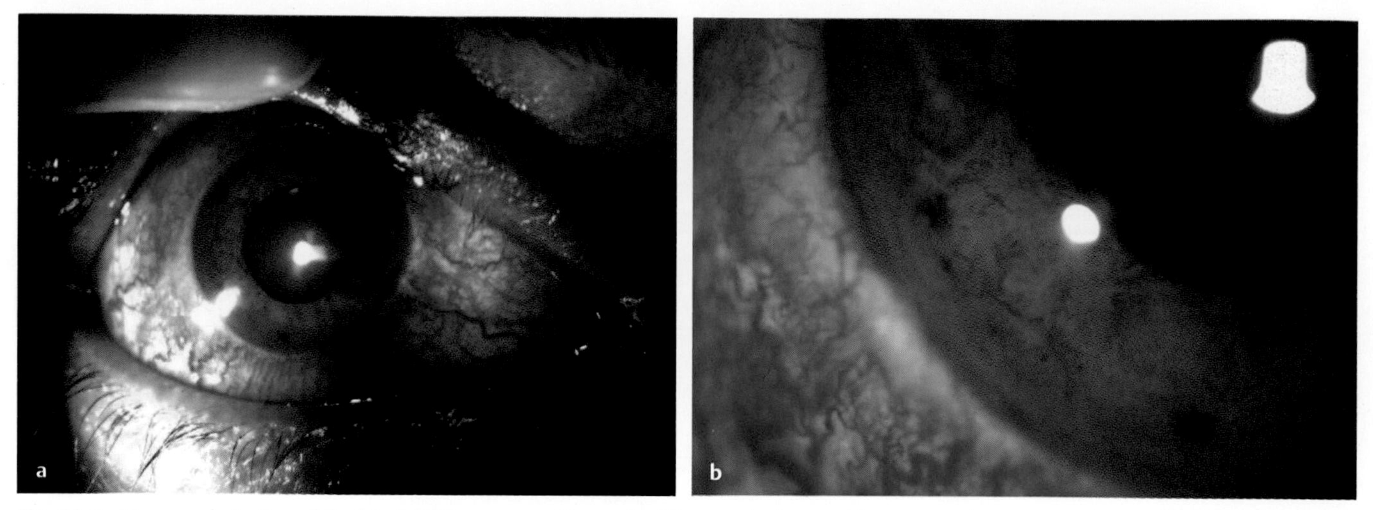

Fig. 18.2 Neovascularization of the iris. **(a)** Ciliary congestion and mild corneal edema with new vessels seen over the iris. **(b)** Magnified view of the relatively fine new vessels that branch irregularly and are not radial as is the normal iris vasculature.

Table 18.1 Clinical presentation and management of the stages of iris neovascularization

Stage of iris neovascularization / Differentiating features	1. Early NVI	2. Open angle stage	3. Angle closure stage
History of proliferative diabetic retinopathy/ Severe NPDR/CRVO/other vascular pathologies	Quiet eye	Painful red eye, headache	Severely painful red eye
Examination	NVI red knuckles at pupillary margin or few, fine vessels crossing the scleral spur at the angle	Ciliary congestion, anterior chamber flare, fine vessels over the iris with or without ectropion uveae	Severe visual loss, ciliary congestion, corneal edema, anterior chamber flare, iris neovascularization with large angry vessels, ectropion uvea, closed angle
IOP	Normal/borderline	Moderate rise	Very high IOP with poor response to medications
Management	Full PRP and augmentation as required. Review for glaucoma	Glaucoma medications + anti-VEGF + full PRP	Anti-VEGF + MMC augmented trabeculectomy/drainage device. Later full PRP

Abbreviations: anti-VEGF, anti-vascular endothelial growth factor; CRVO, central retinal vein occlusion; IOP, intraocular pressure; MMC, mitomycin C; NPDR, nonproliferative diabetic retinopathy; NVI, neovascularization of the iris; PRP, panretinal photocoagulation.

Stages of Iris Neovascularization

NVI occurs in clinical stages which progressively affect aqueous outflow and IOP (**Table 18.1**). These stages are:

- Fine, irregular new vessels seen at the pupillary border or angle, NVA, with an *open angle and a normal IOP.*
- Enlarged new vessels seen on the iris, at the angle or pupillary border in the presence of an *open angle, with a normal or raised IOP.*
- Extensive neovascularization with a fibrous membrane over the iris and angle that contracts to cause *secondary angle closure and raised IOP.*

New vessels resolve when the retinal ischemic areas are treated, with ghost vessels remaining. Sometimes large trunk vessels remain visible for a while, after the finer vessels disappear.

In eyes with retinal vasculopathies such as PDR, CRVO, etc., it is important that the anterior segment is examined carefully prior to dilation. *In diabetics with proliferative retinopathy 65% develop NVI and 21% NVG. The fellow eye is always at high risk for NVI. Any ocular surgery increases diabetic retinopathy progression and may precipitate NVI.* In diabetics these new vessels should be looked for and can be detected even in some severe preproliferative diabetic retinopathy eyes, and are almost always present in eyes with PDR.

An *ischemic CRVO* presents with severe visual loss, afferent pupillary defect, extensive retinal hemorrhages, and cotton wool spots (**Fig. 18.3**). In ischemic CRVO eyes,

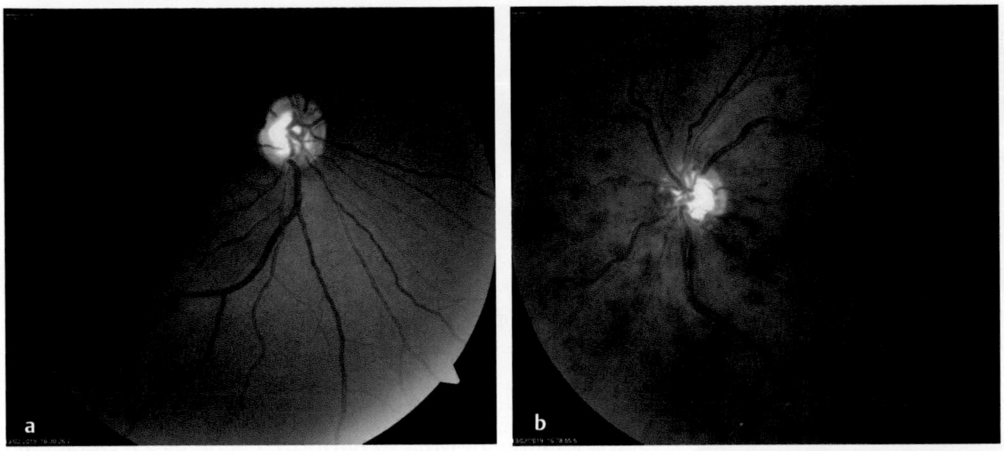

Fig. 18.3 **(a)** Fundus photographs of a patient having left ischemic central retinal vein occlusion (CRVO). The optic nerve head in the right eye has a cup:disc ratio of 0.6 with inferior neuroretinal rim thinning and a possible retinal nerve fiber layer defect at 7 o'clock. **(b)** The left eye optic nerve head similarly has a cup:disc ratio of 0.7 with a possible notch at 5 o'clock, suggesting preexisting glaucoma with extensive retinal hemorrhages.

a mandatory examination of the iris and angle would prevent needless morbidity. *After the occurrence of an ischemic CRVO new vessels in the anterior segment can appear as early as a couple months or later, even up to a few years afterwards.* However, the neovascular glaucoma is frequently seen around 3 months after the occlusive episode and is therefore called 100-day glaucoma. Examination of the optic nerve head commonly shows the presence of *prior glaucomatous neuropathy, which is thought to be one of the causative factors for CRVO.* Both primary open-angle glaucoma (POAG) and primary angle-closure glaucoma (PACG) can predispose to the occurrence of CRVO. *At initial examination the IOP in CRVO eyes may be low, and rise later, so that a regular follow up for glaucoma is important in all CRVO eyes.* The Central Vein Occlusion Study reported that in eyes with an *ischemic or indeterminate CRVO diagnosed by >10 disc diameters of nonperfused areas, there is a 45% chance of developing NVG.* The most important risk factor for developing rubeosis is a poor visual acuity of <6/60, with 31% having NVI/NVA. It is important to remember that 34% of initially nonischemic CRVO become ischemic over 3 years.

Eales' disease presents as retinal periphlebitis in young males, progressing to neovascular fronds, vitreous hemorrhage, and tractional retinal detachment. *Neovascular glaucoma is seen in late stages of the disease, and can be seen in up to 80% of cases if not treated early.* Eales' disease is thought to be due to hypersensitivity to tubercular protein.

Ocular ischemic syndrome is seen in elderly patients with severe carotid artery stenosis, hypertension, diabetes, and ischemic heart disease. This presents with amaurosis fugax, transient ischemic attacks, gradual or acute visual loss, and a dull ache. *Dilated retinal veins and narrowed arteries and retinal hemorrhages are common. Neovascularization of the retina is only seen in about a third of such eyes, whereas iris neovascularization is present in over two-thirds.* An obstruction of the ipsilateral carotid,

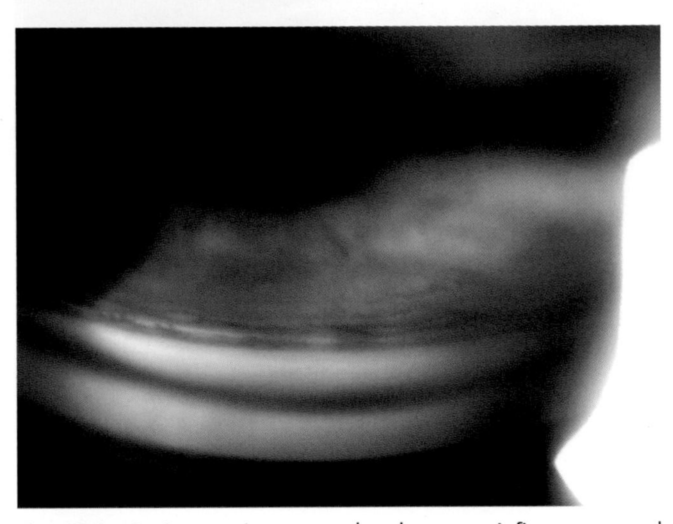

Fig. 18.4 Gonioscopy in neovascular glaucoma. A fine new vessel seen crossing scleral spur and passing over the trabecular meshwork (Stage 1).

90% or greater, is commonly associated with NVG. NVG in such eyes has increased IOP in 50%, while some eyes with ocular ischemia may present with extensive NVI and NVA, but a normal IOP. Fluorescein angiography shows delayed choroidal filling and arteriovenous transit in such eyes. *Such patients should undergo a carotid endarterectomy if the carotid occlusion is >70%.*

Differential diagnosis of NVI includes essential iris atrophy, pseudoexfoliation, and Fuch's heterochromic iridocyclitis where iris stromal atrophy may expose normal iris vessels. In light colored irides, blue or grey, normal iris vessels can be visualized.

Gonioscopy can show the earliest new vessels, and the diagnosis is made when these can be seen to cross the scleral spur, as some anomalous iris vessels may be seen in developmental glaucomas. Initially the angle may be open; however, contraction of the fibrovascular membrane over the iris closes the angle completely in late stages of NVG (**Figs. 18.4–18.6**).

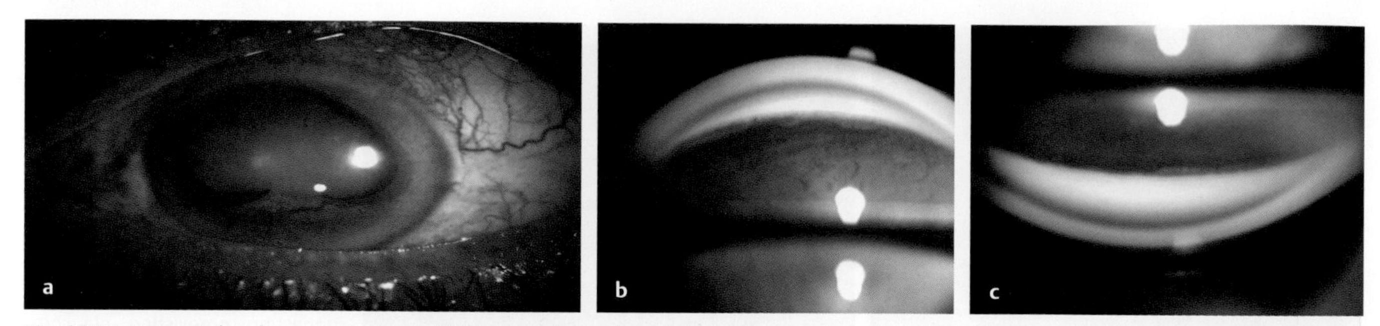

Fig. 18.5 Neovascular glaucoma, Stage 3. **(a)** Corneal edema, large iris vessels, and ectropion uveae. **(b, c)** Gonioscopy showing new vessels in the angle with areas of angle closure.

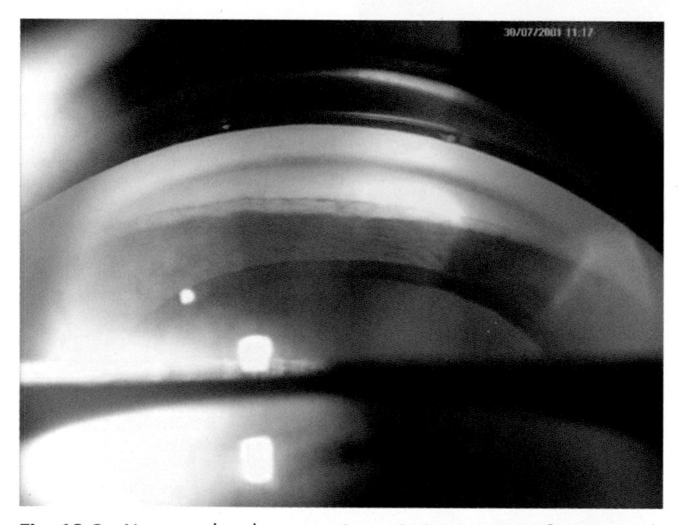

Fig. 18.6 Neovascular glaucoma, Stage 3. Gonioscopy of an eye with extensive ectropion uveae, showing a completely closed angle.

Management

The management of NVI/NVG is aimed at an early management of the primary retinal pathology and control of IOP (**Flowchart 18.1**).

Therapy of NVI with an open angle is aimed at a rapid control of IOP, and evaluation of retinal status, so that adequate panretinal photocoagulation (PRP) can be performed and augmented as quickly as possible. Retinal angiography would guide photocoagulation of ischemic areas and assure that these are adequately lasered. A full PRP, 2000 spots of 500 to 800 µm, applied to the retina beyond the temporal arcades leads to regression of retinal and iris new vessels over weeks. Further augmentation is often required over time.

In patients with significant corneal edema precluding photocoagulation, lowering of IOP with maximal medical therapy is urgently required. Injecting anti-VEGFs—bevacizumab/ranibizumab or aflibercept, intracameral or intravitreal—provides some additional lowering of IOP, and a window of time to perform a good PRP if the media clears. PRP should be done as quickly as possible, but would still take 4 to 6 weeks to act. However, larger new vessel trunks, ghost vessels, and membranes may persist, with continued need for glaucoma medications (**Fig. 18.7**).

In patients having severe neovascular glaucoma, very high IOPs, dense corneal edema, and a totally closed angle, anti-VEGF therapy and maximal medical therapy for glaucoma have to be administered immediately. β-blockers, alpha-agonists, and carbonic anhydrase inhibitors show some lowering of IOP, while prostaglandins and pilocarpine are contraindicated, as they increase the aqueous reaction seen and have not been found to lower the IOP significantly, with angles almost completely closed. Oral acetazolamide and IV mannitol may be used as temporizing measures prior to surgery. Intracameral/vitreal bevacizumab is given in a dose of 1.25 mg/0.05 mL, after aspirating aqueous. This results in a partial fall in IOP and regression of the NVI within 2 to 3 days. In such severe situations, a PRP may still not be possible, and a mitomycin C (MMC) augmented trabeculectomy/drainage device should be placed as soon as possible to reduce IOP to "target" depending in the patient's severity of optic nerve head damage (**Fig. 18.8**). *After 3 to 4 weeks PRP must be started and completed in sittings.*

Glaucoma drainage implants were the mainstay of therapy for NVG before the advent of anti-VEGF agents and MMC. However, there is only a 50% success even at 2 years, with about 25% showing a fall in vision, 8 to 10% phthisis, and 5% corneal decompensation.

Following control of IOP, the effect of anti-VEGF on the new vessels will continue for a couple of months, providing a window of opportunity to treat and monitor the retinal pathology carefully. If this is not properly done, the NVG will reappear and further damage the optic nerve.

In Eales' disease, together with PRP and anti-VEGF, it is also important to treat any active vasculitis and vitreous hemorrhage.

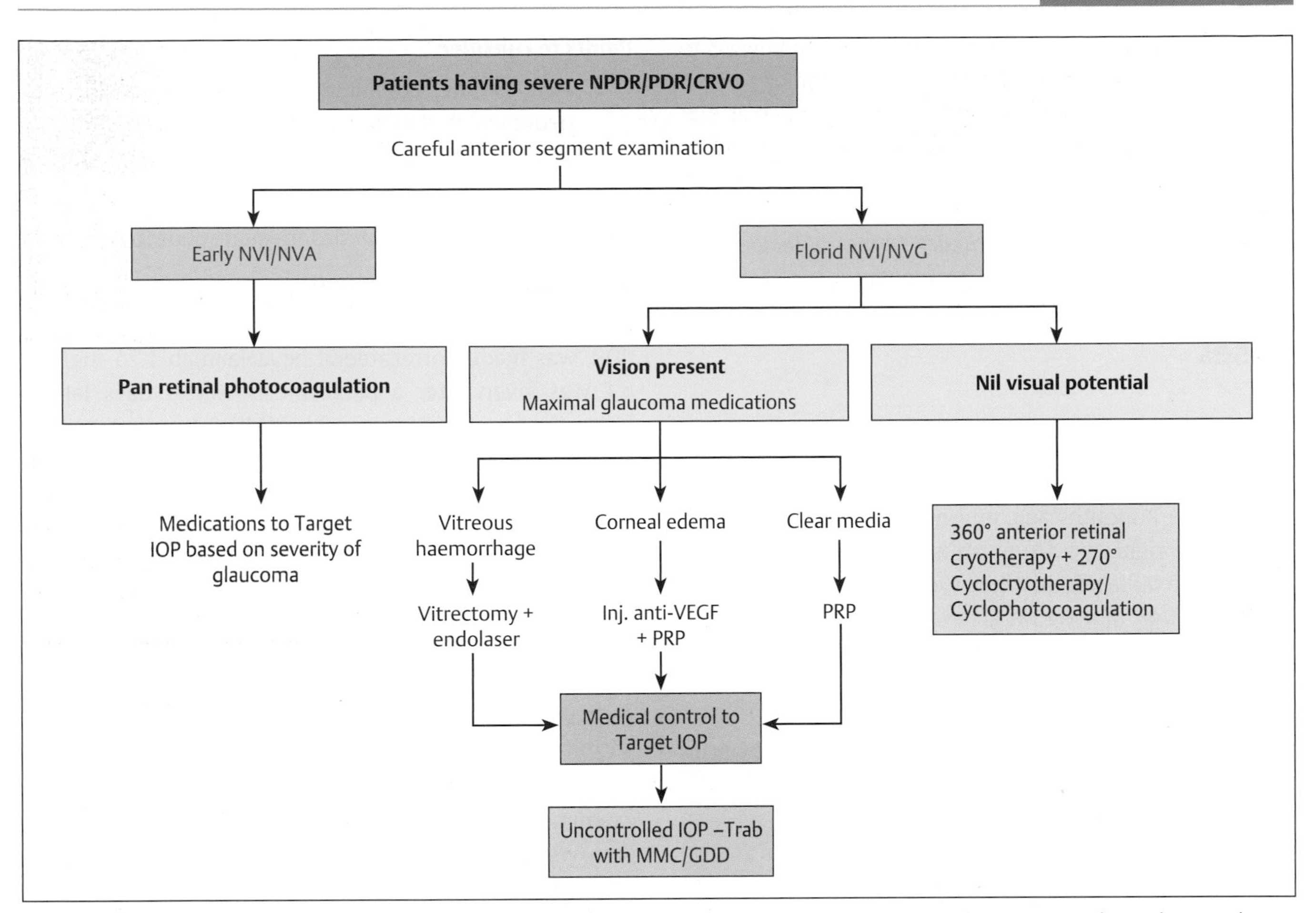

Flowchart 18.1 Algorithm depicting the steps involved in the management of neovascular glaucoma (NVG). CRVO, central retinal vein occlusion; IOP, intraocular pressure; MMC, mitomycin C; NPDR, nonproliferative diabetic retinopathy; NVA, new vessels seen at the pupillary border or angle; NVG, neovascular glaucoma; NVI, neovascularization of the iris; PDR, proliferative diabetic retinopathy; PRP, panretinal photocoagulation.

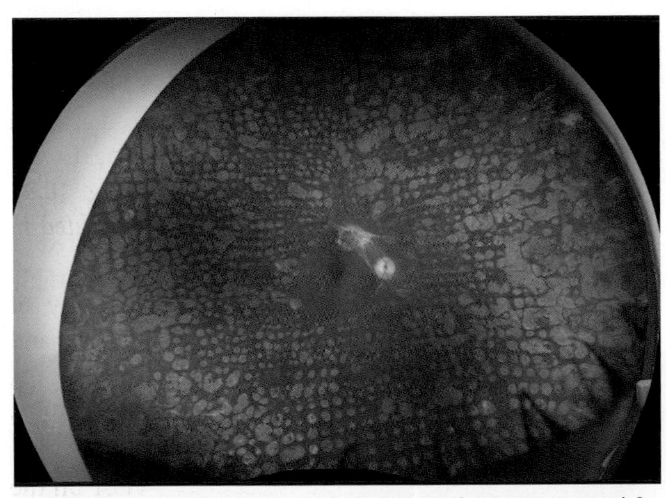

Fig. 18.7 A complete panretinal photocoagulation as required for neovascular glaucoma.

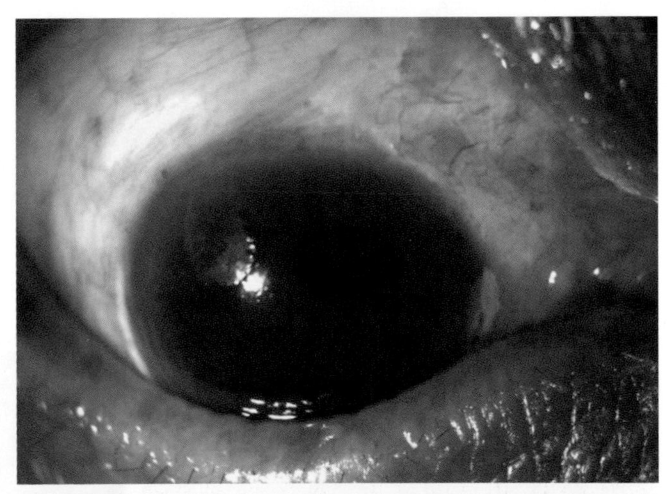

Fig. 18.8 Diffuse bleb 4 years after a mitomycin C (MMC) augmented trabeculectomy for neovascular glaucoma.

Prevention and Prognosis

Early detection of NVI/NVE is the key to prevention of potentially sight-threatening NVG. Therefore, an undilated slit lamp biomicroscopy of the pupillary margin and gonioscopic evaluation of the anterior chamber angle should be done in all cases of PDR and central retinal venous occlusion. Iris fluorescein angiography could be done in severe NPDR or more. Follow-up should be for glaucoma as well as the retinal status periodically.

The long-term success for IOP control is good over 5 to 10 years; however, the primary retinal pathology needs to be treated repeatedly and systemic factors such as diabetes and hypertension managed well. *The prognosis for control of IOP is now good with the use of anti-VEGF therapy and trabeculectomy with MMC. However, visual prognosis is guarded/poor due to the primary retinal pathology and presenting glaucomatous optic neuropathy.*

Cases

Case 1

A 65-year-old, known diabetic for 12 years, lost vision in the left eye 2 months ago, and now complains of severe pain in the right eye. On examination there was corneal edema with bullae in the right eye, NVI seen in both eyes. IOP was 44/46 mm Hg on all available topical glaucoma medications. Vision was 1/60 in the right eye and no PL in the left.

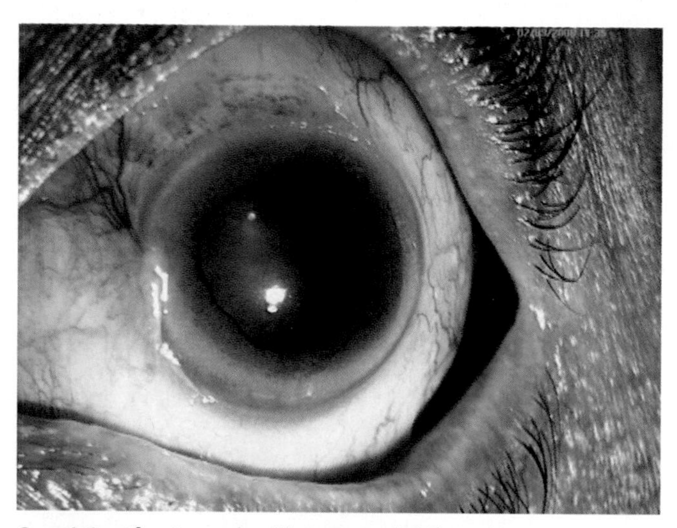

Case 1-1 After 6 months of bevacizumab followed by a mitomycin C augmented trabeculectomy, clear media allowing adequate panretinal photocoagulation.

Points to consider

- PDR is the common retinal cause of bilateral neovascular glaucoma.
- 40+ mm Hg unlikely to be controlled on topical medications.
- Corneal edema precludes adequate photocoagulation.

Diagnosis and Management

A diagnosis of neovascular glaucoma, possibly due to PDR, was made. Intracameral bevacizumab 1.25 mg/0.05 mL was given after a paracentesis, and 3 days later a trabeculectomy was done with MMC 0.4 mg/mL applied subsclerally and subconjunctivally. After 6 months IOP in the right eye was 12 mm Hg, with a clear cornea and absence of NVI, and the vision had improved to 6/24 (**Case 1-1**). Patient was advised a PRP and careful review of the diabetic retinopathy and IOP for life.

Case 2

A 42-year-old hypertensive lady was diagnosed to have a CRVO in her right eye 3 months ago. She complained of a sudden blurring of vision with pain yesterday. On examination, mild corneal edema and frank NVI were seen without ectropion uveae. IOP was 32 mm Hg, and gonioscopy showed an open angle with few blood vessels seen crossing scleral spur (**Case 2-1**).

Points to consider

- Duration of symptoms is 1 day.
- Open angle stage of NVI.
- Conservative management can be successful.

Diagnosis and Management

A diagnosis of post-CRVO NVI was made. The IOP was reduced to 14 mm Hg with brimonidine, timolol, and acetazolamide tablets. A PRP was done and augmented to cover 5/8th of the retina. After 6 weeks, the NVI had largely

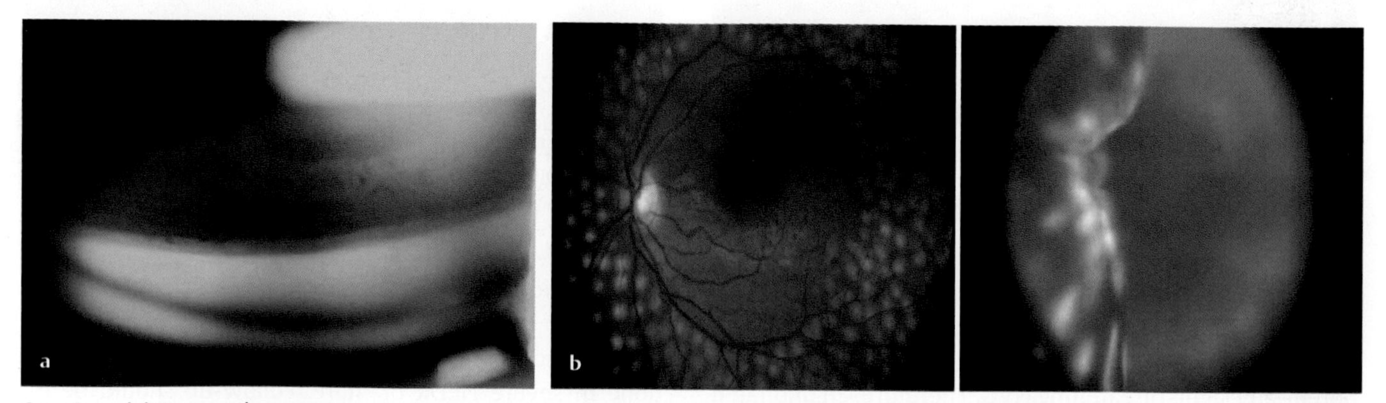

Case 2-1 **(a)** Open angle on gonioscopy showing a few fine vessels crossing the scleral spur. **(b)** Well done panretinal photocoagulation.

resolved, and the patient was taken off acetazolamide. She was advised good control of systemic hypertension, IOP, and retinal pathology.

Case 3

A 63-year-old lady, a known case of PACG on timolol, noticed a sudden diminution of vision in the left eye of 2 weeks duration. On examination, her vision was 6/6 and 3/60, with a shallow anterior chamber and lamellar iridotomies in both eyes. Cup:disc ratio was 0.7 and 0.9, with extensive retinal hemorrhages and cotton wool spots in the left eye. IOPs were 22 and 30 mm Hg. A careful examination of the left pupillary area showed red knuckles of NVI (**Case 3-1**).

Points to consider

- Uncontrolled glaucoma, especially CPACG is a common cause of CRVO in India.

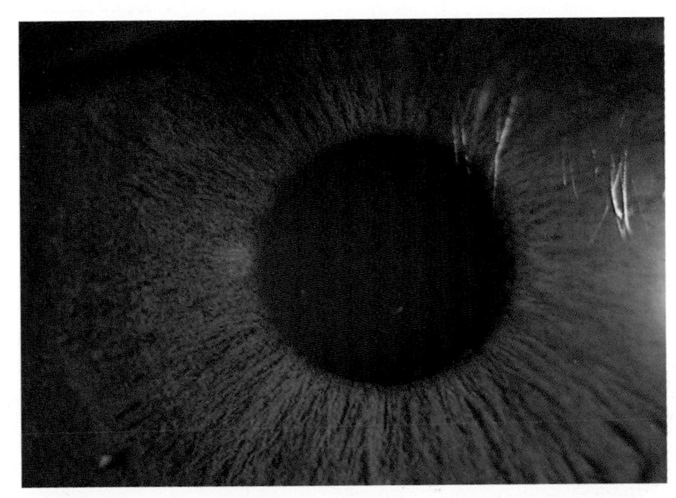

Case 3-1 *Red dots* and fine new vessels present.

- Duration of symptoms is 2 weeks.
- IOP moderately elevated.

Diagnosis and Management

A diagnosis of PACG with left CRVO was made. She was advised to use a timolol–dorzolamide combination twice a day in both eyes and brimonidine twice a day in the left. The laser iridotomies were completed with an Nd:YAG laser, and PRP was done in three sittings. After 2 months the NVI had resolved and IOPs were well controlled at 14/12 mm Hg on the same medications. The left retina continued to show resolution of edema and hemorrhages, and the patient was advised continued review for glaucoma and the retina.

Case 4

A 22-year-old male presented with pain and redness in the right eye of 2 days duration, and a past history of vitrectomy for a vitreous hemorrhage 3 months earlier. On examination, there was corneal edema, NVI, pseudophakia, and an IOP of 44 mm Hg (**Case 4-1**). The anterior segment of the left eye was within normal limits, and the fundus had a few areas of healed peripheral vasculitis.

Points to consider

- Young male.
- Past history of vitreous hemorrhage.
- Neovascularization of iris.

Diagnosis and Management

A diagnosis of Eales' disease with right NVG and pseudophakia was made. The patient was given maximal glaucoma medications and an IV mannitol, followed by inj bevacizumab 1.25 mg intracamerally. After 2 weeks

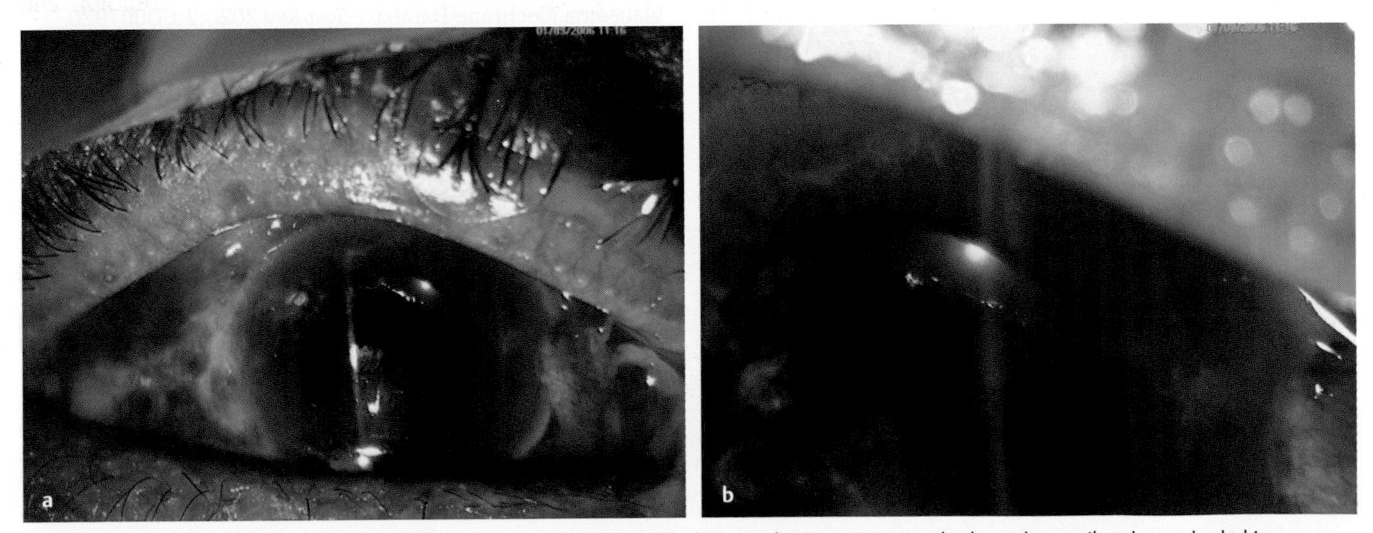

Case 4-1 **(a)** Corneal edema and conjunctival congestion. **(b)** Magnified image showing new vessels along the pupil and pseudophakia.

augmentation of the retinal photocoagulation was done. The patient required timolol–brimonidine combination and brinzolamide twice a day to maintain an IOP of 16 to 18 mm Hg. He was counseled for close review for his glaucoma and retina.

Case 5

A 75-year-old male, hypertensive and smoker, presented with gradual progressive diminution of both eyes over 1 year. He had been diagnosed with glaucoma 2 years ago. On examination, vision was 6/60 and 2/60, with pseudophakia and extensive NVI in both eyes, and an IOP of 24/22 mm Hg on timolol drops. Fundus examination revealed near-total cupping with marked neuroretinal rim pallor in both eyes, with significant arteriolar narrowing and venous dilation (**Case 5-1**).

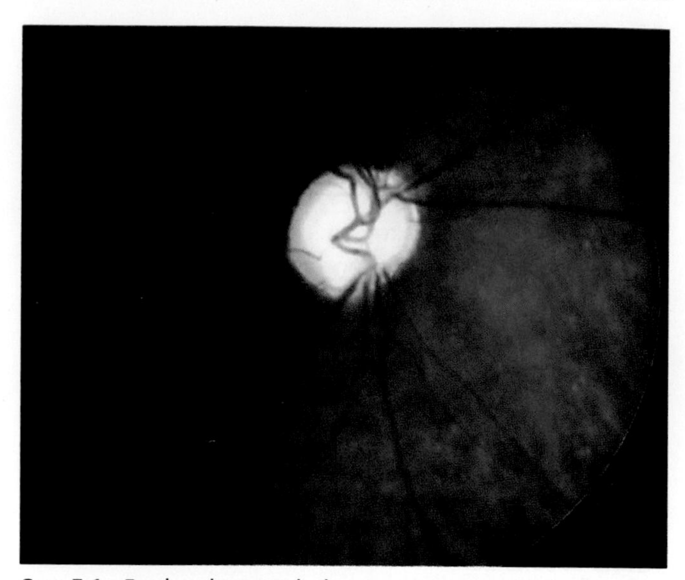

Case 5-1 Fundus photograph showing an average sized optic nerve head having a cup:disc ratio of 0.8:1. Retinal arterioles are very attenuated and veins are mildly dilated.

Points to consider

- Elderly smoker.
- Retinal arteriolar attenuation.
- NVI without significantly high IOPs.

Diagnosis and Management

A possible diagnosis of ocular ischemic syndrome was made, and a carotid doppler showed an obstruction of 80/85% on both sides. Travoprost and dorzolamide drops were added to reduce IOP to 10 to 12 mm Hg and possibly increase ocular perfusion. He was referred for a carotid endarterectomy/stent, which he refused, and was then put on Aspirin. Regular IOP check-ups to maintain an IOP in the low teens and low vision aid trials were advised.

Suggested Readings

Havens SJ, Gulati V. Neovascular glaucoma. Dev Ophthalmol 2016;55:196–204

Higashide T, Murotani E, Saito Y, Ohkubo S, Sugiyama K. Adverse events associated with intraocular injections of bevacizumab in eyes with neovascular glaucoma. Graefes Arch Clin Exp Ophthalmol 2012;250(4):603–610

Liu L, Xu Y, Huang Z, Wang X. Intravitreal ranibizumab injection combined trabeculectomy versus Ahmed valve surgery in the treatment of neovascular glaucoma: assessment of efficacy and complications. BMC Ophthalmol 2016;16:65

Olmos LC, Sayed MS, Moraczewski AL, et al. Long-term outcomes of neovascular glaucoma treated with and without intravitreal bevacizumab. Eye (Lond) 2016;30(3):463–472

Rodrigues GB, Abe RY, Zangalli C, et al. Neovascular glaucoma: a review. Int J Retina Vitreous 2016;2:26

Simha A, Aziz K, Braganza A, Abraham L, Samuel P, Lindsley KB. Anti-vascular endothelial growth factor for neovascular glaucoma. Cochrane Database Syst Rev 2020;2:CD007920

CHAPTER 19

Medical Therapy in Glaucoma

Overview

- Clinical Baseline for Starting Medical Therapy in Glaucoma
- Drug Administration
- Glaucoma Medications
  - Decreased Aqueous Production
  - Increasing Trabecular Outflow
  - Increasing Uveoscleral Outflow
  - Fixed Drug Combinations
- Choice of Medications
  - Glaucoma Therapy in Pregnancy
- Newer Drugs and Newer Delivery Systems
- Nonresponders
- Failure of Medical Treatment
- Neuroprotection
- Stem Cell Therapy
- Cases
- Suggested Readings

Introduction

It has been established by many randomized control trials that lowering intraocular pressure (IOP) helps to stabilize or delay the progression, at any stage, of all types of glaucomas. Initial therapy is generally with medications, topical and, if required, systemic. *The aim of therapy is to prescribe the least number of medications, having the least side effects, to achieve the required "target" IOP for an individual eye, over 24 hours* (**Fig. 19.1** and **Flowchart 19.1**).

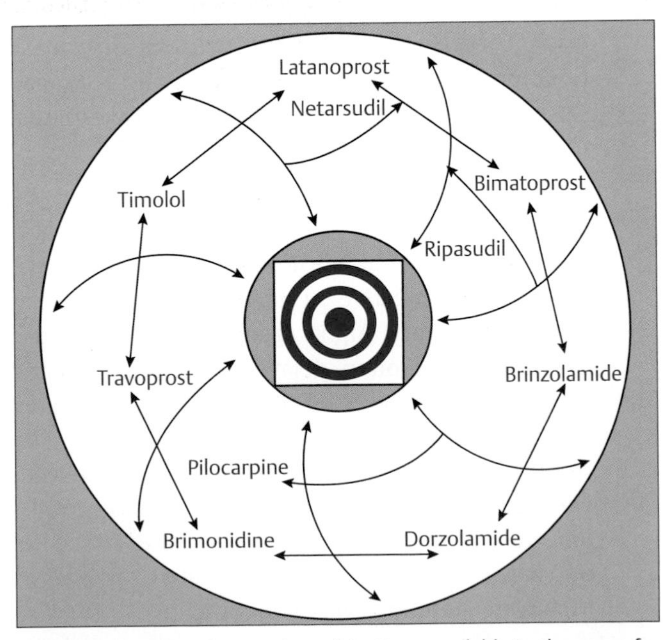

Fig. 19.1 Permutations and combinations available in the quest for medical control of intraocular pressure (IOP).

Clinical Baseline for Starting Medical Therapy in Glaucoma

Knowing baseline IOP, that is, IOP at which glaucomatous damage was seen to occur without any glaucoma medication, is important. Ideally a diurnal phasing, from early morning to late night, provides information about the time at which the IOP is highest, peak IOP, and the height of peak IOP which is the highest IOP that needs to be controlled to "target." Thereafter on medications, the IOP at the time

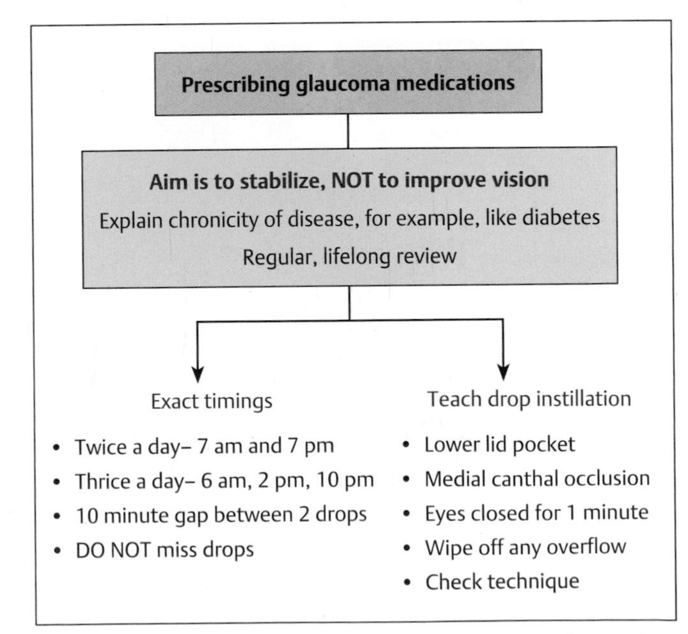

Flowchart 19.1 Systematic algorithm to enhance understanding, compliance, and adherence to glaucoma medical therapy.

of the peak can be rechecked to best ascertain good IOP control. *As a rule of thumb, it is generally seen that a baseline IOP of <30 mm Hg can be lowered to target IOP with topical medications alone.*

It is important to take a good history of systemic diseases and medications, as there may be an *overlap of effect as in medications for systemic hypertension*, or glaucoma medications may be contraindicated as in chronic obstructive airway disease, which is common in the elderly.

Drug Administration

The best way of administering medications needs to be explained to every patient. This includes cleaning of hands before opening the bottle, and tilting the head back or lying down, and then pulling out the lower eyelid to form a pocket into which the drop can be instilled. This allows medication to be retained in the conjunctival sac. Any overflow should be immediately cleaned with a tissue, as it may cause irritation or discoloration around the eye (**Fig. 19.2**). Closing the eye and applying gentle pressure at the inner canthus for a minute decreases systemic absorption of medications.

Patients should also be made to understand that if a drop is to be used thrice a day, it must be put at 8-hour intervals to cover 24 hours of the day, for example, 6 am, 2 pm, and 10 pm. Twice a day drops should be used every 12 hours, 7 am and 7 pm or 6 am and 6 pm, as convenient for the patient, and once a day drops should be used at the same time every day.

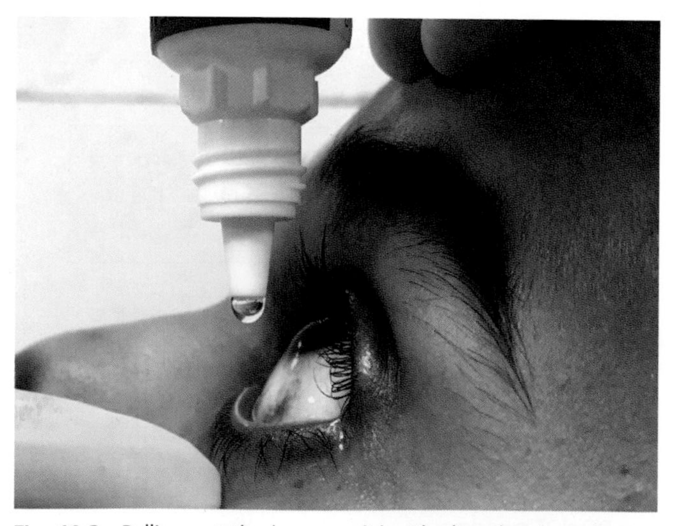

Fig. 19.2 Pulling out the lower eyelid with clean hands to form a pocket into which the drop is put, making sure the eyelids or eye is not touched. The bottle should be securely closed.

Glaucoma Medications

Table 19.1 lists the mode of action, effect on IOP, side effects, and contraindications of some of the commonly used glaucoma medications.

Glaucoma medications work in a number of ways, the principle being (**Table 19.1**):

- Decreased aqueous production.
- Increased aqueous outflow—via trabecular outflow or uveoscleral outflow.

Decreased Aqueous Production

Some of the medications which cause reduction in aqueous production are briefly described below.

- *β blockers (BBs)*: Topical BBs work by blocking sympathetic receptors in the ciliary body to reduce the formation of aqueous. Nonselective BB, that is, timolol, blocks both the beta-1 and beta-2 receptors, while a selective BB such as betaxalol blocks only beta-1 receptors. The efficacy of IOP reduction by BB is thought to be 25 to 27%, with twice a day, but rarely by once-a-day dosing. There is less lowering of IOP seen at night. BBs are seen to have a short-term drift and the appearance of long-term tolerance to the drug; therefore, their efficacy must be reassessed over months and years. Systemic BBs have about 75% of the effect of topical BBs, and therefore topical BB should be a last resort for glaucoma, in cardiovascular patients already on systemic BB. *BBs are contraindicated in patients with asthma, chronic obstructive pulmonary disease (COPD), and a heart block.* They also cause depression, and may mask symptoms of a hypoglycemic attack. Topical BBs may cause a dry eye and in some cases corneal anesthesia. Allergy to BB is rare.
- *Alpha 2 agonists*: Brimonidine reduces IOP by decreasing aqueous production, and may also increase uveoscleral outflow. It has been shown to be neuroprotective in acute trauma models of optic nerve injury. Alpha agonists frequently cause drowsiness and often delayed but severe allergic blepharoconjunctivitis. *They are contraindicated in children below 2 years and should be used with caution in children less than 6 years or patients with Parkinsonism, taking monoamine oxidase (MAO) inhibitors.* Brimonidine sustained-release (SR) ocular implant is currently being evaluated, but needs repeat implantation every 6 months.

Table 19.1 Glaucoma medications

Pharmacological group	Name of drug	Approximate % fall in IOP	Mode of action	Ocular side effects	Systemic side effects	Contraindications
Parasympathomimetics	Pilocarpine 2–4%	15–25	↑ conventional outflow	Fluctuating and blurred vision, miosis, brow ache, accommodative spasm	Increased sweating and salivation, urinary frequency, diarrhea, bronchospasm	Uveitis
Adrenergic antagonists						
Nonselective β-blockers (β-1 and β-2)	Timolol 0.25–0.5%	20–30	↓ aqueous production	Stinging, local anesthesia	Bronchospasm, bradycardia, decreased cardiac output, hypotension, depression, impotence, altered lipid profile	Asthma, chronic obstructive pulmonary disease, congestive heart failure, sinus bradycardia, atrioventricular blocks
Selective β-blockers (β-1)	Betaxolol 0.25–0.5%	15–25	↓ aqueous production	Stinging, local anesthesia	Less pulmonary side effects	Sinus bradycardia, atrioventricular blocks
Sympathomimetics						
Selective (α-2)	Brimonidine 0.15%	20–30	↓ aqueous production ? ↑ uveoscleral outflow	Conjunctival blanching, ocular allergy	Drowsiness, fatigue, blood pressure changes	Use of MAO inhibitors, Parkinson's disease, hypertensive crisis
Carbonic anhydrase inhibitors	Dorzolamide 2% Brinzolamide 1%	20–35	↓ aqueous production	Punctate keratitis, ocular allergies	Bitter taste, headache, asthenia, renal calculi	Hypersensitivity to sulphonamides, eye injury
Prostaglandins and hypotensive lipids	Latanoprost 0.005% Bimatoprost 0.03% Travoprost 0.004% Tafluprost 0.0015%	25–35	↑ uveoscleral outflow	Iris pigmentation, punctuate keratitis	Headache, symptoms of upper respiratory tract infection	Ocular infection or inflammation
Rho kinase inhibitors	Netarsudil 0.02% Ripasudil 0.4%	15	↑ conventional outflow ↓ episcleral venous pressure	Conjunctival hyperemia and hemorrhages, cornea verticillata	Nil known	

Abbreviations: IOP, intraocular pressure; MAO, monoamine oxidase.

- *Topical carbonic anhydrase inhibitors (CAIs)*: Dorzolamide and brinzolamide drops inhibit carbonic anhydrase in the ciliary body, slowing bicarbonate production, and decreasing sodium and fluid transport, and therefore aqueous production. *They should not be used in eyes with corneal endothelial dysfunction* as they inhibit carbonic anhydrase which is responsible for fluid transport out of the cornea.
- *Oral carbonic anhydrase inhibitors:* These are used in addition to topical medications, if a designated "target" IOP is not achieved, if patients develop allergies to topical therapy, or if there is an acute rise in IOP as in acute primary angle-closure glaucoma (PACG) or post-traumatic glaucomas. Long-term use is not desirable in view of side effects such as fatigue, loss of appetite, peripheral paresthesias, and nephrolithiasis. Their use is *contraindicated in patients with a history of sulphonamide allergy*.

Increasing Trabecular Outflow

Some glaucoma medications that work by increasing trabecular outflow are briefly described below.

- *Cholinergic agonists*: Pilocarpine is a directly acting miotic agent that pulls the iris away from the trabecular meshwork in angle closure. It also pulls on the sclera spur by contraction of the longitudinal ciliary muscles, stretching trabecular beams and opening spaces available. Induced myopia, headache, cataract formation, and miosis are local effects that make this difficult to use in younger patients. *In older patients the headache wears off after a few days, and they appreciate an increased depth of focus.* It is specifically used to prevent/treat angle closure and is additive to other medications for PACG. Pilocarpine is also used prior to and after a laser iridotomy, or after trabeculoplasty to stretch the iris.
- *Rho-associated protein kinase inhibitors (ROCK inhibitors)*: This group of drugs works by many mechanisms: (i) reversing structural and functional trabecular meshwork changes seen in glaucoma, through calcium-independent regulation of smooth muscle contraction, cell adhesion, cell morphology, and extracellular matrix reorganization. (ii) They also cause vasodilation, and reduce episcleral venous pressure. (iii) They are thought to increase optic nerve head and retinal blood flow, with a possible neuroprotective effect. (iv) After filtering surgery ROCK inhibitors have been reported to decrease fibrosis. *Netarsudil 0.02% is thought to work by inhibiting ROCK and norepinephrine transporter.* It lowers IOP in 2 hours and the effect continues for 24 hours; hence, it is advised once daily. Norepinephrine transporter inhibition leads to vasoconstriction in the ciliary processes reducing aqueous production. Netarsudil 0.02% works well in eyes with both low and high IOPs. It has no systemic side effect and can be used in patients having systemic problems. *Ripasudil 0.4% affects the ROCK system only* and should be prescribed twice a day. They have been shown to work well in open angles, but need evaluation in eyes with angle closure of any kind. *Common side effects are significant hyperemia in about 10 to 60%, small conjunctival hemorrhages, and reversible cornea verticillata.* A combination of netarsudil and latanoprost has been shown to be more effective than either constituent alone.

Increasing Uveoscleral Outflow

Prostaglandin (PG) analogs help in increasing the uveoscleral outflow. Currently available PG analogs are latanoprost (0.005%), bimatoprost (0.03%), tafluprost (0.0015%), and travatoprost (0.004%). These are analogs of endogenous arachidonic acid cyclooxygenase metabolite, $PGF_{2\alpha}$, and esterification of the carboxylic acid occurs in the eye. This leads to activation of matrix metalloproteinases that degrade ciliary muscle extracellular matrix and increase uveoscleral outflow and also has some effect on trabecular outflow. They reduce IOP by 30 to 35% in most patients, with a once-a-day dosage and long-term efficacy. The nocturnal efficacy of PG analogs is greater than BBs. In case one PG analog does not reduce IOP adequately, it is possible to switch to another PG analog, and the efficacy may be better. *The duration of effect is longer than other glaucoma medications, 24 to 60 hours,* and may thus help maintain IOP in case any dose is missed. PGs acting through the uveoscleral *outflow can reduce IOP even from normal levels*, and are therefore the first-line therapy for normal tension glaucoma. *These should be avoided in uveitis, herpetic keratitis, and in pseudophakic patients in whom the posterior capsule is not intact.* Commonly reported ocular changes are hyperemia, a darkening of iris color in light irides, thickening and elongation of lashes, and periocular skin pigmentation. Eyelid and lash changes may reverse after stopping of the medication. Periorbitopathy and fat atrophy can also lead to cosmetic problems with long-term use. Rarely, some patients may develop chronic upper respiratory complaints. The use of PG analogs during pregnancy is not clearly defined.

Punctal plugs impregnated with latanoprost and a canalicular implant of travoprost are being investigated.

Latanoprost bunod 0.024% has a dual action by breaking down into latanoprost acid and nitric oxide within the eye. The latanoprost acid increases uveoscleral outflow and the nitric oxide is thought to relax trabecular meshwork increasing conventional outflow.

Fixed Drug Combinations

The use of glaucoma medications having more than one mode of action has been shown to be additive, and when used as fixed drug combinations, improve compliance, decrease preservative side effects, and are more cost effective. *Prior to using a combination, both components must be individually assessed for efficacy* (**Fig. 19.3**).

Most combinations include timolol, latanoprost, travoprost, bimatoprost, brimonidine, dorzolamide, brinzolamide, and pilocarpine. Brimonidine is available in combination with brinzolamide. Netarsudil in combination with latanoprost has been shown to be more efficacious than latanoprost.

Choice of Medications

The choice of medications depends on the patients' target IOP, baseline IOP, and the efficacy, safety, persistence of effect, convenient dosage, and cost of a drug. Glaucoma is a chronic disease and needs lifelong medication which patients need to understand and be able to afford. It is best to explain its chronicity, using examples of diabetes and hypertension as other diseases that need lifelong treatment (**Flowchart 19.2**).

About 10 % of individuals could be nonresponders to any given glaucoma medication; therefore, it is imperative to *evaluate the efficacy of each drug by looking for a reduction in IOP of at least 15%* before continuing the medication. Subsequently added drugs should also be similarly

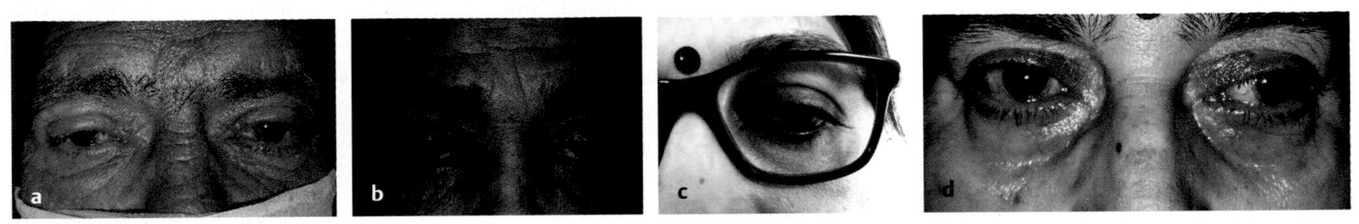

Fig. 19.3 **(a)** Allergic conjunctivitis after use of multiple glaucoma medications. **(b)** Blepharoconjunctivitis 4 months after starting brimonidine. **(c)** Dark and long eyelashes touching the spectacle lens after long-term use of prostaglandins are seen in some patients. **(d)** Redness of the conjunctiva is generally seen with rho-associated protein kinase (ROCK) inhibitors.

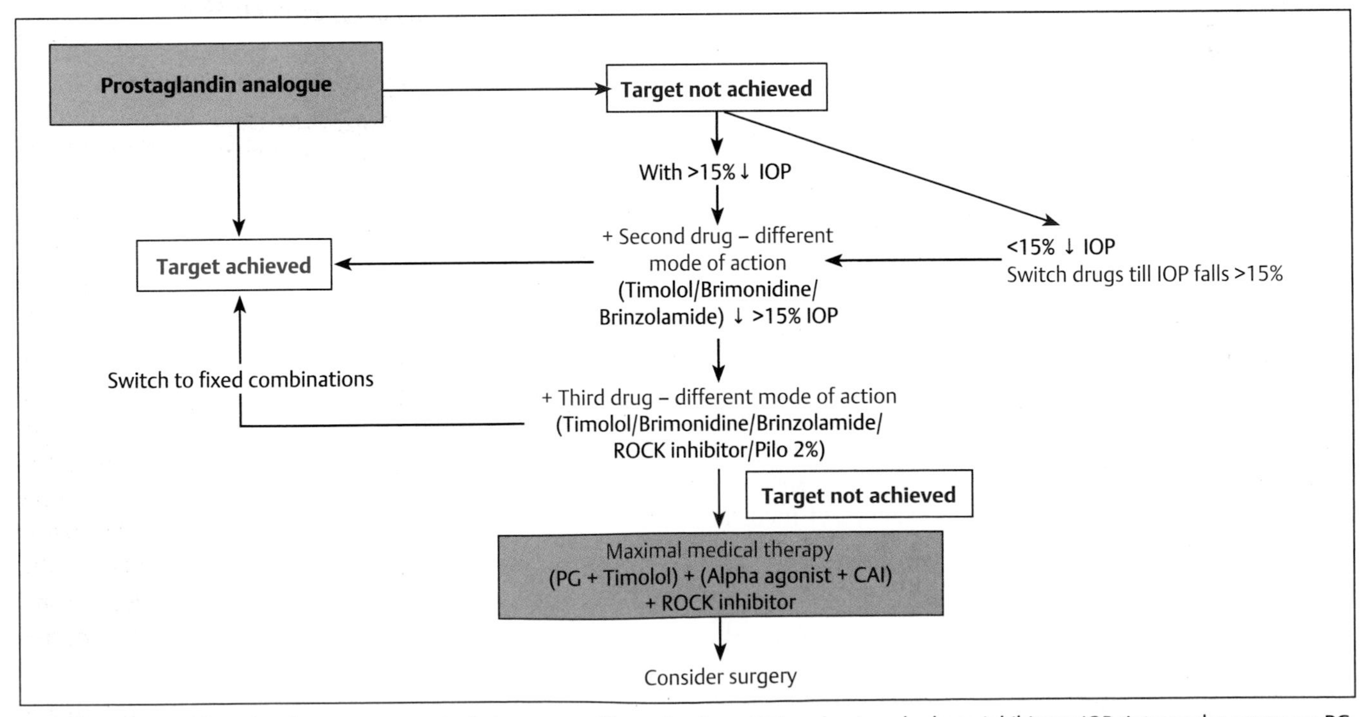

Flowchart 19.2 Algorithm for management of glaucoma with medications. CAI, carbonic anhydrase inhibitors; IOP, intraocular pressure; PG, prostaglandin; ROCK, rho-associated protein kinase.

evaluated, otherwise the patient will have all the side effects of the medications with no ocular benefit. A *unilateral trial* has been suggested, but could be adversely affected by the consensual effect of drugs such as the adrenergics, and the second eye may be left with high IOPs till the drug efficacy is determined in one eye.

In cases where the baseline IOP is less than 30 mm Hg, medication should be started and reassessed in 2 to 3 weeks, before adding a second medication. *With an IOP >30 mm Hg, two or more medications can be prescribed to lower IOP initially together with acetazolamide for 3 days*, and as a *reverse therapeutic trial*, one medication may be reduced to see if it is actually required to achieve target IOP.

First-line treatment should generally be the most effective. *Drugs used as first line are PG analogs, BBs, and alpha agonists.* As PG analogs are likely to produce about a 30% reduction in IOP, they are best tried first, keeping cost in mind or if a lower reduction in IOP is required. *Second-line therapy working through a different mechanism is less effective, but complements first-line therapy to lower IOP further*, and are topical carbonic anhydrase inhibitors, pilocarpine, etc. The response to the second medication added will not be to the same extent, as if it were used alone. The use of a third or fourth drug will have an even smaller IOP lowering efficacy. Therefore, a fourth drug for chronic use may tilt the risk benefit ratio toward greater risk of side effects. Any change in medications should be reviewed for IOP lowering in 3 to 4 weeks.

Once the patient's "target" IOP is reached with drugs the patient can tolerate and use, continuing review is required, as tolerance may develop, or age-related trabecular changes cause the IOP to rise. Those having early glaucomatous damage may be seen every 6 months, while those with moderate glaucoma, a review every 4 months, and those with severe visual field loss, every 3 months till stabilization. Thereafter a visit twice a year should suffice.

In case "target" IOP is not reached or the patient shows progression on perimetry, switching or addition of medications may be done. A repeat tonometry at the point of the peak rise at baseline may help determine if a high IOP is the cause of the progression. Systemic hypotension and sleep apnea should be looked for in patients, especially those with normal tension glaucoma. Failure of medical therapy may be due to a lack of efficacy, lack of compliance, economic compulsions, tolerance over time, or side effects.

Patients already on medication with a lower IOP than required may need a "reverse" trial, reducing one medication for the duration of its washout period, before checking of IOP at the next visit.

The Collaborative Initial Glaucoma Treatment Study (CIGTS) showed that medical therapy was as effective as surgical therapy in the initial stages of glaucoma in maintaining visual fields, even though some patients in both groups continued to show progression.

Maximum tolerated medical therapy is considered to be a combination of all drugs that cause IOP lowering in an individual patient, and do not adversely affect quality of life. If this combination does not achieve IOP lowering to target IOP, lasers or surgery is necessitated.

Glaucoma Therapy in Pregnancy

Glaucoma therapy in pregnancy is still being evaluated, with safety of the child being foremost; however, one-third of women having glaucoma develop very high IOP with progression of the neuropathy during pregnancy.

No definite guidelines are available. The safest drug is brimonidine and can be used in the first and second trimesters, but not in the third trimester or during lactation. Timolol has been thought to be relatively safe at all times, but should be stopped a few days prior to delivery. PGs may cause a miscarriage, and should be avoided as far as possible. Carbonic anhydrase inhibitors should be avoided in the first trimester.

Newer Drugs and Newer Delivery Systems

Latanoprostene bunod, 0.024%, is a novel nitric oxide (NO)-donating PG F2α analog. It breaks down into latanoprost acid and nitric oxide in the eye. It is thought to lower IOP by increasing outflow of aqueous humor through both the trabecular meshwork and uveoscleral routes. The NO-donating moiety causes cytoskeletal relaxation allowing increased aqueous outflow through the trabecular meshwork.

Adenosine receptor agonists: These are shown to lead to cell shrinkage and remodeling of extracellular matrix by matrix metalloproteinases (MMPs) in the trabecular meshwork.

Cannabinoids: Topical and oral drugs acting on cannabinoid receptors reduce aqueous production and have been tried.

Newer drug delivery systems currently under evaluation are punctal plugs, drug eluting rings, nanoparticles, intraocular lenses (IOLs) and contact lenses, and anterior chamber implants. Gene therapy using adenoviral vectors to deliver therapeutic genes into retinal ganglion cells (RGCs) to enhance survival is under investigation.

Nonresponders

There is no agreed definition of nonresponse to glaucoma medications, but it is agreed that there should be a sufficient IOP fall to justify the continued use of the medication. All glaucoma medications show a nonresponse, a *<15% drop of IOP* in 5 to 10% of individuals. PG analogs show nonresponse in about 5% and with timolol, the nonresponse is seen in about 10%. *Nonresponse to available glaucoma medications is greater in children.*

BBs are known to show both early drift of efficacy and late tolerance, with a concomitant rise of IOP. If a patient was well controlled on medications including a BB, and shows a waning efficacy after months to years, the BB should be discontinued for 6 weeks, and replaced with another glaucoma drug in the interim.

Failure of Medical Treatment

Despite a number of pharmacological options, failure of medical treatment is a significant issue not only owing to drug nonresponse and intolerance, but also due to poor patient compliance and persistence. Other causes of failure of medical therapy include lack of diurnal control, and systemic side effects.

Poor compliance in persistent use of medications is very common, being seen in probably about half of individuals on chronic therapy. Patients do not perceive any visual benefit from the drugs, and are not aware of the importance of maintaining a stable IOP. *Understanding that more damage occurs during fluctuation of IOP, as in when a drop is not used, may help motivate patients to use the drugs as prescribed.* Insisting of *an alarm on a smartphone for every time a drop is to be instilled* makes a difference. Including care givers in the discussions ensures that instructions are reinforced at home. Using a QR code can allow the patient or relatives to listen to instructions at their convenience (**Box 19.1**).

Neuroprotection

Medications that do not lower IOP but prevent or delay deterioration or RGC loss are neuroprotective. Many drugs, N-methyl-D-aspartate (NMDA) antagonists such as memantine, nitric oxide synthetase inhibitors, glutamate antagonists, calcium channel blockers, etc., have been tried for a possible neuroprotective effect, but this has not been confirmed.

Brimonidine has been suggested to have a neuroprotective effect, over and above its IOP lowering efficacy, by reducing glutamate-induced excitotoxicity, inhibiting nitric oxide synthase, decreasing oxidative stress, and inhibiting glial activity. This has only been shown in animal models of crush injury.

Nicotinamide, vitamin B3, is a precursor of nicotinamide adenine dinucleotide and could be neuroprotective for ganglion cells, as it decreases mitochondrial dysfunction. It also improves calcium signaling, and reverses endothelin-mediated vasoconstriction.

A polymeric device containing a *human cell line that secretes ciliary neurotrophic factor (CNTF)* has been implanted at the pars plana. CNTF is sequestered in a semipermeable membrane to bypass an immune reaction, and it may enhance survival of RGCs. Similarly, other growth factors and neurotrophins are being studied.

Stem Cell Therapy

Intravitreal stem cell therapy has shown some promise in RGC protection, but the cells did not migrate into the retina. They are, therefore, more likely to be used as a vector for secretion of factors needed to protect/repair dysfunctional RGCs. Mesenchymal stem cells and factors secreted by them provide neuroprotection and immunomodulation.

Stem cells have also been used intracamerally to prevent or modify changes seen in the trabecular meshwork of

Box 19.1 Hand out/instructions on the use of glaucoma medications

- Do not touch the container tip to the eye, eyelid, or other skin.
- Tilt your head back, pull lower eyelid out to form a pocket, and apply one drop.
- Keep your eyes closed. Put pressure on the inside corner of the eye for 1 to 2 minutes to prevent systemic absorption.
- If a drop is prescribed to be used twice a day, that should be every 12 hours, 7 am and 7 pm.
- If a drop is prescribed to be used three times a day, it should be every 8 hours, 6 am, 2 pm, and 10 pm.
- Put an alarm on your phone.
- When multiple drops are used in the same eye, it is important to wait at least 10 minutes between drops.
- Replace cap tightly.
- Keep bottles in a cool place.

glaucomatous eyes. The therapeutic potential of stem cell therapy in glaucoma is still to be validated.

Conclusion

Currently available glaucoma medications are effective in a large proportion of glaucoma patients and are therefore the first line of therapy. Using drugs properly, with nasolacrimal duct block, on time and regularly has been shown to stabilize glaucomatous optic neuropathy in the long-term.

It is important to remember that the *aim of medical therapy is to achieve a target IOP range with least fluctuation, using least possible medications, two to three bottles at most, and with the least disruption to a patient's lifestyle—economic or social—to stabilize the glaucomatous neuropathy present.*

Cases

Case 1

A 46-year-old female came for presbyopic correction, and was found to have a cup:disc ratio of 0.7 in both eyes with inferior neuroretinal rim thinning. There was a definite retinal nerve fiber layer defect in the left eye inferotemporal area and a thin defect in the right eye. IOPs were 18 to 26 mm Hg on diurnal phasing, highest at 7 am. On perimetry there was a superior nasal step in the right eye and a superior arcuate defect in the left eye. Gonioscopy was wide open with moderate trabecular pigmentation (**Case 1-1**).

Points to consider

- Young patient with long life expectancy.
- Mild glaucomatous damage in the right eye and moderate in the left eye.
- A swing of 8 mm in IOP on diurnal.

Diagnosis and Management

A diagnosis of primary open angle with hypertension (POAH) with target IOP of <17 mm Hg in the right eye and <15 mm Hg in the left eye. The patient was started on a PG analog, and after 3 weeks her IOP at 8 am was 16 mm Hg in both eyes. As there was a significant drop of IOP, >15% from baseline, the PG analog was continued. Additionally, timolol, twice a day, was added to the left eye, and the IOPs after 6 weeks were 16 and 12 mm Hg in the right eye and left eye, respectively. The patient was counseled for proper use and timing of drugs, and lifelong review.

Case 2

A 68-year-old man diagnosed to have chronic primary angle-closure glaucoma (CPACG) was on a PG analog, timolol, brimonidine, and pilocarpine in four different bottles, to achieve a target IOP of 12 to 15 mm Hg for the last 2 months. Known to be a mild hypertensive, the patient suddenly developed a hypertensive crisis.

Points to consider

- Is this a side effect of glaucoma therapy?
- Should four bottles be continued?
- Perimetry should be done to determine target IOP.

Diagnosis and Management

On asking about his systemic status, it was learned that he had Parkinsonism and was on MAO inhibitor, selegiline. Brimonidine was stopped, as it is known to interact with MAO inhibitor, and was replaced by brinzolamide.

He was asked to use a PG analog at night, a combination of pilocarpine and timolol, twice a day, and brimonidine, twice a day. This brought his blood pressure (BP) to normal, and also increased compliance as the drops were put only twice a day, at 10 minutes intervals (**Case 2-1**).

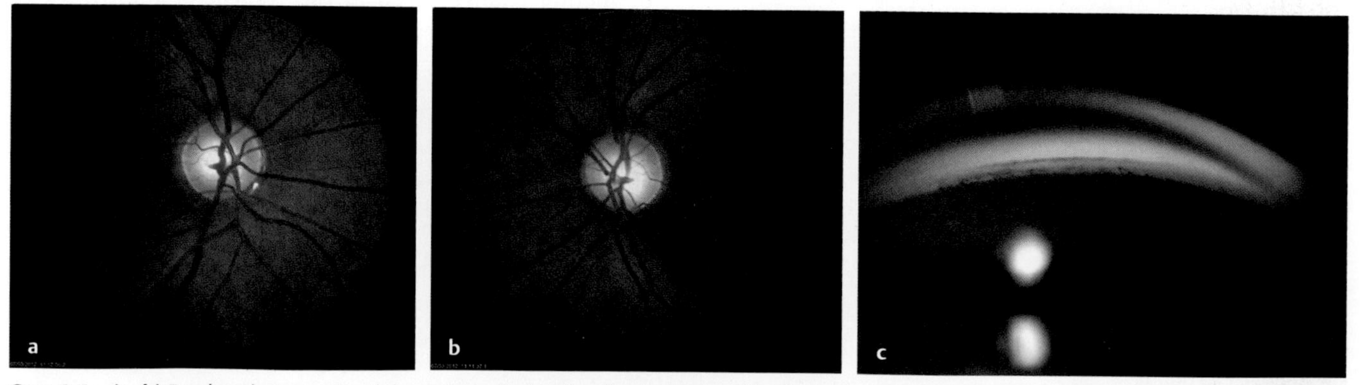

Case 1-1 **(a, b)** Fundus photographs of the optic nerve head and retinal nerve fiber layer showing cup:disc ratio of 0.7 in both eyes, with definite retinal nerve fiber layer defect in the left eye inferotemporal area and a thin defect in the right eye. **(c)** Goniophotograph showing an open angle with moderate pigmentation of trabecular meshwork anterior to Schwalbe's line.

• PG analogue: 9 pm • Timolol: 6 am and 10 pm • Brimonidine: 7 am and 10.30 pm • Pilocarpine: 6 am, 12 noon and 7 pm	→	• PG analogue: 9.20 pm • Timolol/pilo combination: 9 am and 9 pm • Brinzolamide: 9.10 am and 9.10 pm

Case 2-1 Adjusting medications to decrease the number of times medications have to be used.

Case 3

A 70-year-old lady with mild glaucomatous optic neuropathy (GON) due to primary open-angle glaucoma (POAG), baseline IOP of 28 mm Hg, was prescribed the use of PG analog drops at bedtime, with which her IOP was in the range of 15 to 17 mm Hg. On review 3 months later, she wanted to stop the drops as her family felt that her eyelids, especially the lower eyelids, had become darker in color (**Case 3-1**).

Points to consider

- PG analogs are known to cause pigmentation of the eyelids.
- Other first-line drugs can control mild glaucoma but have systemic side effects in the elderly.

Diagnosis and Management

She was advised to use her drops lying down, and keep her eyes closed after instilling just one drop. Immediate wiping of any overflow was explained. At her next review, the irregular pigmentation below the lower eyelid had reduced but hyperpigmentation of both eyelids was still present. Her glaucoma medication was switched first to timolol alone, and then a combination of dorzolamide and timolol, twice a day, to get a similar IOP effect. Her eyelid hyperpigmentation reduced over 2 to 3 months, but did not completely reverse.

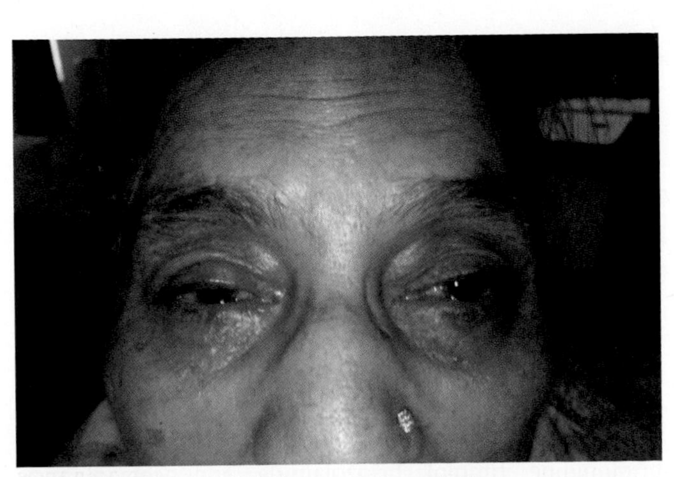

Case 3-1 Bilateral eyelid edema and pigmentation.

Case 4

A 60-year-old lady diagnosed with severe PACG, baseline IOP of 36/32 mm Hg and a cup:disc ratio of 0.8 with generalized thinning and pallor of the neuroretinal rim, underwent an iridotomy under cover of oral acetazolamide. She was advised the use of a PG analog hs and dorzolamide and timolol combination twice a day. After 2 weeks her IOP was 24/20 mm Hg. As her optical coherence tomography showed significant retinal nerve fiber layer damage in both eyes, a moderate glaucoma was diagnosed for which target IOP of 12 to 15 mm Hg had not been achieved (**Case 4-1**). Pilocarpine 2% at 6 am, 2 pm, and 10 pm was added. She called the next day complaining of a mild headache.

Points to consider

- Brow ache is expected to occur with pilocarpine but reduces within a week in older patients.
- Pilocarpine is an effective medication for PACG.
- Its additive effect with PG analogs is questionable.

Diagnosis and Management

She was advised to continue the drops, and advised to report if it got worse. On review 2 weeks later, she said the headaches had stopped after 2 to 3 days, her IOP reduced to 16/14 mm Hg, and she was also finding it easier to read.

Case 5

A 30-year-old lady was diagnosed with traumatic glaucoma following a shuttle cock injury in her left eye 6 months earlier. Her baseline IOP recorded was 32 mm Hg in the presence of angle recession of about 180 degrees, and a cup:disc ratio of 0.7 with inferior neuroretinal rim thinning. She had been using a PG analog for the duration, but complained of darker eyelashes in the left eye (**Case 5-1**).

Points to consider

- PG analogs are known to cause darker, thicker, and longer lashes more visible on unilateral use.
- All PG analogs may have the same effect.
- Significant angle recession with glaucomatous neuropathy requires an IOP of <17 mm Hg.

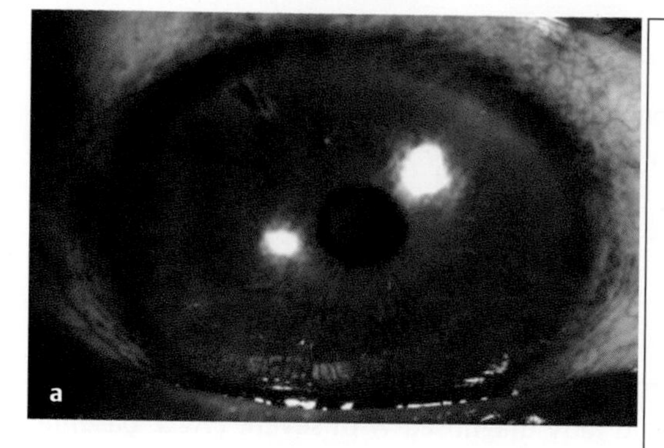

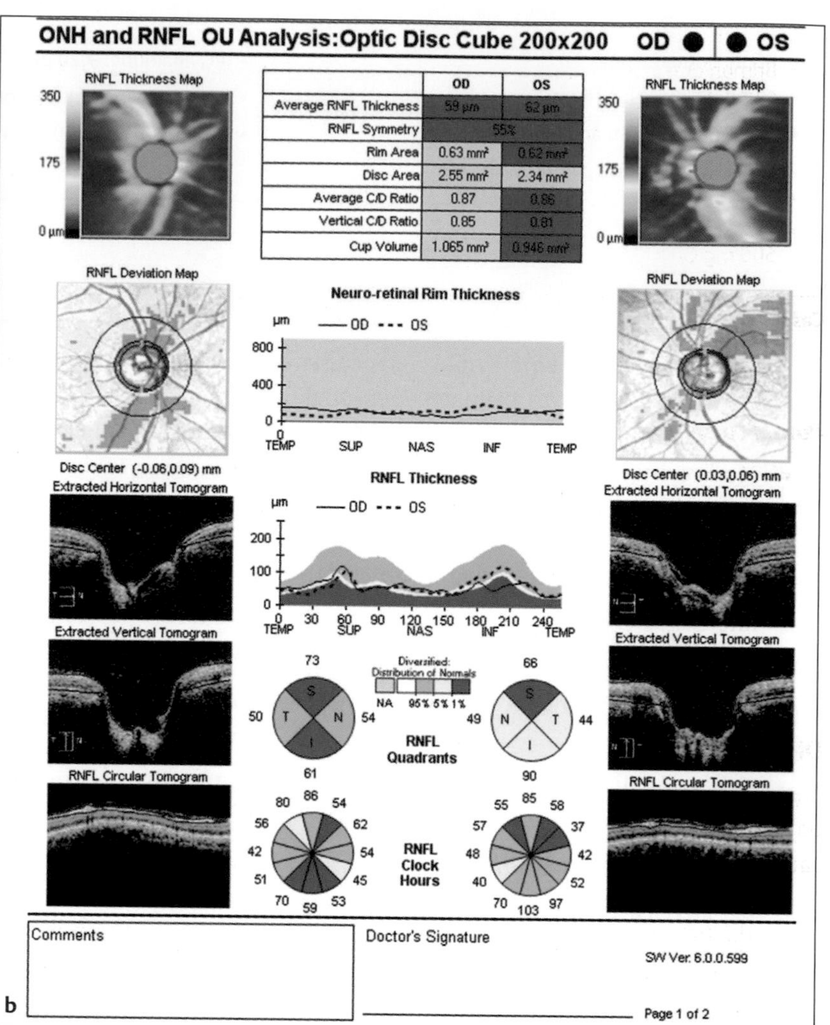

Case 4-1 **(a)** A patent laser iridotomy. **(b)** Optical coherence tomography: Good quality scan showing retinal nerve fiber layer loss at both poles in the right eye and superior pole of the left.

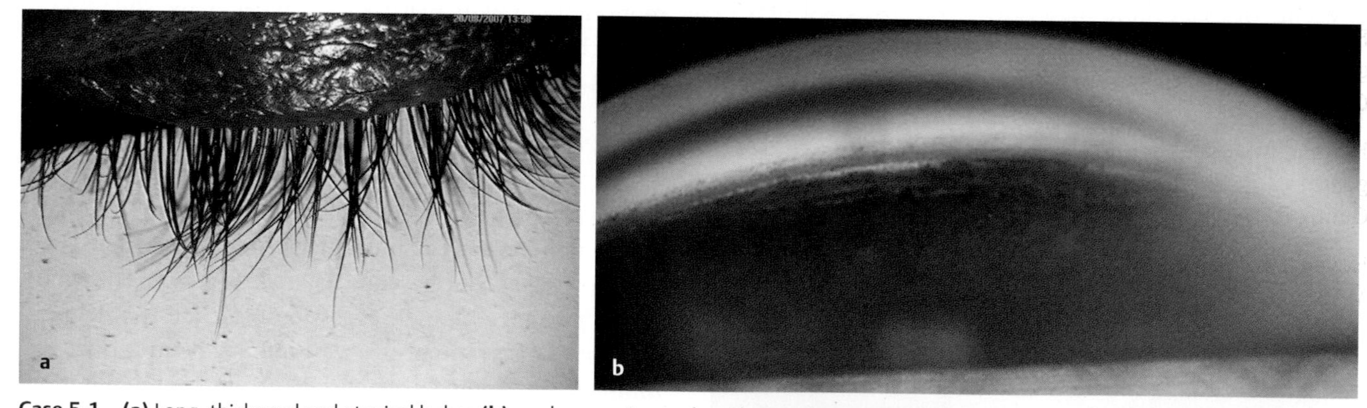

Case 5-1 **(a)** Long, thickened and atypical lashes **(b)** angle recession and moderate pigmentation of the trabecular meshwork.

Diagnosis and Management

The patient was advised to stop the PG analog and was shifted to a dorzolamide–timolol combination twice a day.

Case 6

A 40-year-old man presented with blurring of vision to casualty. He was known to have juvenile open-angle glaucoma (JOAG), cup:disc ratio of 0.7 in both eyes, and was well controlled on a PG analog till 2 months earlier. His IOP in casualty was 50/46 mm Hg with moderate corneal edema. He gave a history of using a steroid cream for 3 weeks, and a diagnosis of JOAG with high steroid response was made. Despite stopping the steroid and using PG analog, brimonidine, timolol, brinzolamide, and acetazolamide (250 mg Q8h), his IOP remained at 30/26 mm Hg.

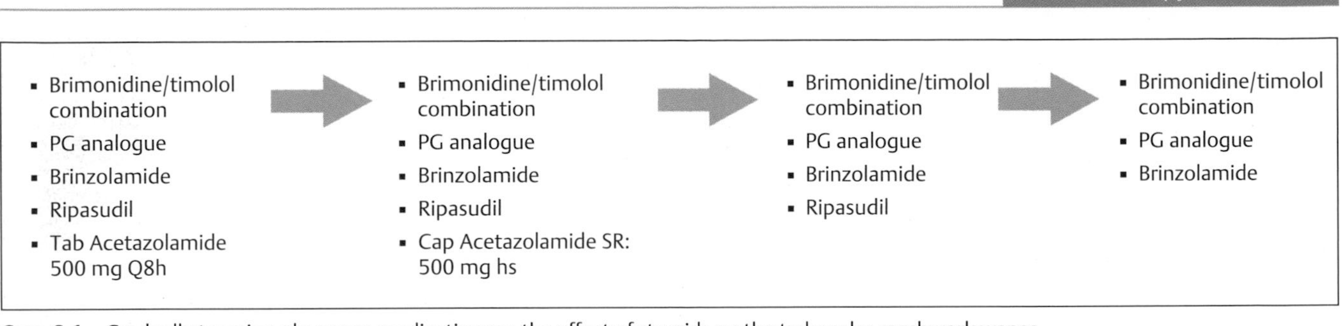

Case 6-1 Gradually tapering glaucoma medications as the effect of steroids on the trabecular meshwork wanes.

Points to consider

- Medications working on both aqueous inflow and uveoscleral outflow have brought the IOP down to 30 mm Hg, but chances of retinal vein occlusion persist.
- Rho kinase inhibitors work to enhance trabecular outflow.
- Filtering surgery could be considered.

Diagnosis and Management

The patient was advised the use of ripasudil 0.4% twice a day in addition, which dropped the IOP to 24/22 mm Hg, causing persistent redness. The patient was reviewed closely, and medications were tapered off over 3 months, ripasudil first, as the steroid effect wore off and the IOP reduced (**Case 6-1**).

Suggested Readings

Bucolo C, Platania CB, Reibaldi M, et al. Controversies in glaucoma: current medical treatment and drug development. Curr Pharm Des 2015;21(32):4673–4681

Harasymowycz P, Birt C, Gooi P, et al. Medical management of glaucoma in the 21st century from a Canadian perspective. J Ophthalmol 2016;2016:6509809

Hedengran A, Steensberg AT, Virgili G, Azuara-Blanco A, Kolko M. Efficacy and safety evaluation of benzalkonium chloride preserved eye-drops compared with alternatively preserved and preservative-free eye-drops in the treatment of glaucoma: a systematic review and meta-analysis. Br J Ophthalmol 2020;104(11):1512–1518

Li T, Lindsley K, Rouse B, et al. Comparative effectiveness of first-line medications for primary open-angle glaucoma: a systematic review and network meta-analysis. Ophthalmology 2016;123(1):129–140

Nayak B, Gupta S, Kumar G, Dada T, Gupta V, Sihota R. Socioeconomics of long-term glaucoma therapy in India. Indian J Ophthalmol 2015;63(1):20–24

Schehlein EM, Novack GD, Robin AL. New classes of glaucoma medications. Curr Opin Ophthalmol 2017;28(2): 161–168

Tang W, Zhang F, Liu K, Duan X. Efficacy and safety of prostaglandin analogues in primary open-angle glaucoma or ocular hypertension patients: a meta-analysis. Medicine (Baltimore) 2019;98(30):e16597

Xing Y, Zhu L, Zhang K, Huang S. The efficacy of the fixed combination of latanoprost and timolol versus other fixed combinations for primary open-angle glaucoma and ocular hypertension: a systematic review and meta-analysis. PLoS One 2020;15(2):e0229682

Xu L, Wang X, Wu M. Topical medication instillation techniques for glaucoma. Cochrane Database Syst Rev 2017;2: CD010520

CHAPTER 20

Laser Therapy in Glaucoma

Overview

- Laser Iridotomy
  - Indications for an Iridotomy
  - Procedure
  - Postlaser Therapy
- Laser Trabeculoplasty
  - Indications
  - Procedure
  - Postlaser Therapy
  - Complications
  - Prognostic Factors
- Laser Iridoplasty
  - Mechanism of Action
  - Indications
  - Procedure
  - Complications
- Cyclophotocoagulation
  - Indications
- Diode Laser Cyclophotocoagulation
  - Mechanism of Action
  - Technique
  - Postlaser Regimen
  - Complications
  - Endocyclophotocoagulation
- Cases
- Suggested Readings

Introduction

Laser procedures in glaucoma provide ophthalmologists with options beyond medications and surgery, and sometimes even the only option. *Patient's acceptance of these procedures is high because they are noninvasive, and generally have few significant side effects.* However, the indications and efficacy should be understood, and the procedures done with care.

Laser Iridotomy

Laser peripheral iridotomy (LPI) is the preferred procedure for treating *angle-closure disease* caused by relative or absolute pupillary block. LPI is indicated for all forms of angle-closure glaucoma, primary angle closure disease at any stage, and secondary angle closure due to pupillary block. It is also a prophylactic measure for high-risk primary angle closure suspects.

LPI eliminates pupillary block by allowing aqueous to pass directly from the posterior chamber into the anterior chamber, bypassing the pupil. This causes the iris to fall back exposing areas of the trabecular meshwork that had iridotrabecular functional apposition, not organic synechiae (**Fig. 20.1**). An iridotomy also prevents further attacks of angle closure, as seen by studies of dark room prone provocative test or mydriatic tests. Laser iridotomy itself is not expected to control intraocular pressure (IOP), as resistance to aqueous outflow and therefore IOP depends on pre-existing damage to outflow channels.

LPI can be performed with an argon laser with a Q-switched Neodymium: Yttrium-Aluminum-Garnet (Nd: YAG) laser or, in certain circumstances, with both, argon followed by YAG laser. *Nd:YAG laser is the most appropriate laser for dark colored irides that are thicker than light irides.* It is a photodisruptive laser where an intense focal laser beam is delivered over a period of nano- or picoseconds causing optical breakdown and a resultant shock wave that disrupts tissue, independent of pigmentation.

Indications for an Iridotomy

- Acute or chronic primary angle closure glaucoma (PACG).
- Primary angle closure (PAC).
- Fellow eyes of patients having primary angle closure disease (PACD).
- Primary angle closure suspects (PACS) with risk factors as follows:
  - Family history of PACD.

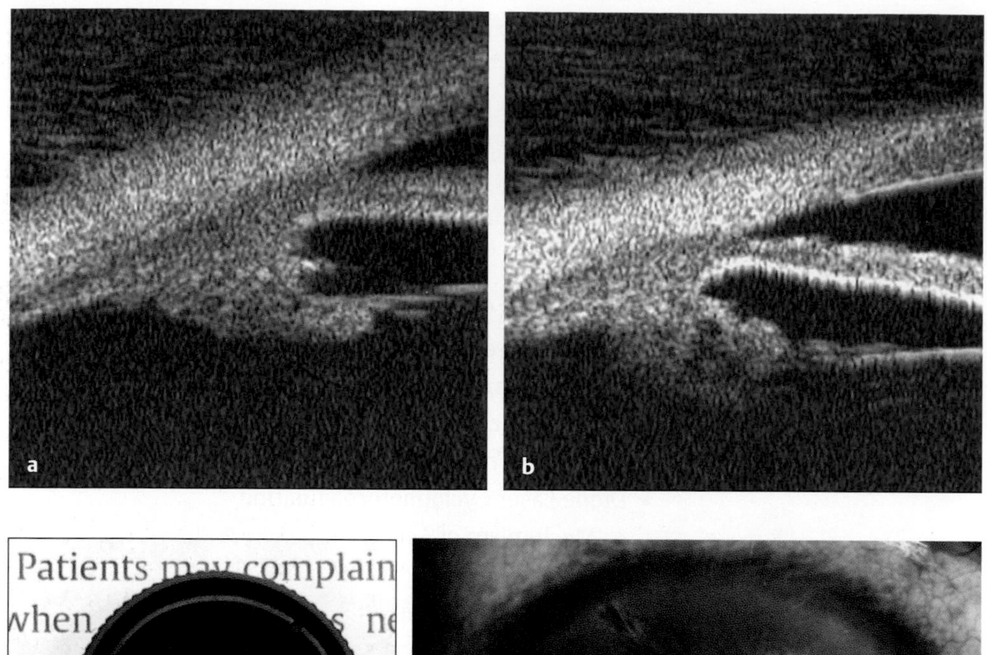

Fig. 20.1 Ultrasound biomicroscopy (UBM) pictures. **(a)** Iridotrabecular contact in primary angle-closure glaucoma. **(b)** After laser iridotomy the iris appears flatter and the extent of iridotrabecular contact has reduced.

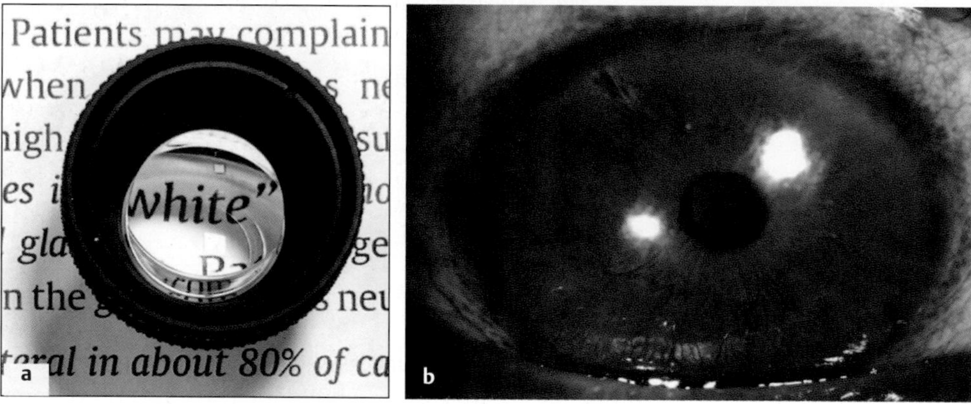

Fig. 20.2 **(a)** Photograph showing Abraham lens with +66D planoconvex decentered lens that focuses the laser beam, increasing power delivered at a point, thereby preventing collateral damage. **(b)** Photograph showing a good position and size of a laser iridotomy.

 - ◦ Frequent dilation required, as in diabetic retinopathy.
 - ◦ Difficulty accessing ophthalmic care, e.g., rural areas.
- Secondary angle closure, e.g., uveitis, aphakic, or pseudophakic pupillary block.
- Combined mechanism glaucoma.
- In eyes with phakic intraocular lenses (IOLs) or anterior chamber IOLs.
- Pigmentary glaucoma, if a reverse pupillary block is demonstrated on ultrasound biomicroscopy (UBM).
- To reach a diagnosis of aqueous misdirection syndrome.

Procedure

The procedure should be discussed and *a written, informed consent taken, explaining that a line of light may be appreciated after the procedure. A history of anticoagulant/aspirin* use should be checked for and they can be stopped after consulting a physician. *Instill one to two drops of pilocarpine 2% 10 to 15 minutes before the procedure to thin out the iris.* Under topical anesthesia and using an iridotomy lens (**Fig 20.2**), a peripheral iris crypt or a thin area is chosen under the upper eyelid, avoiding the 12 o'clock position. *The laser beam is first focused on the iris surface, and then defocused slightly into the iris stroma. An initial energy level of 4 to 6 mJ may be used in one to three pulses per burst.* A gush of pigment and aqueous, with deepening of the anterior chamber, is noted on penetration. The size of the opening is then enlarged with lower energy levels, and a size of about 250 to 400 µm is considered adequate (**Fig. 20.2**). This is approximately four times the size of the aiming beam.

To control inflammation and possible IOP spikes post laser, *administer topical steroids and add one glaucoma medication to those already being taken, for 5 to 7 days post laser.* The eye should be monitored for *IOP spikes 2 to 4 hours post laser*, especially in eyes with advanced glaucomatous optic neuropathy or prior raised IOP. *Eyes with severe glaucoma should get systemic acetazolamide immediately after and for 3 days post laser.* Mild candle wax like iris bleeding can be controlled by gentle pressure with the iridotomy lens.

Postlaser Therapy

- Topical steroids—four times a day for 5 to 7 days.
- Continue antiglaucoma medications.
- Add one glaucoma medication, if the patient is already on glaucoma therapy.
- Tab acetazolamide cover in advanced glaucoma or if IOP is >21 mm Hg.

After 2 to 3 weeks, the patency of an iridotomy is best appreciated when the lens capsule can be seen; however, complete clarity on retroillumination may also be used (**Figs. 20.3–20.6**). *Gonioscopy should be performed to look for areas of residual iridotrabecular synechiae. At least three tonometry readings should be taken, preferably at different times of the day, and a "target" IOP planned according to severity of glaucoma.*

Complications are rare, and include:

- Postlaser IOP spikes of >8 mm Hg in 6 to 10%.
- Glare/thin line of light visible.
- Anterior uveitis.
- Iris bleed.
- Cataract, usually nonprogressive.
- Closure of iridotomy—opening becoming smaller by 50%, within 6 to 8 weeks, after argon iridotomy.
- Pupillary distortion—mostly with argon iridotomy.
- Retinal and corneal burns—rare.
- Corneal endothelial cell loss—only with argon or combined argon and YAG iridotomies.

Laser Trabeculoplasty

The procedure of argon laser trabeculoplasty (ALT) was first described by Weiss and Witter to treat open angle glaucoma. In 1995, Latina and Park popularized the concept of "selective laser trabeculoplasty" (SLT) due its ability to selectively target pigmented trabecular

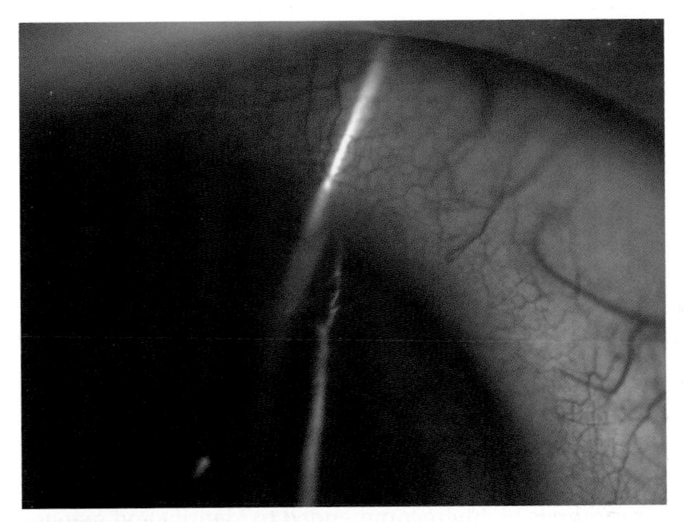

Fig. 20.3 Lens capsule visible through the iridotomy.

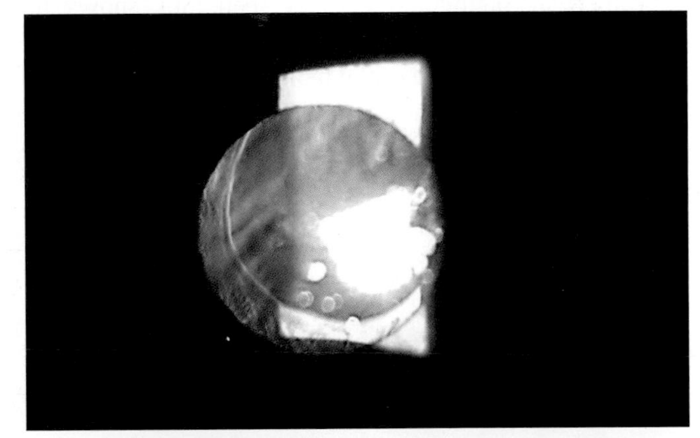

Fig. 20.4 Retroillumination to check for the patency of an iridotomy may be fallacious as this may be present with a lamellar iridotomy too, and needs to be corroborated by a view of the lens capsule through the iridotomy.

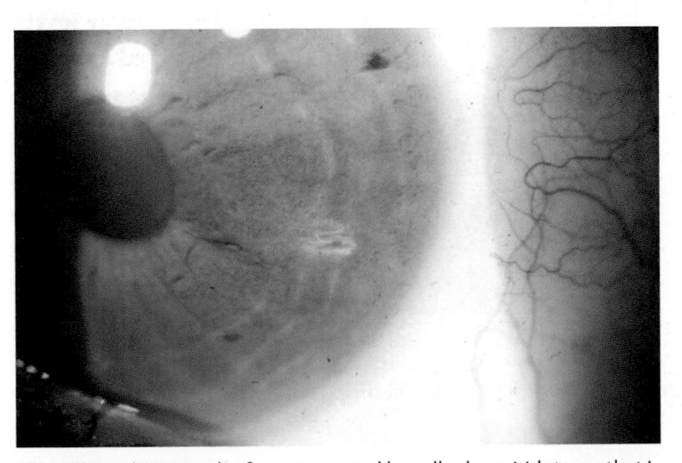

Fig. 20.5 Photograph of an attempted lamellar laser iridotomy that is more central, not midperipheral, and would overlie the lens.

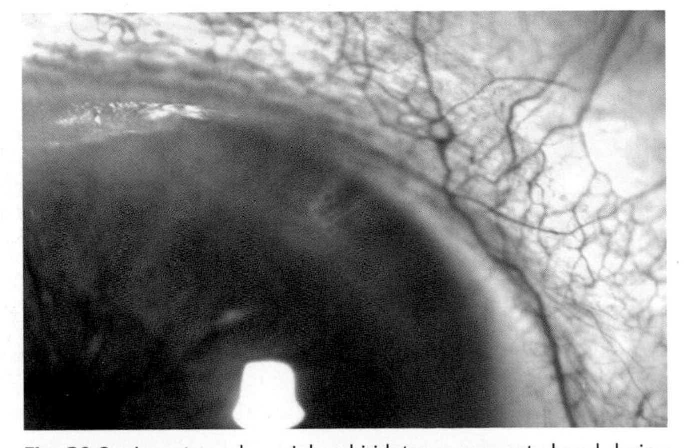

Fig. 20.6 An extremely peripheral iridotomy may get closed during dilation of the pupil.

meshwork cells, minimizing collateral damage. ALT and SLT provide similar results; however, the latter has gained wider acceptance due to its enhanced safety and success of repeat applications.

SLT uses green Q-switched, frequency-doubled neodymium doped yttrium aluminum garnet (Nd:YAG) laser of 532 nm, to cause laser-induced thermal changes to specific pigmented trabecular cells, sparing adjacent tissues within the irradiated field. The pulse duration of SLT is 3 nanoseconds (ns), which is much less than the thermal relaxation time of melanin, 1 µs, that is, the time required for the absorbed energy to dissipate out of the pigmented cells causing damage to surrounding tissue.

Tonographic studies have revealed that laser trabeculoplasty decreases IOP by enhancing aqueous drainage via the conventional pathway, secondary to morphological and biological changes that occur. Morphological changes in argon/diode laser trabeculoplasty are the opening up of spaces due to contraction of trabecular beams. In SLT disruption of trabecular endothelial cells, a decrease in trabecular pigmented cells is seen. SLT shows no disruption or coagulative change in corneoscleral or uveal trabecular beams. Some of the biological changes seen are a modification of trabecular cellular activity resulting in increased cytokine and matrix metalloproteinase secretion, increased cell division and re-population, phagocytosis, and intercellular junction alterations.

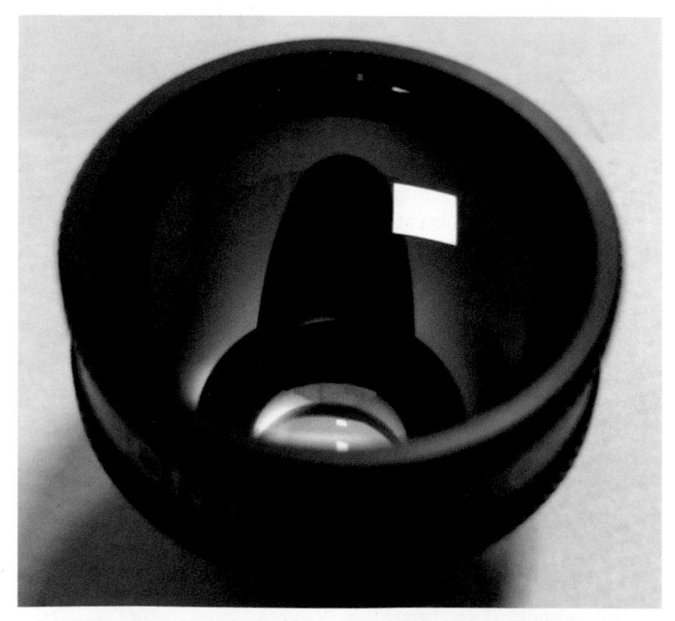

Fig. 20.7 Latina lens for selective laser trabeculoplasty (SLT) consists of a single mirror inclined at an angle of 63 degrees and provides a magnification of 1×.

Indications

Indications for laser trabeculoplasty are the lowering of IOP in all open angle glaucomas, especially:

- Ocular hypertension.
- Pseudoexfoliation glaucoma.
- Pigmentary glaucoma.
- Steroid-induced glaucoma.
- Secondary open angle glaucomas—pseudophakic.

Procedure

A drop of brimonidine 0.2% should be applied 15 minutes before the procedure to prevent any post-SLT IOP spike. For SLT a Latina or Ritch trabeculoplasty lens (**Fig. 20.7**) is used to focus the 532-nm, Q-switched, frequency-doubled Nd:YAG laser beam, set at 400 µm spot size with 1 to 5 ns pulse duration, placed over the entire trabecular meshwork, avoiding Schwalbe's line or ciliary body. The total energy can vary from 0.5 to 1.2 mJ per pulse, starting with 0.4 mJ and titrated in 0.1 mJ steps looking for micro bubbles, champagne bubbles, at which point slowly reduce power. Place 50 contiguous, nonoverlapping adjacent spots over 180 degrees of the trabecular meshwork (**Fig. 20.8**). 180 or 360 degrees can be done at a single sitting.

Argon or diode laser trabeculoplasty uses spots of 50 µm in size, 0.1 s duration, at the junction of the pigmented and nonpigmented trabecular meshwork. Apply 50 spots over 180 degrees, adjusting power till a mild blanching is seen.

Postlaser Therapy

Five days of nonsteroidal anti-inflammatory therapy is generally used. An IOP measurement 1 to 2 hours after the procedure is highly recommended to identify and manage cases of postlaser IOP spike. The first follow-up after SLT can be routinely done 1 to 3 weeks postoperatively, except

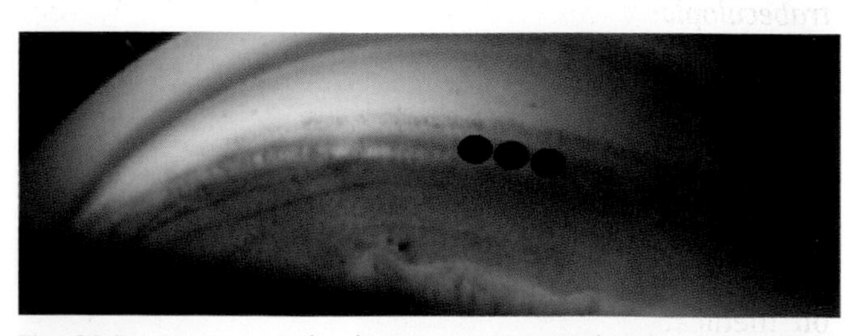

Fig. 20.8 An open angle glaucoma eye treated with selective laser trabeculoplasty (SLT). Nonoverlapping spots of 400-µm diameter are placed over the trabecular meshwork.

for those with significant immediate postlaser IOP spikes and those with severe visual field defects. *The patient must be followed up periodically to ascertain IOP control, as the efficacy of laser trabeculoplasty wanes with time.*

The efficacy and success rates of SLT and ALT are similar, and vary widely with different types of glaucomas. In general, *an IOP reduction of 20 to 30% from baseline, without the addition of any glaucoma medications, is considered as absolute success.*

Complications

SLT employs only 1% of the energy used by ALT, and due to its high tissue selectivity, exhibits a low complication rate. The most common complication is the acute spike in IOP occurring within 2 hours and lasting less than a day. *An IOP rise of ≥5 mm Hg is seen in up to one-third of patients*, and is assumed to be secondary to inflammatory debris blocking the trabecular meshwork. This tendency is higher in pigmentary glaucoma and low in pseudoexfoliation glaucoma. *Uveitis is seen in some eyes after ALT, but in up to 83% eyes treated with SLT.* It is also transient and usually resolves in roughly 5 days. A heavily pigmented trabecular meshwork and past history of ALT offer higher risk to iritis. Treatment with topical steroids or nonsteroidal anti-inflammatory drugs (NSAIDs) may be given. Other rare complications include peripheral anterior synechiae, hyphema, appearance/worsening of cystoid macular edema, choroidal effusion, accidental foveal burns, transient refractive errors, corneal haze, and keratitis.

Repeat SLT is feasible producing similar mean IOP reduction as that of primary SLT. It can be applied to the previously treated area or a new area of the trabecular meshwork, with both giving equal results.

Prognostic Factors

The most significant factor for predicting success of laser trabeculoplasty is a high baseline IOP, although extremely elevated pressures may not be controlled. Laser in Glaucoma and ocular HyperTension (LiGHT) study randomized newly diagnosed patients with primary open angle glaucoma (POAG) or ocular hypertension (OHT) to selective laser trabeculoplasty or medications as first-line therapy. At 3 years, 95% of SLT eyes were at target IOP, with 74.2% off medications. There was a reduced need for filtering surgery.

Laser trabeculoplasty has opened a new treatment possibilities for almost all types of glaucoma with efficacy and safety overall comparable to that of medical management. It has the advantage of being a short, safe, and easy procedure as against life-long medical therapy. *However, not all glaucomas are uniformly amenable to it and the effect wanes with time.*

Laser Iridoplasty

Laser iridoplasty is the technique by which low-energy coagulative laser burns are applied onto the surface of the peripheral iris, such that it does not penetrate but produces a visible tissue contraction, thereby pulling open an occluded/occludable angle.

Mechanism of Action

A laser iridoplasty spot placed on the peripheral iris causes heat-induced collagen shrinkage, and the long-term response is secondary to fibroblastic membrane contraction, pulling the iris root away from the trabecular meshwork, and opening up an appositionally closed angle.

Indications

- Acute angle closure nonresponsive to maximal glaucoma medications.
- Plateau iris syndrome.
- To facilitate laser trabeculoplasty in eyes with narrow angles

Procedure

Topical pilocarpine 2% is applied to attain miosis, exposing the most peripheral part of the iris. In cases of moderate corneal edema, topical glycerine may be used to temporarily clear the haze to enhance visualization. Under topical anesthesia, a Goldmann goniolens or an Abraham lens is placed on the eye. The suggested initial settings are a 200-µm spot size for 0.2 to 3 s with 300 mW power, increased gradually, until a visible iris contraction and deepening of the overlying peripheral anterior chamber is seen. Pigment dispersion or bubble formation from the lasered area warrants a decrease in power/duration. Roughly 10 to 15 spots/quadrant with a gap of one spot distance between each (**Fig. 20.9**) are placed in up to 180 degrees of angle per sitting.

Glaucoma medications are required before and after iridoplasty, based on presenting IOP and severity of glaucomatous neuropathy. Topical steroids four to six times per day are used for 3 to 5 days.

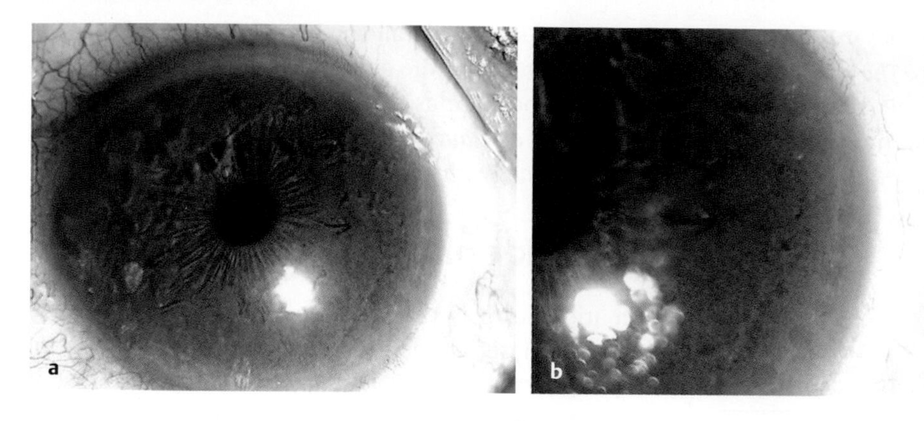

Fig. 20.9 (a, b) Argon laser peripheral iridoplasty: 200 to 500 µm spots of 0.2 to 0.5 s and 400 to 800 mW power, placed at the peripheral-most iris, with separation of two burns width apart.

Complications

Postoperatively mild iritis and an IOP spike may occur transiently. In the long term, pigmented burn marks, focal iris atrophy, and pupillary distortion are seen. Rare cases of pupillary dilatation and resultant photophobia may occur.

Cyclophotocoagulation

Cyclodestructive procedures are restricted to eyes with refractory or end-stage glaucomas which are some of the most difficult to control with conventional glaucoma filtration surgery. *Laser applications to the ciliary body, transsclerally or internally, are used to damage the pigmented ciliary epithelium, decreasing aqueous production.* However, it is commonly associated with uveitis and cystoid macular edema and therefore is used largely in eyes with poor vision or those that are nonseeing.

Many different types of lasers have been used, with the diode being the most frequent, but micropulse lasers have now been introduced.

Indications

- Very advanced glaucomas with poor visual potential.
- Refractory glaucomas—neovascular and inflammatory glaucoma, glaucoma associated with corneal transplantation, silicone oil-induced glaucoma, etc.
- In urgent situations, where eyes have dangerously elevated IOP—malignant glaucoma, early postvitreoretinal surgery, etc.
- For pain relief in eyes with no visual potential.

Diode Laser Cyclophotocoagulation

DLCP is a technique used to ablate the ciliary body using a laser directed through the sclera.

Mechanism of Action

Diode laser transscleral cyclophotocoagulation is known to achieve its IOP-lowering effect via two independent mechanisms: (i) by direct *thermal destruction of the ciliary epithelial cells that produce aqueous*, and (ii) by inducing *inflammation that may in turn lead to decreased aqueous production and/or increased uveoscleral outflow*. The former mechanism should produce relatively permanent IOP reduction, while the latter may result in transient IOP reduction that disappears as the inflammation clears.

The 810-nm semiconductor diode laser appears to offer a better method of cycloablation with potentially fewer complications as there is better absorption of this wavelength by the pigmented tissues of the ciliary body causing coagulation necrosis of the ciliary body stroma. The glaucoma probe handpiece footplate that comes in contact with the sclera is arched spherically to match the scleral contour. The anterior, curved edge of the footplate is designed to overlie and match the surgical limbus during laser application. *The probe handpiece has a fiberoptic tip which protrudes 0.7 mm beyond the contact surface. The protruding fiberoptic indents the conjunctiva and the sclera to enhance laser light transmission.*

Technique

An informed consent is important, and should clearly state the indication for cyclophotocoagulation and emphasize that the procedure is not for visual improvement. Local anesthesia by peribulbar injection of lignocaine hydrochloride (2%) in combination with bupivacaine hydrochloride (0.5%) is necessary for this painful procedure. The G-probe is placed with its edge at the limbus and is automatically centered 1.2 mm posterior to the limbus in the region of the ciliary body. In eyes with scarred or stretched limbus it is best to *transilluminate the sclera posterior to the limbus to identify the dark demarcation just behind the limbus, which is the anterior edge of the ciliary body.* Care is taken to apply the G-probe to the limbus indenting properly to ensure that the G-probe surface contour matches the scleral curvature and *the posterior angulation is correctly oriented to protect the lens in phakic eyes from laser damage.* The laser is applied at an initial power of 1750 mW, for a duration of 2 s, and power is gradually increased, watching out for a "pop" sound, suggestive of tissue disruption. At this point the power is reduced by increments of 250 mW till no pop is heard. Each laser application is spaced approximately 2 mm apart. About 20 applications are required to cover 270 degrees (**Fig. 20.10**).

The 3 and 9 o'clock meridians are spared to prevent damage to anterior ciliary arteries. More frequent phthisis occurs with 360-degree photocoagulation, so a quadrant is usually spared at the first sitting. Also, in case DLCP does not reduce IOP enough, a quadrant is available for further filtering surgery.

Postlaser Regimen

Topical steroids and cycloplegics, along with oral analgesics, are prescribed as required. In patients on oral acetazolamide before laser treatment, it is continued for a period of 1 week after laser treatment also. At 1 week post laser treatment oral acetazolamide can be discontinued if the IOP is <22 mm Hg, with continuation of topical IOP-lowering medications depending on the response. Review at 4 weeks provides information on IOP-lowering efficacy of the DLCP. After 4 weeks, if the IOP under medical treatment is persistently high on two consecutive visits separated by an interval of at least 1 week, a second session can be repeated in the inferior 180/270 degrees.

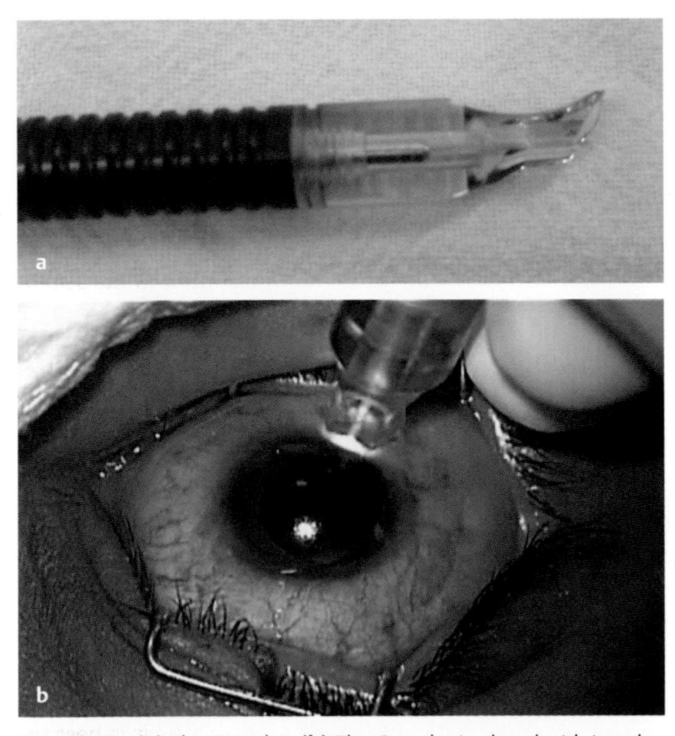

Fig. 20.10 **(a)** The G-probe. **(b)** The G-probe is placed with its edge at the limbus and is automatically centered 1.2 mm posterior to the limbus in the region of the ciliary body. (The images are provided courtesy of Dr Dewang Angmo, AIIMS, New Delhi, India.)

Complications

Complications seen include pain, intraocular hemorrhage, prolonged ocular inflammation, hypotony, visual loss, postoperative pain, and often the need for retreatment in 3 to 6 months. Hypotony may occur in a few patients, and phthisis has been reported in about 2%. Atonic pupil has also been reported in 28 to 50% and there is high risk of corneal graft failure seen.

Micropulse transscleral cycloablation appears to produce less damage to the surrounding tissues of the ciliary body, as it works in short bursts with rest times between pulses. High-intensity focused ultrasound for cycloablation is also being studied.

Endocyclophotocoagulation

This utilizes a 810-nm laser, through the limbal or pars plana approach, directly visualizing and photocoagulating ciliary processes. This is commonly used in conjunction with phacoemulsification, with a significant reduction in IOP with glaucoma medications, but is accompanied by a reported fall in vision of more than two lines in 1%, and cystoid macular edema in 0.7%.

Conclusion

Lasers are an important part of the armamentarium for glaucoma treatment today. The therapeutic status for lasers in glaucoma has increased over the years, as they are noninvasive, safer than incisional procedures, and efficacious in specified types and severities of glaucoma. *If not counseled adequately, patients may consider the laser therapy to be definitive for glaucoma, and become lax with medications and review.* It is important to use them judiciously, in appropriate eyes, and maintain a long-term review.

Cases

Case 1

A 40-year-old female presented with acute painful diminution of vision in left eye for 1 week, associated with headache and colored haloes. On examination, her baseline IOP was 24 mm Hg OD and 38 mm Hg OS. The anterior chamber was shallow in both eyes **Case 1-1a** with pupillary ruff atrophy in both eyes. Right eye had sectoral iris atrophy and a fixed dilated nonreacting pupil and circumcorneal congestion. Gonioscopy of left eye showed occludable angles with goniosynechia and right eye extensive synechial angle closure. Fundus examination revealed a cup:disc ratio near-total cupping in the right and 0.6 in the left eye (**Case 1-1b**).

Points to consider

- Total synechial closure indicates severe dysfunction of trabecular meshwork.
- Fluctuations in IOP due to intermittent angle closure are damaging to the optic nerve.
- Laser iridotomy would prevent further angle closure but not control chronically raised IOP.

Diagnosis and Management

A diagnosis of primary angle-closure glaucoma in both eyes was made. The patient underwent an Nd:YAG iridotomy after control of IOP with timolol–pilocarpine combination, and brinzolamide–brimonidine combination twice a day. In view of severe glaucomatous neuropathy in the left eye, systemic acetazolamide was given in addition to earlier topical drops for 3 days. An applanation phasing and perimetry at 3 to 4 weeks would allow an assessment to see if "target" IOP of 15 to 17 mm Hg in the lefteye and 10 to 12 mm Hg in the right have been achieved. Lifelong review was emphasized.

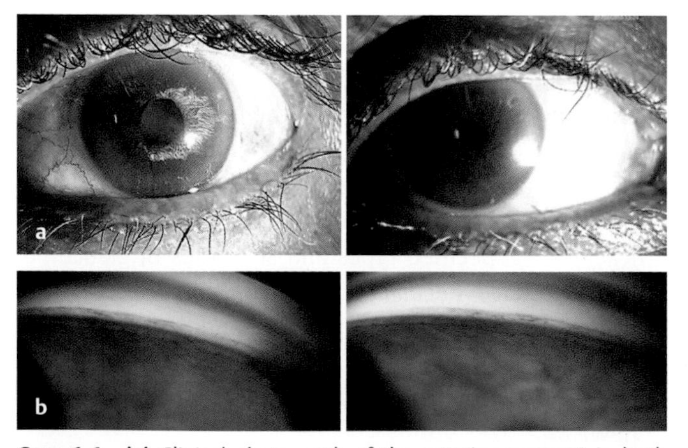

Case 1-1 **(a)** Clinical photograph of the anterior segment in both eyes showing shallow anterior chambers, pupillary ruff atrophy in the right eye, and sectoral iris atrophy in the left eye. **(b)** Gonioscopic appearance in the right eye of peripheral anterior synechiae and a densely pigmented trabecular meshwork. The left eye had a totally closed angle, and pigmentation seen is anterior to Schwalbe's line.

Case 2

A 47-year-old male presented with pain, redness, and watering over 2 months. On examination, baseline IOP was 36 mm Hg right eye and 38 mm Hg left eye. Anterior chamber was deep in both eyes (**Case 2-1**). Gonioscopy showed: Open angles with increased pigmentation and concave iris configuration in both eyes. Fundus revealed right eye: 0.3:1 and left eye: 0.4:1.

Points to consider

- Densely pigmented trabecular meshwork in an open angle.
- Concave iris configuration.
- Young male.

Diagnosis and Management

A diagnosis of pigment dispersion with ocular hypertension was made. The patient underwent 360 degrees SLT

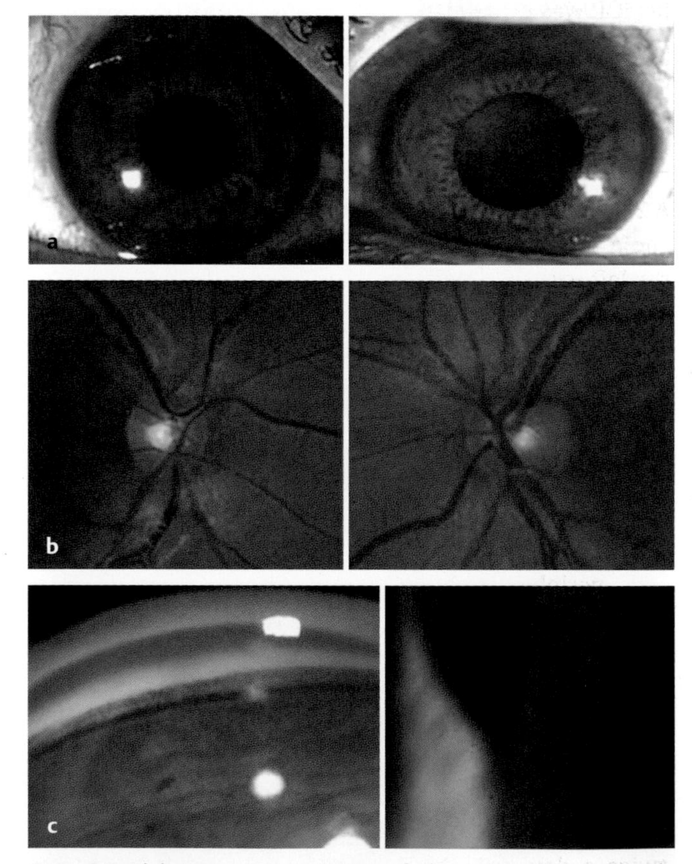

Case 2-1 **(a)** Dense pigmentation of the trabecular meshwork. **(b)** Krukenberg's spindle, linear pigment deposition in the central cornea. **(c)** Cup:disc ratio of 0.4 in both eyes, with normal neuroretinal rim color. (The images are provided courtesy of Dr Dewang Angmo, AIIMS, New Delhi, India.)

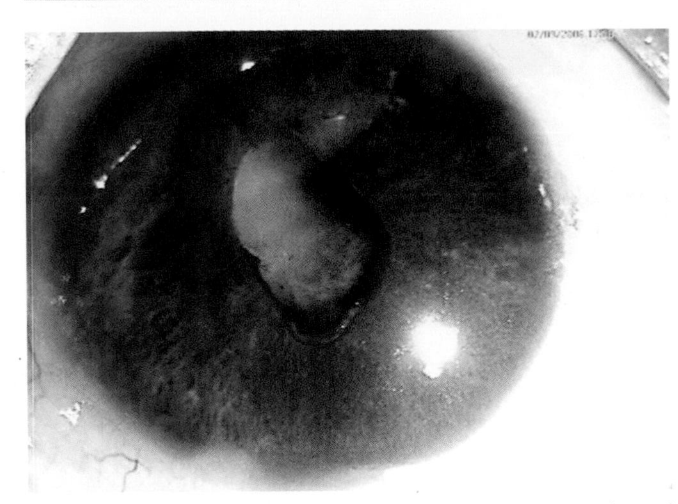

Case 3-1 Diode laser cyclophotocoagulation (DLCP) being performed in an eye with uveitic glaucoma.

in two sittings after medical control of IOP on four topical drugs. Over the next 3 months his IOP was well controlled and glaucoma medications were tapered. After 6 months his IOP was controlled to target 16/18 mm Hg on timolol twice a day alone. Lifelong follow-up was advised as the efficacy of the laser can wane over time.

Case 3

A 27-year-old female diagnosed as uveitic secondary glaucoma with a complicated cataract complained of pain in the left eye. On examination, visual acuity was 6/12 in the right eye; hand movements close to face and projection of rays inaccurate in the left eye, baseline IOP was 24 mm Hg right eye and 38 mm Hg OS. Anterior chamber was shallow in both eyes, with extensive posterior and peripheral anterior synechiae.

Points to consider

- Inaccurate projection of light, and extensive peripheral anterior synechiae.
- Risk of failure of filtering surgery.
- Possible decompensation of the cornea.

Diagnosis and Management

The patient underwent left eye: 270 degrees DLCP (**Case 3-1**) and an Nd:YAG iridotomy for the right eye, and after 6 months, her IOP was 16 mm Hg/18 mm Hg on timolol twice a day in both eyes and additional brinzolamide-brimonidine combination in the left.

Suggested Readings

Cai W, Lou Q, Fan J, Yu D, Shen T, Yu J. Efficacy and safety of argon laser peripheral iridoplasty and systemic medical therapy in Asian patients with acute primary angle closure: a meta-analysis of randomized controlled trials. J Ophthalmol 2019;2019:7697416

Chen MF, Kim CH, Coleman AL. Cyclodestructive procedures for refractory glaucoma. Cochrane Database Syst Rev 2019;3: CD012223

Chi SC, Kang YN, Hwang DK, Liu CJ. Selective laser trabeculoplasty versus medication for open-angle glaucoma: systematic review and meta-analysis of randomised clinical trials. Br J Ophthalmol 2020;104(11):1500–1507

Fleck BW. How large must an iridotomy be? Br J Ophthalmol 1990;74(10):583–588

Gazzard G, Konstantakopoulou E, Garway-Heath D, et al. Selective laser trabeculoplasty versus drops for newly diagnosed ocular hypertension and glaucoma: the LiGHT RCT. Health Technol Assess 2019;23(31):1–102

Gupta V, Ghosh S, Sujeeth M, et al. Selective laser trabeculoplasty for primary open-angle glaucoma patients younger than 40 years. Can J Ophthalmol 2018;53:81–85

Heijl A, Peters D, Leske MC, Bengtsson B. Effects of argon laser trabeculoplasty in the Early Manifest Glaucoma Trial. Am J Ophthalmol 2011;152(5):842–848

Lam DSC, Tham CCY, Congdon N. Peripheral iridotomy for angle-closure glaucoma. In: Shaarawy trabecular meshwork, Sherwood MB, Hitchings RA, Crowston JG, eds. Glaucoma. China: Saunders; 2009. Vol. 2: 61–69

Latina MA, Park C. Selective targeting of trabecular meshwork cells: in vitro studies of pulsed and CW laser interactions. Exp Eye Res. 1995 Apr;60(4):359–71

Michelessi M, Bicket AK, Lindsley K. Cyclodestructive procedures for non-refractory glaucoma. Cochrane Database Syst Rev 2018;4:CD009313

Bayliss JM, Ng WS, Waugh N, Azuara-Blanco A. Laser peripheral iridoplasty for chronic angle closure. Cochrane Database Syst Rev. 2021 Mar 23;3:CD006746

Robin AL, Eliassi-Rad B. Laser iridotomy. In: Morrison JC, Pollack IP, eds. Glaucoma: Science and Practice. New York, NY: Thieme; 2003:439–445

Song J. Complications of selective laser trabeculoplasty: a review. Clin Ophthalmol 2016;10:137–143

Wise JB, Witter SL. Argon laser therapy for open-angle glaucoma. A pilot study. Arch Ophthalmol. 1979 Feb;97(2):319–22

Zhang L, Weizer JS, Musch DC. Perioperative medications for preventing temporarily increased intraocular pressure after laser trabeculoplasty. Cochrane Database Syst Rev 2017;2: CD010746

Zhou R, Sun Y, Chen H, Sha S, He M, Wang W. Laser trabeculoplasty for open-angle glaucoma: a systematic review and network meta-analysis. Am J Ophthalmol. 2020 Sep 1:S0002-9394(20):30412–8

CHAPTER 21

Diagnosing and Managing Progression in Glaucoma

Overview

- Ideal Test for Detecting Glaucoma Progression
- Frequency of Testing and Review
- Quantification of Progression
- Identifying Progression
  - Clinical Evaluation
  - Disc Photography
  - Perimetry
  - Optical Coherence Tomography of Retina and Optic Nerve Head
  - Combined Structural and Functional Assessment
- Management of Progression in Glaucoma
  - General Risk Factors
  - Ocular Risk Factors
- Cases
- Suggested Readings

Introduction

Glaucoma is a chronic, progressive optic neuropathy with characteristic changes in the retina and optic nerve, resulting in corresponding visual field loss. *The goal of glaucoma therapy is to stabilize glaucomatous neuropathy and prevent further loss and visual morbidity within a patient's lifetime.* Therapy is aimed at reducing intraocular pressure (IOP) to a level commensurate with optic nerve head damage, *maintaining quality of life at a sustainable socioeconomic expense.*

Diagnosis of change is a prerequisite for the diagnosis of glaucoma, and identifying early progression is the cornerstone of management of glaucoma, so that therapy can be modified to prevent further loss. Perimetry is a psychophysical test and therefore inherently variable, additionally, *glaucomatous change on imaging and perimetry is unpredictable, linear in some patients, and with an erratic rate of change in some.*

Rates of change in primary open-angle glaucoma (POAG) eyes are generally slow, but there is a subset of individuals in whom progression can be much faster, leading to significant visual morbidity. Availability and use of effective glaucoma medications and safer surgery have decreased the occurrence of blindness due to glaucoma, and earlier identification of progressors, both slow and fast, would allow physicians to further decrease visual morbidity associated with glaucoma over time.

Detecting progression in glaucoma is difficult because of many reasons such as ongoing age-related ganglion cell loss, absence of objective and sensitive diagnostic techniques, and individually variable rate and pattern of progression among patients. There are also few long-term studies in different kinds of glaucoma that have arrived at definitive end points and definitions of progression. Studies have shown that morphological changes on the optic nerve head and retinal nerve fiber layer commonly occur prior to detectable perimetric loss, however, it is also seen that in some patients functional glaucomatous deficits can occur before structural change. *The World Glaucoma Association suggests that both functional and structural testing would allow earlier detection of change in more individuals, as some may progress on optic nerve head morphology first and others on perimetry first.* Correlation between structural and functional changes may also not be universal, as the *pathogenesis of glaucomatous optic neuropathy in different patients may result from permutations of ischemia, excitotoxicity, alterations in ocular perfusion pressure, and genetic predisposition to mechanical damage.* Age-related neural loss and the intertest/intratest variability further confound any analysis for progression.

Ideal Test for Detecting Glaucoma Progression

Ideal test for detecting glaucoma progression should:

- Distinguish test variability from progression.
- Be sensitive to very localized changes.
- Be sensitive to subtle changes.
- Provide an analysis of change with every test performed.

Clinically, each ophthalmologist has to make an informed decision on the effectiveness of therapy initiated in terms of a "target" IOP, risk of progression in a given individual, and structural and functional parameters over time. *Any suspicion of structural or functional change on a test in a patient needs to be repeated for confirmation, and correlated with clinical features.* Further, the appropriate change in therapy would differ based upon an assessment of benefit versus risk to an individual patient.

Frequency of Testing and Review

Frequency of testing and review of any test used for detecting progression in glaucoma should increase in eyes with:

- Greater severity of glaucomatous neuropathy.
- Inability to achieve target IOP in the long term.
- Fast rate of progression on perimetry and/or imaging.
- Presence of greater number of risk factors for progression.

In an eye with visual field defects in both hemispheres, and those where the defect is approaching fixation, where possible progression is highlighted on perimetry, or where target IOP is not achieved, a review every 3 months is necessary. In patients with mild glaucomatous optic neuropathy (GON) or those with moderate but stable perimetry with well-controlled IOPs to target, the review may be every 6 months.

For standard achromatic perimetry (SAP), Bengtsson et al estimated the rate of age-related loss as being 0.6 to 0.7 dB per decade, greater peripherally than centrally, and defined visual field progression based on three contiguous abnormal loci, to be associated with a mean deviation reduction by 2.26 dB.

The Advanced Imaging for Glaucoma study reported that a focal loss of ganglion cell complex (GCC) was the strongest single predictor for visual field (VF) progression, followed by any focal loss of peripapillary retinal nerve fiber layer. The combination of GCC focal loss volume with increasing age and decreasing central corneal thickness (CCT) was evaluated as a composite index called the "glaucoma composite progression index," which further improved the prediction of progression. *They considered an mean deviation slope of more than −0.5 dB/year or VF index of more than −1%/year as diagnostic of fast progressors.*

Quantification of Progression

Quantification of progression has been largely done in two ways:

- **Event-based analysis:** This looks for change by predefined criteria for progression, designated as an event, that vary with the tests studied. With respect to visual fields, an event is highlighted if a change from two baseline fields is significantly higher than test-retest variability at a given locus.
- **Trend-based analysis:** This describes linear change of parameters over time, and can represent both global change or at each location (**Flowchart 21.1**).

Identifying Progression

Various ways in which progression can be identified are:

- Clinical evaluation.

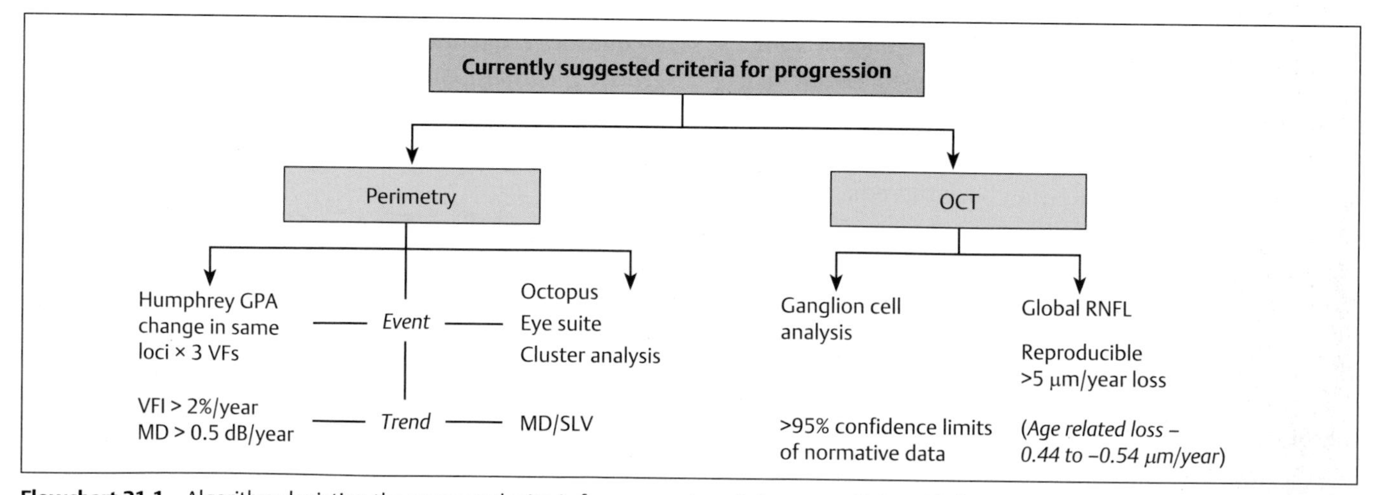

Flowchart 21.1 Algorithm depicting the suggested criteria for progression of glaucoma. GPA, guided progression analysis; MD, mean deviation; OCT, optical coherence tomography; RNFL, retinal nerve fiber layer; VFI, visual field index; VFs, visual fields.

- Photography.
- Perimetry.
- Imaging—optical coherence tomography and confocal scanning laser ophthalmoscopy.
- Combined structural and functional assessment.

The relationship between changes in structure and function differ in different patients, and therefore a combination of both diagnostic techniques, together with the clinical picture, is more likely to permit earlier diagnosis of change, i.e., progression.

A broken stick model of change is being used to describe the nonlinearity of the relationship between structure and function of the optic nerve in glaucoma. This was used to quantify the retinal nerve fiber layer loss at which visual field loss becomes detectable, after which functional tests may correlate with change. *In early glaucoma, imaging of the ganglion cell complex may highlight changes better than perimetry, and in severe glaucomatous damage, evaluation with 10-2 fields and ganglion cell complex may show up changes in the residual central field/retina* (**Flowchart 21.2**).

Clinical Evaluation

A good clinical examination and manual record of optic nerve head and retinal nerve fiber layer loss may be the only possible way to evaluate change in some situations. This examination should be performed with a dilated pupil, and after a laser iridotomy in primary angle-closure glaucoma (PACG) eyes. The use of a 78 or 90D at the slit lamp provides a stereoscopic view of the optic nerve head, permitting easy identification of the contour cup, small changes in the neuroretinal rim and retinal nerve fiber layer, and disc hemorrhages, etc. A careful diagram of the disc with any associated loss of retinal nerve fiber layer or hemorrhages may allow a gross comparison over time, but will not pick up early, subtle changes (**Figs. 21.1** and **21.2**).

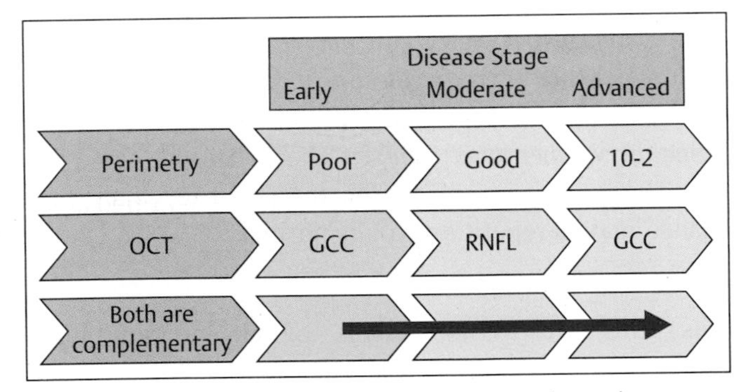

Flowchart 21.2 Best diagnostic technique to evaluate change over time in different severities of glaucoma. GCC, ganglion cell complex; OCT, optical coherence tomography; RNFL, retinal nerve fiber layer.

Disc Photography

Optic nerve head photography gives a permanent record of the disc and retinal nerve fiber layer, and changes in the neuroretinal rim, cup, or retinal nerve fiber layer can be identified on serial photography. The use of stereophotography permits better evaluation, but needs more expensive cameras. The ready availability and falling prices of fundus cameras make photography an important tool in the diagnosis and management of glaucoma. Photographs also highlight retinal nerve fiber layer loss around the disc, which can be serially assessed to diagnose progression (**Fig. 21.1**). Large randomized trials have used stereophotographs and dedicated "Reading" centers to assess change, but this was still subjective and subtle changes could not be detected.

The presence of the following characteristic features observed on examination, serial optic disc stereophotography or photographs, can indicate glaucoma progression:

- Increase in cup:disc ratio.
- Progressive neuroretinal rim loss.
- Increase in beta zone parapapillary atrophy.
- Presence of one or more disc hemorrhages.
- Appearance of retinal nerve fiber layer defects or widening of pre-existing retinal nerve fiber layer defects.

Fig. 21.1 Optic nerve head photograph of a patient having primary open-angle glaucoma (POAG). **(a)** Generalized thinning of the neuroretinal rim, with significant pallor and neuroretinal rim loss around 7 o'clock, accompanied by a wedge-shaped retinal nerve fiber layer defect. There is associated peripapillary atrophy, both alpha and beta zones, and baring of the circumciliary vessel seen. **(b)** After 8 years further extension of the thinning and pallor of the neuroretinal rim is seen extending from 6 to 7 o'clock with widening of the peripapillary atrophy.

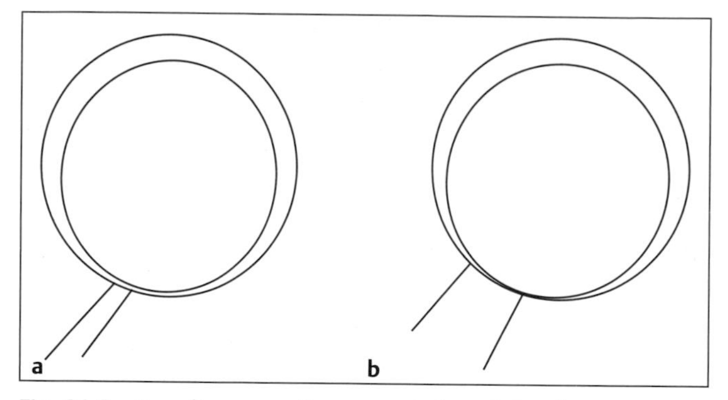

Fig. 21.2 Easy diagrammatic representation of the changes seen in **Fig. 21.1.** **(a)** Optic nerve head of a patient having primary open-angle glaucoma (POAG) at presentation. **(b)** After 8 years.

- Change in position of the vessels at the optic disc, e.g., baring of circumlinear vessels.

Perimetry

Standard achromatic perimetry, white on white, is the most common method of assessing functional changes in glaucoma, providing retinal sensitivity measurements at each locus. These can be compared over time, individually or against age-matched normative controls, to determine significant change over time.

Patterns of progression reported in order of frequency are:

- Deepening of existing defects.
- Expansion of defects.
- New defects.
- Second hemifield being affected.

Changes on review are evaluated in different ways, clinical evaluation, event- or trend-based analyses, as seen on Humphrey field analysis (HFA), guided progression analysis (GPA), and EyeSuite of Octopus, while scoring systems have been used in large-scale trials such as Advanced Glaucoma Intervention Study (AIGS) and Collaborative Initial Glaucoma Treatment Study (CIGTS).

Clinical comparison using individual fields or an overview printout can be done to assess obvious changes over time, but will not be able to pick out early, small but significant changes. It is useful for a general assessment, and can be quickly correlated with other ocular or systemic changes in the patient's presence. It is likely to be affected by the physician's expertise and training, and is subjective.

Criteria suggested by Zeyen and Caprioli to diagnose progression on individual fields are:

- *New defect:*
  - >10 dB loss in two or more contiguous points.
  - >5 dB loss in three or more contiguous points in a normal hemifield.
  - 10 dB difference at horizontal midline in two or more adjacent locations.
- *Progression of defect:*
  - Deepening by 10 dB.

Validated change can be assessed only against reliable baseline fields. *A good baseline of two reliable fields is essential for future comparison of visual fields to monitor for progression.* Due to the known learning curve for perimetry, two to three fields may have to be done initially before a reliable baseline can be set up. Unreliable fields will lead to an erroneous interpretation later. *The most important factors in obtaining reliable fields are a proper explanation of the test to the patient and monitoring by a trained technician.* If there are obvious learning defects, high false positive/negative errors (>15%), significant fixation losses (>20%), rim artifacts, scotoma due to drooping eyelids, and inadequate refractive correction, these examinations should be removed from any progression analyses. *Reestablish a new baseline after a significant therapeutic intervention such as cataract or any other ocular surgery.*

True progression should be differentiated from changes due to variability or fluctuation between tests. Fluctuation varies among patients and among sectors in the same visual field, and usually increases with severity of disease. *Progression on perimetry can only be confirmed if visual field defects are reproducible on at least two consecutive examinations, and there is clinical correlation with disc and retinal nerve fiber layer changes.* This is because some loci may show values reaching the threshold for change by chance, and on repetition will be normal.

Event-Based Analysis

This uses prespecified levels of change to define progression. A comparison is made of sensitivity values on a visual field, against a baseline of two reliable fields, to identify a change significantly higher than test-retest variability, at a $p < 0.05$, for a given locus. This is marked by an open triangle. *A significant change in the same three loci on two fields is labelled as possible progression, with a half black triangle, and if present on three consecutive fields as likely progression, with a black triangle, in the GPA of HFA.* This is based upon the findings of the Early Manifest Glaucoma Trial (EMGT). Event analysis has been thought to diagnose change earlier than trend-based analysis. As the patient's own responses are compared over time, it is not affected by age and differences in individual responses. *However, it does not take into account changes such as caused by cataracts, etc., that may have occurred over time, and is unable to distinguish glaucomatous loss from that due to other causes.*

Trend-Based Analysis

This uses linear regression of all available sequential global indices, visual field index (VFI), or individual locus sensitivity over a period of review to determine rates of loss. *The use of sequential fields provides a better picture of change, with an improvement in specificity and sensitivity. A minimum of five examinations over 3 years is required for this assessment.* It also provides an extrapolated projection of change for the next 5 years. A significant disadvantage is the fact that visual field loss is not always linear, and episodic or curvilinear changes may be missed. Changes in mean deviation over time may not reflect localized change, while pattern standard deviation (PSD) would reflect this only up to a moderate loss. In severe glaucoma, PSD may even show a decline and VFI could show variability.

This rate of progression is still being evaluated for threshold of significance over time, compared to changes with age and baseline damage. Aging produces a change of mean deviation of around 0.1 dB per year, and VFI of around 1% per year. Progression may be diagnosed with an mean deviation change of 0.5 dB per year, and a VFI change of 2% per year. Fast progressors have been variously described as those showing an mean deviation change of >1 dB per year and VFI deterioration of >5%. Catastrophic progressors are those with an mean deviation change of >2 dB per year.

VFI represents visual function as a percentage, with 100% being a normal age-adjusted visual field and 0% perimetric blindness. The central field is more heavily weighted, using five concentric rings of increasing eccentricity, and the percentage of loss is based on comparison with controls—pattern deviation in earlier loss, and total deviation for defects beyond −20 dB. VFI may miss early changes, but appears to be less influenced by progression of cataract, and hence may help determine progression in the elderly.

The GPA on Humphrey field analyzer averages the values of two reliable baseline fields, and compares them to every subsequent field, to highlight pointwise differences, beyond 95% confidence limits for intertest variability in stable glaucoma patients. This therefore provides a good assessment of actual glaucomatous progression. *There is a possibility of false positive diagnosis of progression if intertest variability is very high.*

The GPA printout on Humphrey field analyzer provides two baseline fields on top and the most recent inferiorly, with event analysis highlighting loci having a significant depression as triangles—open, half black, and fully black. Between them is a VFI plot recording trend over time. Rate of progression is provided as change of VFI per year, identifying "slow" and "fast" progressors. The VFI bar is a histogram of the patient's current visual field status and a projection for 5 years, with the underlying provision that the rate of change will remain linear and the same. High sensitivity and specificity have been found for GPA diagnosis of "likely progression" (**Figs. 21.3–21.6**).

Octopus perimeters have EyeSuite progression analysis using global trend analysis, corrected cluster trend analysis, and polar trend analysis. Global trend analysis looks at the global indices for stability, change, and rate of change. *The cluster trend analysis assesses cluster-specific progression within 10 nerve fiber bundle regions. Polar trend analysis facilitates the detection of spatially corresponding structural changes on the optic nerve head and visual field changes* (**Figs. 21.7** and **21.8**).

Pointwise Linear Regression

Pointwise linear regression assesses change over time at each locus, providing spatial information, a rate of change, and its level of significance. Therefore, *it is more likely to pick up early progression that may be present in only a few loci, as well as change in advanced glaucoma when threshold sensitivity approaches 0 dB.* However, this analysis does not factor in diffuse glaucomatous loss, media changes, and effects of aging on retinal sensitivity. This has been widely studied using PROGRESSOR software. Similar evaluations are being assessed, looking for change in the same two to three points or a cluster of points on consecutive fields.

A Glaucoma Rate Index (GRI) has been suggested, looking at VF locations with exponential decay or exponential improvement models. Each test location status is graphically represented as worsening, improving, or stable. Further the eyes can be classified as fast or slow progressors for appropriate therapy.

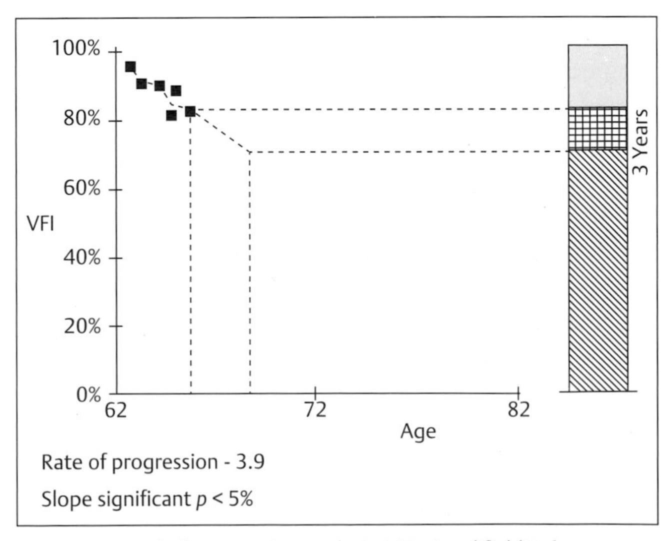

Fig. 21.3 Guided progression analysis. VFI, visual field index

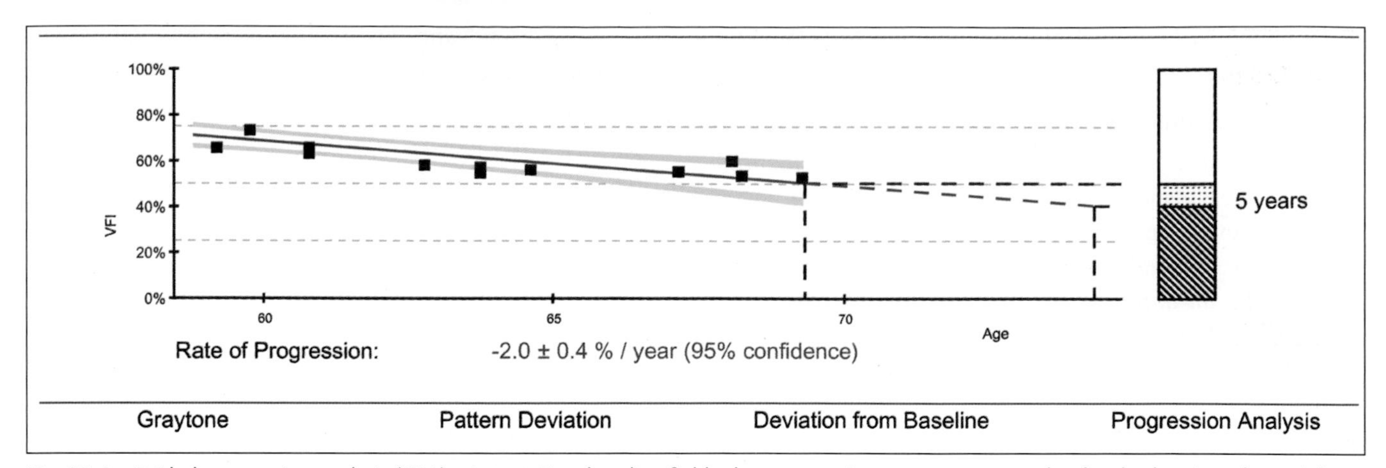

Fig. 21.4 Guided progression analysis (GPA) printout. Two baseline fields show a superior arcuate scotoma that has broken into the periphery, with a large inferior nasal step. Visual field index (VFI) trend analysis shows a downward slope, rate of progression of −2.0 dB per year, and change probability plot, event analysis, at last visit highlighting 12 loci of significantly depressed sensitivity seen in three fields at the same points. The GPA alert in *red* has labeled this as "likely progression."

Identifying Progression in Advanced Glaucoma

In advanced glaucomas there is an increased variability in responses, and there may be great unreliability when test locations have a sensitivity below 15 to 19 dB. *Changing the stimulus size from size III to V helps, as it has a dynamic range with low test-retest variability and perimetric contrast sensitivity increases with a size V stimulus.* Standard automated perimetry size V has eight distinct steps for change, with a floor of around 4 to 8 dB, and thus there is less variability of responses below 15 dB. *Changing the strategy to 10-2 improves detection of central field loss as it tests 68 locations in the central 10-degree field which are 2 degrees apart, thus increasing the likelihood of detecting central functional loss in these severely affected patients.* The use of kinetic perimetry can be considered in patients with advanced glaucoma and poor vision.

Frequency of Perimetry for Diagnosing Progression

Progression on perimetry occurs as a deepening or expansion of a prior scotoma, or development of a new scotoma. However, small defects or a generalized loss of sensitivity can occur as well. It is difficult to determine the frequency of testing in individual eyes, and the ophthalmologist needs to take into account the stage of glaucoma, proximity of visual field defect to fixation, reliability of perimetry done, life expectancy, and other systemic risk factors for progression.

To acquire the number of fields required for analysis and identification of fast progressors, two to three fields need to be done per year in the first 2 years. Variables such as pupil size, ambient light, etc., should be reduced. Thereafter fast progressors would need a change in therapy, a new baseline, and 6 monthly fields. Annual fields should suffice for slow progressors.

The frequency of follow-up of visual fields should be based on the extent of pre-existing damage, life expectancy of the patient, control to target IOP, presence of other risk factors, and structural progression as below:

- In low-risk/stable patients, at least one visual field per year.
- In moderate risk—two fields a year.
- In high risk but well-controlled IOP—two to three visual fields per year.
- In case of possible progression repeat fields within 1 to 3 months to validate the change.

Perimetric changes are not linear, and sudden changes can occur for which the ophthalmologist must stay alert. *Any perimetric change has to be correlated with optic nerve head appearance, as other pathologies such as anterior ischemic optic neuropathy (AION), retinal vascular occlusions, and pituitary adenomas can also lead to visual field changes over time.*

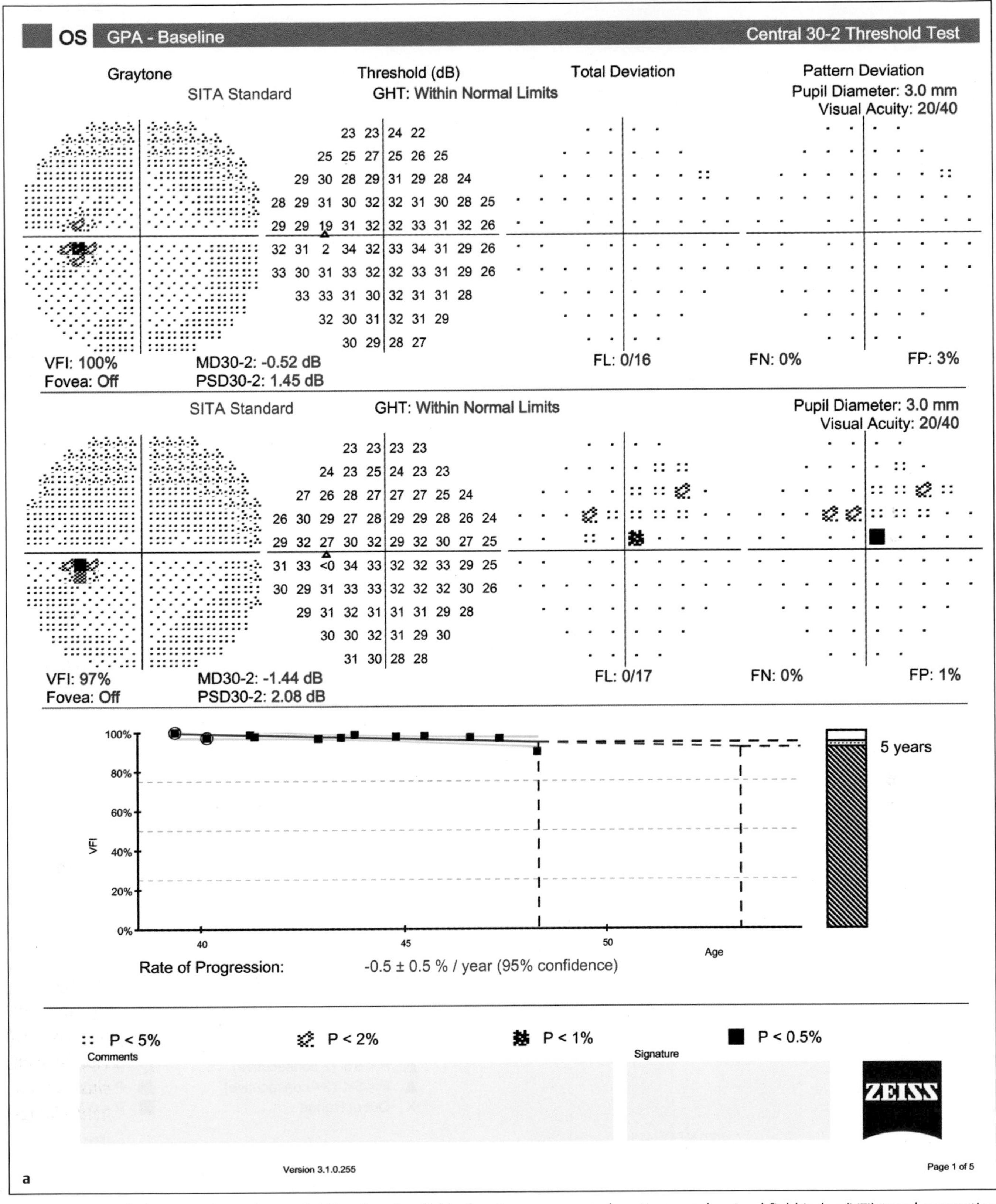

Fig. 21.5 A guided progression printout. **(a)** Two baseline fields showing a paracentral scotoma, and a visual field index (VFI) trend suggesting stability; rate of progression −0.5%/year. *(Continued)*

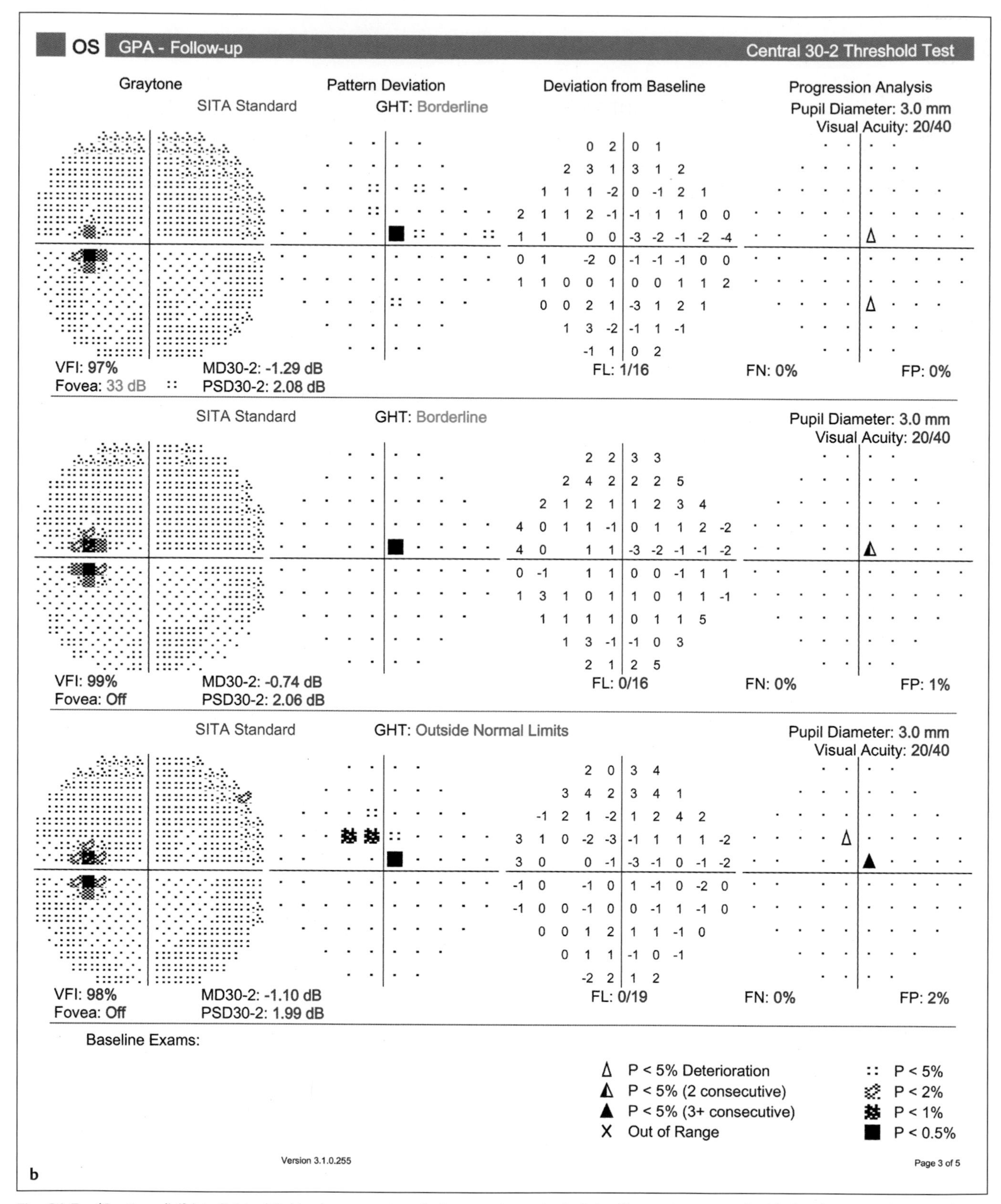

Fig. 21.5 *(Continued)* **(b)** Individual fields show event analysis; one to two loci of significant change are highlighted as triangles, but this is not progression as three loci are not affected.

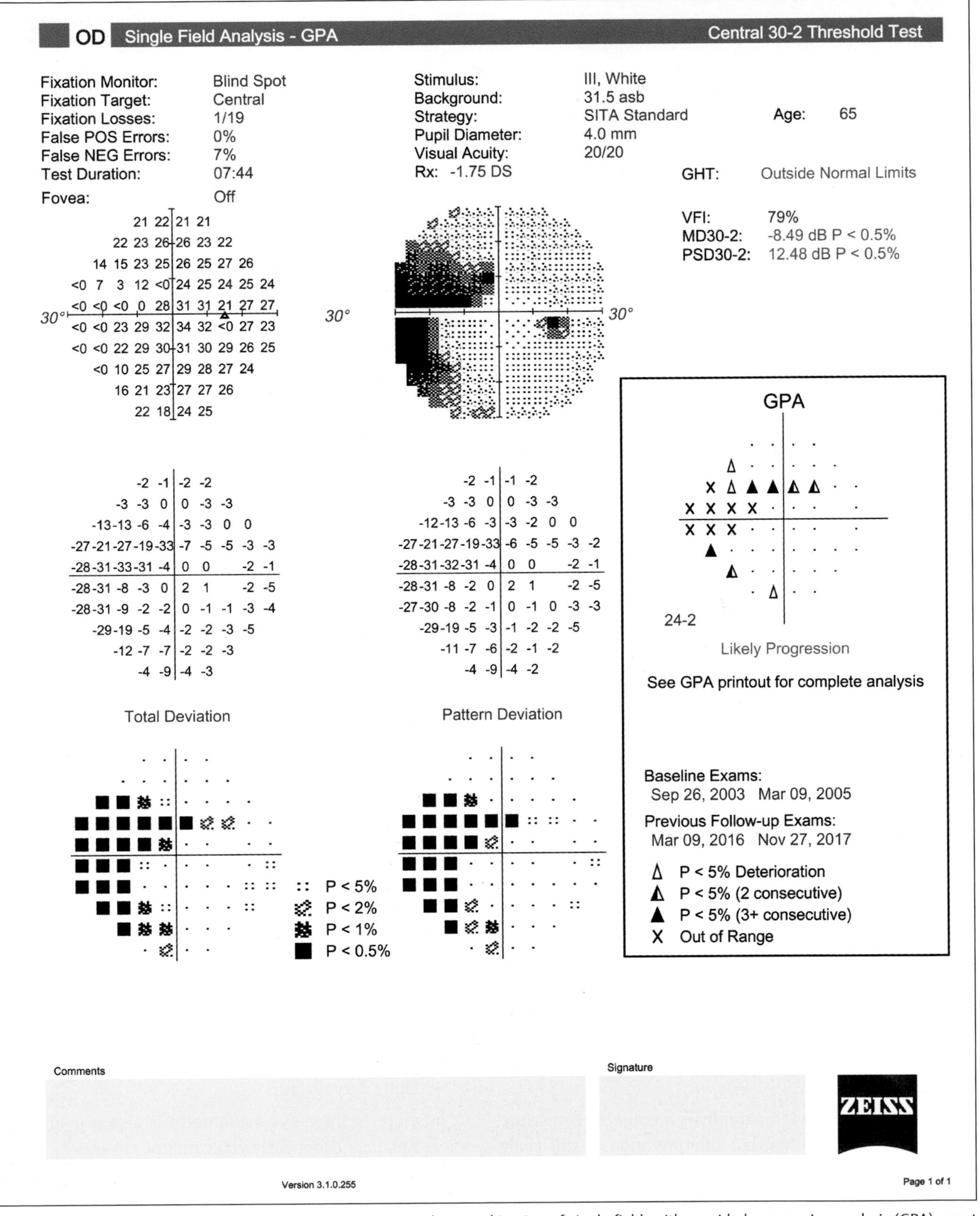

Fig. 21.6 Humphrey field analysis (HFA) printouts now provide a combination of single field, with a guided progression analysis (GPA) event analysis as well.

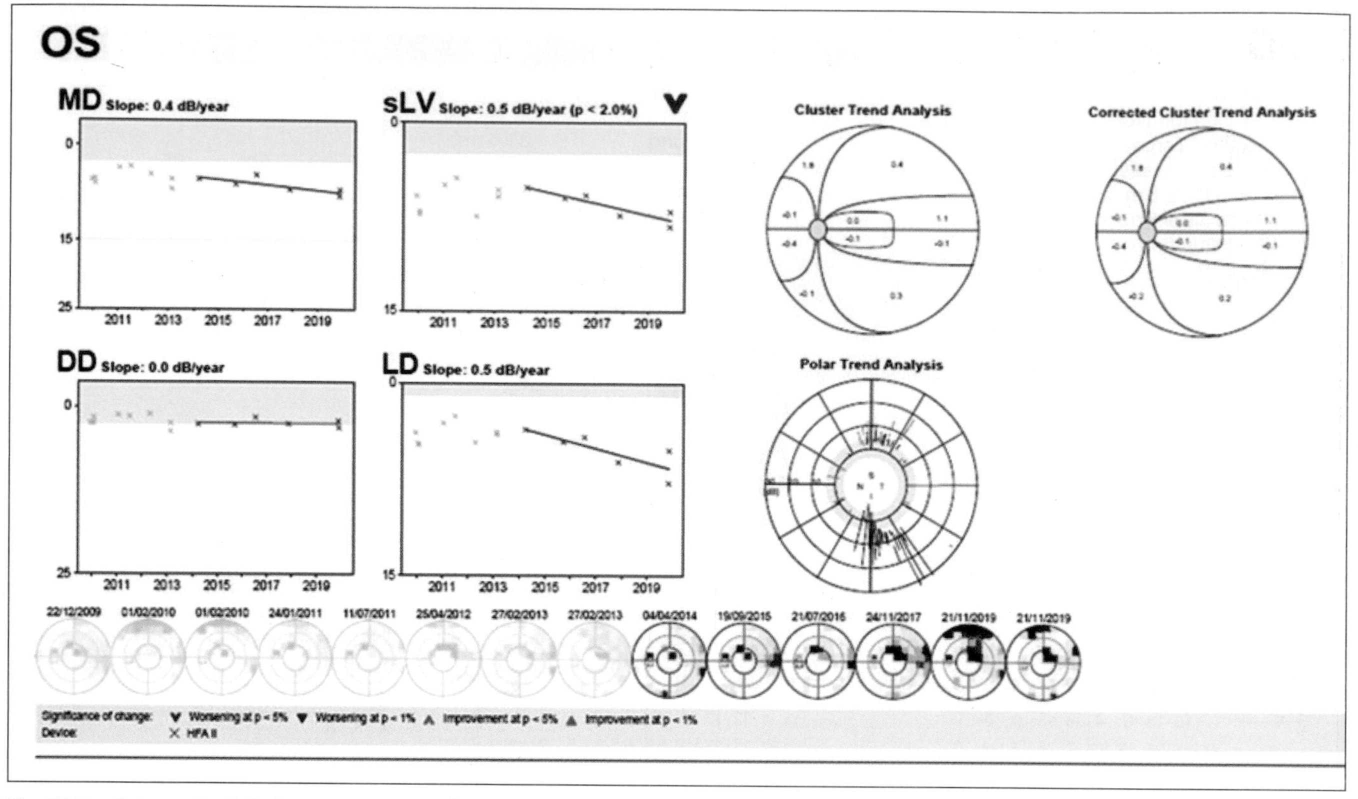

Fig. 21.7 Octopus EyeSuite for progression analysis.

Optical Coherence Tomography of Retina and Optic Nerve Head

As structural loss occurs before a visual field defect in many eyes, it has been suggested that optical coherence tomography abnormalities could precede visual field loss by 3 to 4 years in POAG suspects. Spectral domain optical coherence tomography provides the high resolution necessary for detecting early structural progression at the optic nerve head, retinal nerve fiber layer, and macula. With a faster scanning speed, eye tracking, and better axial resolution, spectral domain optical coherence tomography has less movement artifacts and less variability. This is seen to occur uniformly and affects all retinal layers, allowing evaluation of individual retinal layers. *Intertest variability may still affect the detection of smaller, sectoral changes if present.*

Optical coherence tomography is an objective measure of changes in glaucoma, but *interpretation is still being evaluated, with no consensus on end points of progression or age-related changes. Different machines have different ways of measurement and varying normative data, and cannot be interchanged or compared.* Interpretation has to be done keeping in mind the clinical picture of the eye, as optical coherence tomography cannot distinguish other ocular diseases or age-related changes from glaucoma. Edema, inflammation, epiretinal membranes, etc., can cause retinal nerve fiber layer, disc, and macular distortion and artifacts on optical coherence tomography that may not permit proper segmentation.

Optical coherence tomography abnormalities in glaucoma are assessed at:

- Retinal nerve fiber layer.
- Macula for ganglion cells.
- Optic nerve head.

A measure of inter-eye asymmetry is also provided as a means of diagnosing early glaucomatous changes.

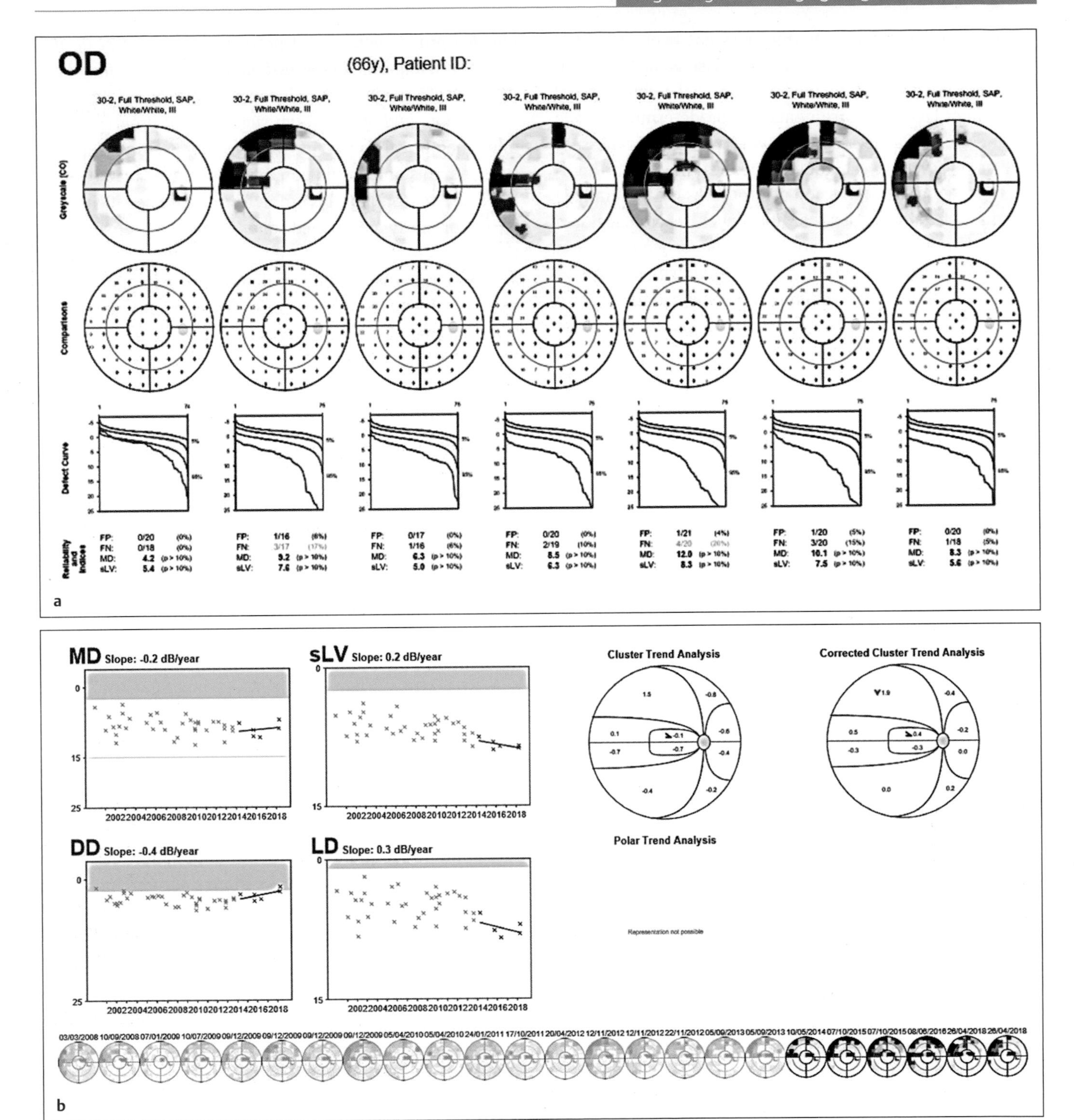

Fig. 21.8 (a, b) Octopus EyeSuite showing progression over time. Trend analysis to the left shows a gradual decline in mean deviation and SLV. The diffuse defect (DD) is within normal limits, but localized defect (LD) shows a significant loss. The area of loss is highlighted on the corrected cluster trend analysis with a *black arrow* in the superior temporal area.

Retinal nerve fiber layer thickness has been evaluated for a while, but average or quadrant-wise values have not been found to correlate well with visual fields. Retinal nerve fiber layer measurements at a predetermined circle around the optic nerve head provide average thickness, as well as thickness of each quadrant. Focal thinning is highlighted in guided progression printouts, as is a generalized thinning of the retinal nerve fiber layer. *It was suggested that a thinning by 5 µm may be specific for glaucomatous progression, but this has not been validated. Progressive retinal nerve fiber layer thinning may be a biomarker for a higher risk of visual field progression, compared with those without progressive thinning.*

Macular scans highlight retinal ganglion cell loss in glaucoma, as this area contains more than 50% of the retinal ganglion cells. The macula is avascular with a multilayered structure that is easily interpreted. It also has less interindividual variability as compared to optic nerve head and retinal nerve fiber layer parameters. *It has been reported that macular retinal nerve fiber layer + ganglion cell layer (GCL) + IPL thickness, retinal nerve fiber layer thickness, and total macular thickness are better at diagnosing early glaucomatous change* (i.e., a change from suspect to glaucoma). *Similarly, in advanced glaucoma when the loss of retinal nerve fiber layer has reached "floor level," macular scans may help detect change over time.* However, other macular diseases occur around the same age as glaucoma, diabetic macular edema, age-related macular degeneration, and epiretinal membranes, and therefore macular scans cannot be used for detecting glaucomatous progression in such patients.

Optical coherence tomography parameters on the optic nerve head are disc and rim area, cup:disc ratio, and rim width. *Bruch's membrane opening (BMO)–minimum rim width (MRW) is thought to reflect structure–function relationships better, measuring rim from the actual outer border to the inner limiting membrane, the point where axons traverse the edge of the disc.* A loss of about 25% at this point has been reported to result in visual field loss.

In optical coherence tomography machines, the software analyzes sequential scans to detect progressive changes, again either as an event or a trend. As in perimetry, event analysis compares at least two subsequent optical coherence tomography scans to two baseline tests, and when the difference crosses a predetermined threshold, greater than possible test-retest variability, progression is diagnosed. *If the change is seen for the first time, this is highlighted in yellow with a diagnosis of possible progression, and if present on the next scan, it is colored red and called progression. A retinal nerve fiber layer decrease of 5 µm in a sector is considered to be suspicious for progression, and of 7 to 8 µm suggestive of progression.* As only one optical coherence tomography is compared with baseline, this analysis is possible with fewer tests, but for the same reason may be prone to inaccuracies if the scan is not properly performed, and aligned. To ensure that the same areas are compared, eye tracking is employed and post processing with realignment of images can be done. *A difference of 9 µm in average retinal nerve fiber layer thickness between eyes is suggestive of early glaucoma* (**Figs. 21.9** and **21.10**).

Trend analysis looks at the change in quantitative parameters over time, generating a rate of change. All optic disc, retinal nerve fiber layer, or macular parameters can provide a slope of change, which may or may not be statistically significant. *The first scan at which a significant slope is seen is highlighted in yellow, and if present after the next examination, it is colored red.* The diagnosis of progression becomes more clinically relevant if the confidence intervals provided are tighter. Unlike event analysis, a large number of scans have to be available for trend analysis which makes it less prone to an outlying scan with artifacts, but would also be less likely to pick up very early progression (**Fig. 21.11**).

The macula has less interindividual variability as compared to retinal nerve fiber layer or optic nerve head, and has very few large vessels. Asymmetry across the horizontal meridian of more than 5 µm is suggestive of a suspect developing early glaucoma, while a ganglion cell inner plexiform layer (GCIPL) thickness change of more than 4 µm over time is possible glaucomatous progression. This change at the macula is seen as an arcuate defect on both thickness and change maps (**Fig. 21.12**). RTVue optical coherence tomography also provides global and focal loss volume to pick up early changes.

Diagnosis of progression on optical coherence tomography has to take into account *age-related thinning* of both retinal nerve fiber layer and macula. A thinning of retinal nerve fiber layer by 0.2 to 0.5 µm per year has been reported, with thicker baseline retinal nerve fiber layer eyes showing a greater decrease. Macular thickness reduces by about −0.25 µm annually. *Rate of change on progression has also been suggested to be larger in suspects and eyes with mild glaucoma than those having severe glaucoma due to the fact that fewer fibers remain.*

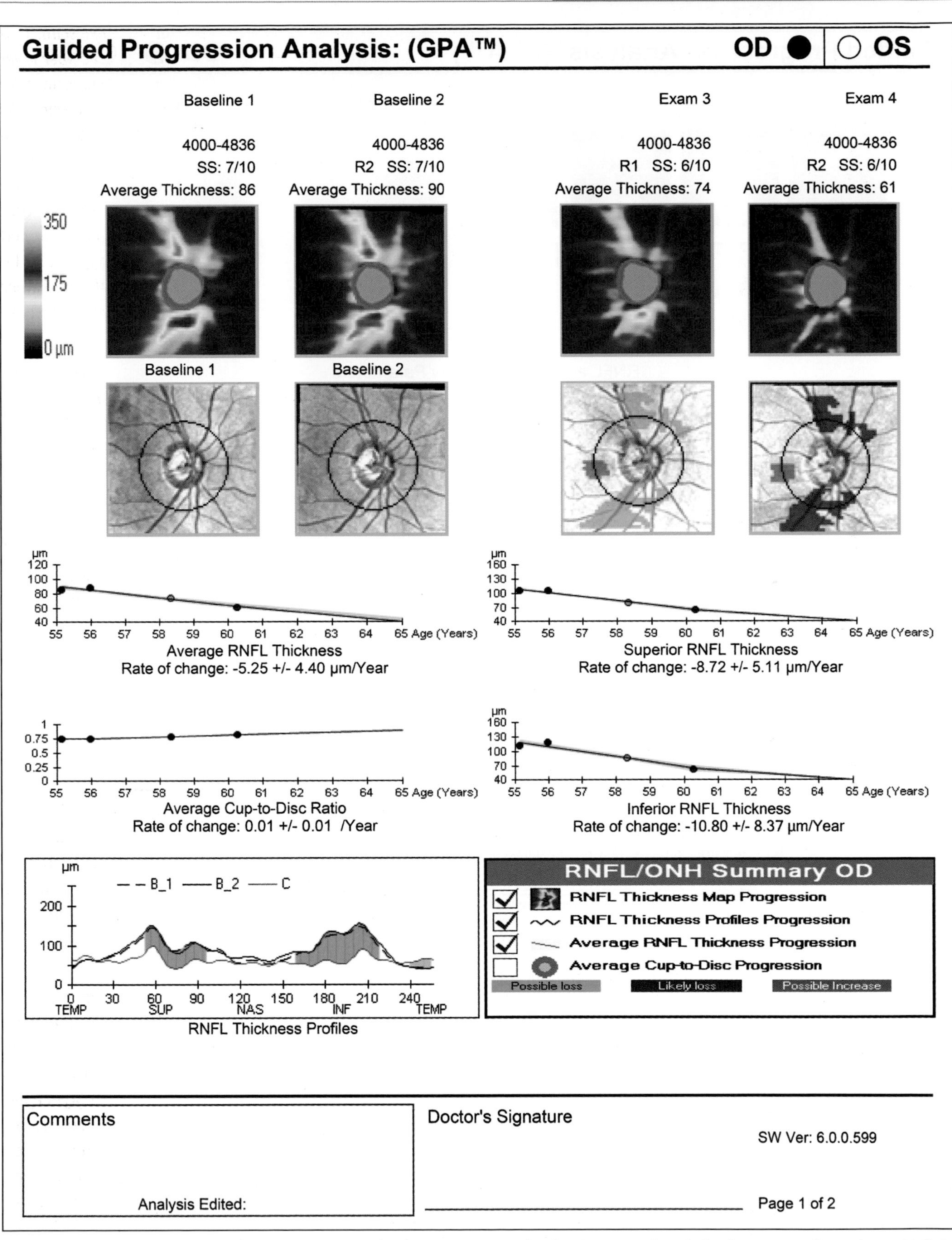

Fig. 21.9 Guided progression analysis on Cirrus optical coherence tomography showing a trend analysis of average and superior and inferior retinal nerve fiber layer, as well as cup:disc ratio. Loss in significant areas, akin to event analysis, is highlighted in the gray scale fundus picture images, and the TSNIT graph. *Yellow* represents possible loss, *red* is likely loss, and *purple* highlights a possible increase.

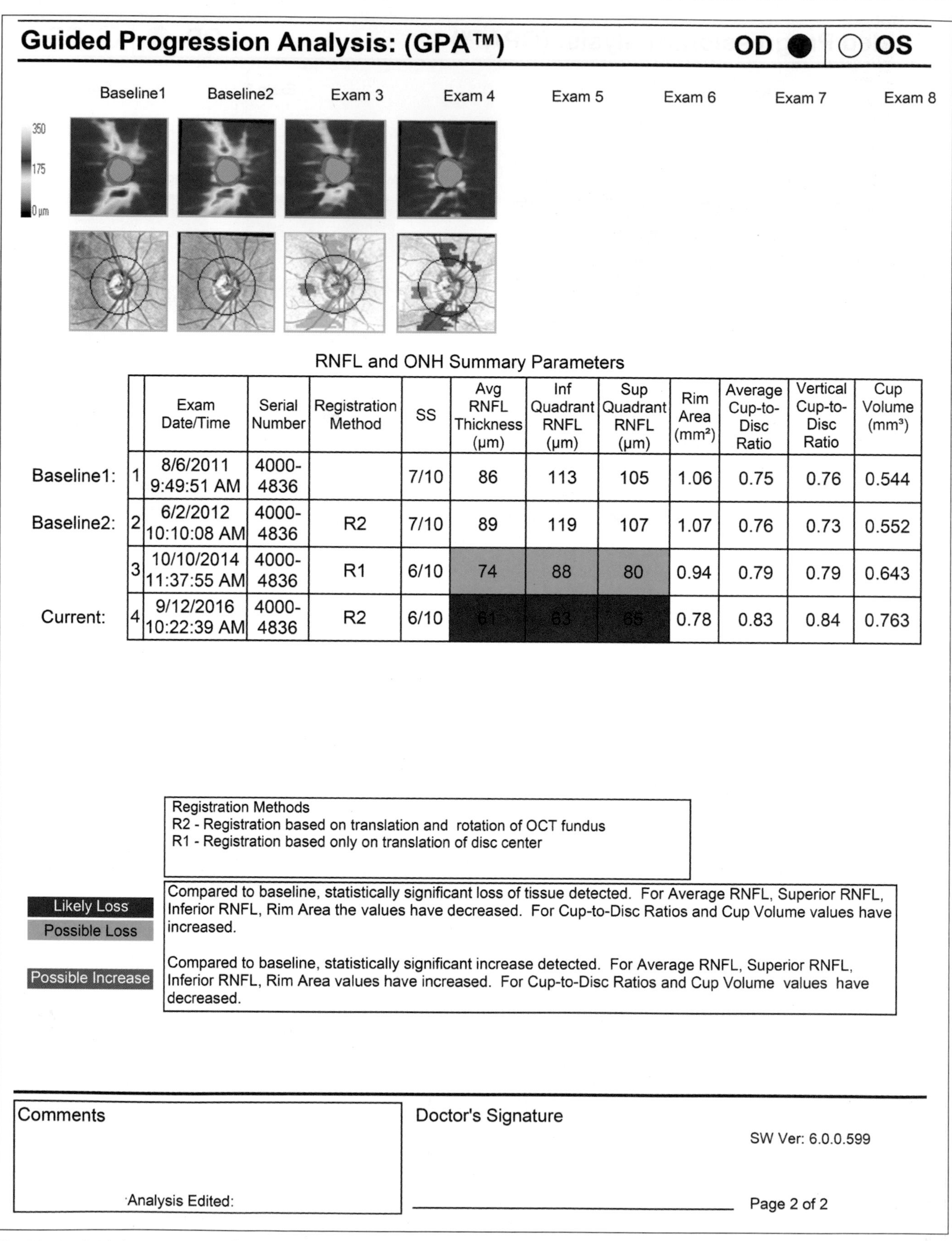

Guided Progression Analysis: (GPA™) OD ● ○ OS

Baseline1 Baseline2 Exam 3 Exam 4 Exam 5 Exam 6 Exam 7 Exam 8

350
175
0 µm

RNFL and ONH Summary Parameters

		Exam Date/Time	Serial Number	Registration Method	SS	Avg RNFL Thickness (µm)	Inf Quadrant RNFL (µm)	Sup Quadrant RNFL (µm)	Rim Area (mm²)	Average Cup-to-Disc Ratio	Vertical Cup-to-Disc Ratio	Cup Volume (mm³)
Baseline1:	1	8/6/2011 9:49:51 AM	4000-4836		7/10	86	113	105	1.06	0.75	0.76	0.544
Baseline2:	2	6/2/2012 10:10:08 AM	4000-4836	R2	7/10	89	119	107	1.07	0.76	0.73	0.552
	3	10/10/2014 11:37:55 AM	4000-4836	R1	6/10	74	88	80	0.94	0.79	0.79	0.643
Current:	4	9/12/2016 10:22:39 AM	4000-4836	R2	6/10	61	63	65	0.78	0.83	0.84	0.763

Registration Methods
R2 - Registration based on translation and rotation of OCT fundus
R1 - Registration based only on translation of disc center

Likely Loss
Possible Loss

Compared to baseline, statistically significant loss of tissue detected. For Average RNFL, Superior RNFL, Inferior RNFL, Rim Area the values have decreased. For Cup-to-Disc Ratios and Cup Volume values have increased.

Possible Increase

Compared to baseline, statistically significant increase detected. For Average RNFL, Superior RNFL, Inferior RNFL, Rim Area values have increased. For Cup-to-Disc Ratios and Cup Volume values have decreased.

Comments

Analysis Edited:

Doctor's Signature

SW Ver: 6.0.0.599

Page 2 of 2

Fig. 21.10 Guided progression analysis on Cirrus optical coherence tomography highlighting significant qualitative and quantitative changes on each test.

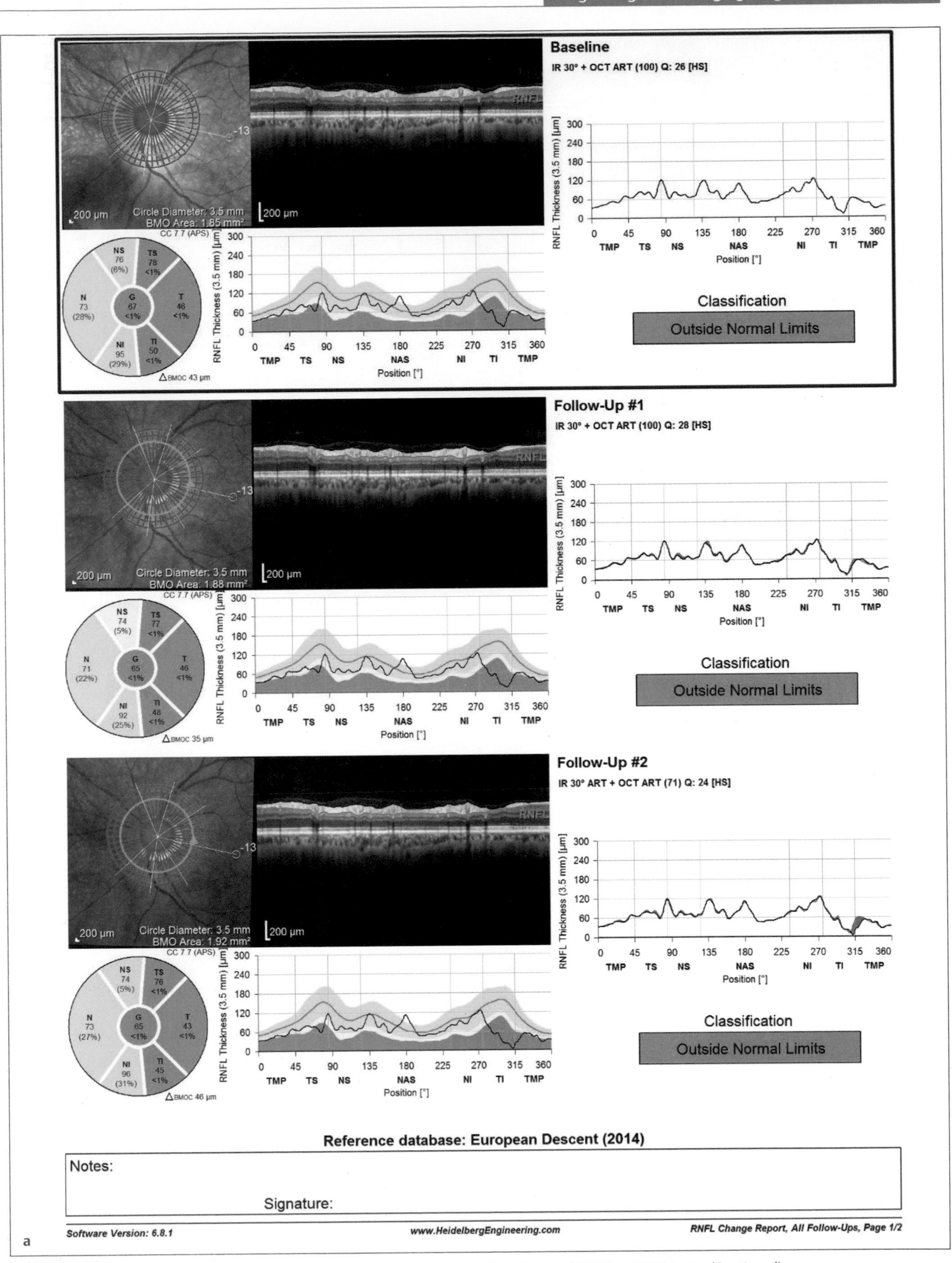

Fig. 21.11 Spectralis tracking laser tomography analysis. **(a)** Overview of baseline and 2016 to 2017 tests. *(Continued)*

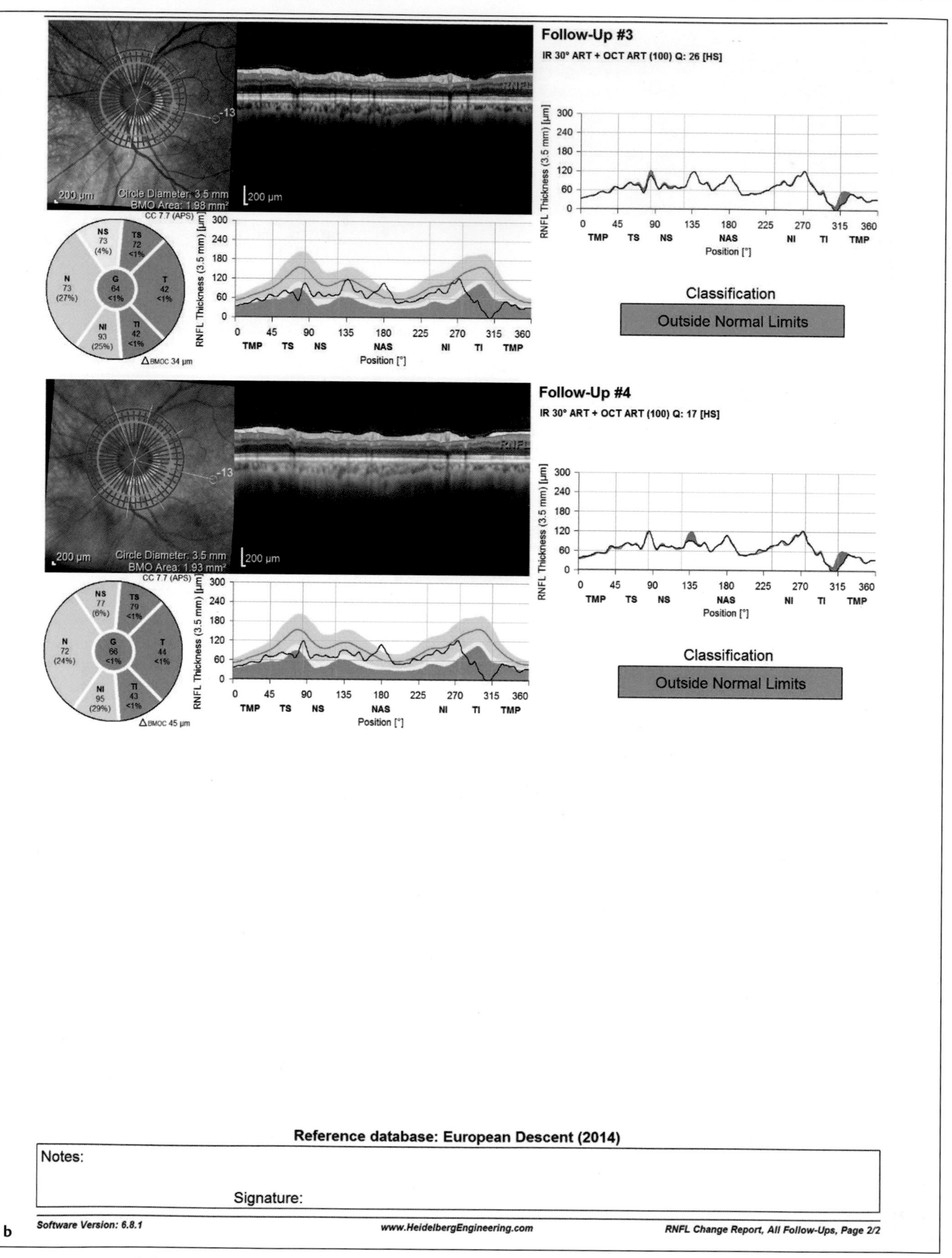

Fig. 21.11 *(Continued)* **(b)** Overview of further 2017 tests.

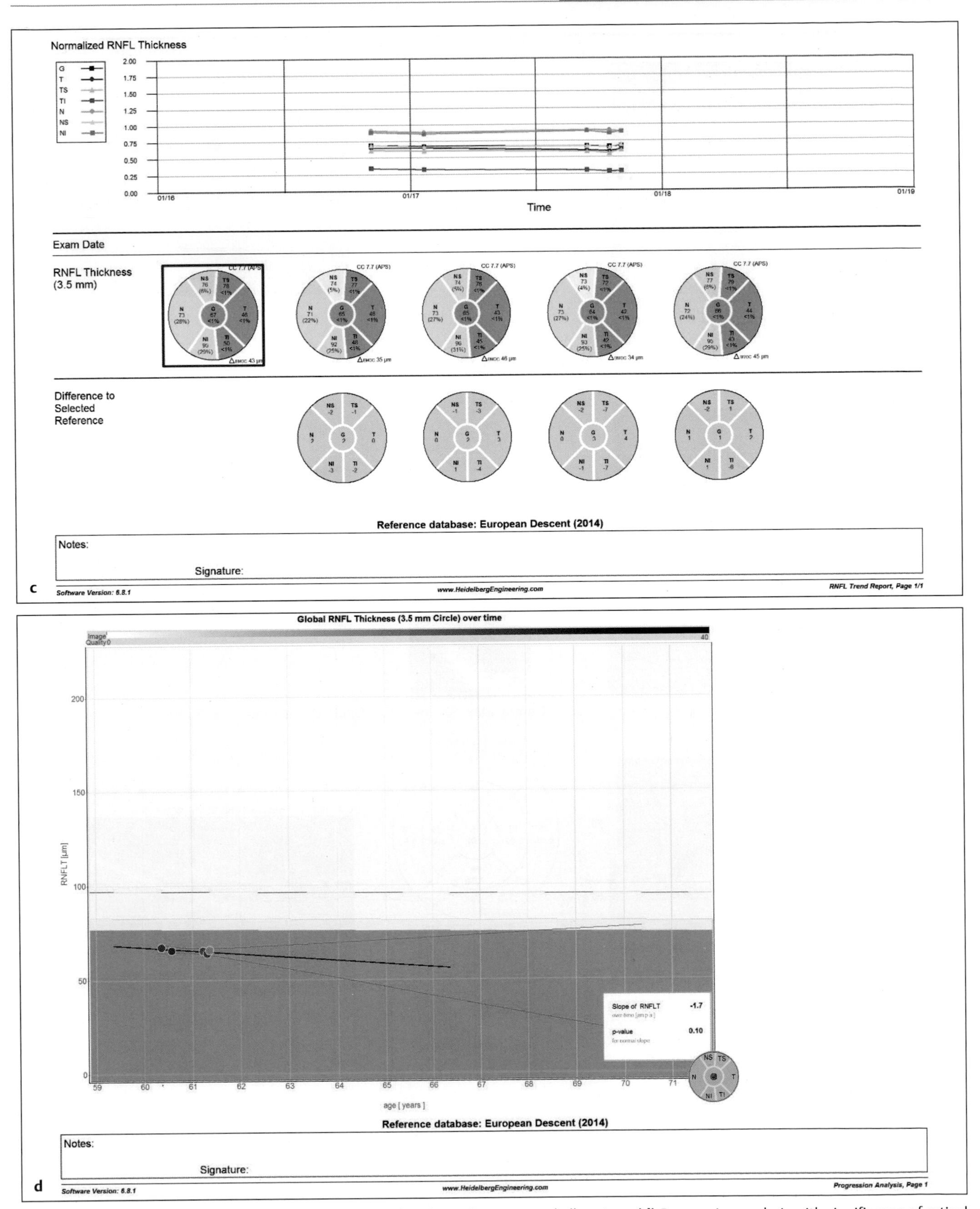

Fig. 21.11 *(Continued)* **(c)** Retinal nerve fiber layer trend analysis of average and all sectors. **(d)** Progression analysis with significance of retinal nerve fiber layer thickness change over time.

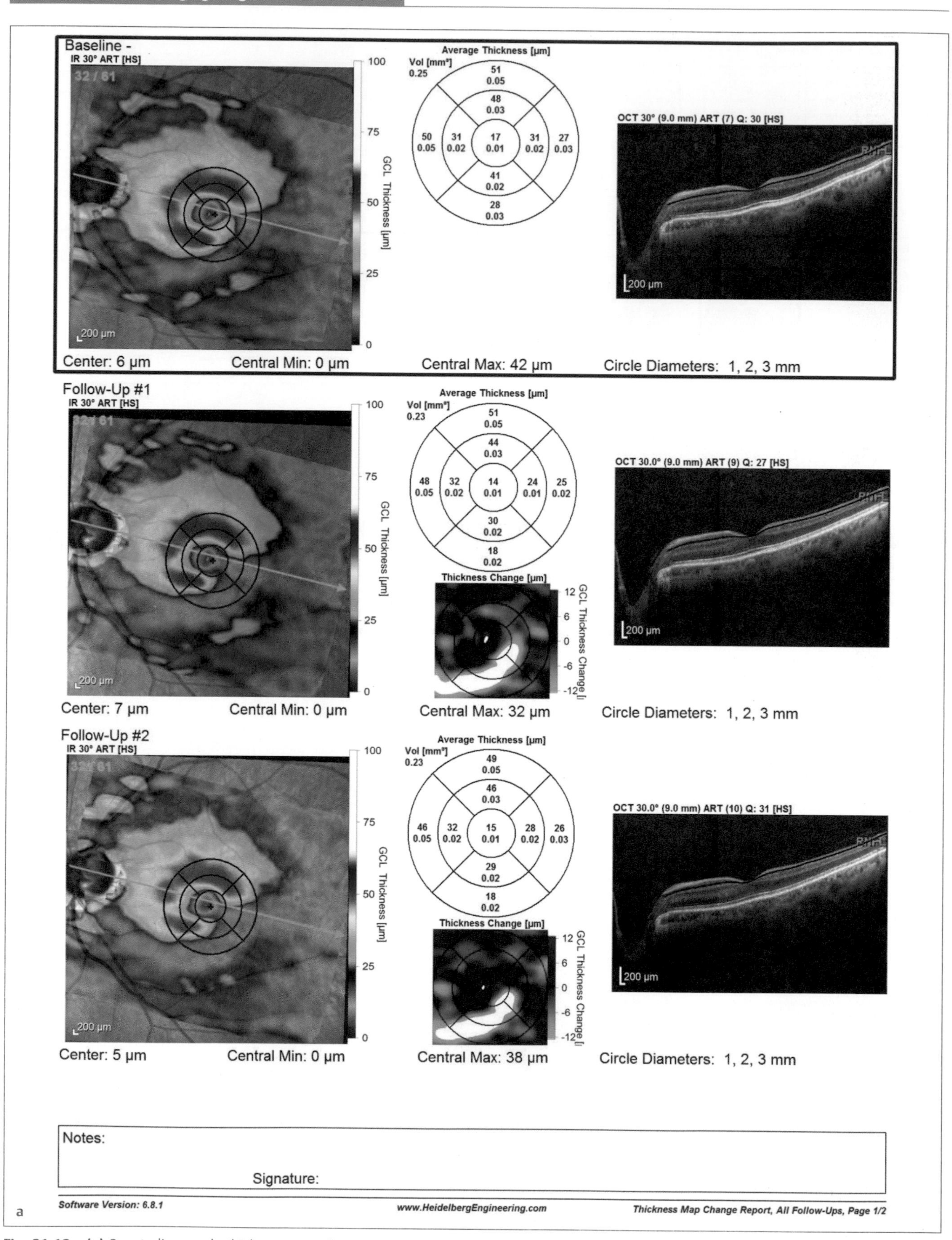

Fig. 21.12 **(a)** Spectralis macula thickness map change report providing information about thickness and volume, and a map of ganglion cell layer (GCL) thickness change over time. *(Continued)*

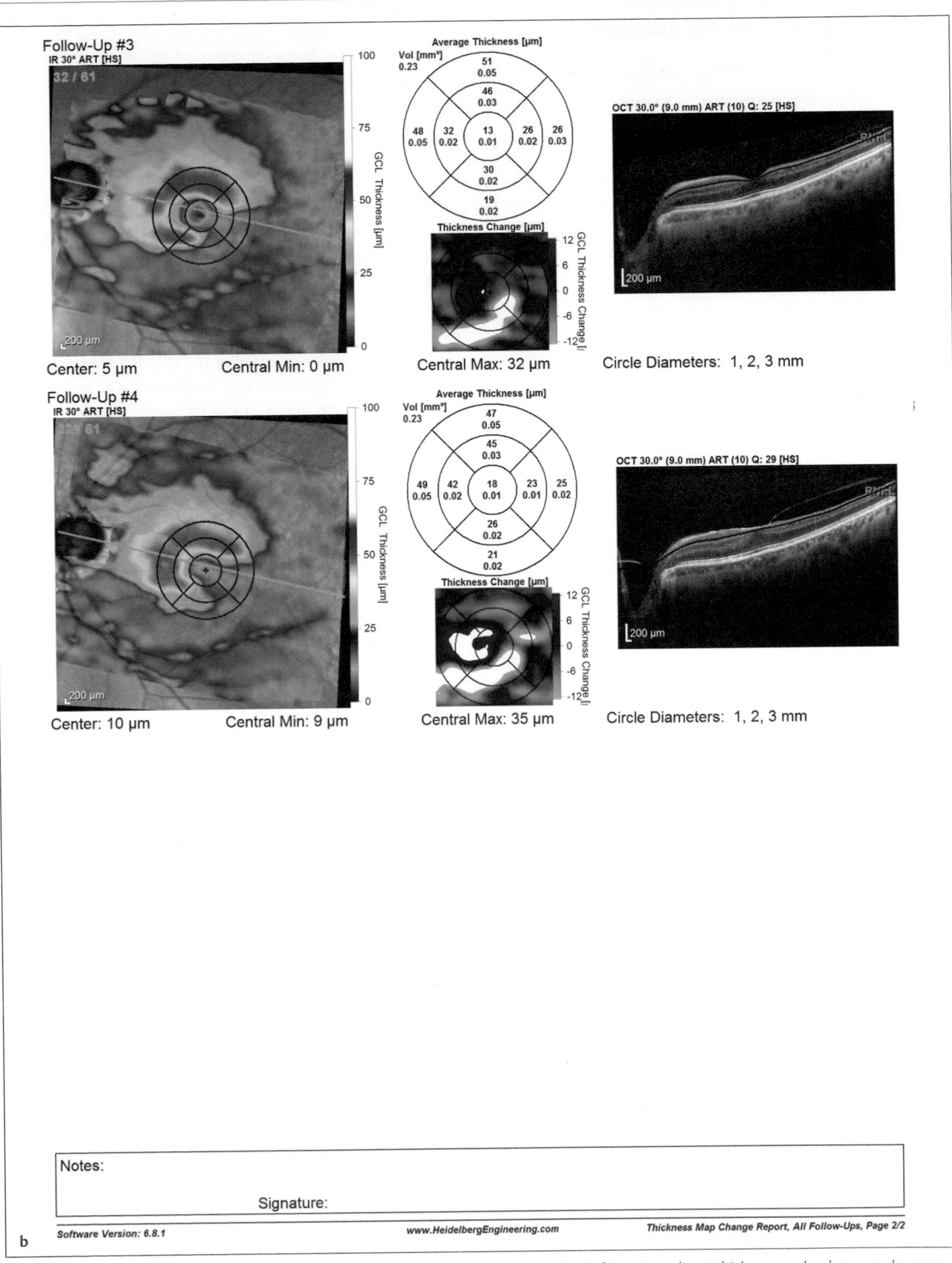

Fig. 21.12 *(Continued)* **(b)** Spectralis macula thickness map change report providing information about thickness and volume, and a map of ganglion cell layer (GCL) thickness change over time.

Combined Structural and Functional Assessment

Models combining functional and structural loss in glaucoma patients have been suggested, as some patients are seen to progress initially with either or both. The Hood Glaucoma report anatomically aligns optical coherence tomography scans and 10-2 and 24-2 visual field points to identify subtle changes in retinal nerve fiber layer over time. Many researchers are looking at ways to combine structure and function into one metricand a single printout. The polar trend analysis on Octopus perimeters combines pointwise linear regression analysis of focal defects with optical coherence tomography–based nerve fiber analysis at the disc margin.

Management of Progression in Glaucoma

Ophthalmologists should be looking out for known risk factors for progression among their patients.

General Risk Factors

- Strong family history.
- Socioeconomic status.
- Extremes of age—elderly and the young.
- Cardiovascular disease—systemic hypotension, transient ischemic attacks (TIA), migraine.
- Steroid use.

Ocular Risk Factors

- Severe glaucoma at baseline.
- Intervisit IOP fluctuations.
- Thin cornea.
- Disc hemorrhage.
- Myopia.
- Pseudoexfoliation.

Putting together structural and functional evaluations, clinical features, imaging, and perimetry, changes are likely to be seen as deepening or expansion of an existing loss and later as new areas of loss. It is incumbent on the ophthalmologist to look more carefully in such areas to pick up early changes. *Any test showing change needs to be repeated to see if it is reproducible, and then if it can be corroborated with other tests and clinical examination.* Changes due to other diseases or artifacts must be ruled out.

As already stated there are no universally accepted defined thresholds for progression or of target IOP. The ophthalmologist has to take into consideration many factors for determining progression to be present, and factors such as stage of the disease, age, systemic status, and socioeconomics, etc., to decide on further action (**Flowchart 21.3**).

The importance of both the mean IOP on review and high intervisit fluctuations in IOP has been shown in progression of glaucomatous eyes. It is therefore important to reduce fluctuations in IOP by better compliance and timely use of medications as per the drug's known duration of action. Medications prescribed to be used thrice a day must be put at 8-hour intervals to cover the day, for example, 6 am, 2 pm, and 10 pm, twice a day drops every 12 hours, 7 am and 7 pm or 6 am and 6 pm as convenient to the patient, and once a day drops at the same time every day.

Slow rates of progression, mean deviation change of <1 dB per year or a rate of progression on trend analysis of <1 to 4% per year, especially in older patients with mild to moderate glaucoma may not need a drastic change in therapy, but would warrant a closer review with repeat optical coherence tomography and perimetry (**Fig. 21.13**). In younger patients, juvenile open-angle glaucoma with such changes, target IOP range must be lowered, as increasing life expectancy means that there is a greater possible progression over time.

Rapid rates of progression, mean deviation change >1.5 dB or >2 dB per year or a rate of progression on trend analysis of >4 to 5% per year, especially in severe glaucoma, patients with a family history of glaucoma blindness, or in young patients, should lead to a lowering of "target" IOP with additional medications or surgery.

A new baseline should be marked out for perimetry and optical coherence tomography so that further rates of change or increases in perimetric loci affected can be easily seen, and the efficacy of changes in therapy evaluated.

Additionally, other systemic factors for vascular perfusion such as systemic hypotension, sleep apnea, history of transient ischemic attacks, etc., must be investigated and treated.

Bayesian modeling, big data analysis, machine learning, and artificial intelligence are all being used to determine actual change from variability. The search for better perimetry and imaging in glaucoma continues with analysis of small changes over time becoming possible and also more reproducible. Clinical examination, fundus photographs, perimetry, and imaging need to be put together so that the efficacy of therapy or its modifications can stabilize glaucoma.

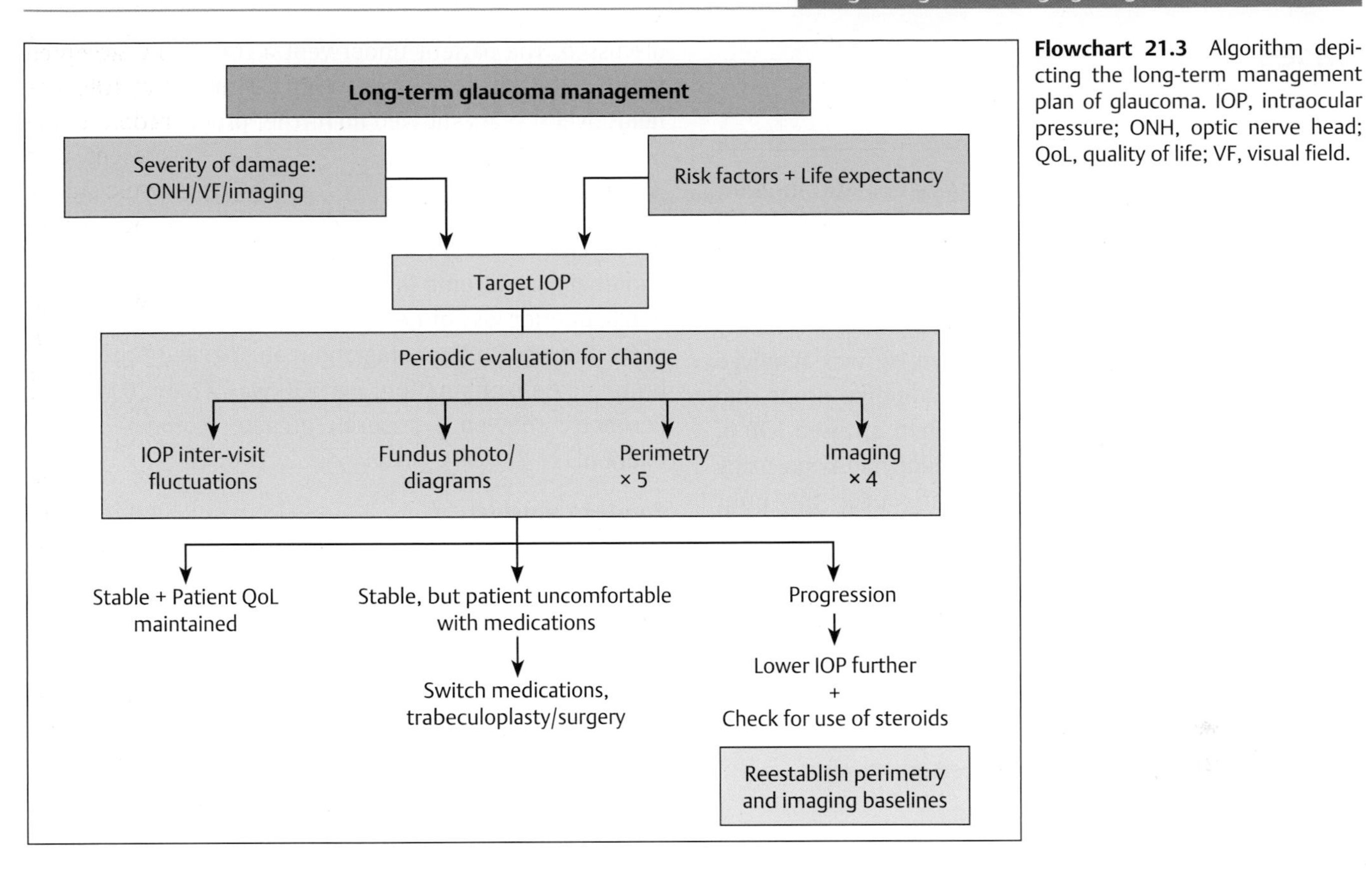

Flowchart 21.3 Algorithm depicting the long-term management plan of glaucoma. IOP, intraocular pressure; ONH, optic nerve head; QoL, quality of life; VF, visual field.

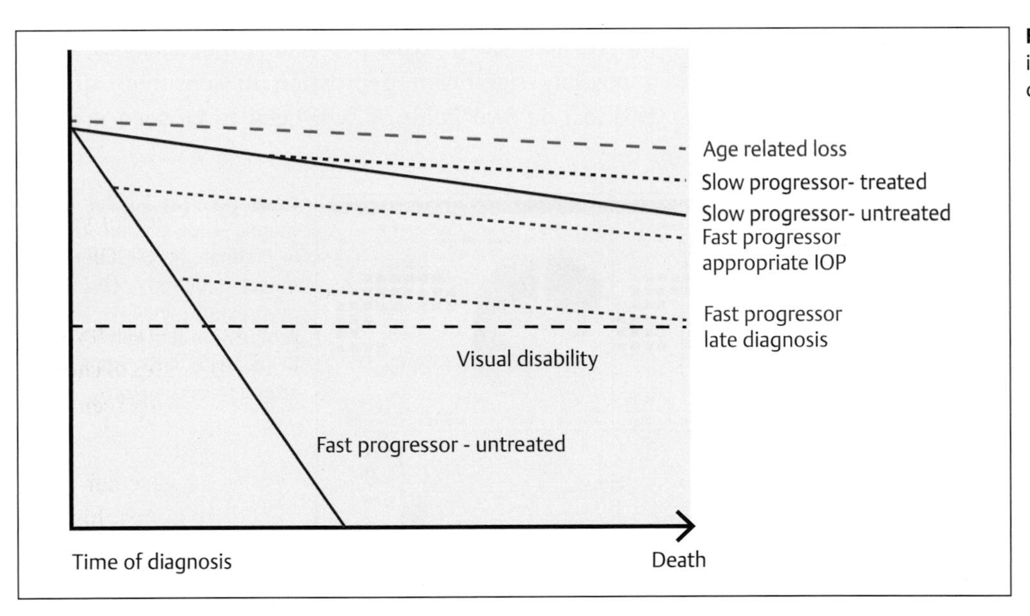

Fig. 21.13 Effect of therapeutic intervention on the rate of glaucoma progression.

Cases

Case 1

A 50-year-old lady was diagnosed to have PACG in 2006, with an IOP of 28 mm Hg in the left eye. There was a superior arcuate scotoma, with a large inferior nasal step which had not reached the blind spot. Fundus photos showed a retinal nerve fiber layer defect both superiorly and inferiorly. A target IOP of <15 mm Hg was achieved using a prostaglandin analog and brimonidine drops, and the patient was stable for 5 years, when a raised IOP of 22/24 mm Hg was recorded. The patient had been using steroid inhalers for chronic bronchitis over the prior 3 months. IOP remained at 20/22 mm Hg despite the addition of brinzolamide. An enlargement of the superior retinal nerve fiber layer defect was seen on fundus photographs, with an increased visual field defect and inferior arcuate scotoma. Rate of progression -2%/year (**Case 1-1**).

Points to consider

- Target IOP could not be achieved on steroids.
- A β-blocker could not be added.
- Chronic bronchitis would need steroids in the future too.

Diagnosis and Management

In view of the possible need for long-term steroids, options of further increasing medications or surgery were discussed. The patient underwent a trabeculectomy after which the IOP remained between 12 and 14 mm Hg and fields over 9 years showed no further progression.

Case 2

A 55-year-old lady was diagnosed to have iridocorneal endothelial syndrome in the left eye, with a cup:disc ratio of 0.8, inferior loss of neuroretinal rim, and a baseline IOP of 34 mm Hg. On a prostaglandin analog, and timolol and brimonidine combination, her IOP was 22 to 20 mm Hg. Perimetry showed a superior arcuate scotoma close to fixation.

Points to consider

- The patient has moderate glaucoma.
- There is corneal endothelial dysfunction.
- Rho kinase inhibitors were too expensive, and not available in her town.

Diagnosis and Management

A target IOP of <15 mm Hg was considered appropriate and trabeculectomy with mitomycin C (MMC) was performed. The IOP in the left eye has remained <15 mm Hg over 11 years, off glaucoma medications. On guided progression analysis, trend analysis of VFI shows stability with rate of progression being −0.3% per year. Event analysis shows a possibly significant depression in sensitivity at only two loci on two fields. It will need to be seen if this is

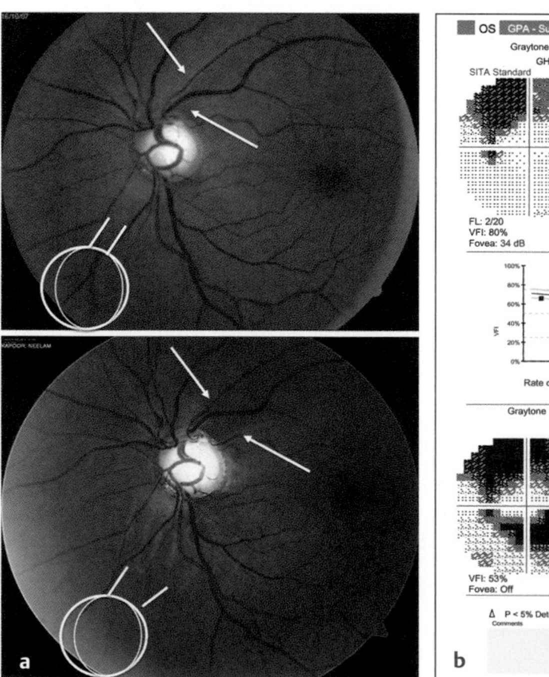

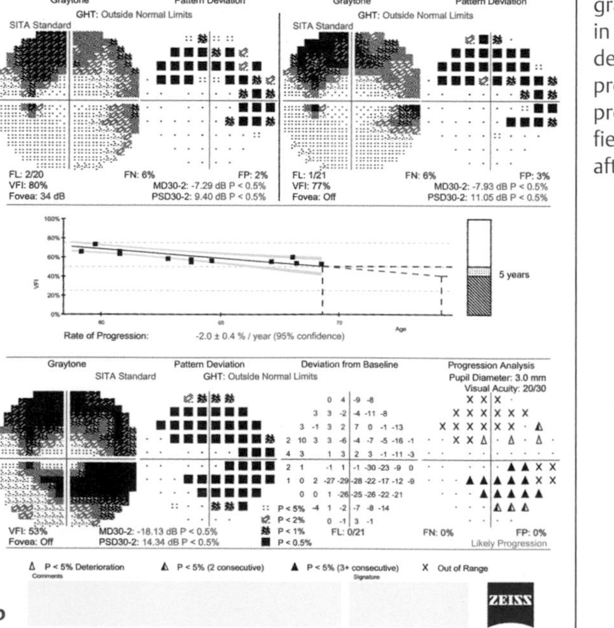

Case 1-1 **(a)** Fundus photographs showing an increase in retinal nerve fiber layer defect superiorly. **(b)** Guided progression analysis showing progression at the fifth and sixth fields, with later stabilization after a trabeculectomy.

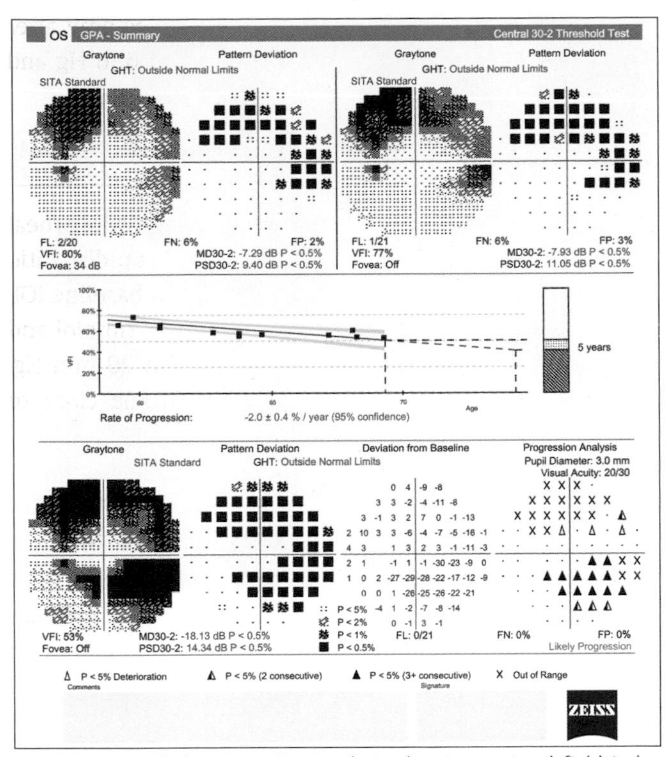

Case 2-1 Guided progression analysis showing a visual field index (VFI) rate of progression of −2% per year. Event analysis shows a possibly significant depression in sensitivity at many loci, filled and half-filled triangles.

reproduced on a third field, so that the IOP could be further lowered (**Case 2-1**). The patient has been advised to review every 6 months.

Case 3

A 50-year-old myopic male was found to have an IOP of 28/30 mm Hg, an open angle, and large optic nerve heads with a cup:disc ratio of 0.8 in both eyes. Perimetry was within normal limits. CCT was 540 µm in both eyes (**Case 3-1**).

Points to consider

- Myopia is a risk factor for progression.
- IOPs are high in both eyes.
- Already thin neuroretinal rim.

Diagnosis and Management

A diagnosis of POAG suspect was made, and the high risk of progression to visual filed defects was explained. On a prostaglandin analog and timolol, his IOP was maintained at <18 mm Hg, and over 6 years optical coherence tomography in both eyes shows no significant change in trends of retinal nerve fiber layer and cup:disc ratio, and no area of focal loss.

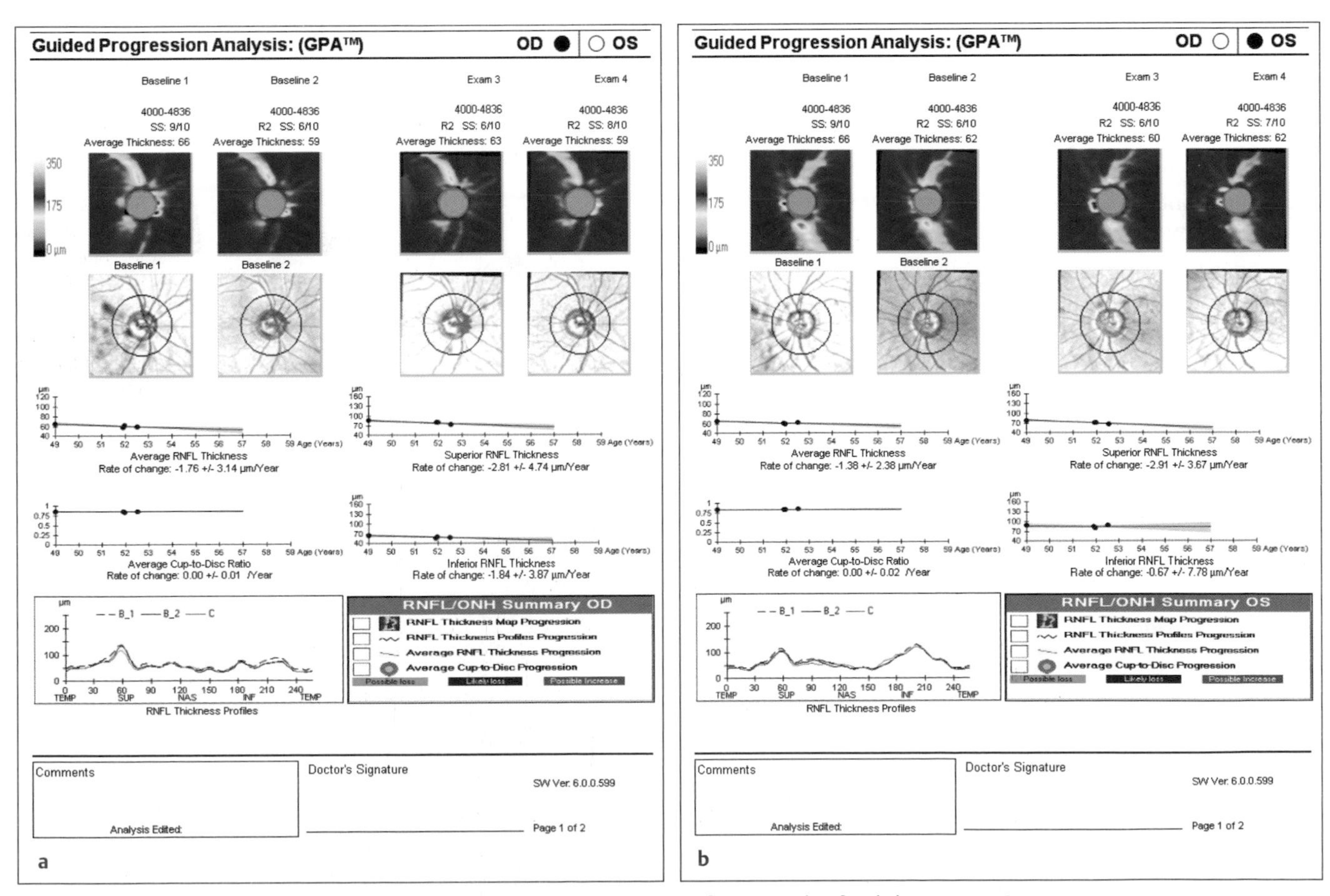

Case 3-1 **(a, b)** Stable optical coherence tomography parameters—no significant trend or focal change over 6 years.

Case 4

A 64-year-old male was diagnosed to have POAG in his only eye on the basis of a cup:disc ratio of 0.8, with thinning of the neuroretinal rim all around, and a loss of neuroretinal rim both inferiorly and superiorly. There was extensive beta zone peripapillary atrophy as well. The Octopus field showed a superior arcuate scotoma, and an inferior nasal step. Polar analysis highlighted areas of expected neuroretinal rim loss, which corresponded with the clinical findings (**Case 4-1**). The other was lost in a road traffic accident.

Points to consider

- Moderate glaucoma.
- The superior arcuate scotoma is very close to fixation, and any extension would affect central vision.
- Only seeing eye.

Diagnosis and Management

The target IOP was set to <12 mm Hg and the patient was reviewed regularly thereafter for 10 years, and showed stability on EyeSuite—mean deviation and diffuse defect trend analysis and on cluster analysis. However, an increase in localized defect is seen in the superior periphery, which was due to retinal photocoagulation done for a retinal break.

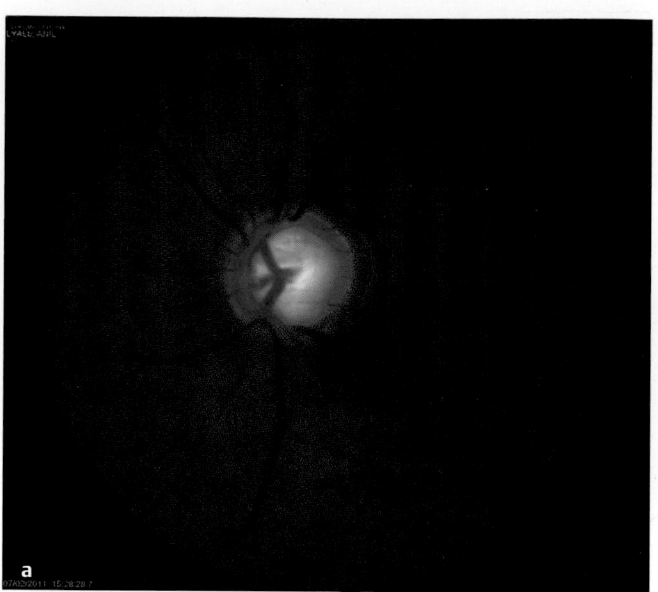

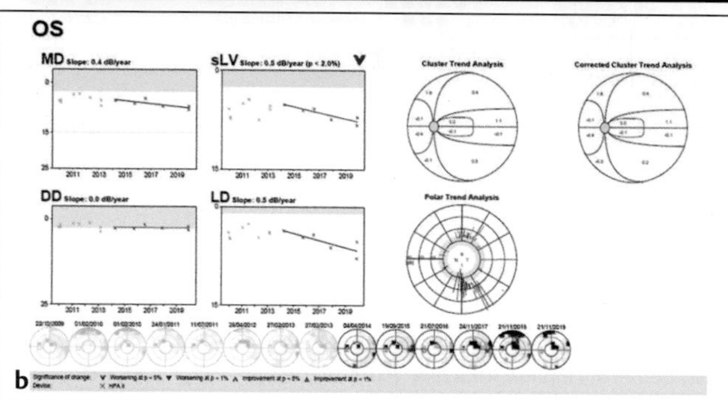

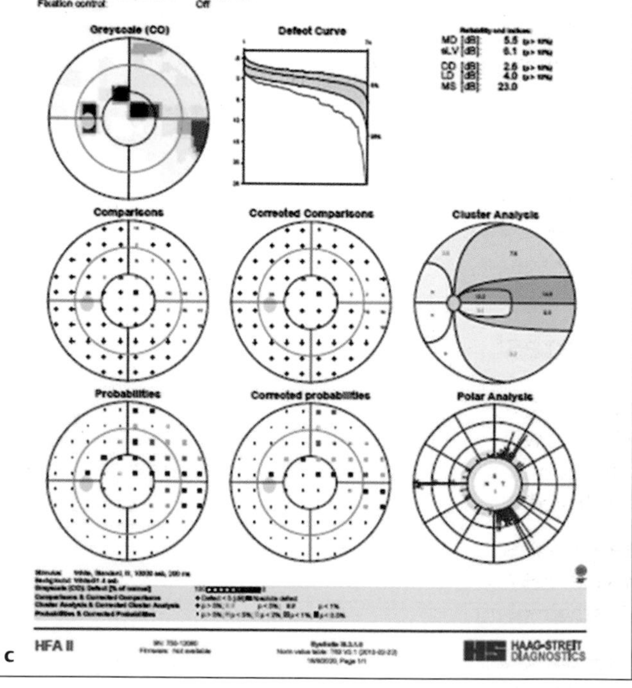

Case 4-1 (a–c) Octopus perimetry, EyeSuite, showing a stable mean deviation and diffuse defect trend analysis. A localized defect is seen in the superior periphery.

Case 5

A 56-year-old patient was diagnosed to have PACG, with an occludable angle having more than 180 degrees of peripheral anterior synechiae, cup:disc ratio of 0.7, and a baseline IOP of 36 mm Hg in the right eye. Perimetry showed a few inferior paracentral defects. After an iridotomy, the IOP was reduced to 16 mm Hg on a combination of a prostaglandin analog and timolol. The patient continued medications and review for 2 years. But on taking a second opinion, was advised that two medications were not required. He returned 4 years later with an IOP of 28 mm Hg on timolol and had developed a superior hemispheric field defect. Optical coherence tomography showed the development of retinal nerve fiber layer loss at both poles on all trend and event analyses (**Case 5-1**).

Points to consider

- Lifelong use of medications to achieve a target IOP is essential.
- Repeated perimetry and imaging are required to detect changes.
- PACG progresses faster than POAG.

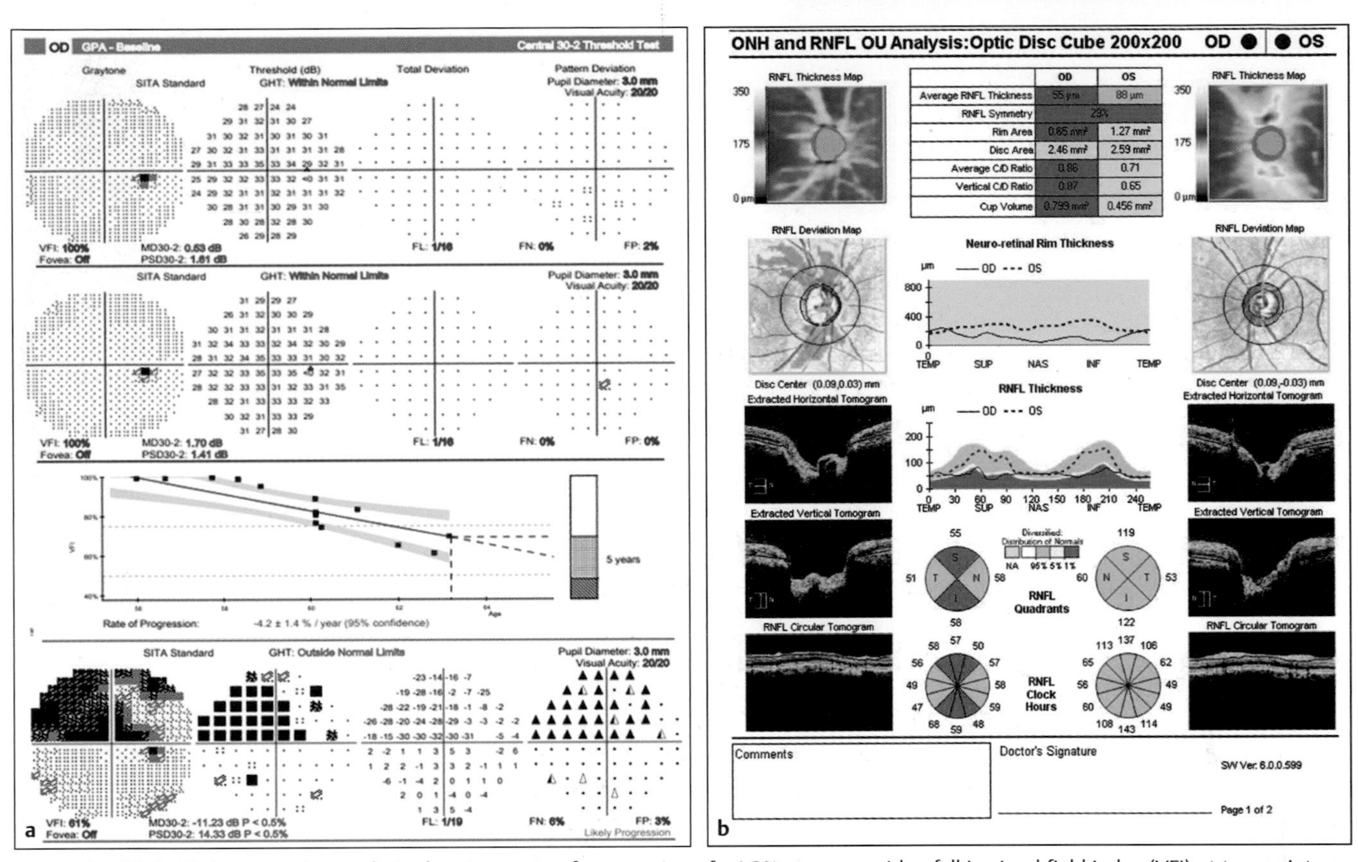

Case 5-1 **(a)** Guided progression analysis showing a rate of progression of –4.2% per year, with a fall in visual field index (VFI) at two points on review. **(b)** Optical coherence tomography of the same patient highlighting the significant change on trend analysis and focal loss as "likely loss" in *red*.

Diagnosis and Management

In view of progression of field defects to moderate stage of PACG, the IOP was lowered to <15 mm Hg with a prostaglandin analog and timolol. However, the optical coherence tomography repeated after 3 year showed a further area of "likely progression," and the IOP was lowered to <12 mm Hg using a prostaglandin analog with a combination of dorzolamide and timolol. Baselines of both perimetry and imaging were reset to detect even the slightest change.

Suggested Readings

Belghith A, Bowd C, Medeiros FA, Balasubramanian M, Weinreb RN, Zangwill LM. Learning from healthy and stable eyes: a new approach for detection of glaucomatous progression. Artif Intell Med 2015;64(2):105–115

Bengtsson B, Patella VM, Heijl A. Prediction of glaucomatous visual field loss by extrapolation of linear trends. Arch Ophthalmol 2009;127(12):1610–1615

Caprioli J, Zeyen T. A critical discussion of the rates of progression and causes of optic nerve damage in glaucoma: International Glaucoma Think Tank II: July 25-26, 2008, Florence, Italy. J Glaucoma. 2009 Aug;18(6 Suppl):S1-21

Giangiacomo A, Garway-Heath D, Caprioli J. Diagnosing glaucoma progression: current practice and promising technologies. Curr Opin Ophthalmol 2006;17(2):153–162

Grewal DS, Tanna AP. Diagnosis of glaucoma and detection of glaucoma progression using spectral domain optical coherence tomography. Curr Opin Ophthalmol 2013;24(2):150–161

Medeiros FA, Zangwill LM, Alencar LM, et al. Detection of glaucoma progression with Stratus optical coherence tomography retinal nerve fiber layer, optic nerve head, and macular thickness measurements. Invest Ophthalmol Vis Sci 2009;50(12):5741–5748.

Musch DC, Gillespie BW, Lichter PR, Niziol LM, Janz NK; CIGTS Study Investigators. Visual field progression in the Collaborative Initial Glaucoma Treatment Study the impact of treatment and other baseline factors. Ophthalmology 2009;116(2):200–207

Rossetti L, Goni F, Denis P, Bengtsson B, Martinez A, Heijl A. Focusing on glaucoma progression and the clinical importance of progression rate measurement: a review. Eye (Lond) 2010;24(Suppl 1):S1–S7

Sharma P, Sample PA, Zangwill LM, Schuman JS. Diagnostic tools for glaucoma detection and management. Surv Ophthalmol 2008;53(Suppl1):S17–S32

CHAPTER 22

Trabeculectomy and Its Modifications

Overview

- Trabeculectomy
  - Indications
  - Preoperative Measures
  - Surgical Procedure
  - Trabeculectomy Modifications
  - Postoperative Care
  - Early Postoperative Complications
  - Late Complications
- Cases
- Suggested Readings

Introduction

The management of glaucoma patients with advanced damage or very high intraocular pressures (IOPs) frequently necessitates surgical options. *This reduction of IOP by surgery entails a diversion of aqueous through an alternative pathway, or by increasing the efficacy of existing channels.* There is currently a plethora of surgeries being done, many still investigational.

The ideal glaucoma surgery would:

- Not damage existing aqueous outflow.
- Provide alternate channels.
- Enhance existing ones.
- Be predictable.
- Be adjustable for the target IOP needed for each individual.
- Have few postoperative interventions.
- Avoid thin-walled blebs.
- Last for 10 to 20 years as glaucoma is a chronic disease.
- Be easily taught/performed.
- Allow further surgery if required, in the patient's lifetime.
- Be cost effective.

Advantages of glaucoma surgery are many, as it lowers IOP significantly, while negating compliance issues in a chronic disease such as glaucoma:

- It significantly decreases diurnal fluctuations in IOP.
- Patient compliance is not an issue.
- It is more cost effective than long-term medications.
- Patients avoid the numerous side effects of glaucoma medications.
- Collaborative Initial Glaucoma Treatment Study (CIGTS) has shown less glaucoma progression over time in surgical versus medically treated primary open-angle glaucoma (POAG) patients.

None of the currently available surgeries can tick all the criteria above, and those that are validated and more accepted will be detailed in this book (**Tables 22.1** and **22.2**).

Trabeculectomy

Trabeculectomy has remained the gold standard for glaucoma surgery, and with its many modifications has

Table 22.1 Pathways utilized in different glaucoma surgeries

Pathway addressed	Surgery
Subconjunctival space	▪ Trabeculectomy ▪ Drainage devices ▪ Ex-PRESS shunt ▪ XEN gel stent
Trabecular meshwork bypass	▪ iStent ▪ Hydrus ▪ OMNI
Trabecular ablation	▪ Trabectome
Schlemm's canal dilation	▪ Viscocanalostomy
Suprachoroidal space	▪ MINIject

Table 22.2 Comparing generally reported outcomes and expected postoperative interventions, which vary with the type of glaucoma and success criteria

Glaucoma surgery	Success rates over >3 years	Postoperative review and manipulations	Complications	Other comments
Trabeculectomy	50–80%	6–8 weeks	Shallow anterior chamber, hypotony	
Drainage devices	40–70%	6–8 weeks	Hypertensive phase, corneal decompensation	
Laser trabeculoplasty	30–40%	No	10% per year failure	
Minimally invasive glaucoma surgeries	Long-term unavailable	4–8 weeks	Blockage, Malposition	Commonly done with cataract surgery
Cyclophotocoagulation—Diode/Micropulse	20–30%, proportional to baseline IOP	2–3 weeks	▪ Efficacy for 3–4 months only ▪ Repeat required ▪ Chances of pthisis	

Abbreviation: IOP, intraocular pressure.

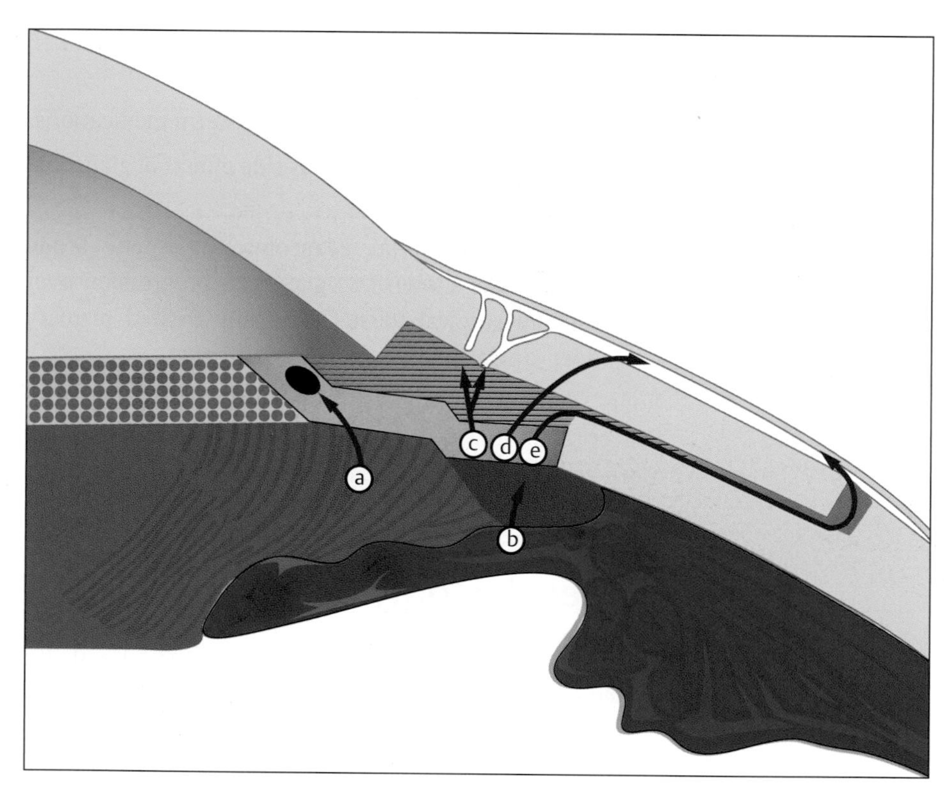

Fig. 22.1 Possible routes of aqueous outflow in a trabeculectomy. **(a)** Through cut ends of Schlemm's canal. **(b)** Cyclodialysis. **(c)** Through vessels and lymphatics in sclera. **(d)** Diffusion through sclera. **(e)** Subconjunctival drainage.

become safer and more effective over time. It was *described by Cairns and modified by Watson*, at a time when free filtering surgeries were causing many complications, such as shallow anterior chambers and thin-walled blebs. The initial concept was that excising a part of the trabecular meshwork would leave the cut ends of the Schlemm's canal open allowing aqueous egress. The formation of a bleb in a significant number of patients suggested that subconjunctival drainage played a part.

It is now suggested that a trabeculectomy lowers IOP by many means (**Fig. 22.1**):

- Subconjunctival drainage with aqueous being absorbed by episcleral and conjunctival vessels.
- Drainage through vessels/lymphatics in the sclera.
- Diffusion through the scleral base.
- Marginal cyclodialysis.
- Drainage through Schlemm's canal.
- Drainage through newly formed aqueous veins.
- Diffusion through the conjunctiva to tear film.

Indications

Indications for a trabeculectomy in any glaucoma are:

- IOP uncontrolled on maximal tolerated medical therapy, leading to a risk of progression.

- Low "target" IOP required for advanced glaucomatous neuropathy, which cannot be achieved medically.
- Inability to afford medication in the long term.
- Physical difficulty in instilling drops.
- Side effects with most glaucoma medications.

Preoperative Measures

Counseling: It is essential to discuss the outcome of the surgery with *the patient who should understand that the healing response of each patient varies, and therefore the final IOP cannot always be guaranteed to be the "target" desired.* The consent form should state that the surgery is being done for control of IOP only, and *there will not be any improvement in vision. In fact, it should be emphasized that there will be blurring of vision for a few weeks, which will return to preoperative levels in 6 to 8 weeks.* It should also be adequately explained that the surgery is only a part of the therapy, and *manipulations and medications over the next 6 to 8 weeks will also determine the outcome.*

Any *blood thinners should be stopped* prior to surgery, ecosprin, a week earlier, and clopidogrel, 5 days earlier. In the quest for a quiet eye prior to surgery, pilocarpine and prostaglandin analogs could be stopped; however, as the IOP is generally uncontrolled, this is not always possible. *If the conjunctiva is congested, a few days of a mild steroid such as fluorometholone may improve the success of the filtering surgery.*

A trabeculectomy should not be attempted in eyes with extremely high IOPs, and it is advisable to lower the IOP as much as possible with maximal medical therapy prior to undertaking surgery. Intravenous (IV) mannitol or Diamox given half an hour before surgery is also very important in decreasing the volume of the vitreous and lowering IOP in eyes with primary angle-closure glaucoma (PACG) or advanced glaucoma. This decreases the possibility of suprachoroidal hemorrhage, malignant glaucoma, and repeated intraoperative shallowing of the anterior chamber. *If the IOP remains high even after oral Diamox and IV mannitol, repeated paracentesis should be done over 2 to 5 minutes before making the sclerostomy.*

Surgical Procedure

The procedure itself has remained close to the original description, with wound modulation using antifibroblastic agents added, and safety enhanced with releasable/adjustable sutures.

A trabeculectomy is generally done under peribulbar block to get some preoperative lowering of IOP and good akinesia with anesthesia; however, it can also be done under topical anesthesia.

The eye is rotated downwards using a superior rectus bridle or a cornea traction suture. The superior rectus muscle is grasped with superior rectus forceps or fixation forceps about 10 mm posterior to the limbus, and a 6–0 Vicryl suture is passed through the muscle tendon. For clear cornea traction, a 6-0 polyglactin suture is passed at 12 o'clock, 1 mm anterior to the limbus with a wide bite of approximately 4 mm.

The site of surgery is currently debatable; 12 o'clock has a wider limbus but can compromise any second filtering surgery if required, as conjunctiva is affected on both sides. *A superior nasal site allows for virgin conjunctiva at a 12 o'clock site for a repeat filtering surgery, and is also distant enough from a temporal cataract incision to permit continued bleb function.*

A conjunctival flap is raised by making an incision 6 to 8 mm above the limbus to keep it as remote as possible from the scleral incision in *limbus-based flap*, or as a peritomy at the limbus for a *fornix-based flap*. Trauma to the conjunctiva should be minimized by using a nontoothed forceps and blunt dissection, avoiding button holing and bleb leaks. The conjunctiva and tenon's flap is dissected in one layer, leading to visibility of the episcleral vessels at first incision, with later extension of the incision for adequate visualization of the surgical area (**Fig. 22.2**).

A 4 × 4 mm rectangle is marked on the sclera with a scratch incision, posterior to the insertion of the conjunctiva, and the proposed edges are gently cauterized. *The depth of the superficial flap is determined at one corner to approximately half to two-thirds thickness by identifying a*

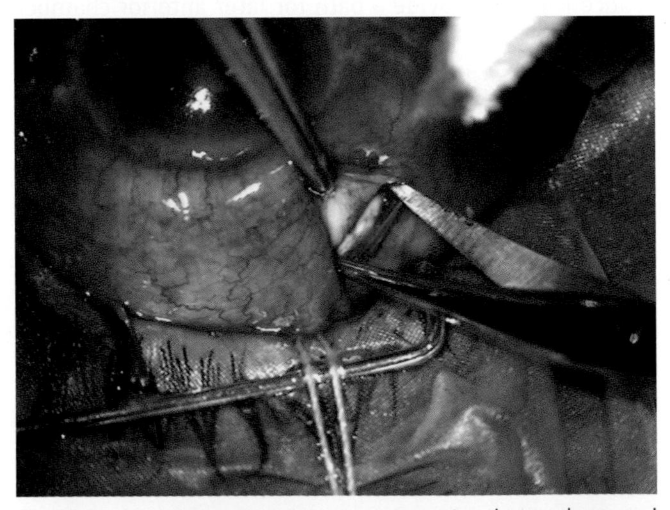

Fig. 22.2 Superior rectus traction suture rotating the eye down, and a conjunctival incision made 8 mm from the limbus, going down to the sclera, with visibility of the episcleral vessels.

change to a bluish hue of the dissected base from the white of the full-thickness sclera (**Fig. 22.3**). At this depth the scleral fibers left will prevent the formation of staphyloma, while permitting some diffusion of aqueous. The superficial scleral flap is dissected toward the limbus, stopping 1 mm posterior to it. Care should be taken to avoid premature perforation as the application of antifibroblastic agents may then have to be abandoned. The size and shape of the scleral flap and sclerostomy vary considerably among surgeons. The shape may be triangular, rectangular, w shaped, or trapezoid, but this has not been shown to affect IOP outcomes.

Antifibroblastic agents, e.g., mitomycin C (MMC), should be applied judiciously, with minimum dose and duration, assessed preoperatively, and during surgery, for a given patient. *MMC can be applied either before making the superficial scleral flap or afterwards. The application should be over a wide area and as posterior as possible.* The dose and duration of application vary from surgeon to surgeon; however, the maxim should be the minimum deemed necessary. *A rule of thumb for primary adult glaucomas: POAG and PACG use 0.1 to 0.2 mg/mL for 1 minute subcojunctivally (***Fig. 22.4***). A dose of 0.4 mg/mL could be used for children less than 6 months, as also in refractory glaucomas such as neovascular, post penetrating keratoplasty (PK), or after vitreoretinal (VR) surgery.* In cases of repeat surgeries and refractory glaucomas where scleral scarring is seen, MMC application both subscleral and subconjunctival may be more effective. The conjunctival edge should be protected from MMC, especially in fornix-based trabeculectomies. Any surface MMC should be washed out with copious irrigation of balanced salt solution (BSS) or saline.

A *paracentesis using a 26/30-gauge needle* is done to reduce IOP and provide a path for later anterior chamber reformation (**Fig. 22.5**). Air or viscoelastic may be injected to keep the anterior chamber formed. A rectangle of the deeper sclera of about 3 × 1 mm is outlined under the superficial flap by a blade to leave a shelf of deeper sclera of at least 0.5 mm on either side (**Fig. 22.6**).

Two radial entries into the anterior chamber at either edge of the marked ostium further lower IOP, and when the eye is seen to be soft, first the anterior and later the posterior sides are cut with an angled Vannas scissor (**Fig. 22.7**). The sclerostomy may also be made using a trabeculectomy punch, starting with an anterior incision at the scleral flap hinge, with an average of two punches for an opening of 1.5-mm diameter. *The deepest layer of the trabeculum must be excised, along with any membrane present that may provide a scaffold for later fibrosis. A gush of aqueous should be seen with iris presenting at the window made.*

A broad basal iridectomy of the width of the ostium is made by placing scissors parallel to the limbus (**Fig. 22.8**).

The scleral flap is sutured with a combination of fixed and releasable or adjustable sutures (**Fig. 22.9**). *The conjunctiva and tenon's flap should be sutured with care to provide a watertight closure of the wound* (**Fig. 22.10**). This should be examined carefully for any point of leakage.

Manipulations in the anterior chamber should be minimized and the anterior chamber should be maintained throughout the procedure to reduce cataract progression and endothelial cell loss. At the end, the pupil should be round, and the iridectomy visible, preempting any internal blockage of ostium, and the anterior chamber should be returned to its preoperative depth using air, viscoelastics, or BSS.

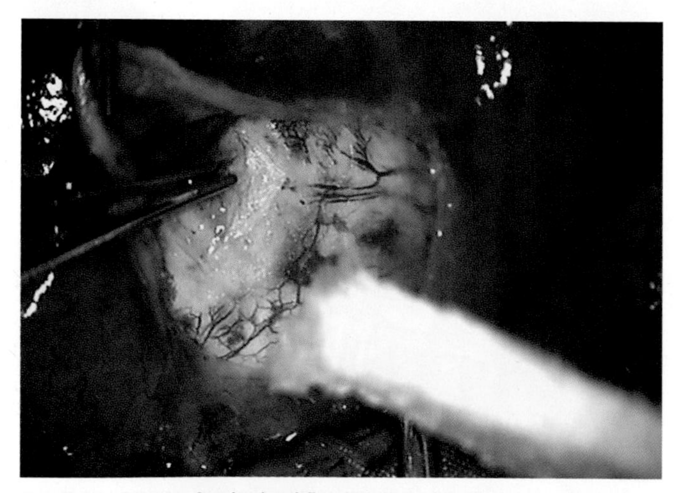

Fig. 22.3 A superficial scleral flap has been marked out with scratch incisions. One corner of the flap is dissected to half/two-thirds thickness so that a bluish hue of the underlying uvea is seen.

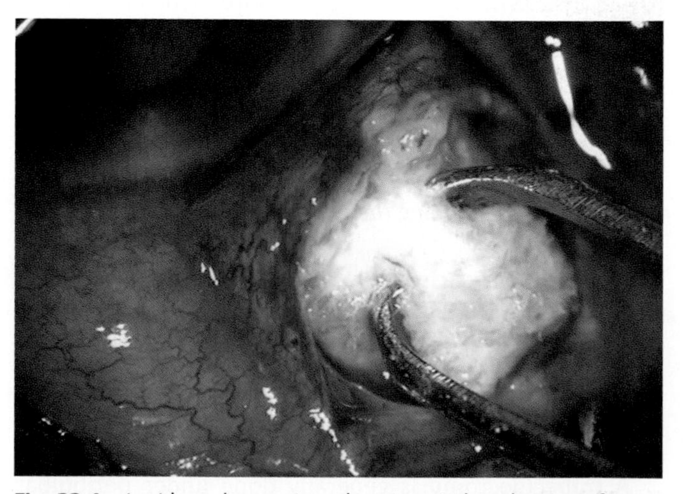

Fig. 22.4 A wide and posterior subconjunctival application of mitomycin C (MMC).

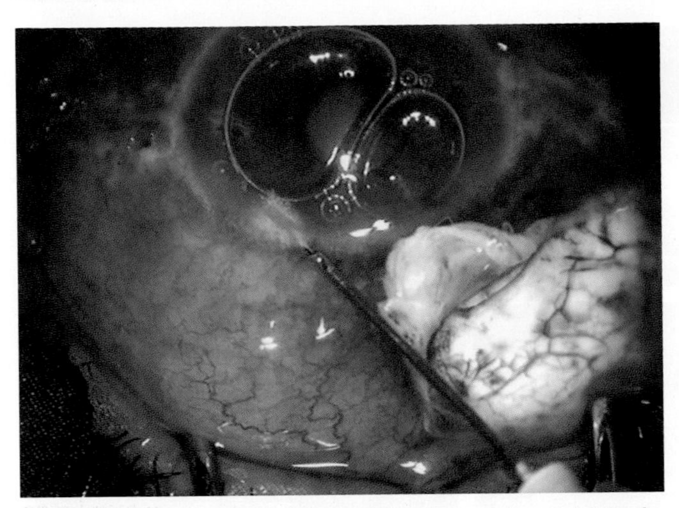

Fig. 22.5 A paracentesis is done and air injected to maintain the anterior chamber during surgery.

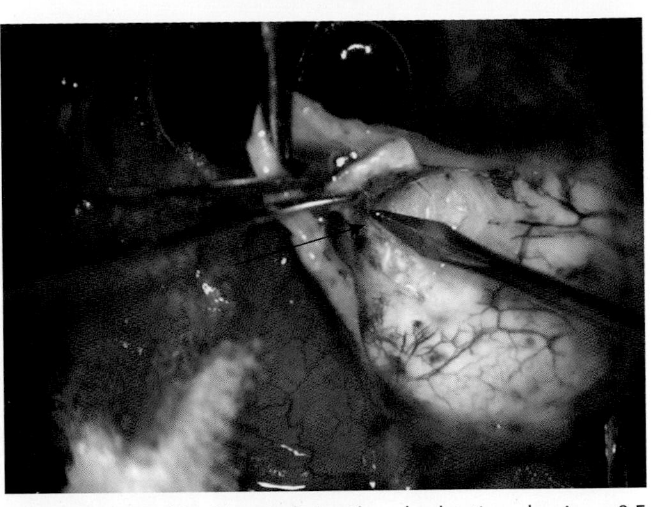

Fig. 22.6 Scratch incision outlining the scleral ostium, leaving a 0.5 mm shelf on either side (*black arrow*).

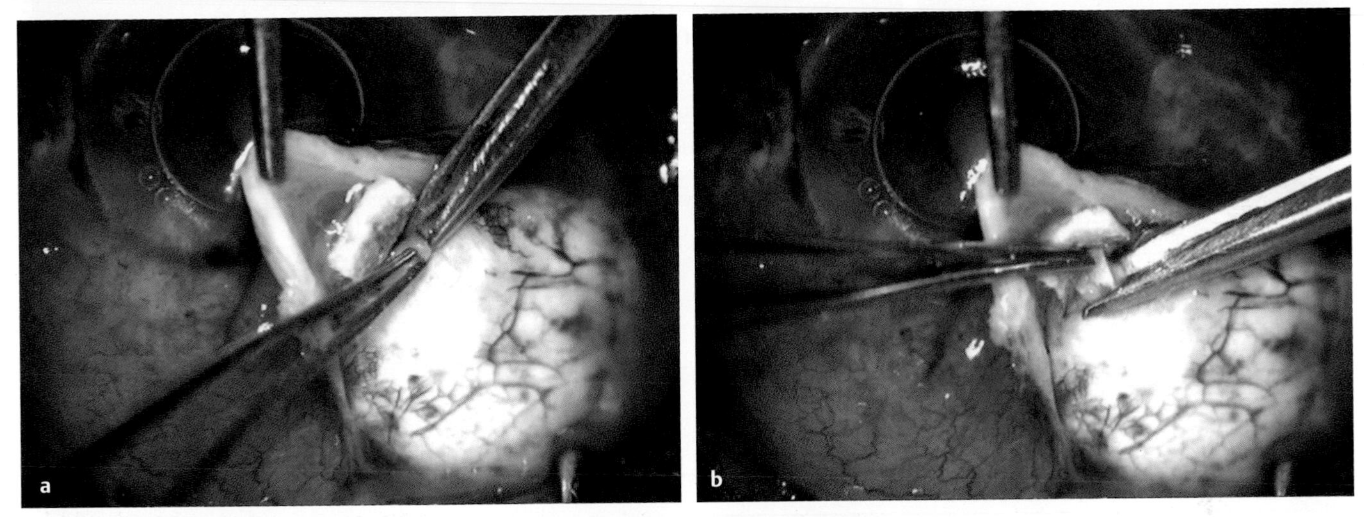

Fig. 22.7 **(a, b)** Excising the sclera first anteriorly then posteriorly to make a 3 × 1 mm ostium.

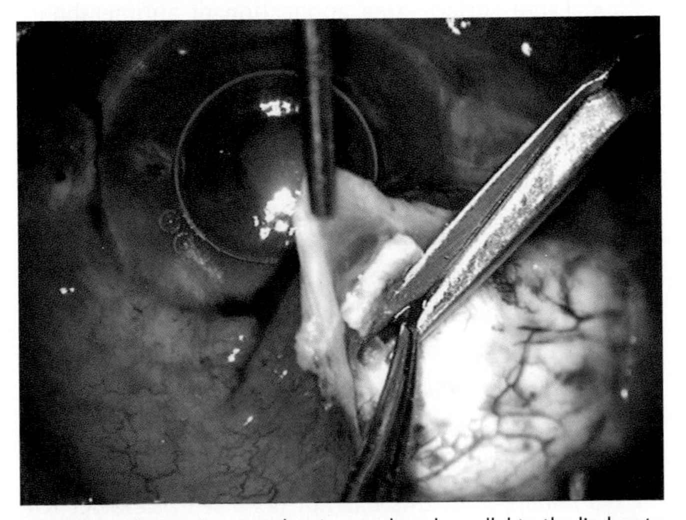

Fig. 22.8 The iris is cut with scissors placed parallel to the limbus to form an iridotomy wider than the ostium.

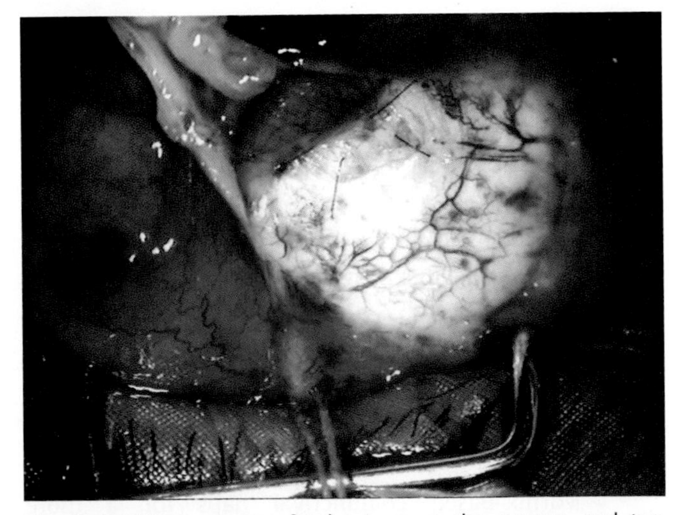

Fig. 22.9 There are two fixed sutures at the corners, and two releasable sutures adjacent to the limbus.

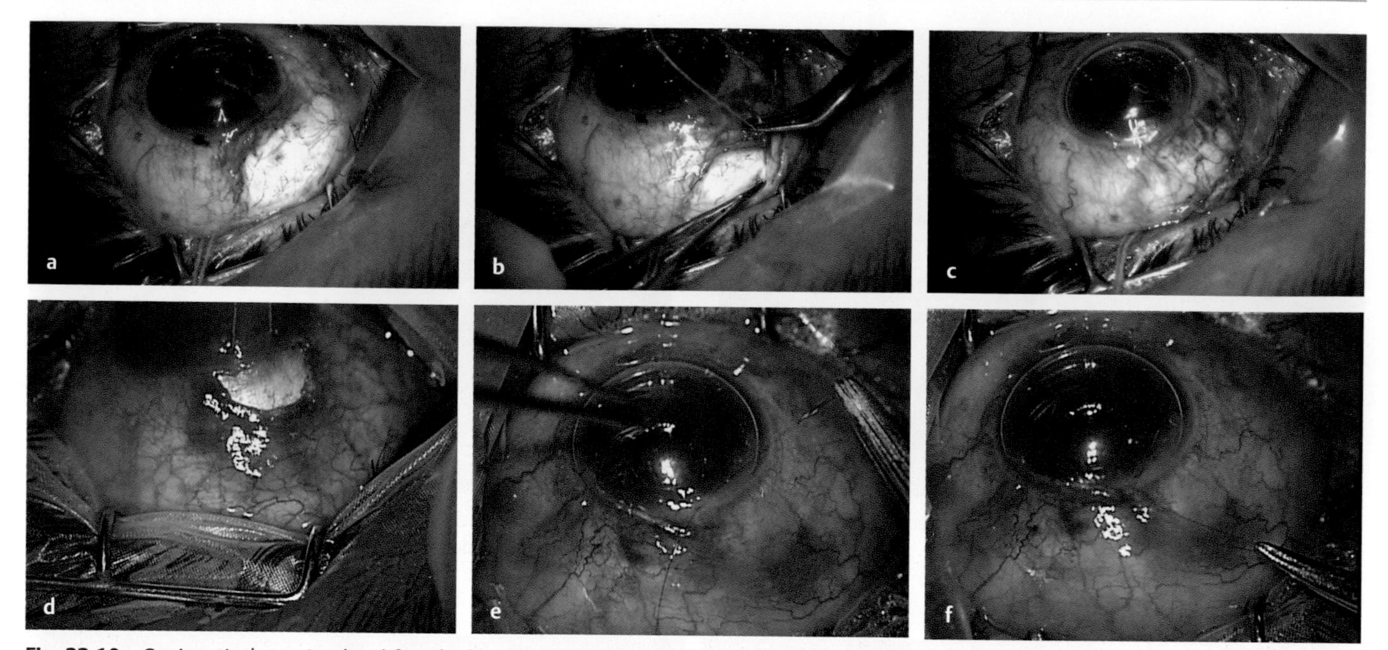

Fig. 22.10 Conjunctival suturing **(a–c)** for a limbus-based flap, and **(d–f)** for a fornix-based flap.

Table 22.3 Comparison between limbus-based and fornix-based conjunctival flaps

Limbus-based conjunctival flaps	Fornix-based conjunctival flaps
Rare leak from wound	Early microleaks common
More anterior, relatively avascular blebs Postoperative globe massage can be done	More posterior blebs Globe massage may disrupt wound
Larger area of dissection Thin conjunctivas may button hole	Smaller area of dissection Button holes are less common

Trabeculectomy Modifications

Over decades, there have been many modifications to the original technique, designed to decrease complications and increase efficacy.

- **Conjunctival flap:** This may be either limbus based or fornix based (**Fig. 22.10**). It is thought that a fornix-based flap provides a more posterior bleb, safer in the long term, but prone to early leaks, while a limbus-based flap rarely has an early postoperative leak, but has anterior blebs. Long-term IOP control with both has been shown to be largely equivalent (**Table 22.3**).
- **Safer surgery technique:** *Moorfields* suggested modifications in trabeculectomy steps to decrease postoperative problems (**Fig. 22.11**). These are as listed below:
  - Fornix-based conjunctival flaps for a more posterior and diffuse bleb.
  - Superficial scleral flap side incisions should stop 1 mm short of the limbus to direct aqueous posteriorly.
  - Large surface area application of antimetabolite posteriorly.
  - Anterior segment infusion cannula used to maintain the anterior chamber.
  - Sclerostomy punch of 0.5 mm.
  - Releasable and adjustable sutures.
- **Antifibroblastic agents:** *5-Fluorouracil* is a pyrimidine analog antimetabolite, blocking DNA synthesis at the S phase of cell proliferation. This may be used as *a 5-mg subconjunctival injection* for 2 weeks, but causes a significant keratopathy. It may also be *applied topically during surgery, 50 mg/mL for 5 minutes*, but this has not been seen to lower IOP significantly in the long term.

Mitomycin C is an antibiotic and antifibrotic agent isolated from *Streptomyces caespitosus*, and affects all phases of the cell cycle. It has been used in concentrations of 0.1 to 0.5 mg/mL, applied for 1 to 5 minutes, either subconjunctivally or subsclerally. The risk of later bleb thinning and avascularity can be reduced by minimizing the dose and duration of exposure. *For primary adult glaucomas a dose of 0.1 or 0.2 mg/mL for 1 minute subconjunctival works well.*

- **Buried knots of 10/0 fixed scleral sutures** prevent suture ends puncturing the conjunctiva and causing bleb failure/bleb leak (**Fig. 22.12**).
- **Releasable and adjustable sutures:** Shallowing of the anterior chamber after surgery is the commonest problem encountered, and a *tight closure of the superficial scleral flap over the sclerostomy determines aqueous egress and anterior chamber depth, before remodeling of the episcleral tissue occurs weeks after surgery*. These sutures also control IOP, preventing hypotony and its attendant problems of choroidal effusion, macular edema, and cataractogenesis. To maintain control on postoperative aqueous outflow through the trabeculectomy, surgeons resort to various techniques: tight scleral flap closure followed by laser suture lysis, release of externalized sutures, and loosening of adjustable sutures.
  - **Tight scleral flap sutures:** These can be applied and lysed using a frequency doubled YAG laser, 50- to 100-µm spots, at 300 mW. Visualization of the suture in the early postoperative period can be hampered by conjunctival edema and vascularity, which can be reduced using the edge of a four-mirror gonioscope or a special lens such as the Blumenthal or Ritch lens. Complications such as conjunctival burns, holes, and inability to lyse the sutures in cases have made this less popular over time.
  - **Adjustable sutures:** These were described as part of the "safe" surgery described by Khaw et al, where 10-0 sutures with four throws, but no knots, can be manipulated postop through intact conjunctiva. These manipulations have attendant complications, namely, buttonholing and/or disinsertion of the conjunctival flap. Also, adjustment is only possible in the immediate postoperative period, before episcleral tissue proliferation, as this later prevents both suture visualization and manipulation.
  - **Releasable sutures:** Interrupted, externalized scleral flap sutures, which can be removed at any point of time, on the slit lamp, also called releasable sutures, are now frequently used. Many techniques have been described.

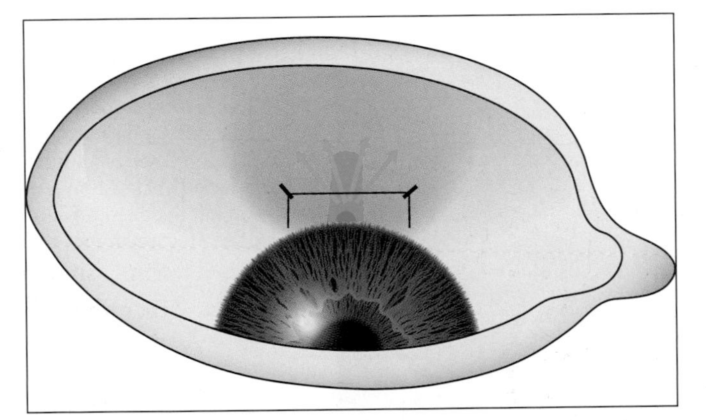

Fig. 22.11 Moorfields safer surgery technique fornix based conjunctival flap and wide MMC application.

A "Box" type suture (**Figs. 22.13** and **22.14**), starting at the cornea, is passed through the limbus in line with and into the scleral shelf on either side of the scleral ostium, close to the posterior end of the limbus. The needle is then taken through the superficial scleral flap to closely approximate

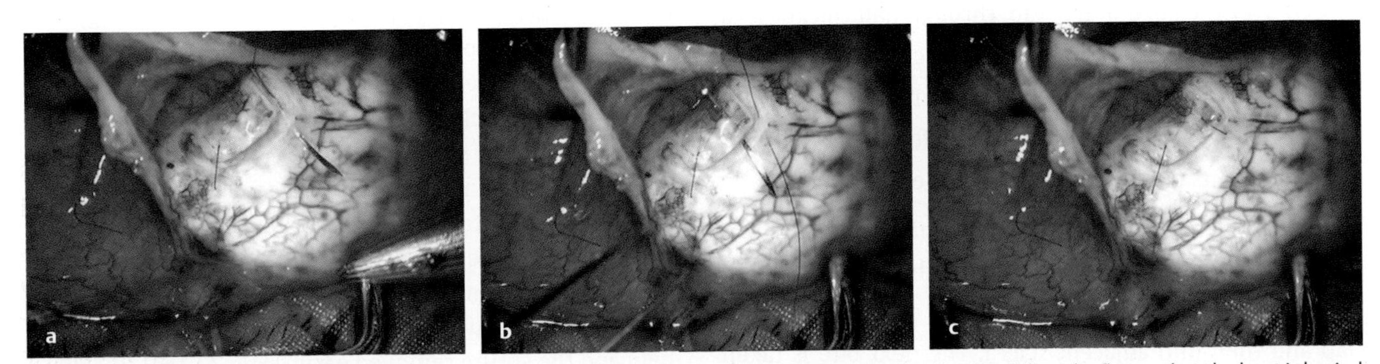

Fig. 22.12 (a–c) Techniques of burying fixed posterior corner sutures—first bite through the scleral bed and then the flap so that the knot is buried between the superficial and deep sclera.

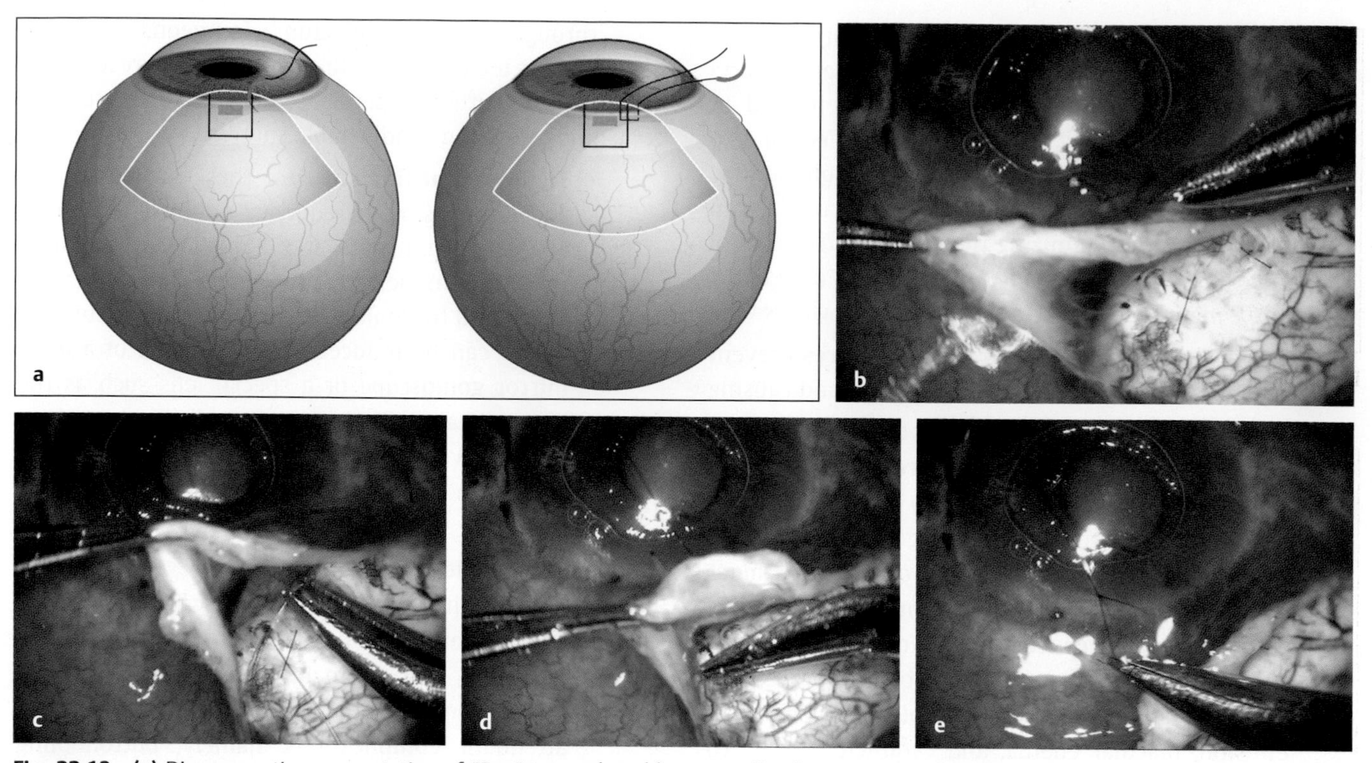

Fig. 22.13 **(a)** Diagrammatic representation of "Box" type releasable suture. **(b–e)** "Box" type releasable suture technique. **(b)** The needle is passed from the limbal cornea into the scleral shelf on either side of the scleral ostium. **(c)** The needle is then taken through the superficial scleral flap to closely approximate the shelf and superficial scleral tissues. **(d)** The suture is now passed over the edge of the flap through half thickness of the adjacent sclera back across the limbus to the cornea. **(e)** The two ends are tied and the knot buried.

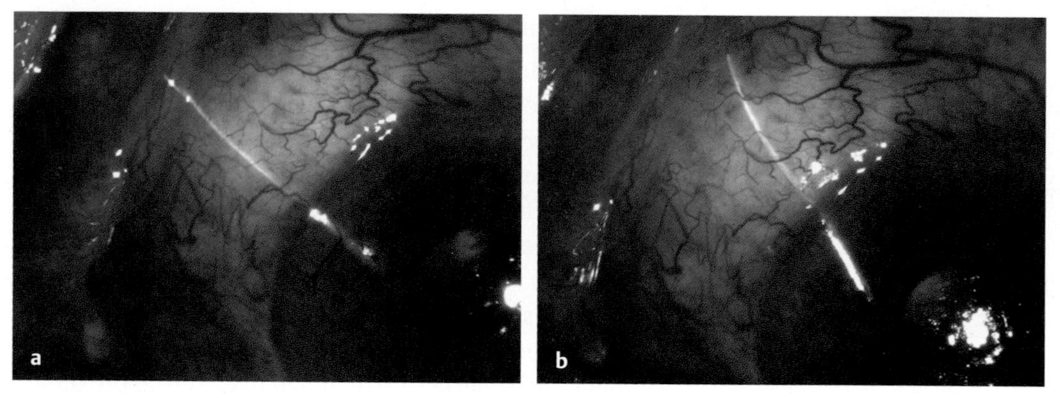

Fig. 22.14 **(a)** A vascularized bleb 2 weeks after surgery with a formed anterior chamber and a "Box" type releasable suture at 10 o'clock. **(b)** Elevation and extension of the bleb toward 9 o'clock after releasing the suture.

the shelf and superficial scleral tissues. The suture is now passed over the edge of the flap, through half thickness of the adjacent sclera, 1 mm from the trabeculectomy incision back across the limbus to the cornea, where the two ends are tied and the knot buried. This differs from Wilson's technique in its direct effect on the flap edge.

Wilson described a mattress type scleral flap suture where the suture is passed from clear cornea through the limbus to intact sclera. It is passed through the edge of the scleral flap and then into adjacent sclera. The next bite is taken into adjacent sclera and back under the limbus to clear cornea to be tightly tied (**Fig. 22.15**).

Releasable sutures described by Kolker et al and Cohen and Osher are popular as they do not pass through the conjunctiva, and patient comfort is better as there is no knot on the cornea. The suture is passed from sclera to the edge of the scleral flap, either at the apex or sides of a scleral flap. The suture is then passed through the base of the scleral flap across the limbus to clear cornea. A loop from the initial bite is tied using a quadruple throw. Kolker suggested that the end on the cornea can be passed back into the cornea and cut flush to avoid windscreen wiper keratopathy. At any point in time the corneal loop can be held and the suture removed easily (**Fig. 22.16**).

Releasable sutures can be removed under topical anesthesia at the slit lamp 1 to 4 weeks after surgery, and if

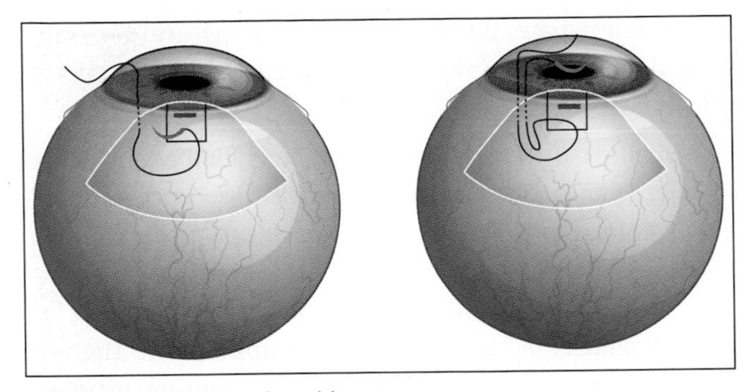

Fig. 22.15 Wilson's releasable suture.

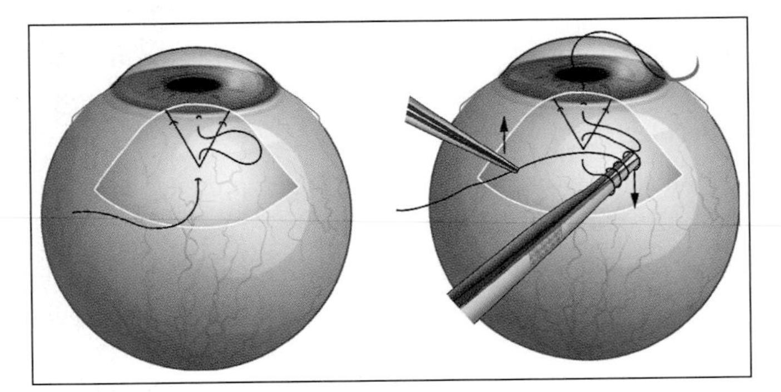

Fig. 22.16 Diagrammatic representation of releasable suture of Kolker et al and Cohen and Osher.

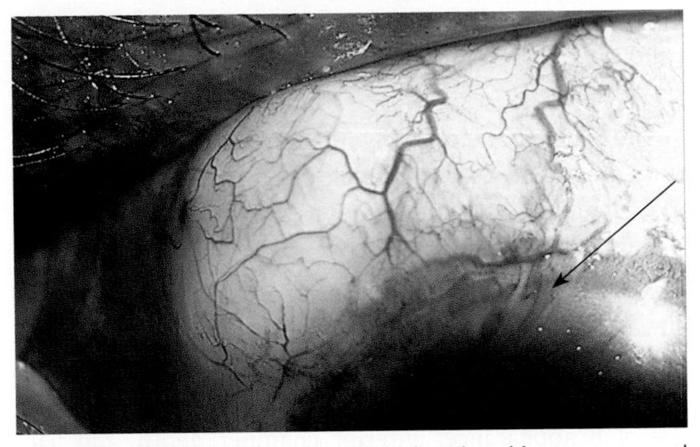

Fig. 22.17 An elevated over-filtering bleb. Releasable suture removal should be deferred.

Table 22.4 Indiana Bleb Appearance Grading Scale

Bleb features	Grading
Height	H: 0–4, flat → high
Extent	E: 0–3, <1 → >4 clock hours
Vascularity	V: 0–4, avascular → extensive vascularization
Leak on Seidel's test	S: 0–2, none → streaming

MMC has been used even up to 6 weeks. Suture removal is indicated when the bleb appears flatter than expected, or is very vascular and congested, but only when the anterior chamber is well formed (**Fig 22.14**). A very high IOP may also be an indication for suture removal. *It is best to avoid suture removal for the first few days after surgery, as no episcleral remodeling has occurred and even minor pressure on the eye may result in a flat anterior chamber.* Topical glaucoma medications may lower the IOP and allow suture release to be postponed. *Releasable sutures should be removed one at a time, with a gap of a few days, to prevent a shallow anterior chamber and hypotony.*

In the presence of a shallow anterior chamber or over-filtering bleb suture removal should be deferred (**Fig. 22.17**).

These additional sutures may themselves cause problems such as foreign body sensations, suture-related infections, and fibrosis. Inadvertent early removal may result in hypotony and a shallow anterior chamber. The looped sutures may get embedded in fibrosis, making removal difficult and sometimes leading to breakage of the suture.

Postoperative Care

Trabeculectomy surgery in itself is only half the story, as adjusting postoperative medications, timing of suture removal, and managing early bleb failure continue for at least 6 weeks.

Advice on discharge includes:

- Antibiotic + steroid drops tapering over 4 to 6 weeks, depending on the bleb inflammation, IOP, and risk factors for failure.
- Tropicamide drops once a day to dilate fully.
- Antibiotic + steroid ointment at night.
- *Fellow eye should not be on any aqueous suppressant.*
- Eye pad should be used at night for 1 week to prevent inadvertent rubbing of the eye.

The filtering bleb has to be examined closely at all visits to look for evidence of functionality or problems, current or likely. *Early diagnosis of failure and appropriate timing of interventions are important for the long-term viability of a trabeculectomy.* Many classifications have been suggested to allow a clinical estimate of function of which the *Indiana Bleb Appearance Grading Scale* (IBAGS) is the easiest to use (**Table 22.4**).

Moorfields Bleb Grading System additionally looks at differences in vascularity and area, central to periphery of the bleb, and the presence of a subconjunctival bleed. Currently gradings using anterior segment optical coherence tomography (ASOCT) are being proposed based on bleb size, bleb wall reflectivity, internal morphology, intrascleral lake, scleral flap, and ostium, but need more validation in differentiating working and nonfunctioning surgeries.

Different problems may manifest at times, and the surgeon should be on the look out for the common ones that manifest at different postoperative time points (**Table 22.5**).

On the first postoperative day, the bleb should be mildly elevated and diffuse with IOPs normal/borderline high to prevent hypotony. Suture removal/adjustment/lysis can be done over the following 2 to 3 weeks, depending upon the bleb appearance, anterior chamber depth, and IOP. Over the next few weeks the bleb becomes diffuse, mildly elevated, and relatively avascular (**Fig. 22.18**).

Early Postoperative Complications

The IOP and bleb should be assessed to look for a bleb leak, over-filtration or very tight scleral sutures, clots at the bleb site, or even tight conjunctival suturing as the cause. Immediate postoperative problems are generally related to a shallow anterior chamber or abnormal IOP (**Flowchart 22.1**).

A shallow anterior chamber can be graded as suggested by *Spaeth, into grade 1 with peripheral iridocorneal touch alone, grade 2 with iridocorneal touch up to the pupil, or grade 3 with lenticular corneal touch.* Managing shallow anterior chambers after a trabeculectomy requires an early diagnosis of the cause, so that appropriate therapy is instituted as quickly as possible, preventing needless corneal endothelial cell loss and cataractogenesis (**Fig. 22.19**).

Combinations of clinical features provide a framework for management of a shallow anterior chamber following trabeculectomy.

- *A shallow anterior chamber in the presence of a low IOP and no bleb leak:*
    - A grade 1 shallow anterior chamber responds well to conservative management. A cycloplegic

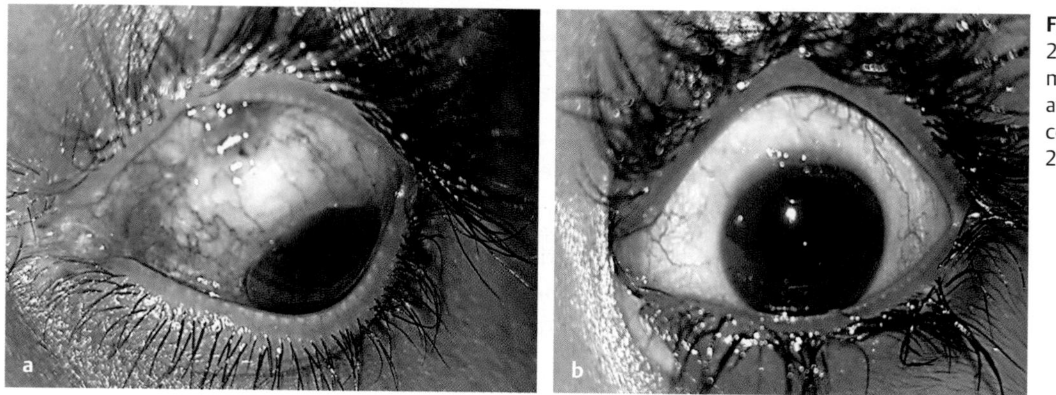

Fig. 22.18 **(a)** Filtering bleb 2 weeks after surgery, diffuse, mildly elevated, and relatively avascular. The suture line is still congested. **(b)** Filtering bleb 2 weeks after surgery.

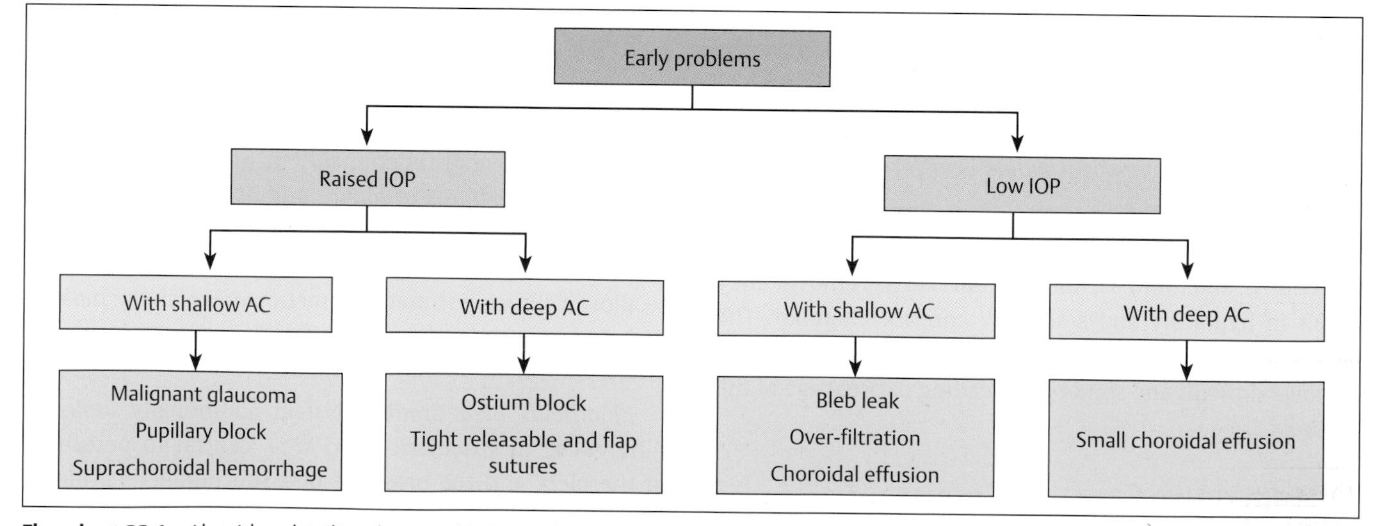

Flowchart 22.1 Algorithm detailing the most likely condition underlying IOP and anterior chamber abnormalities soon after a trabeculectomy. AC, anterior chamber; IOP, intraocular pressure.

Table 22.5 Post-trabeculectomy problems possible at different times and their management

	Cause	Diagnosis	Intervention
		Early	
↓ IOP	Over-filtering bleb	▪ ↑ height and extent of bleb shallow anterior chamber grade 1 or 2 ▪ Shallow anterior chamber grade 3	Pressure bandage and cycloplegia × 24 hours; if persists—anterior chamber reformation ▪ anterior chamber reformation, ± resuturing of scleral flap
	Conjunctival leak	Seidel's +ve, DM folds, shallow/flat anterior chamber	▪ Purse string suture ▪ Bandage CL if near limbus ▪ Conjunctival flap advancement
	Choroidal detachment	Shallow anterior chamber, choroidal mounds on indirect/USG	▪ Difluprednate, cycloplegia, systemic steroids ▪ If no resolution, scleral suturing
↑ IOP	Tight sutures	Deep anterior chamber, flat bleb	Release suture/Laser suturolysis
	Blocked/Small scleral ostium	Flat/localized bleb, subconjunctival clot, peaked pupil	Bleb massage, miotics, glaucoma medications
	Suprachoroidal hemorrhage	Pain, diminution of vision, dark choroidal mounds limited by vortex veins	Control IOP medically, drain if retinal surfaces touch, 7–10 days later
	Malignant glaucoma	Pain, diminution of vision, flat anterior chamber	▪ Atropine and aqueous suppressants topical and systemic ▪ Break vitreous face – YAG laser or vitrectomy + phaco
Hyphema		Blurring of vision	Resolves spontaneously
		Intermediate	
↑ IOP	Hypertensive phase of bleb	4–6 weeks, vascularized bleb	Continue topical steroids + glaucoma meds
	Encysted bleb	Well-demarcated localized raised bleb	▪ Needling ▪ MMC application
	Subconjunctival fibrosis	Tortuous, "corkscrew" vessels overlying a flat bleb	▪ MMC application ▪ Continue topical steroids + glaucoma meds
	Steroid-induced IOP rise	Unremarkable bleb	Low dose/stop steroids or NSAIDs
↓ IOP	Choroidal detachment	Hypotony maculopathy	Resuture scleral flap if medications have failed
		Late	
↑ IOP	Subconjunctival fibrosis	Vascularized flat bleb	Glaucoma medications to target IOP, or repeat filtering surgery
	Scleral block/scarring	Flat bleb, ostium blocked on gonioscopy	▪ Glaucoma medications to target IOP ▪ YAG laser to reopen ostium or repeat filtering surgery
↓ IOP	Avascular/thin bleb	Sweating on fluorescein examination, or transparent conjunctiva, scleral melt, hypotonic maculopathy	Bleb-sparing conjunctival exchange
	Traumatic rupture of bleb	Seidel's +ve, choroidal folds	Conjunctival advancement flap
Infections	Blebitis		Concentrated antibiotic drops, IV antibiotics
	Endophthalmitis		Intravitreal antibiotics and early vitrectomy
Dysesthetic bleb			Bleb revision
Accelerated cataractogenesis	Over-filtration	Shallow anterior chamber, hypotony, macular edema	Bleb-sparing conjunctival exchange ± partial blebectomy

Abbreviations: CL, conjunctival leak; DM, Descemet's membrane; IOP, intraocular pressure; MMC, mitomycin C; NSAIDs, nonsteroidal anti-inflammatory drugs; USG, ultrasonography.

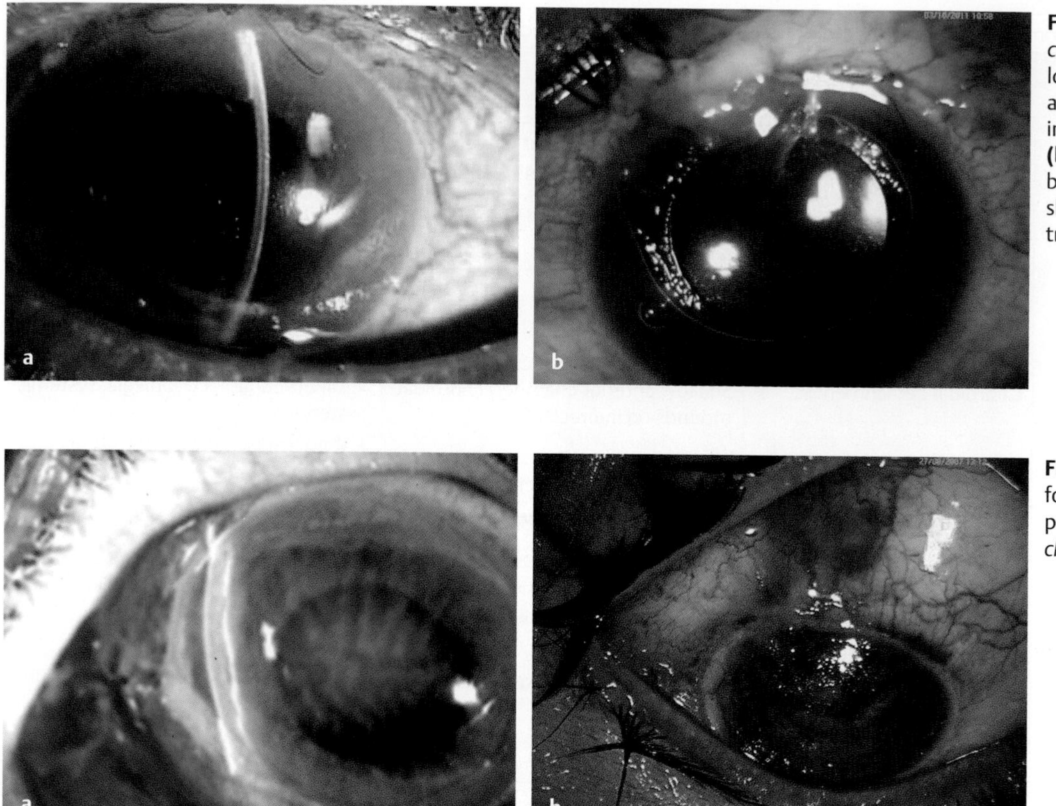

Fig. 22.19 A shallow *anterior chamber* in the presence of a low intraocular pressures (IOP) and no bleb leak. **(a)** Extensive iridocorneal touch, grade 2. **(b)** An entrapped, immobile air bubble highlights a significantly shallow *anterior chamber* after trabeculectomy.

Fig. 22.20 **(a, b)** Descemet's folds seen in an eye with prolonged shallow *anterior chamber* with over filtration.

helps relax the ciliary body and move the lens iris diaphragm posteriorly. Additionally, cycloplegics dilate the iris, which then partially blocks the scleral ostium. Topical steroids should be reduced. A pressure bandage may be used additionally to mechanically flatten the bleb and prevent aqueous outflow.

 - A low IOP with more significant anterior chamber shallowing is seen in about 1% of patients, more often in PACG eyes. This should be taken up for an anterior chamber reformation, with air, BSS, or viscoelastics as early as possible.

- *A shallow anterior chamber with low IOP due to a bleb leak:* Immediately postoperatively a bleb leak may be seen from the edges of a fornix-based flap or a conjunctival buttonhole, and is initially treated conservatively with a pressure bandage or a bandage contact lens. If it persists to the second day, resuturing after scraping the limbal area in case of a leak or else a 10/0 monofilament purse string suture around a buttonhole tethered to the episclera is required. Anterior chamber reformation is done thereafter with air or a viscoelastic.
- *A shallow anterior chamber associated with choroidal effusion and hypotony* generally occurs with an IOP of <6 mm Hg, and needs to be managed as per the cause, if known and discussed above. Choroidal capillaries allow transudation of fluid due to the pressure gradient produced by a low IOP. This tends to occur in 1 to 2% of eyes, especially if the IOP was not lowered preoperatively, and in the presence of postoperative inflammation. Nanophthalmos, Sturge–Weber syndrome, and eyes having a caroticocavernous fistula are more prone to develop choroidal effusions. Choroidal effusions are also more common in patients with myopia, collagen disease, or a thin sclera. *They are recognized by noting a poor glow from the retina, and smooth mounds visible peripherally on distant direct examination.* The patient may have refractive changes due to the forward movement of the lens iris diaphragm, or may have significant visual loss of the effusion. Ultrasonography (USG) is diagnostic, showing dome-shaped retinal mounds with an underlying echolucent space. An associated serous retinal detachment may be seen in some eyes.

Prolonged hypotony with a grade 2 or 3 anterior chamber can lead to corneal decompensation, Descemet's folds, and cataractogenesis (**Fig. 22.20**). Early restoration of the anterior chamber is very important. Systemic and frequent topical steroids and atropine ointment are required to help resolve the effusion. *Difluprednate drops appear to work better than betamethasone or dexamethasone* (**Fig. 22.21**). When the IOP rises to around 7 to 9 mm Hg, these tend to resolve. If a couple of anterior chamber reformations over a few days does not lead to at least a grade 2 shallow chamber and some elevation of IOP, resuturing of the scleral flap should be done. *Bleb resuturing* is also indicated if there is an over-filtering bleb or a significantly shallow anterior chamber. Compressive sutures using 9/0 or 10/0 monofilament over the bleb have been described and are effective in some cases, but may rupture the bleb. Choroidal effusions take a few weeks to resolve, and *need to be drained only if they are very large, "kissing choroidals" or there is prolonged corneolenticular touch* (**Fig. 22.22**). Drainage of the effusion is imperative in "kissing" choroidals or grade 3 shallow anterior chamber and should be considered in large nonresolving effusions lasting over months.

Drainage of the effusion is done 4 to 5 mm from the limbus in the quadrant with the highest dome seen. An anterior chamber maintainer is placed to increase IOP and a 2 to 3 mm radial scleral incision is carefully made to reach the suprachoroidal space, when the fluid will be seen to egress (**Fig. 22.23**). Drainage may also be done with a 26-gauge needle passed tangentially into the sclera. Gentle pressure around the eye with a cotton bud and an increase in anterior chamber pressure will permit drainage of the fluid, as much as possible, with an easily formed anterior chamber. The sclerotomy should be left open and conjunctiva closed over it.

Choroidal effusions can be prevented by the use of IV mannitol half an hour prior to surgery, and by preventing postoperative hypotony with tight scleral flap closure and releasable sutures. In inflamed eyes, systemic steroids may be started preoperatively.

- *A high IOP with a formed anterior chamber* on the first postoperative day may be caused by tight scleral sutures or a clot, and should ideally be treated conservatively with gentle globe massage, and if required oral glycerol and topical glaucoma medications (**Fig. 22.24**). Globe massage is done to permit flow from under the scleral flap to the subconjunctival space, and therefore aims to separate the superficial and deep sclera. Applying two forefingers on either side of the bleb alternately in a seesaw fashion pushes the scleral bed back, allowing aqueous flow to occur, and breaking any adhesions that may be forming (**Fig. 22.25**). Some surgeons use pressure inferiorly to force aqueous upwards, and through the ostium, but this needs far more pressure on an operated eye, which is best avoided.

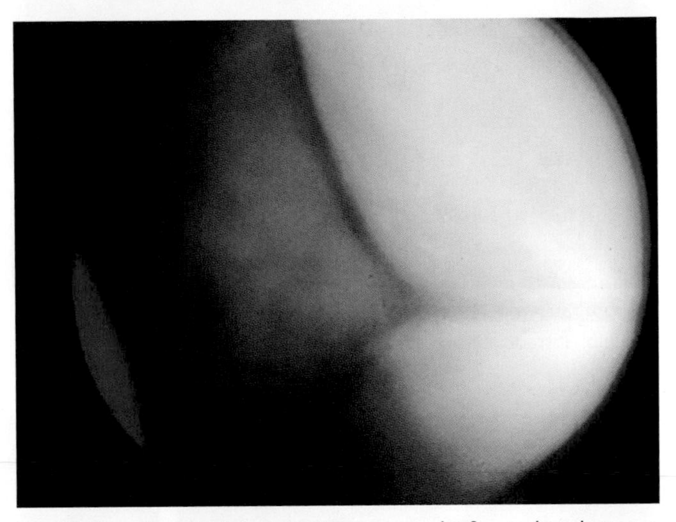

Fig. 22.21 Choroid detachment seen a week after trabeculectomy. Conservative management should suffice in this eye.

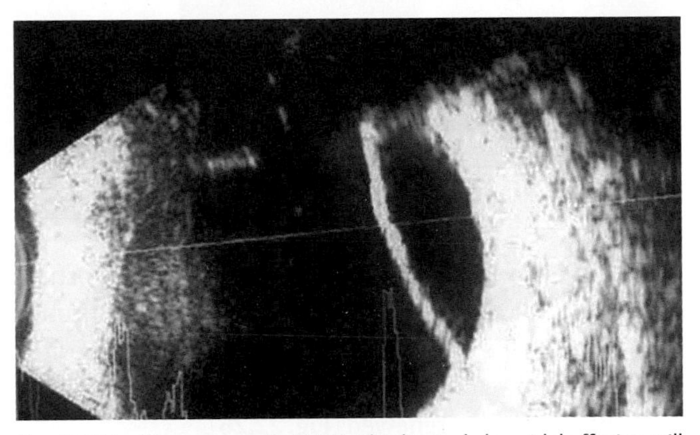

Fig. 22.22 *Ultrasonography (USG)*. This limited choroidal effusion will resolve with conservative management.

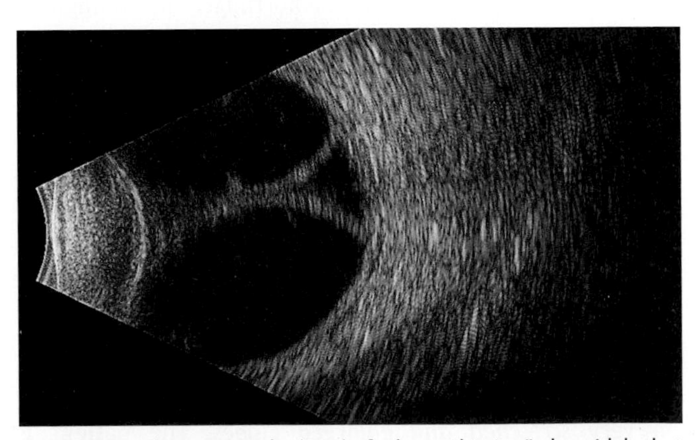

Fig. 22.23 *Ultrasonography (USG)* of a large "kissing" choroidals that would need to be drained.

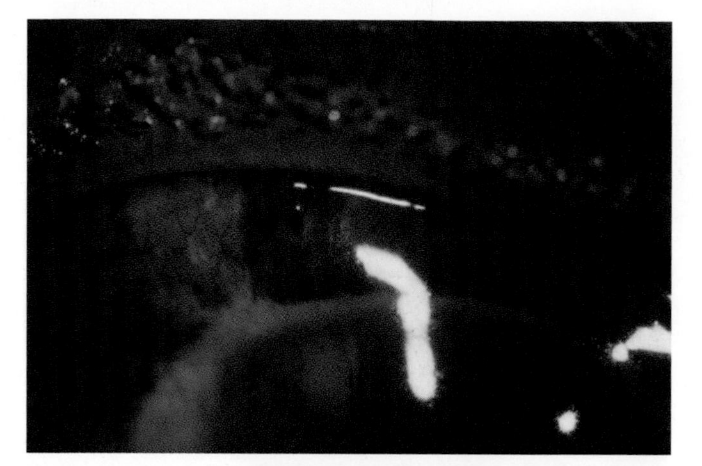

Fig. 22.24 Subconjunctival clot preventing aqueous outflow, leading to a high intraocular pressure (IOP).

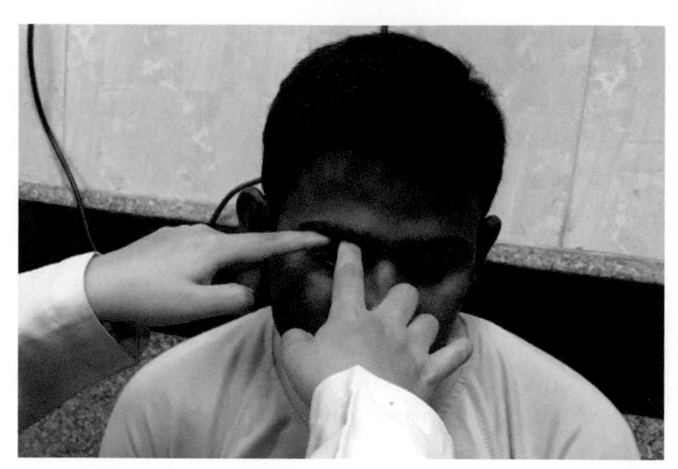

Fig. 22.25 Globe massage by placing the two forefingers on either side of the bleb.

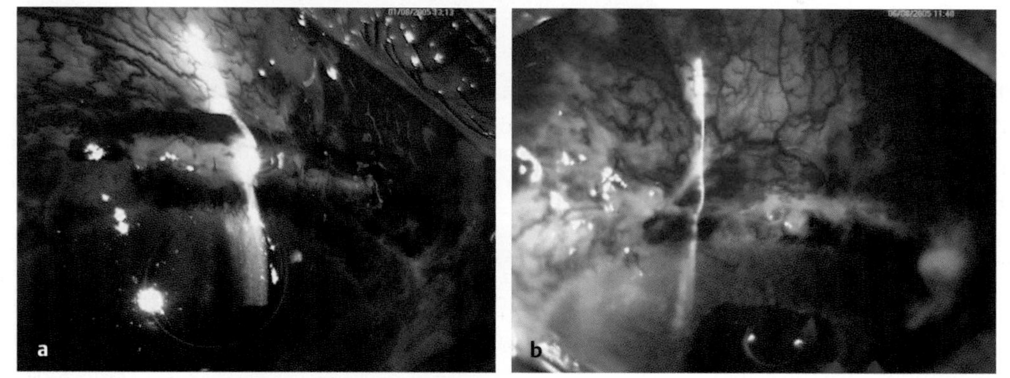

Fig. 22.26 **(a)** Peaked iris blocking the scleral ostium. **(b)** Intracameral pilocarpine pulled the iris out and *anterior chamber* could be reformed later.

Iris or even the lens may block the scleral ostium and also cause a high IOP. Anatomic reconstitution of the anterior chamber using miotics, iris repositor, etc., and reforming the anterior chamber may allow function to be renewed (**Fig. 22.26**).

- *Cases with a high IOP having a shallow anterior chamber should prompt an examination for pupillary block, suprachoroidal hemorrhage, or malignant glaucoma.*

Pupillary block may occur if a lamellar iridectomy happened and therefore air or the lens blocks the pupil, and will resolve with a laser iridotomy if the cornea is clear enough. Removing an excess of air or doing a surgical iridectomy may be necessary if the cornea is hazy.

Suprachoroidal hemorrhages tend to occur in 1 to 6% of trabeculectomy eyes, when high IOPs are suddenly lowered by trabeculectomy, *especially in elderly atherosclerotic individuals, aphakes, vitrectomized eyes, or after surgery on very stretched and enlarged globes.* The patient is seen to complain of eye pain, headache, and nausea on postoperative review, and would have a very high IOP. It is best treated conservatively if present in the periphery as the blood will first clot, then lyse and be absorbed. Where the IOP becomes medically uncontrolled or very large bullae with retina-to-retina touch occur, drainage of the suprachoroidal hemorrhage may be undertaken through a radial sclerotomy 4 to 5 mm from the limbus, overlying the most elevated quadrant, after waiting at least 7 to 14 days (**Figs. 22.27** and **22.28**). An anterior chamber maintainer would push back the lens iris diaphragm and increase drainage from the sclerotomy. Preventive measures include preoperative lowering of IOP, intraoperative use of air/viscoelastics to maintain the anterior chamber, and preplaced scleral sutures to quickly close the eye.

Aqueous misdirection syndrome, ciliolenticular block, or malignant glaucoma occurs due to aqueous moving posteriorly into the vitreous cavity, pushing the lens iris diaphragm forward, thus blocking aqueous outflow. On examination a very shallow anterior chamber with very high IOPs is generally seen either intraoperatively or early postoperatively (**Fig. 22.29**).

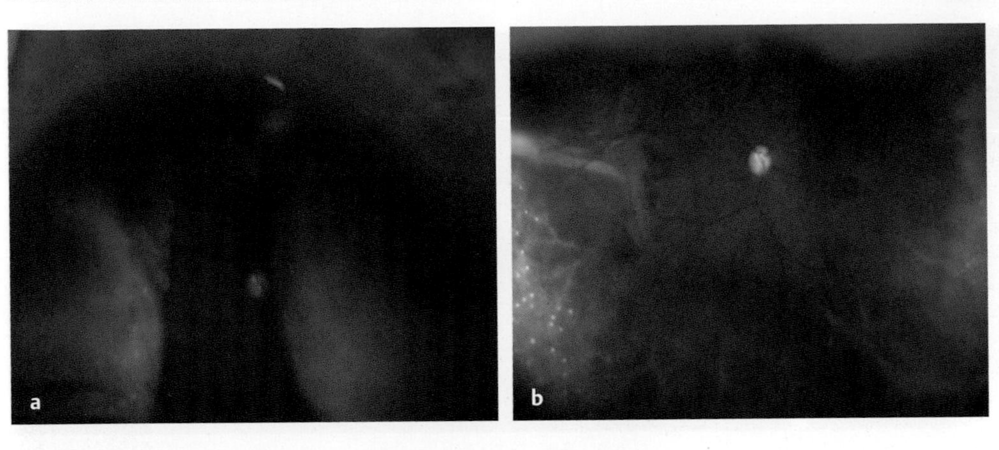

Fig. 22.27 (a) Optos fundus showing a large suprachoroidal hemorrhage, seen as dark retinal bullae. **(b)** After drainage resolution and flattening, the retina is seen.

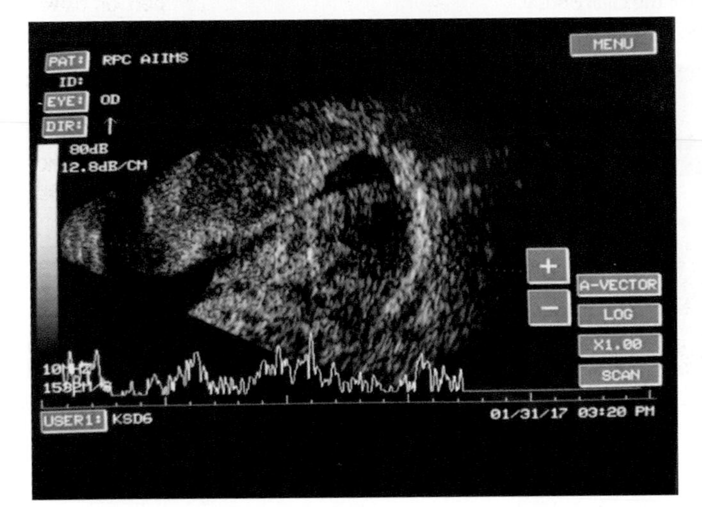

Fig. 22.28 *Ultrasonography (USG)* of a suprachoroidal hemorrhage showing echogenic retinal mounds.

Aqueous misdirection does not respond to routine glaucoma medicines, and a decrease in aqueous formation with cycloplegia is the mainstay of initial medical therapy. Cycloplegia pulls on the zonules, moving the lens back. Cycloplegia and mydriasis are important, and higher doses of phenylephrine and atropine 1 to 2% are advocated. Full doses of acetazolamide, timolol, and brimonidine should be immediately started to reduce aqueous production so that further fluid build-up in the posterior segment is halted. IV mannitol adds to the effect of these medications by decreasing vitreous volume. Topical steroids help reduce inflammation and the ciliary effusion present. The anterior chamber may form and IOP fall on these medications in 3 to 5 days in some patients, and these need to be continued for months with a gradual taper.

The long-term use of topical atropine, even for years, is recommended. *If medical therapy fails to lower IOP, a hyaloidotomy with Nd:YAG laser or surgery may be attempted; however, a lensectomy and anterior hyaloidotomy is often required.* Sectoral cyclophotocoagulation may help by temporarily decreasing aqueous production.

Malignant glaucoma may be prevented by lowering the IOP significantly in predisposed eyes such as PACG and nanophthalmic eyes prior to surgery. It tends to occur in the second eye as well.

Late Complications

Failure of Surgery

Failure occurs due to a block of the scleral ostium inside the anterior chamber, at the sclera or outside, e.g., subconjunctival causes. The internal block can be due to iris, vitreous, or even lens plugging the ostium (**Fig. 22.30a**). A block at the sclera is commonly due to lamellar scleral dissection or a pre-existing membrane at the trabecular meshwork as in uveitis, neovascular glaucoma, or due to postoperative fibrosis (**Fig. 22.30b**). Subconjunctival fibrosis tends to occur over time, and is the predominant cause of failure in adults. This can result in an encysted bleb or a flat vascularized bleb (**Fig. 22.30c**). *Diagnosis of impending failure by looking for the presence of "corkscrew" vessels around or over the bleb may allow timely interventions.* Topical application of MMC 0.4 mg/mL for 3 minutes on alternate days, three to four times, sometimes reduces vascularity and with bleb massage permits some bleb function (**Fig. 22.31**). Hypertensive phase of a bleb may occasionally be seen as a gradual but significantly elevated and congested bleb, which resolves on topical steroids (**Fig. 22.32**).

Late Bleb Dysfunction

Trabeculectomy bleb epithelium tends to become thinner with time, and more so after the use of adjuvant antifibrotic agents, avascular and leaking blebs have become more common. These may occur months or years after the

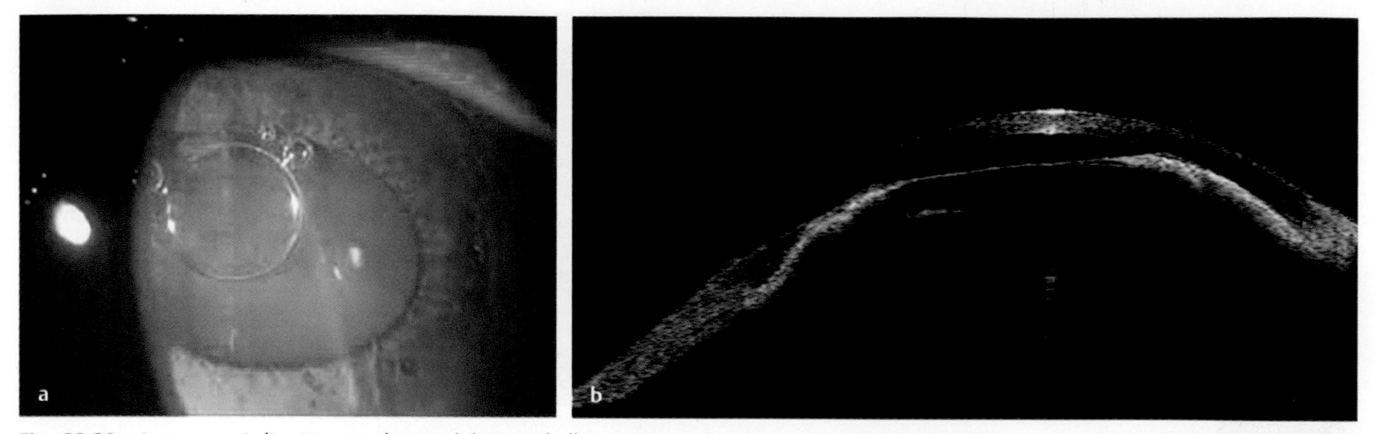

Fig. 22.29 Aqueous misdirection syndrome. **(a)** Very shallow anterior chamber with a high intraocular pressure (IOP). **(b)** Anterior segment optical coherence tomography showing a flattening and anterior rotation of the ciliary body.

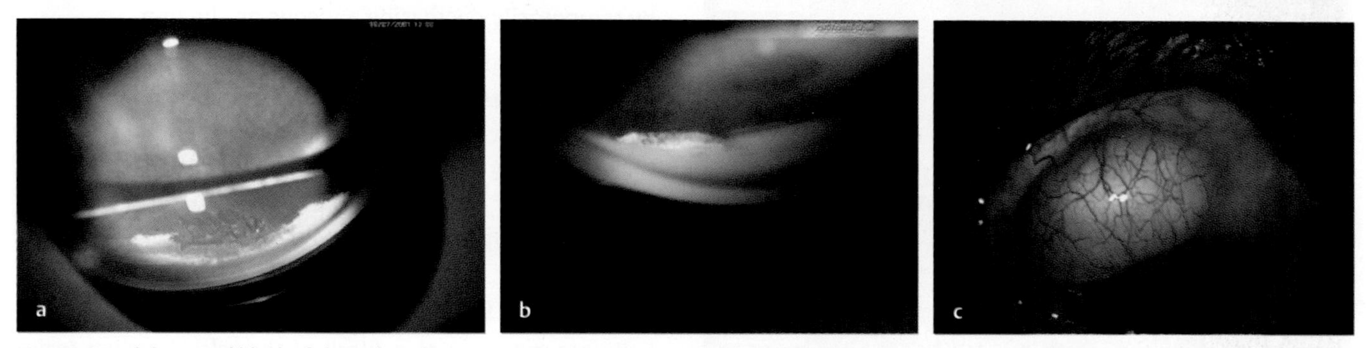

Fig. 22.30 **(a)** Internal block of the trabeculectomy ostium by iris tissue. **(b)** Scleral fibrosis closing a trabeculectomy ostium. **(c)** Subconjunctival fibrosis after trabeculectomy—an encysted bleb in which a needling may break the surrounding fibrous capsule and lower intraocular pressure (IOP).

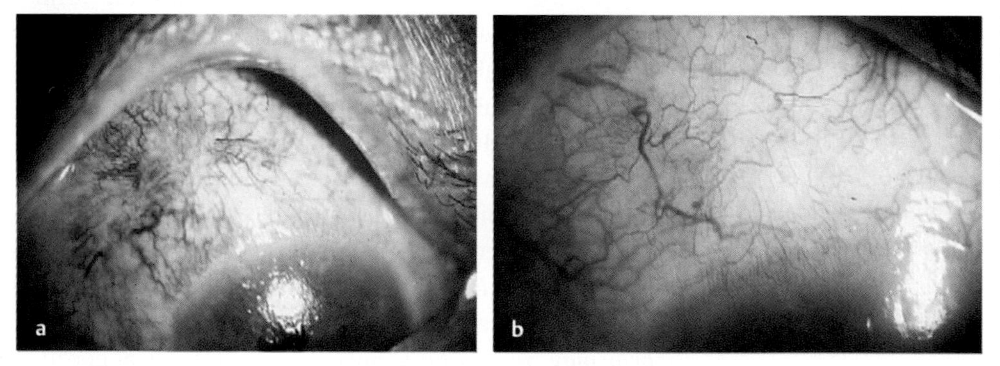

Fig. 22.31 **(a)** "Corkscrew" vessels around and over the bleb which should not be treated with needling. Three topical applications of mitomycin C (MMC) were done. **(b)** Decreased vascularity and moderate function of the bleb after 4 months.

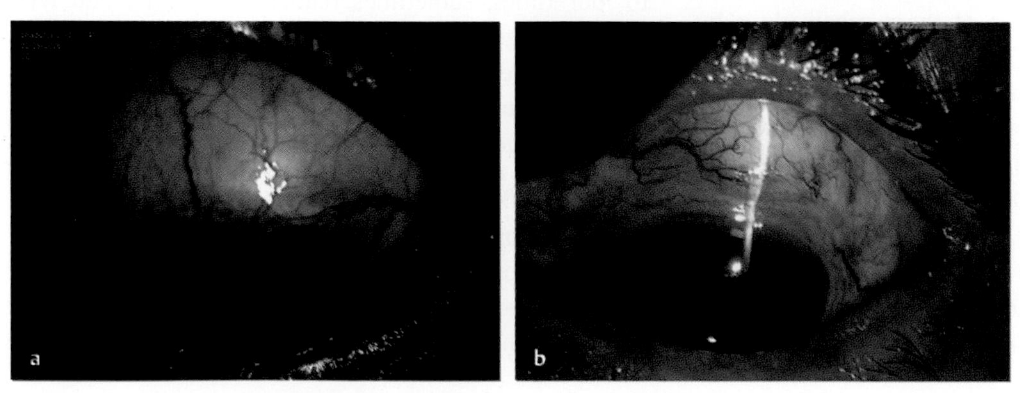

Fig. 22.32 **(a, b)** Hypertensive phase of a bleb around 4 to 6 weeks after trabeculectomy, with shelving edges unlike the sharp borders of an encysted bleb. These resolve with steroids and time in most cases.

surgery. After 5 years, 18 to 20% of eyes may be expected to develop some susceptibility of the blebs. Conservative therapy of aqueous suppressants and bandage contact lenses with systemic antibiotic cover may be tried in small or intermittent leaks with a careful review.

Definite leaks lead to shallowing of the anterior chamber and hypotonic maculopathy (**Figs. 22.33** and **22.34**). *The presence of a frank leak in an avascular, sweating or thin bleb requires removal of the unhealthy epithelium by epithelium peeling and replacement with fresh adjacent conjunctiva.* This permits the underlying bleb to continue to function, so that additional glaucoma medications are generally not required (**Figs. 22.35** and **22.36**). Excision of the bleb with anterior mobilization of the conjunctiva and tenon has been described, but frequently results in a raised IOP requiring glaucoma medications and even a repeat trabeculectomy.

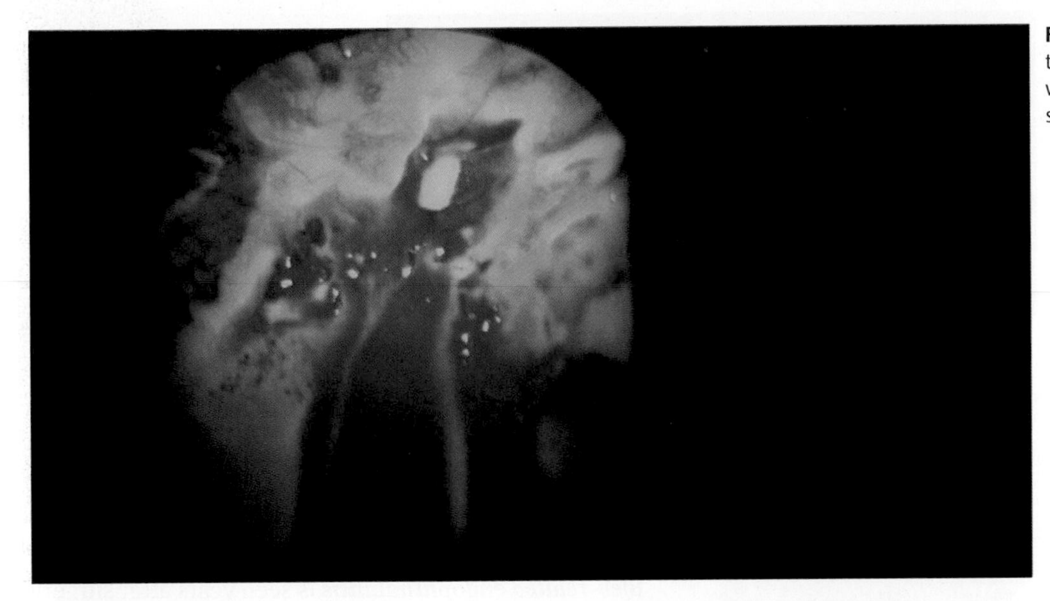

Fig. 22.33 Aqueous flow from the bleb leak seen as a dark stream within the green fluorescein-stained tear film.

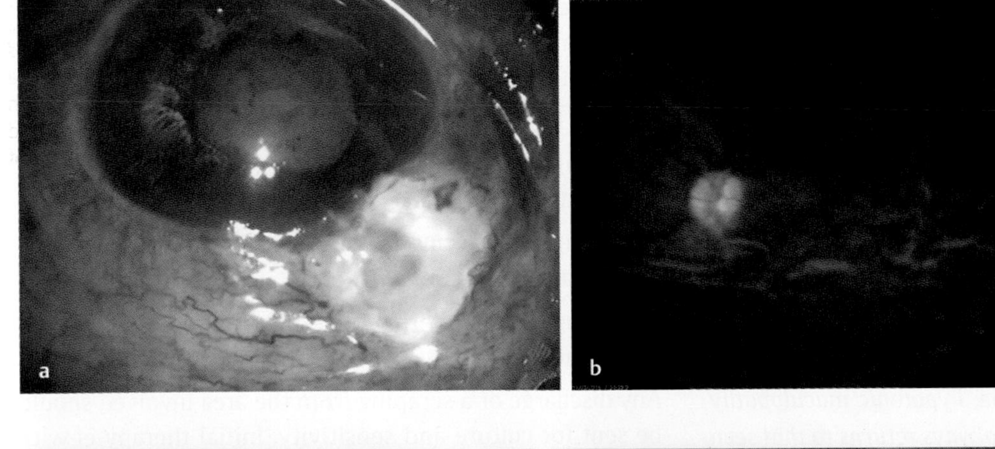

Fig. 22.34 **(a)** A thin, avascular bleb with an intraocular pressure (IOP) of <5 mm Hg. **(b)** Hypotonic maculopathy.

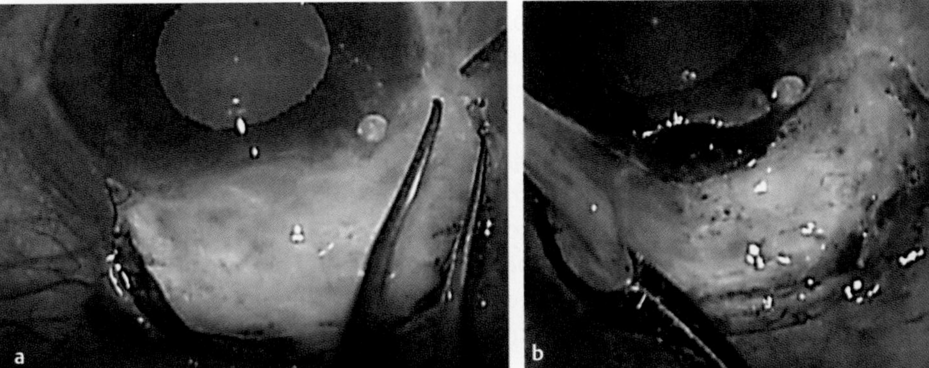

Fig. 22.35 Intraoperative photos of a thin-walled bleb: **(a)** and **(b)** after peeling off the epithelium with retained bleb tissue. The adjacent conjunctiva is then dissected and brought forward to cover the defect.

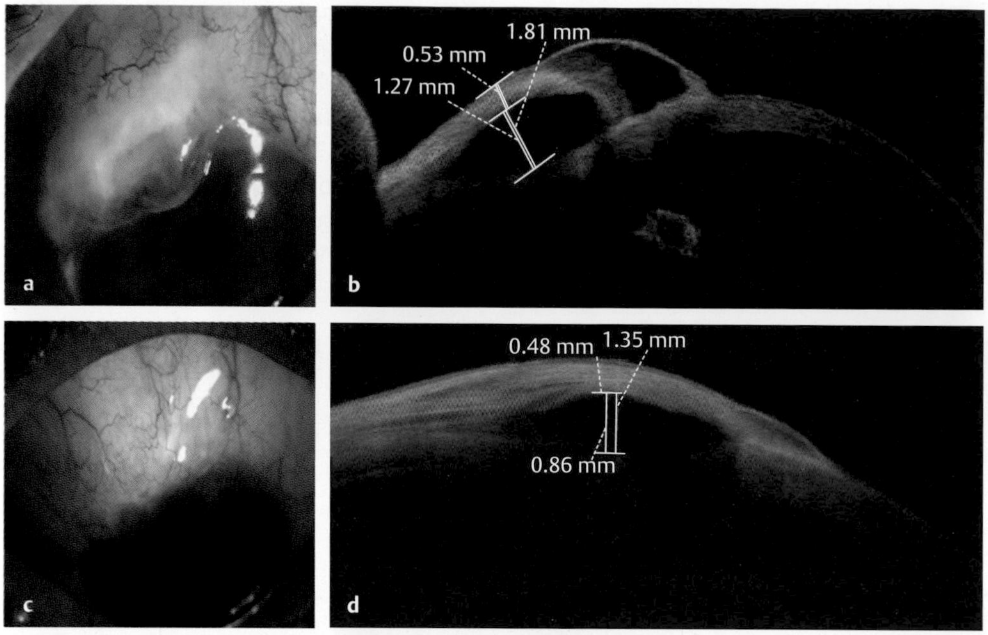

Fig. 22.36 (a, b) Preoperative photos and anterior segment optical coherence tomography (ASOCT) of a thin-walled bleb. **(c, d)** After 5 years of bleb-sparing epithelial exchange surgery, the mean intraocular pressure (IOP) is 12 mm Hg.

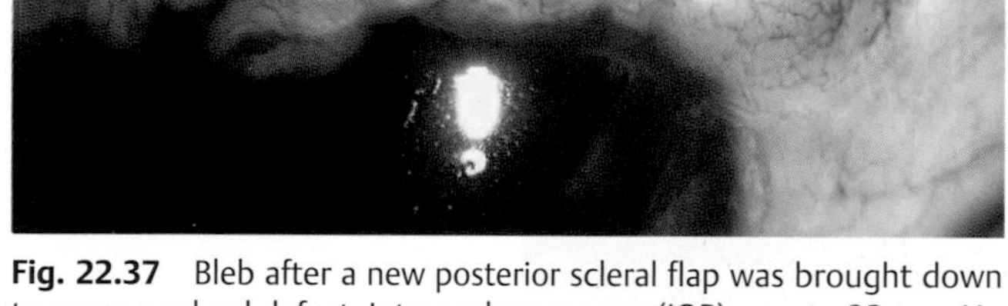

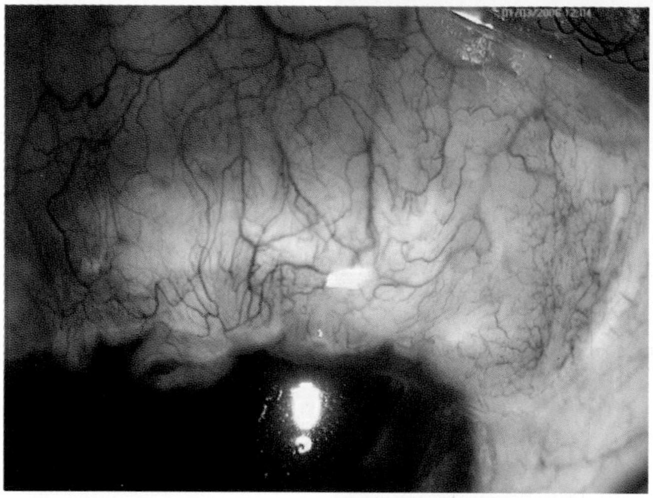

Fig. 22.37 Bleb after a new posterior scleral flap was brought down to cover a scleral defect. Intraocular pressure (IOP) rose to 32 mm Hg and was controlled on medications.

As the IOP rises after bleb revision, hypotonic maculopathy resolves and visual acuity almost always returns to that seen prior to trabeculectomy.

In eyes with thinning of the sclera or sclerolysis in an eye with hypotony, a scleral flap from the posterior sclera may be inverted to cover a scleral defect. This is frequently followed by a rise in IOP, and further glaucoma medications may be required (**Fig. 22.37**).

Blebitis is any inflammation noted around a filtering bleb and should be treated as an ophthalmic emergency to prevent infection within the bleb or its progression to endophthalmitis. The use of broad-spectrum antibiotic drops, especially concentrated tobramycin and cephazoline drops, will control early infection. A bleb revision should be scheduled after 4 to 6 weeks to prevent any recurrence of bleb infections.

Bleb-related endophthalmitis is seen years after surgery or as a consequence of trauma. As the pathogens have easy access to both the anterior chamber and through the iridectomy to the posterior chamber and vitreous, this is more difficult to treat and often results in loss of vision.

It can be graded into three stages:

- Stage 1: Purulent bleb with or without anterior chamber reaction.
- Stage 2: Purulent bleb with moderate anterior chamber reaction.
- Stage 3: Endophthalmitis: Marked anterior chamber reaction, vitritis.

Any discharge or a scraping from the area involved should be sent for culture and sensitivity. Initial therapy is with topical moxifloxacin and concentrated tobramycin and cephazoline drops hourly, and oral and IV antibiotics. Intracameral and subconjunctival antibiotic injections should also be given in stages 1 and 2. *In stage 3, the presence of even minimal vitreous exudates on USG would necessitate an early vitrectomy to preserve vision.* Intravitreal antibiotics may give some relief in early vitritis, but early vitrectomy gives the best results. The prognosis in such eyes remains grim, especially in the presence of a coagulase positive Staph or Strep infection (**Figs. 22.38** and **22.39**).

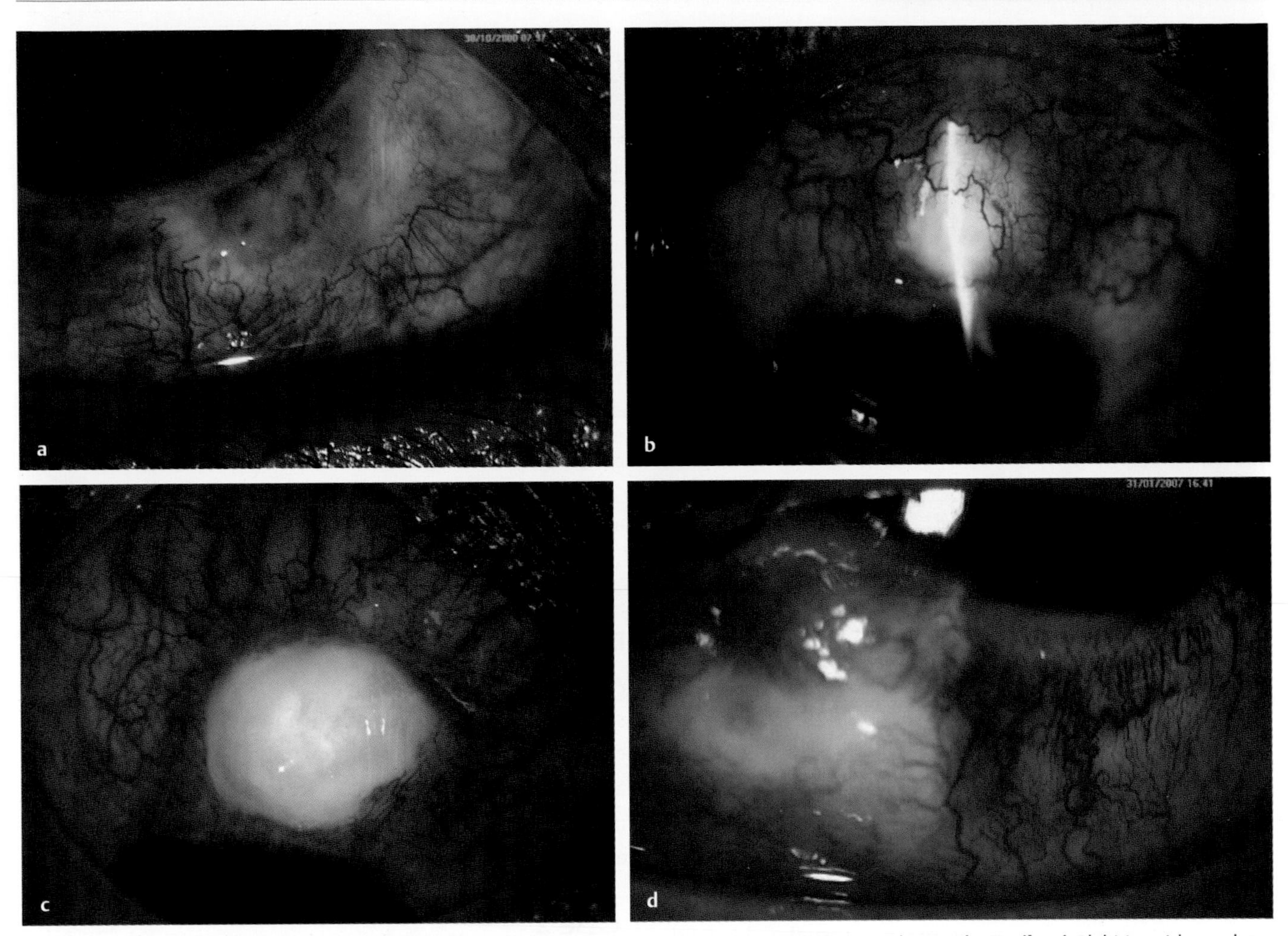

Fig. 22.38 **(a)** Early diagnosis of blebitis should be made in the presence of congestion in a predisposed eye. **(b, c)** Blebitis, with exudates within the bleb and congestion all around. Anterior chamber is quiet. **(d)** An inferior trabeculectomy with bleb-related endophthalmitis, wherein a hypopyon can be seen.

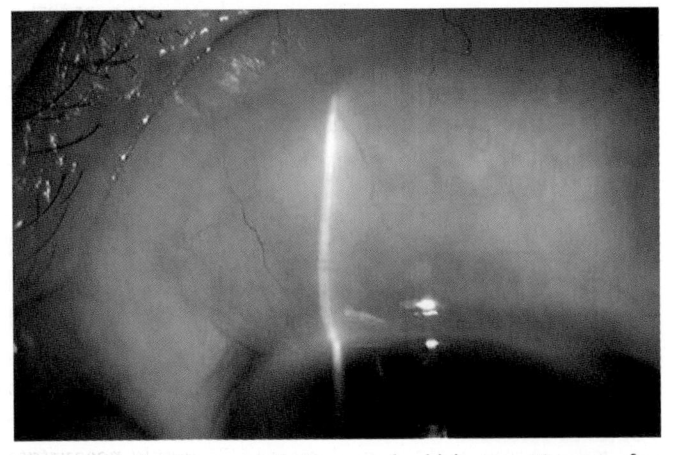

Fig. 22.39 A diffuse, relatively avascular bleb seen 10 years after trabeculectomy.

Chronic hypotony may be due to a cyclodialysis cleft created during the trabeculectomy or following trauma, and is diagnosed on ultrasound biomicroscopy (UBM) or ASOCT. Conservative therapy with atropine and steroids may resolve small clefts by apposing peripheral iris to the cleft. Photocoagulative laser or cryotherapy applications to the cleft area may help adhesions to form. A surgical closure of the cleft may be undertaken to suture the disinserted ciliary body to the sclera if hypotonic maculopathy persists over months.

Trabeculectomy has been evaluated against medications and different glaucoma surgeries in many studies (**Table 22.6**).

Table 22.6 Evaluation of trabeculectomy against medic ations and various other glaucoma surgeries

Study	Trabeculectomy	Eyes operated	Success	Comments
Collaborative Initial Glaucoma Treatment Study (CIGTS)	Trabeculectomy vs. target IOP on medications	POAG, pigmentary and pseudoexfoliation glaucomas	Trabeculectomy lower IOPs, 14–15 vs. 17–18 mm Hg VF effect similar 21% of trabeculectomy and 25% of medically treated patients progressed in 8 years	Trabeculectomy better in advanced glaucomas
Primary tube versus trabeculectomy, PTVT study	Trabeculectomy with 0.4 mg/mL MMC × 2 minutes versus Baerveldt	POAG	Trabeculectomy lower IOPs better at 3 years	Further surgery often required after Baerveldt, hypotony common after trabs
Tube versus trabeculectomy study (TVT)	Trab with 0.4 mg/mL MMC × 4 minutes versus Baerveldt shunt	Pseudophakia with glaucoma or failed trabeculectomy		↑ meds in Baerveldt eyes for 2 years

Abbreviations: CIGTS, Collaborative Initial Glaucoma Treatment Study; IOP, intraocular pressure; MMC, mitomycin C; POAG, primary open angle glaucoma; TVT, tube versus trabeculectomy; VF, visual field.

Conclusion

Trabeculectomy has been shown to work well, reaching target levels of IOP without medications in 60 to 70% of eyes over more than 20 years, and in over 90% with adjunctive glaucoma medications. *It requires postoperative medications and manipulations over 6 to 8 weeks for best results, and a lifelong review for later changes that may occur.* Care during surgery decreases the occurrence of postoperative problems, stabilizing visual fields and maintaining vision in the long term.

Trabeculectomy is still a benchmark for other surgeries, but the steps need to be adjusted by the surgeon for a given patient. There is a learning curve to this surgery, but the long-term results have been repeatedly shown to be good in all kinds of glaucomas.

Cases

Case 1

A 65-year-old male diagnosed with POAG was found to show progression while on four topical medications. An selective laser trabeculoplasty (SLT) was performed, but the IOP remained between 18 and 22 mm Hg after 3 months. He underwent a trabeculectomy with releasable sutures and was asked to review for suture removal a week later.

Points to consider

- Anterior chamber should be well formed.
- The bleb should not be high and extensive.
- IOP should not be < 6mm Hg.

Diagnosis and Management

As the IOP was 10 mm Hg with a significantly elevated bleb, suture removal could lead to further egress of aqueous, causing a shallow anterior chamber (**Case 1-1**). He was asked to review again after a week, and informed that only one suture would be released at a time, and the second at a subsequent visit.

Case 2

A 14-year-old girl with aniridia and bilateral subluxation of cataractous lenses in an enlarged eye was reviewed after a successful trabeculectomy for her worse eye done 1 year earlier. In view of IOPs in the better eye, ranging from 24 to 28 mm Hg with vision of 6/18, a cup:disc ratio of 0.8, and biarcuate scotomas on Goldmann perimetry, a trabeculectomy in the second eye was done. The anterior chamber was maintained through the surgery, and two fixed sutures and two releasable sutures were applied. On the first postoperative day the IOP was recorded to be 30 mm Hg and one releasable suture was removed. The next day she complained of severe pain and loss of vision, and a shallow anterior chamber was seen.

Points to consider

- Enlarged eye with thin sclera.
- Suture released on first postoperative day when no fibrosis has occurred.
- IOP lowered from 30 to 10 mm Hg by releasing a suture.

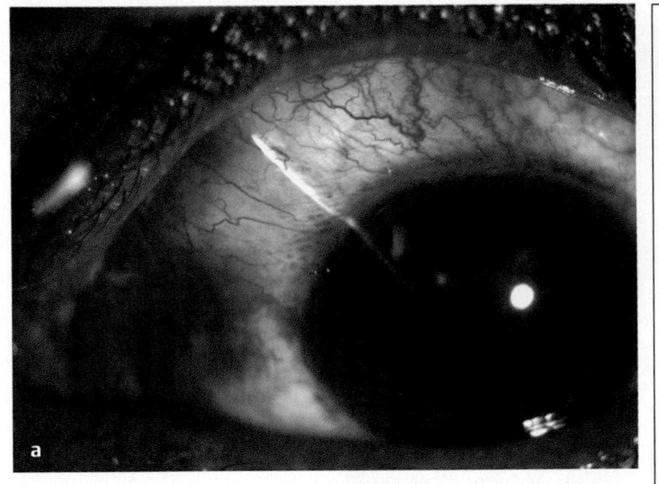

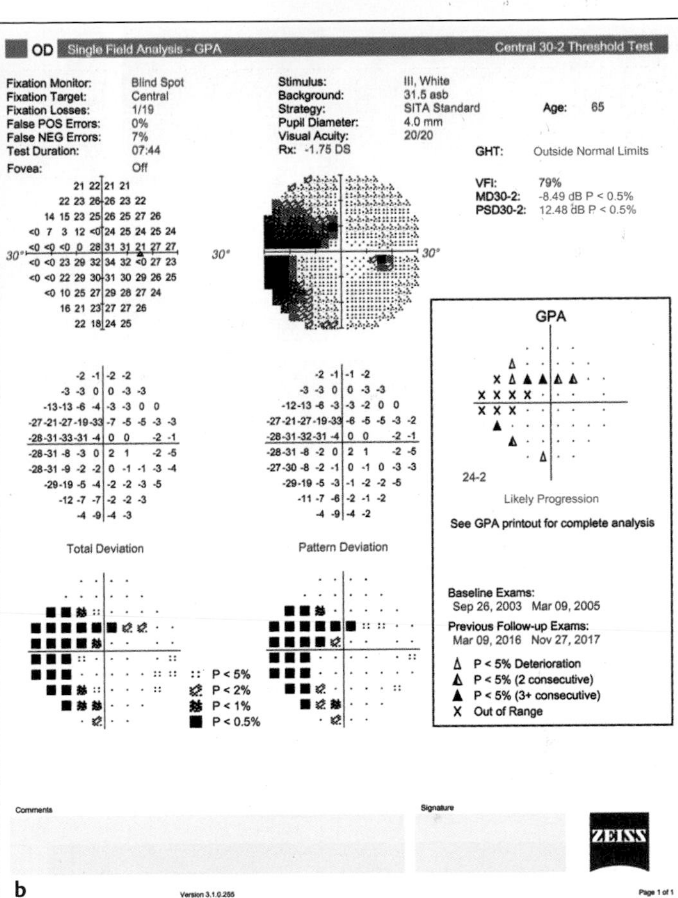

Case 1-1 **(a)** Diffuse and elevated bleb. **(b)** Superior arcuate scotoma with a large inferior nasal step. Progression is shown by the fully black triangles.

Diagnosis and Management

A suprachoroidal hemorrhage was suspected and seen on USG (**Case 2-1**). On the fifth postoperative day retinal contact was seen, so a resuturing of the bleb and two sclerotomies, 4 mm behind the limbus over pars plana in the inferior quadrants, were made. After deepening the anterior chamber with BSS, some blood was seen to come out and the mounds became smaller. On the 12th day, as the mounds persisted, drainage through the sclerotomies was again attempted, and a significant amount of liquified blood could be removed. The patient was kept on oral and topical antibiotics and steroids, and over the next 3 months, the vision returned to 6/18 and the visual field was as in preoperative assessment.

Case 3

A 60-year-old male with POAG underwent a trabeculectomy as he was allergic to almost all glaucoma medications. Post surgery, his IOP ranged between 10 and 16 mm Hg for 6 weeks, when he complained of pain in the eye. His IOP had risen to 30 mm Hg on topical steroids given four times a day.

Points to consider

- The bleb appears very sharply defined and localized.
- There is severe congestion around the bleb.
- The bleb was elevated.

Diagnosis and Management

A diagnosis of an encysted bleb was made (**Case 3-1**). Needling was done after 0.04% MMC application for 3 minutes to the surface of the bleb. Postoperative treatment with topical antibiotics–steroid combination was given for 3 weeks in tapering doses. After 2 months the IOP was 14 mm Hg on dorzolamide–timolol combination drops twice a day, well within target IOP. He has been perimetrically stable since then for 6 years.

Case 4

A 40-year-old lady with prior vitreoretinal surgery had uncontrolled IOPs of 36 to 40 mm Hg on maximal medical

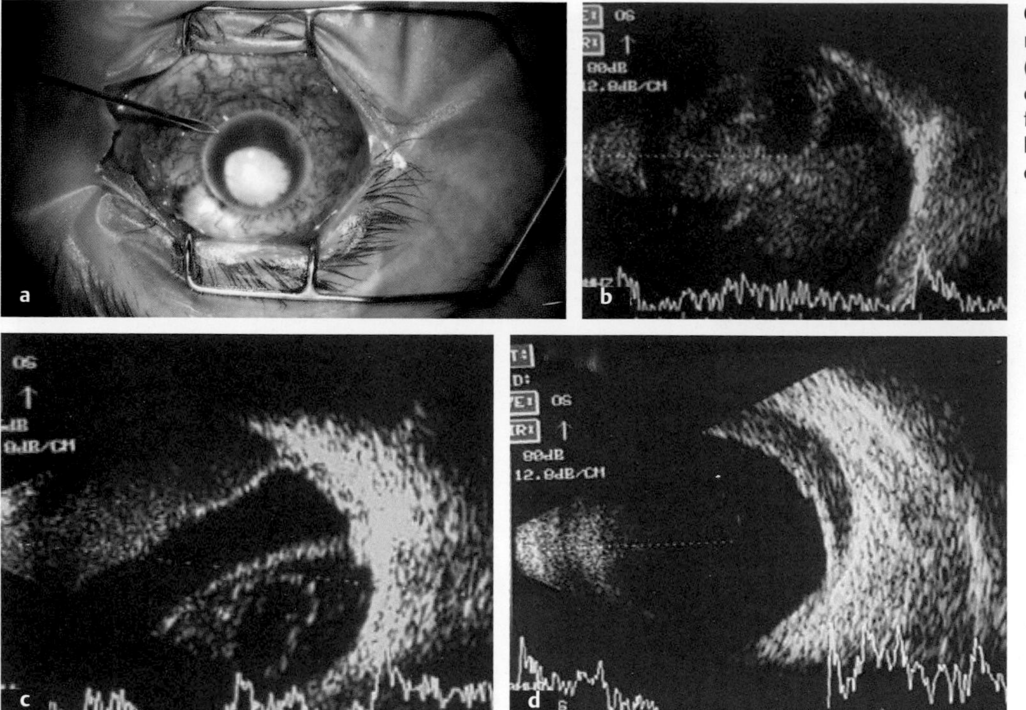

Case 2-1 **(a)** Subluxated cataractous lens. **(b)** Ultrasonography (USG) showing massive suprachoroidal hemorrhage. **(c)** After first drainage. **(d)** After the clot had lysed and could be fully drained.

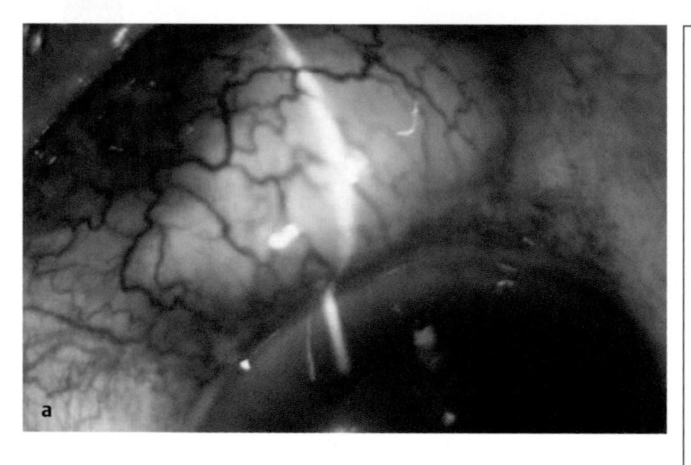

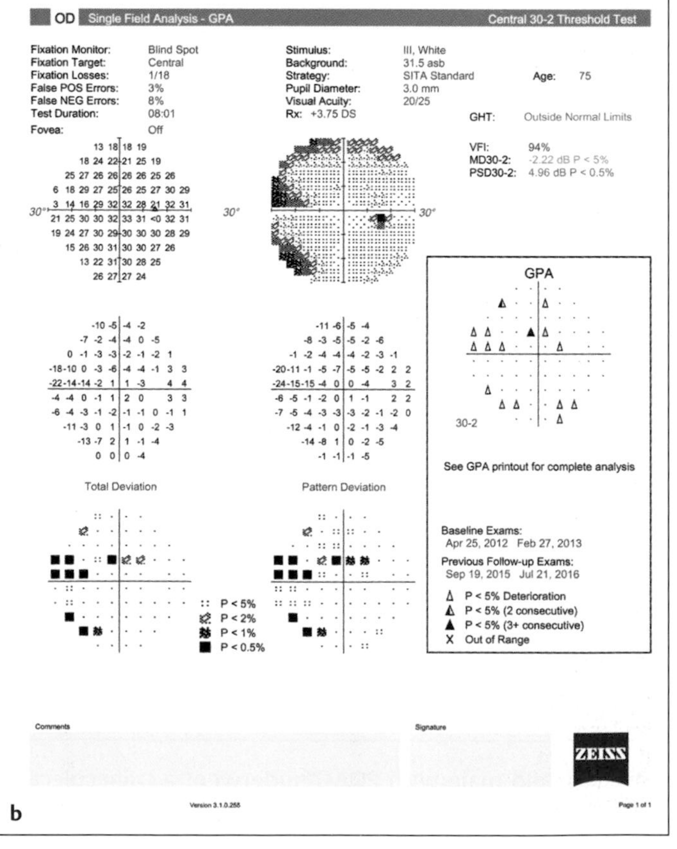

Case 3-1 **(a)** Encysted bleb with sharp edges and significant elevation. **(b)** Perimetry showing stability over the next 6 years at a target intraocular pressure (IOP) of <15 mm Hg.

therapy. Silicon oil removal had been done by the surgeon, but the IOP remained uncontrolled. She was advised a trabeculectomy, and was explained a guarded prognosis for both IOP control and possible retinal problems after surgery. On the table, the first step was a complete wash-out of silicon oil in the anterior chamber by irrigation and aspiration. After dissecting the superficial scleral flap, MMC 0.02% was applied subconjunctival and subscleral for a minute each, in view of the fibrosis present. The IOP reduced to 12 to 14 mm Hg in the first week postoperatively, but rose again to 24 mm Hg after 6 months, with a localized bleb (**Case 4-1**).

Points to consider

- Localized and thin-walled bleb.
- Silicon oil is present within the bleb.
- IOP may be controlled with medications.

Diagnosis and Management

A diagnosis of an encysted bleb was made. The fibrosis could be related to the prior surgery and the silicon oil present within the bleb. Needling of the bleb could be done, but may lead to further fibrosis. As the IOP was 12 to 14 mm Hg on Travatan–timolol combination, the patient is being regularly reviewed. A bleb revision would be done in view of the thinned bleb wall.

Case 5

A 56-year-old lady with a history of unilateral headache and eye pain for a month was diagnosed to have acute PACG. On examination there was a shallow anterior chamber, corneal edema, and areas of iris atrophy with an IOP of 44 mm Hg. Visual acuity was 3/60, with projection inaccurate in one quadrant. On maximal medical therapy and after giving IV mannitol, an iridotomy was tried but remained lamellar and the IOP ranged from 28 to 34 mm Hg (**Case 5-1**).

Points to consider

- A shallow preoperative anterior chamber would be prone to further shallowing after trabeculectomy.
- Cataract surgery could be done first, but there was a chronically uncontrolled IOP suggesting significant trabecular meshwork damage.
- Combined surgery—cataract with a trabeculectomy may not lower IOP sufficiently.

Diagnosis and Management

A diagnosis of acute angle closure glaucoma progressing to chronic PACG was made. Trabeculectomy was done with care—IV mannitol preoperatively to deturgese the vitreous and lower IOP, paracentesis on the table prior to removing the scleral ostium, and tight releasable sutures at the limbus. The anterior chamber was similar to preoperative on the first postoperative day with an IOP of 22 mm Hg. The pupil was dilated with tropicamide daily and releasable sutures were only removed 10 and 14 days after surgery. A year after surgery, IOP off medications was 14 mm Hg, the bleb was relatively avascular and mildly elevated. Visual acuity had improved to 6/18, with inaccurate projection in one quadrant. There was no accelerated cataractogenesis or corneal decompensation.

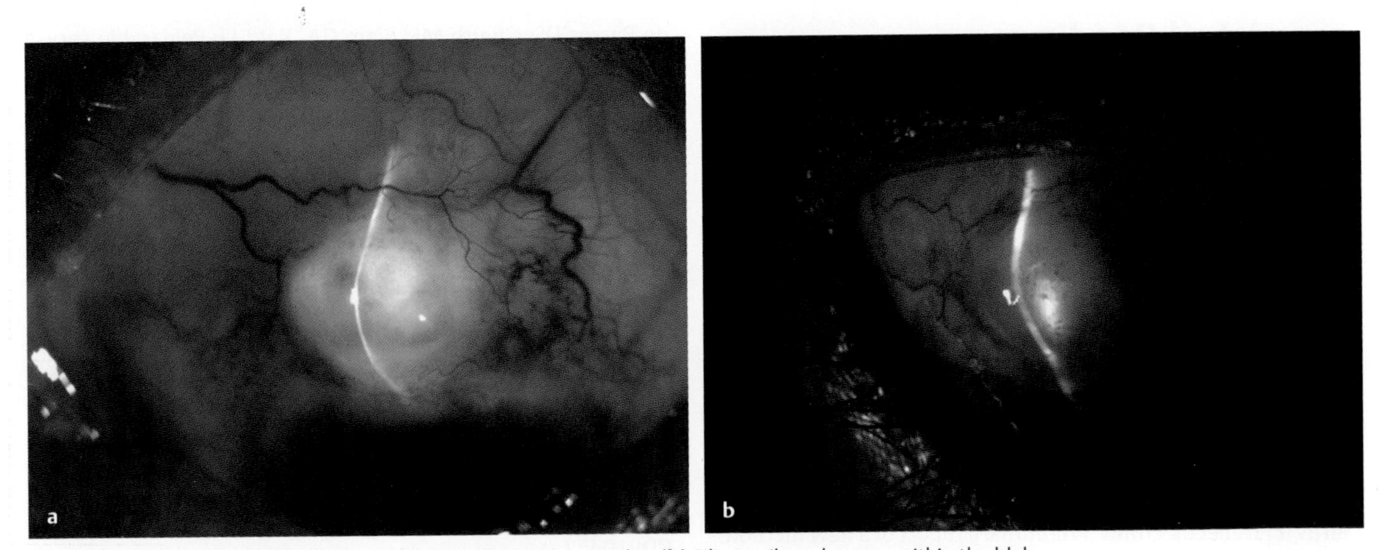

Case 4-1 **(a)** Localized and elevated with vascularization around it. **(b)** Silicon oil can be seen within the bleb.

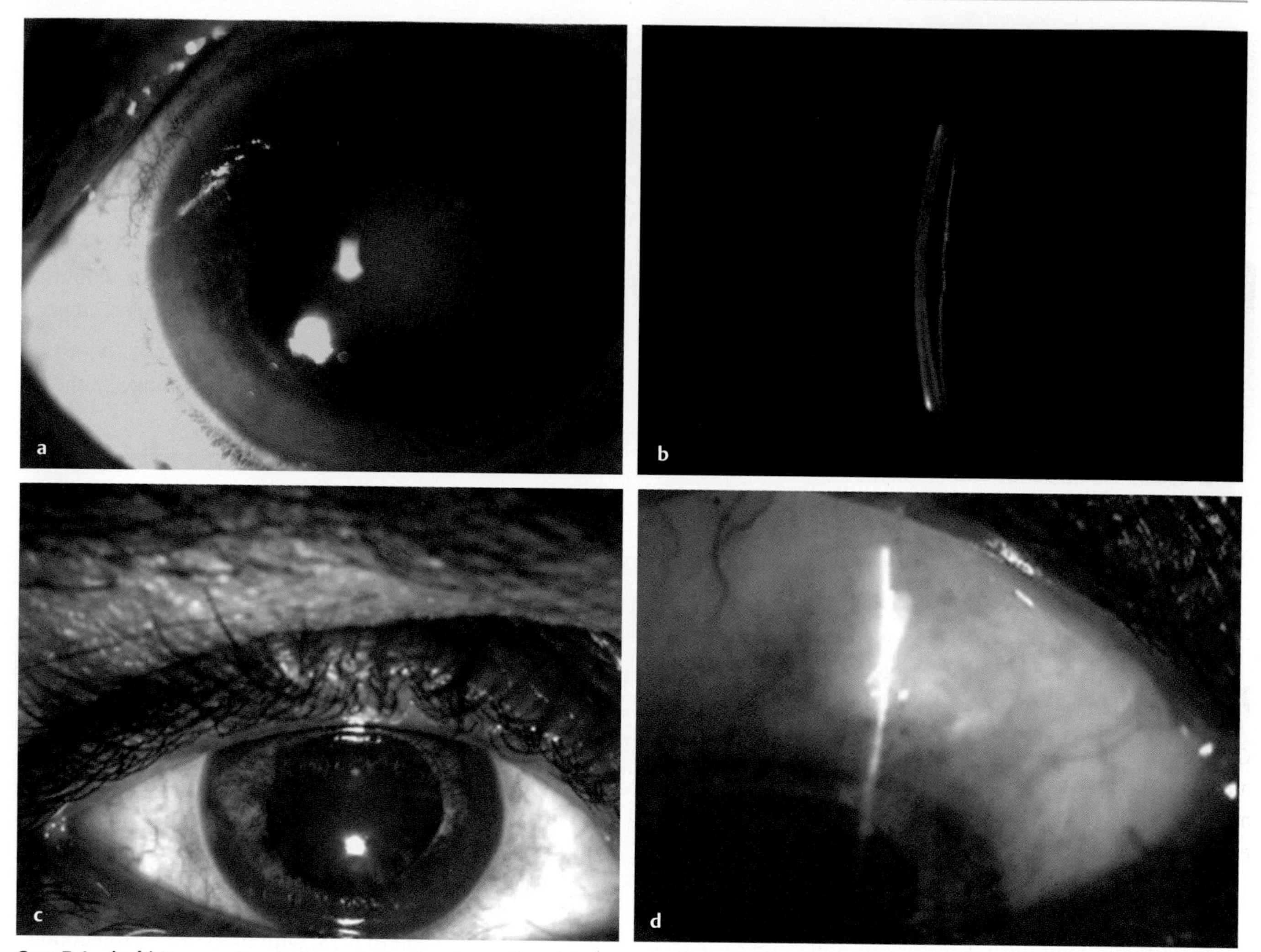

Case 5-1 **(a, b)** Preoperative shallow anterior chamber with mid dilated, nonreacting pupil. **(c)** After 1 year of trabeculectomy, sector iris atrophy is seen with no significant cataract. **(d)** Mildly elevated diffuse bleb.

Suggested Readings

Almatlouh A, Bach-Holm D, Kessel L. Steroids and nonsteroidal anti-inflammatory drugs in the postoperative regime after trabeculectomy—which provides the better outcome? A systematic review and meta-analysis. Acta Ophthalmol 2019; 97(2):146–157

Al-Haddad CE, Abdulaal M, Al-Moujahed A, Ervin AM, Ismail K. Fornix-based versus limbal-based conjunctival trabeculectomy flaps for glaucoma: findings from a Cochrane Systematic Review. Am J Ophthalmol 2017;174:33–41

Cabourne E, Clarke JC, Schlottmann PG, Evans JR. Mitomycin C versus 5-fluorouracil for wound healing in glaucoma surgery. Cochrane Database Syst Rev 2015;(11):CD006259

Cairns JE. Trabeculectomy. Preliminary report of a new method. Am J Ophthalmol. 1968 Oct;66(4):673–9

de Barros DS, Gheith ME, Siam GA, Katz LJ. Releasable suture technique. J Glaucoma. 2008 Aug;17(5):414–21

Grover DS, Kornmann HL, Fellman RL. Historical considerations and innovations in the perioperative use of mitomycin C for glaucoma filtration surgery and bleb revisions. J Glaucoma 2020;29(3):226–235

Khaw PT, Chiang M, Shah P, Sii F, Lockwood A, Khalili A. Enhanced trabeculectomy: the Moorfields Safer Surgery System. Dev Ophthalmol 2012;50:1–28

Stewart RH, Kimbrough RL, Bachh H, Allbright M. Trabeculectomy and modifications of trabeculectomy. Ophthalmic Surg 1979;10(1):76–80

Wang X, Khan R, Coleman A. Device-modified trabeculectomy for glaucoma. Cochrane Database Syst Rev 2015;12(12): CD010472

Watson PG. Surgery of the glaucomas. Br J Ophthalmol. 1972 Mar;56(3):299–306

CHAPTER 23

Glaucoma Drainage Devices

Overview

- Principle
- Types of Implants
- Indications for Using Glaucoma Drainage Devices
- Contraindications for Using Glaucoma Drainage Devices
- Surgical Procedure
  - Surgical Steps for a Valved Glaucoma Drainage Device
  - Surgical Procedure for a Nonvalved Glaucoma Drainage Device
- Postoperative Course
- Complications of Glaucoma Drainage Devices
- Randomized Control Trials
  - Tube versus Trabeculectomy Study
  - Ahmed Baerveldt Comparison Study
  - Primary Tube versus Trabeculectomy Study
- Cases
- Suggested Readings

Introduction

Glaucoma drainage devices (GDDs) act by creating an alternate pathway for aqueous outflow, by channeling aqueous through a tube from anterior chamber to an external reservoir in the subconjunctival space.

GDDs have an important role in management of complicated and refractory glaucoma, both as a primary as well as a secondary surgical procedure where trabeculectomy has either failed or is likely to have very low chances of success.

Principle

Following implantation of GDDs, a fibrous capsule forms around the end plate over a period of several weeks and the tube directs aqueous from the anterior chamber to the space between the end plate and surrounding nonadherent fibrous capsule. *Aqueous passes through the capsule by passive diffusion and is absorbed by periocular capillaries and lymphatics.* It is the fibrous capsule around the end plate that offers the major resistance to aqueous flow with drainage implants. *The tube is generally placed in the anterior chamber, but can be placed at the pars plana using a bent extension to the tube, a pars plana clip.*

Types of Implants

A GDD could be nonvalved or valved.

- **Nonvalved implants**: These devices consist of a silicone tube attached to an end plate of different sizes around which a bleb forms (**Fig. 23.1**). Ridges have been introduced to increase tissue resistance mechanisms and limit aqueous flow.

Molteno implants have been in use since 1969, and have a silicon tube attached to a single or double polypropylene plate.

Baerveldt implants have a silicon tube attached to a wide, barium impregnated silicon plate of differing areas—250 mm^2, 350 mm^2, or 500 mm^2. An Indian version, the Aurolab aqueous drainage implant (AADI), is available.

Other devices such as the express shunt have also been used, but have not been found to be effective or safe as they are metallic, and tend to burrow through adjacent tissues, appearing to hang into the anterior chamber or become subconjunctival (**Fig. 23.2**).

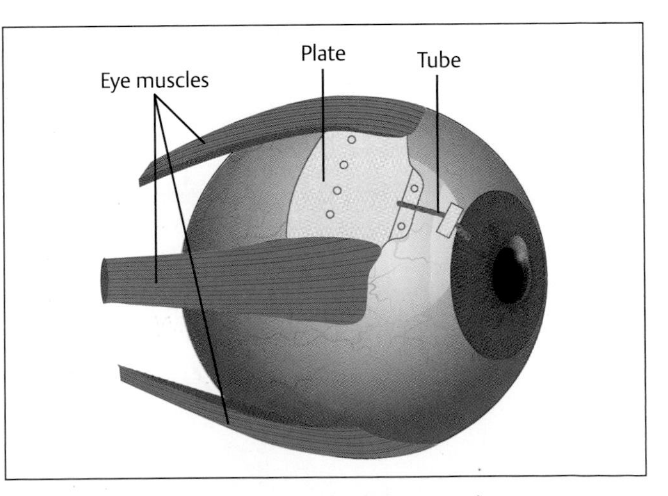

Fig. 23.1 Baerveldt device: Nonvalved glaucoma drainage.

- **Valved implants**: These allow only a unidirectional flow from the anterior chamber to the subconjunctival space, with a predefined opening pressure (**Fig. 23.3**).

Ahmed glaucoma valve (AGV) consists of a silicone tube connected to a silicone elastomer valve within a polypropylene or silicone body. The silicone body has been reported to have better long-term success, with fewer complications than the earlier polypropylene. The valve is designed to open when intraocular pressure (IOP) is 8 to 12 mm Hg. The valve is formed by thin silicon elastomer membranes stretched across a tube which has an internal opening larger than the exterior, creating a pressure differential, and allowing aqueous outflow. This comes in a pediatric size as well.

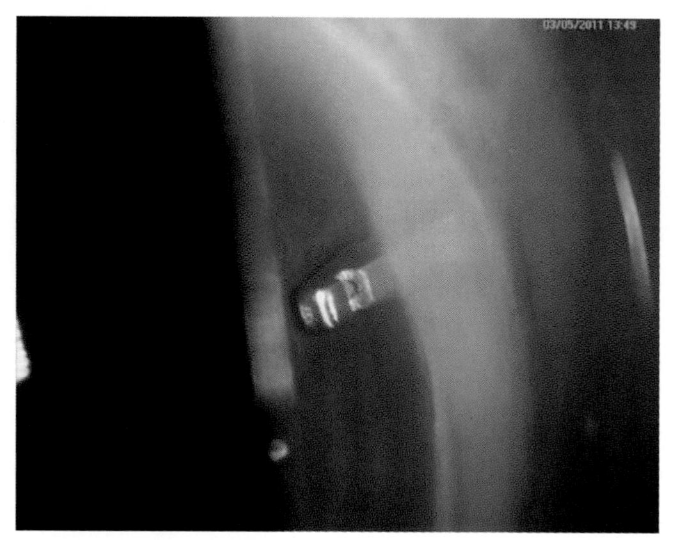

Fig. 23.2 Migration of express shunt into the eye.

Indications for Using Glaucoma Drainage Devices

Some indications for using GDDs:

- Multiple failed trabeculectomies.
- Secondary glaucomas such as:
  - Neovascular glaucoma.
  - Uveitic glaucoma.
  - Fibrous or epithelial downgrowth.
  - Prior penetrating keratoplasty, retinal surgery (pars plana vitrectomy or scleral buckling procedure).
- Refractory infantile glaucoma.
- Iridocorneal endothelial syndrome.
- Cicatricial diseases of the conjunctiva (e.g., Stevens-Johnson syndrome, ocular cicatricial pemphigoid).

Contraindications for Using Glaucoma Drainage Devices

Absolute contraindications for using GDDs are:

- Eyes with severe scleral or sclero-limbal thinning.
- Extensive fibrosis of conjunctiva.
- Ciliary block glaucoma.

Relative contraindications for using GDDs are:

- Vitreous in anterior chamber.
- Intraocular silicone oil implant, where if required, the GDD is placed in inferotemporal quadrant.

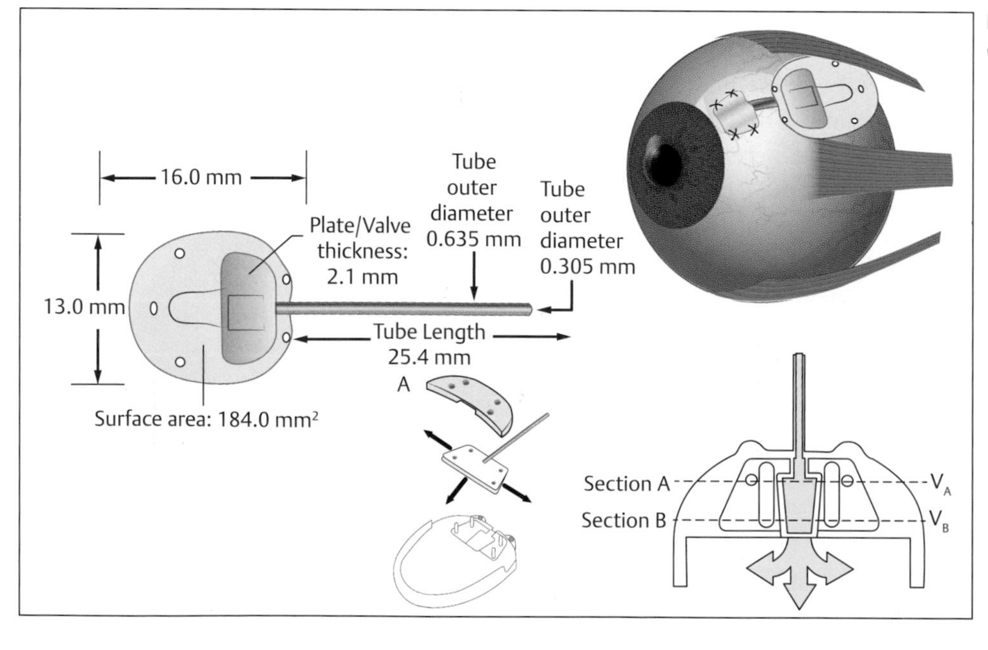

Fig. 23.3 Valved glaucoma drainage device—Ahmed glaucoma valve.

Surgical Procedure

Surgical Steps for a Valved Glaucoma Drainage Device

Flowchart 23.1 provides the management algorithm for using GDDs. A fornix-based conjunctival flap is made in the superotemporal quadrant between the recti muscles to expose the sclera (**Fig. 23.4a**). Blunt dissection between tenon and episclera with Westcott scissors is done up to the limbus, with radial relaxing incisions on one or both sides of the conjunctival flap improving surgical exposure. *The AGV tube is irrigated with balanced saline solution to prime the valve mechanism.*

The body of the implant is then tucked posteriorly into subtenon space (**Fig. 23.4b**) keeping the *anterior border positioned 8 to 10 mm posterior to the limbus.* The implant is sutured to sclera with nonabsorbable 8-0 through the

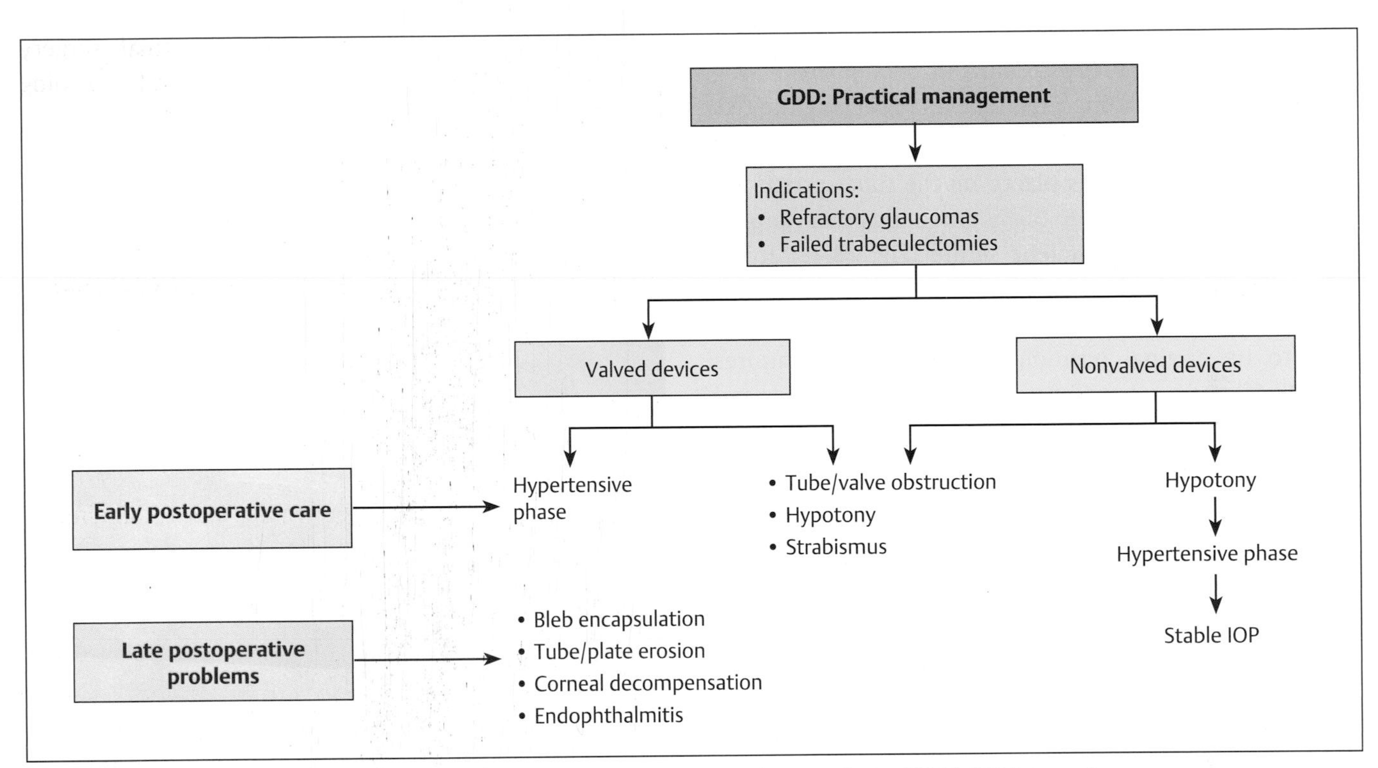

Flowchart 23.1 Algorithm depicting the practical management of glaucoma drainage device (GDD). IOP, intraocular pressure.

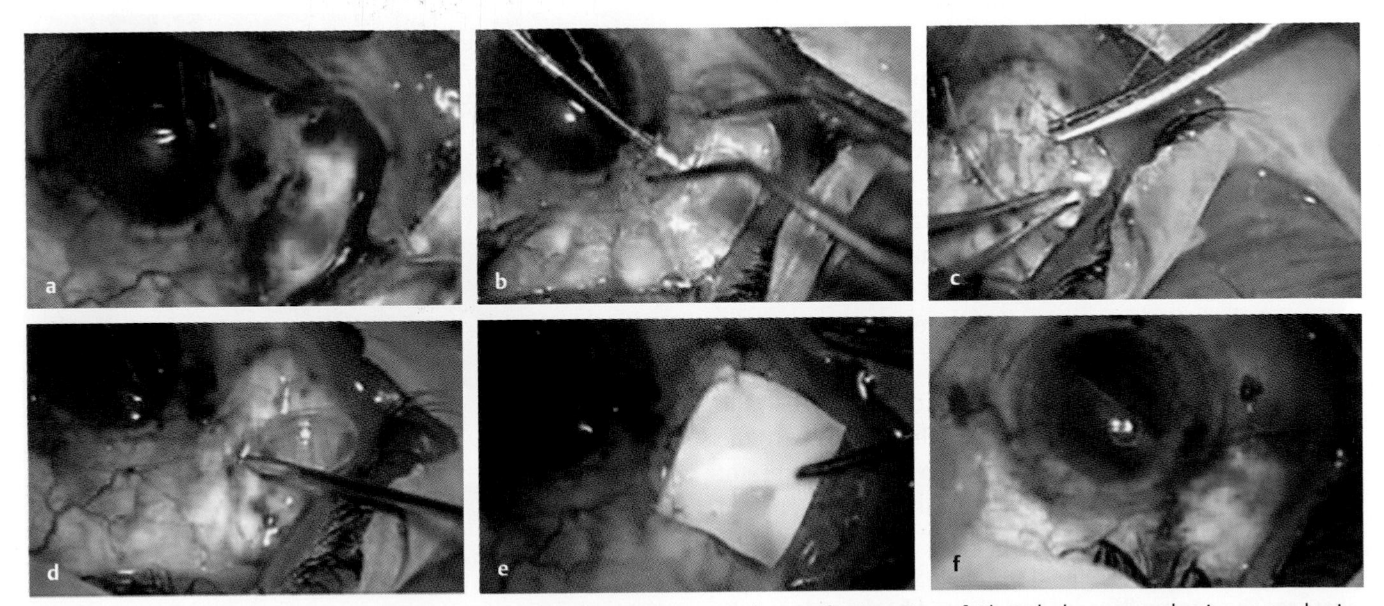

Fig. 23.4 **(a–f)** Intraoperative clinical photographs showing various surgical steps for insertion of Ahmed glaucoma valve in an eye having glaucoma following penetrating keratoplasty. (The images are provided courtesy of Dr Dewang Angmo, AIIMS, New Delhi, India.)

anterior positional holes of the plate (**Fig. 23.4c**). Some surgeons prefer a trabeculectomy like partial thickness flap, under which the tube is placed.

A needle track is made with a 23-gauge needle at the limbus beneath the scleral flap, if made. This should be *parallel, but anterior, to the iris and away from the corneal endothelium.* The tube of the AGV implant is trimmed so that the bevel of it faces the corneal endothelial surface and when subsequently inserted into the anterior chamber, a *2 to 3 mm length enters the anterior chamber* (**Fig. 23.4d**). The use of a needle creates an opening just enough for the silicon tube, thereby leading to a watertight seal, preventing leakage around the tube and reducing the risk of postoperative hypotony.

A scleral patch graft is placed on the tube so that the anterior edge is adjacent to the limbus and is then sutured to the sclera with 8-0 prolene suture (**Fig. 23.4e**). Inject 0.5 cc of a viscoelastic solution into the anterior chamber to avoid early hypotony. The conjunctiva is sutured back to its original position using 8-0 Vicryl sutures (**Fig. 23.4f**) and a subconjunctival injection of steroids and antibiotics is given. No adjunctive metabolites are usually used as they have not been shown to improve outcomes (**Figs. 23.5–23.7**).

Surgical Procedure for a Nonvalved Glaucoma Drainage Device

For a Baerveldt glaucoma implant (BGI) or AADI, the superior and lateral recti muscles are hooked. The 350-mm^2 implant is placed beneath the muscle bellies of the superior and lateral recti muscles, and secured using two interrupted 8-0 nylon sutures through fixation holes. The tube is placed as done for the AGV.

To avoid ocular hypotony in the early postoperative stage after placement of a BGI, a combination of an incomplete occlusion stent and a ligature is performed. A 3-0 Supramid thread is inserted through the silicone lumen to serve as an incomplete occlusion stent. To facilitate removal of this stent, the end of the thread is externalized underneath the conjunctiva in the inferotemporal fornix. Further, a constrictive absorbable 6-0 Vicryl suture is tied around the tube close to the plate.

To avoid elevation of IOP before dissolution of the ligature suture, a fenestration may be created in the extraocular portion of the tube to allow slight egress of aqueous. The fenestration of 1 to 2 mm may be created with a 15-degree micro-sharp blade in a longitudinal fashion on the tube, proximal to the absorbable occluding ligature. The conjunctiva is then sutured back in place.

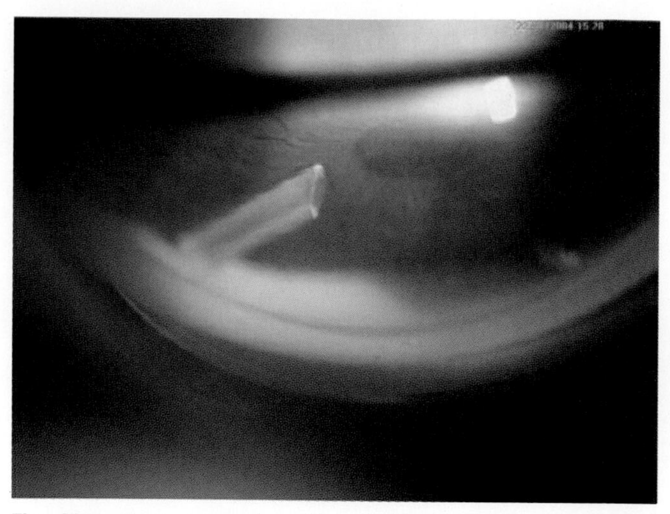

Fig. 23.5 Gonioscopy of an Ahmed glaucoma valve tube placed parallel to the iris, and midway between the iris and cornea.

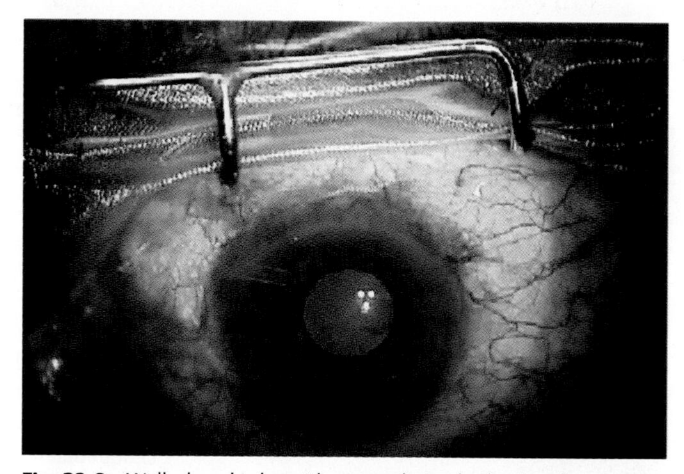

Fig. 23.6 Well-placed tube with a vascularized scleral graft.

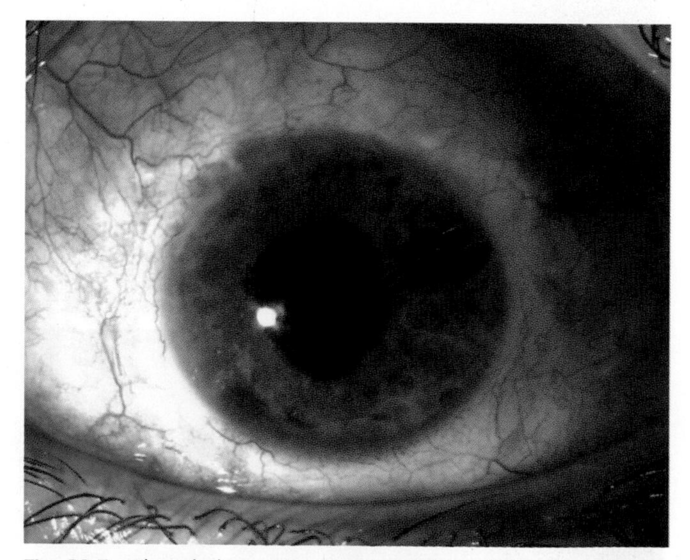

Fig. 23.7 Ahmed glaucoma valve placed through the pars plana in an aphakic eye. There is a flat vascularized capsule, with tube touching the iris.

Postoperatively, topical eye drops containing 0.5% moxifloxacin and 1% prednisolone acetate are prescribed, and tapered slowly over a period of 4 to 8 weeks. Glaucoma medications are adjusted on the basis of IOP and the clinical status of the eye. Patients are examined frequently for 1 month after surgery, and thereafter every 3 months.

Postoperative Course

Postoperative management course includes managing the following:

- *Hypotensive stage*: Initially there is low IOP, diffuse and thick-walled bleb with minimally engorged blood vessels, lasting for 7 to 10 days.
- *Hypertensive stage*: An inflamed and dome-shaped bleb, with high IOP, up to 50 mm Hg, is seen around 4 to 5 weeks. Fibrous tissue in the bleb capsule leads to this, and can last for about 4 to 6 months.
- *Stable stage*: Stabilization of IOP occurs 3 to 6 months after surgery, with a well-circumscribed and moderately vascular bleb.

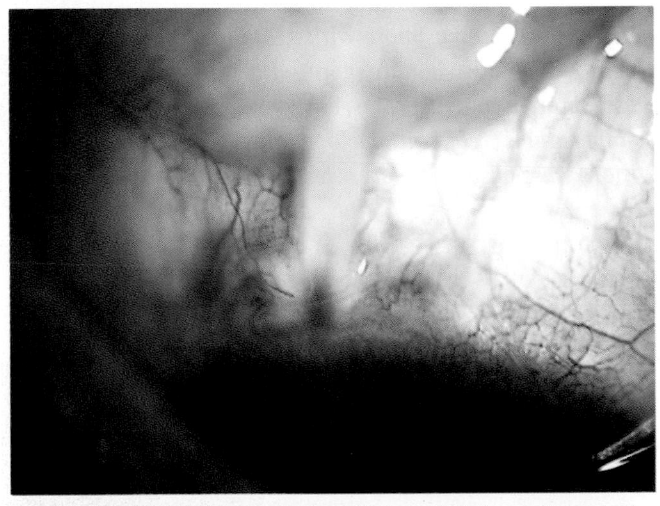

Fig. 23.8 Ahmed glaucoma valve. Plate and bleb are closer to the limbus than 8 mm away, and tube exposure is seen at the limbus.

Complications of Glaucoma Drainage Devices

Intraoperative complications to avoid are tube malposition, scleral perforation, and vitreous prolapse.

Postoperative complications:

- Early:
  - Hypotony due to overfiltration, wound leaks, or choroidal effusions can lead to hypotonic maculopathy, corneal decompensation, accelerated cataract formation, and discomfort.
  - Tube obstruction may be caused by blood, fibrin, vitreous, or iris or may be related to a tight external ligature around the tube.
  - An overhanging bleb can occur due to a thick patch graft or anterior placement of the plate, resulting in chronic dellen formation and ocular irritation.
- Late:
  - Exposure of the tube or plate has been reported to occur in 5 to 30% of patients (**Figs. 23.8** and **23.9**).
  - Bleb encapsulation around the plate leads to a high IOP.
  - Tube retraction.
  - Tube migration into the anterior chamber/extrusion is seen in 10 to 15% cases, more commonly in children (**Fig. 23.10**).
  - Diplopia/ocular motility disturbances usually occur with larger plates, and is significantly higher with a Baerveldt type implant than with AGV or Molteno implant. This extraocular muscle imbalance with diplopia results from mass effect of plate and its surrounding bleb on adjacent extraocular muscle. Other possible causes include Faden effect, entrapment of superior oblique muscle, fat fibrosis syndrome, or pseudo-Brown's syndrome.

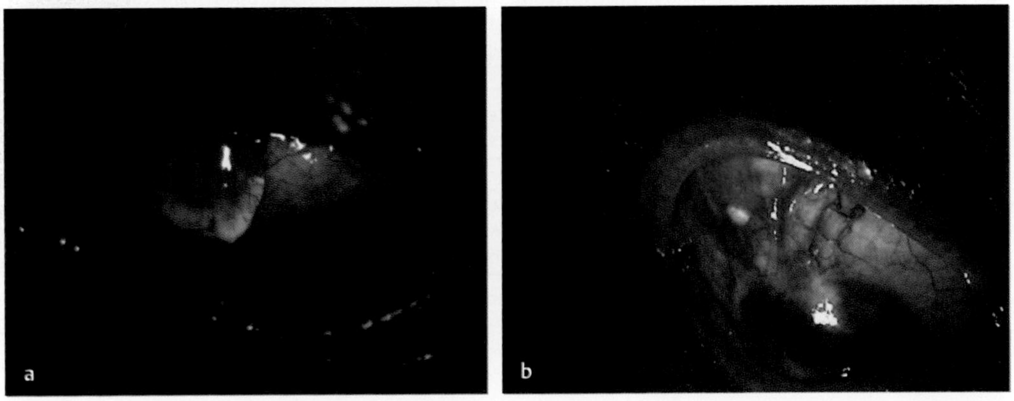

Fig. 23.9 **(a)** Exposure and extrusion of the scleral graft placed over the tube of a drainage implant. **(b)** Re-exposure of the plate of a Baerveldt type implant, despite conjunctival advancement.

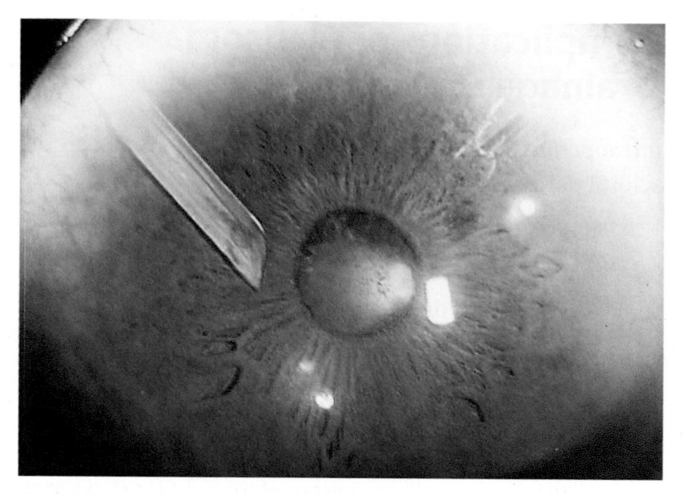

Fig. 23.10 Tube of drainage implant touching the iris and causing chronic uveitis.

- Corneal endothelial loss has been seen to continue over time (10–30% cases).
- Endophthalmitis.

Randomized Control Trials

Table 23.1 provides a brief summary of some randomized control trials (RCT) of glaucoma drainage devices.

Tube versus Trabeculectomy Study

Tube versus Trabeculectomy Study (TVT study) was a 5-year multicentric RCT of outcomes of 350 mm² Baerveldt implant and trabeculectomy with mitomycin C (MMC) 0.4 mg/mL for 4 minutes in 212 eyes with a failed trabeculectomy or pseudophakia.

The mean final IOP was similar, 14.4 ± 6.9 and 12.6 ± 5.9 mm Hg in the tube and trabeculectomy groups, respectively, as were the number of glaucoma medications at 5 years. The cumulative probability of failure during 5 years of follow-up was significantly different, 29.8 and 46.9% in the tube versus trabeculectomy groups. The rate of reoperations for glaucoma was significantly different, 9 and 29% in the tube and trabeculectomy groups.

Failures and reoperations after trabeculectomy were mostly related to hypotony, and probably caused by the high dose and duration of MMC used.

Ahmed Baerveldt Comparison Study

This was a multicentric, randomized controlled clinical trial in 276 cases of refractory glaucoma, majority with either primary open-angle glaucoma (POAG) or neovascular glaucoma (NVG). Among the subjects 42% had previously failed trabeculectomy. The mean baseline IOP was 30 mm Hg.

At 5 years, the mean IOP was significantly lower in AGV eyes, 12.7 ± 4.5 mm Hg versus 14.7 ± 4.4 mm Hg, while the number of medications was similar. The cumulative probability of failure was similar at 44.7 and 39.4% in the AGV and BGI groups.

IOP reduction was more with AGV in the immediate postoperative period whereas more with BGI in the long term. Postoperative complications: early and serious postoperative complications (reoperations to manage complications, loss of vision) were observed more with Baerveldt group.

Primary Tube versus Trabeculectomy Study

This was an RCT of Baerveldt implants versus trabeculectomy (MMC 0.4 mg/mL × 2 minutes) as a primary option in POAG eyes.

Table 23.1 Randomized control trials of the drainage devices and minimally invasive surgeries

Study	Methodology	Summary
TVT	Baerveldt: 350 mm² vs. trabeculectomy (0.4 mg/mL mitomycin-C × 4 minutes)	Similar IOP lowering over 5 years: 14.4 ± 6.9 mm Hg in the tube group and 12.6 ± 5.9 mm Hg in the trabeculectomy ↑ postoperative manipulation in trabeculectomy
Primary TVT	Primary Baerveldt:350 mm² vs. trabeculectomy (0.4 mg/mL mitomycin-C × 2 minutes)	3 years IOP reduction 46% after trabeculectomy vs. 39% Failure 33% in tubes vs. 28% for trabeculectomy
Ahmed–Baerveldt comparison study	Ahmed FP7 glaucoma valve vs. Baerveldt 101–350 glaucoma implant	5 years IOP: 14.7 ± 4.4 mm Hg AGV vs. 12.7 ± 4.5 mm Hg Baerveldt Failures 44.7% in the AGV group and 39.4% Baerveldt persistent hypotony, explantation of implant, or loss of light perception double in Baerveldt

Abbreviations: AGV, Ahmed glaucoma valve, IOP, intraocular pressure; TVT, tube versus trabeculectomy.

At 3 years, the mean IOP was significantly higher at 14.0 ± 4.2 mm Hg in the tube group and 12.1 ± 4.8 mm Hg in the trabeculectomy group. The number of glaucoma medications was also significantly higher in the tube group. Serious complications requiring reoperation or producing loss of two or more Snellen lines were statistically similar in the two groups.

Trabeculectomy with MMC was more effective at reducing IOP than a Baerveldt tube shunt implantation in POAG eyes as a first surgery.

Conclusion

GDDs are competing with trabeculectomy in the control of IOP in refractory glaucomas, but long term data of achievement of target IOP, reoperations, and endothelial dysfunction over time is still awaited.

Cases

Case 1

A 32-year-old male who sustained an injury with a tennis ball in his left eye underwent vitreoretinal surgery with encirclage and silicone oil for a vitreous hemorrhage and retinal detachment. After 3 months an IOP of 38 mm Hg was recorded, and timolol–brimonidine combination, a prostaglandin analog, and brinzolamide were started, but the IOP remained at 28 mm Hg. Gonioscopy showed an angle recession of 180 degrees and emulsified silicon on the trabecular meshwork. Silicone oil removal was done, but the IOP remained around 26 to 28 mm Hg (**Case 1-1**).

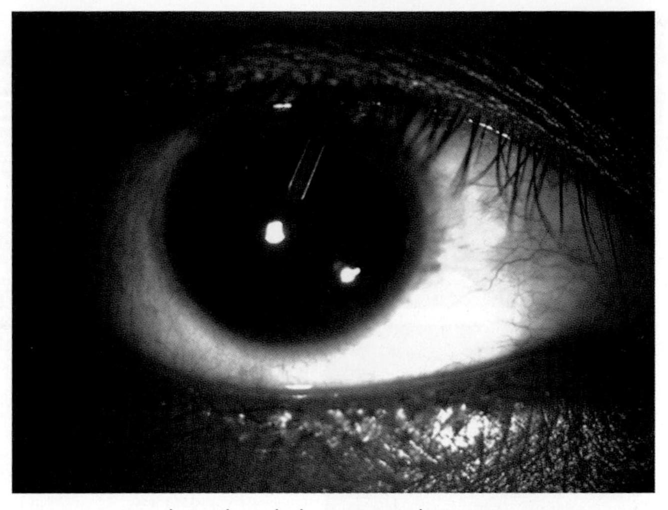

Case 1-1 Pars plana Ahmed Glaucoma implant.

Points to consider

- Traumatic angle recession.
- Trabecular block with silicone oil microdroplets.
- Encirclage and vitreoretinal surgery cause a lot of conjunctival scarring.

Diagnosis and Management

A diagnosis of mixed glaucoma caused by angle recession and silicon oil droplets was made. An Ahmed glaucoma valve implant was putthrough the pars plana in the superotemporal quadrant, with the plate 8 mm away from the limbus, and a donor scleral patch graft over the extraocular tube. The IOP reduced to 8 mm Hg in the first week after surgery, and then rose to 28 mm Hg after 2 weeks. There was continued inflammation and vascularity over the plate and a hypertensive phase was recognized. Topical steroids were continued and timolol–brimonidine combination drops and brinzolamide drops were added. At 4 months, the inflammatory response had resolved, and glaucoma medications could be tapered down to only timolol twice a day for an IOP of 16 mm Hg.

Case 2

A 24-year-old male was diagnosed to have juvenile open angle glaucoma, with two failed trabeculectomies in both eyes. On examination, gonioscopy showed an open angle with closure of the internal trabeculectomy ostium by fibrous tissue. His cup:disc ratio was 0.7 and 0.8, with an IOP of 32 mm Hg in both eyes on all topical glaucoma medications (**Case 2-1**).

Points to consider

- Target IOP should be <15 mm Hg.
- His life expectancy is at least 50 years.
- Scleral fibrosis may be overcome by a drainage device.

Diagnosis and Management

An Ahmed glaucoma valve was inserted in the left eye, and after 6 months, IOP was 20 mm Hg off medications, and 14 to 16 mm Hg after timolol twice a day was prescribed. The other eye was on five glaucoma medications for a similar IOP.

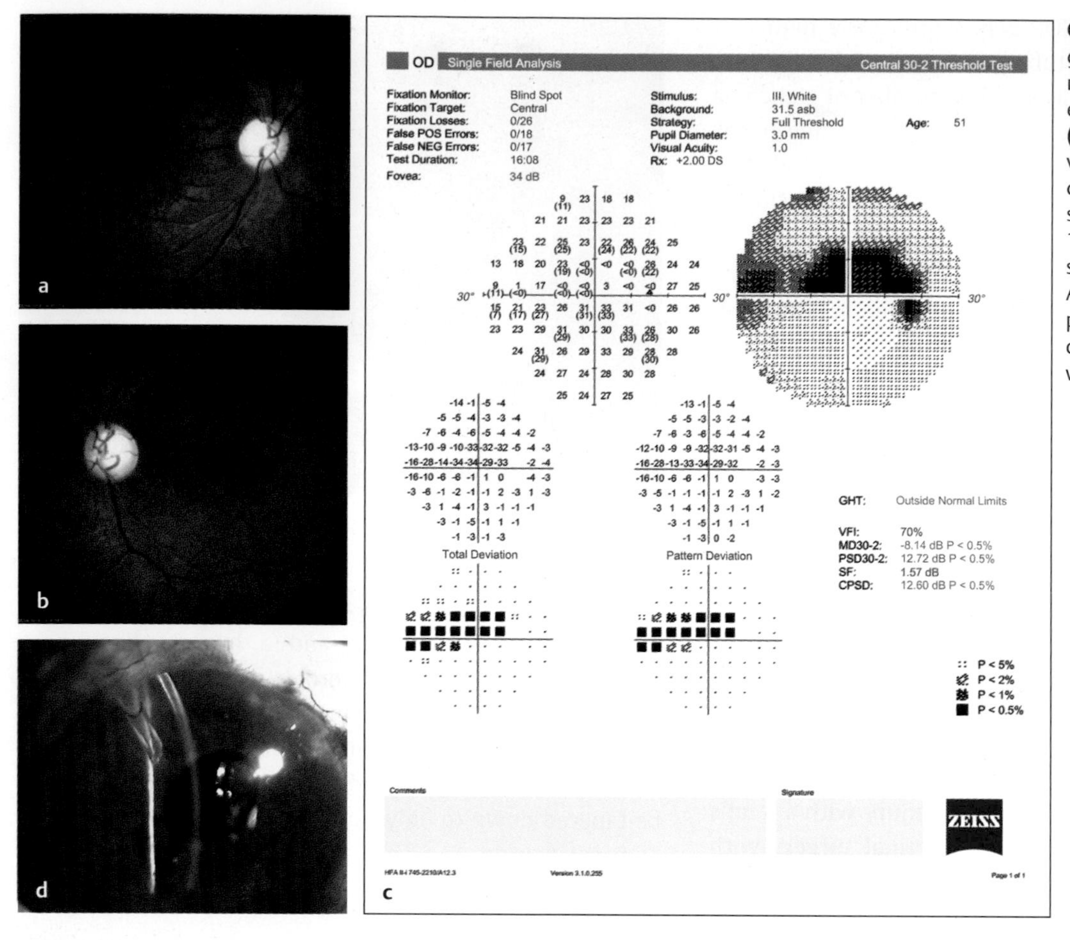

Case 2-1 **(a, b)** Fundus photographs showing a cup:disc ratio of 0.7 and 0.8 in the right eye and left eye, respectively. **(c)** Reliable perimetry with a visual field index of 70%, mean deviation of −8 dB, pattern standard deviation (PSD) of 12 dB, and a superior arcuate scotoma. **(d)** Functioning Ahmed Glaucoma implant tube properly placed away from the cornea and also not in contact with the iris.

Suggested Readings

Budenz DL, Barton K, Gedde SJ, et al; Ahmed Baerveldt Comparison Study Group. Five-year treatment outcomes in the Ahmed Baerveldt comparison study. Ophthalmology 2015;122(2):308–316

Foo VHX, Htoon HM, Welsbie DS, Perera SA. Aqueous shunts with mitomycin C versus aqueous shunts alone for glaucoma. Cochrane Database Syst Rev 2019;4:CD011875

Gedde SJ, Feuer WJ, Lim KS, et al; Primary Tube Versus Trabeculectomy Study Group. Treatment outcomes in the primary tube versus trabeculectomy study after 3 years of follow-up. Ophthalmology 2020;127(3):333–345

Gedde SJ, Schiffman JC, Feuer WJ, Herndon LW, Brandt JD, Budenz DL; Tube versus Trabeculectomy Study Group. Treatment outcomes in the tube versus trabeculectomy (TVT) study after five years of follow-up. Am J Ophthalmol 2012;153(5):789–803.e2

Hong CH, Arosemena A, Zurakowski D, Ayyala RS. Glaucoma drainage devices: a systematic literature review and current controversies. Surv Ophthalmol 2005;50(1):48–60

Tseng VL, Coleman AL, Chang MY, Caprioli J. Aqueous shunts for glaucoma. Cochrane Database Syst Rev 2017;7:CD004918

Wang B, Li W. Comparison of pars plana with anterior chamber glaucoma drainage device implantation for glaucoma: a meta-analysis. BMC Ophthalmol 2018;18(1):212

Wang S, Gao X, Qian N. The Ahmed shunt versus the Baerveldt shunt for refractory glaucoma: a meta-analysis. BMC Ophthalmol 2016;16:83

CHAPTER 24

Other Glaucoma Surgeries

Overview

- Nonpenetrating Glaucoma Surgeries
- Minimally Invasive/Microinvasive Glaucoma Surgeries
  - Types of Implants
- Cases
- Suggested Readings

Introduction

The current management of glaucoma entails medical/laser/surgical therapy to reach target intraocular pressure (IOP) and prevent progression of optic nerve head damage. *Nonpenetrating glaucoma surgery (NPGS) and minimally invasive glaucoma surgery (MIGS) have been designed to bridge the gap between medical and surgical therapy, with fewer complications but less IOP reduction, which may suffice in early open-angle glaucoma.*

Nonpenetrating Glaucoma Surgeries

Nonpenetrating glaucoma surgeries (NPGSs) were devised and introduced to prevent the common complications of trabeculectomy, such as a shallow anterior chamber, hypotony, bleb leaks, etc. Many variations of this surgery avoiding entry into the anterior chamber have been proposed and tried with limited indications.

The principle of deep sclerectomy is to create a superficial scleral flap with very guarded aqueous outflow via a trabeculo-Descemet's window. The aqueous then flows into a subscleral lake and intrascleral and episcleral vascular channels (**Fig. 24.1**). *In canaloplasty, Schlemm's canal is additionally dilated.* The superficial flaps are tightly closed, avoiding shallow anterior chamber or hypotony.

Advantages of NPGS are:

- Minimal effect on vision.
- Safe for end-stage glaucoma.
- Diffuse and shallow blebs.

Disadvantages are:

- Higher final IOP.
- Difficult learning curve.
- Prolonged surgical time.
- Generally require later Nd:YAG goniopuncture.
- Additional cost of implants.

Indications for NPGS therefore are:

- One-eyed patients.
- Patients at a high risk of choroidal effusions or suprachoroidal hemorrhage, e.g., nanophthalmos, Sturge-Weber syndrome.
- Patients at high risk of postoperative hypotony, e.g., young high myopes.

Contraindications are patients with scleral ectasia or scleral thinning or patients with trabecular damage as in synechial closure, prior trabeculoplasty, angle recession, etc.

Deep sclerectomy is similar to trabeculectomy in that a conjunctival flap is raised and a partial thickness scleral

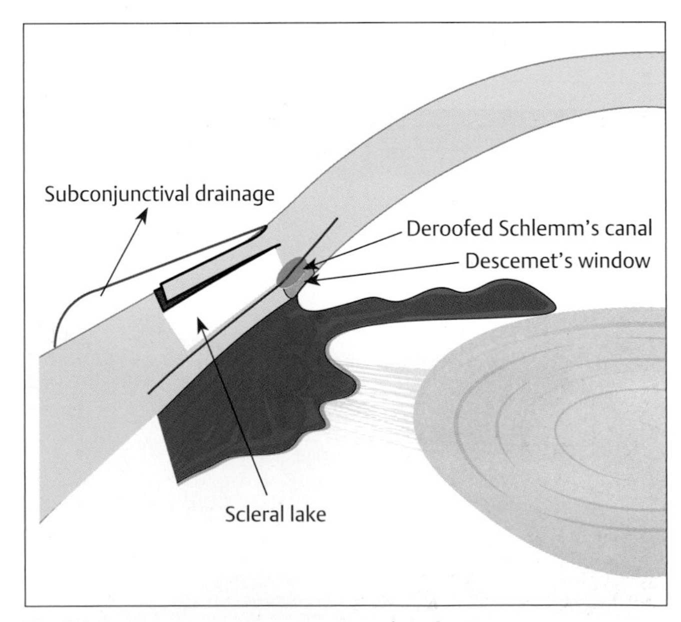

Fig. 24.1 Nonpenetrating surgery modes of action.

flap dissected at the limboscleral junction. The dissection of the flap is extended into the peripheral cornea. A deeper sclerokeratectomy is then done to form a subscleral space between the scleral bed and superficial scleral flap. Careful dissection of the juxtacanalicular tissue and stripping of the inner wall of Schlemm's canal expose the anterior trabecular meshwork and peripheral Descemet's membrane. The deeper subscleral lake permits slow absorption of aqueous without bleb formation.

Viscocanalostomy was described to enhance aqueous flow through Schlemm's canal. First, a superficial scleral flap and deeper space are dissected as described in deep sclerectomy above (**Fig. 24.2**). In addition, high-viscosity hyaluronate is injected into Schlemm's canal, leading to dilation of the canal and collector channels, as well as some breaks in the inner wall of Schlemm's canal, which increase aqueous outflow.

Minimally Invasive/Microinvasive Glaucoma Surgeries

Minimally invasive glaucoma surgeries (MIGSs) have been described by the United States Food and Drug Administration (FDA) as *an implant used with either an ab interno or ab externo approach, associated with little or no scleral dissection, and minimal or no conjunctival manipulation* (**Fig. 24.3**).

The ab interno approach without scarring the conjunctiva has made these techniques popular. These devices are also thought to overcome the side effects associated with prolonged use of medications and several complications related totrabeculectomy/aqueous shunt surgery (**Flowchart 24.1**).

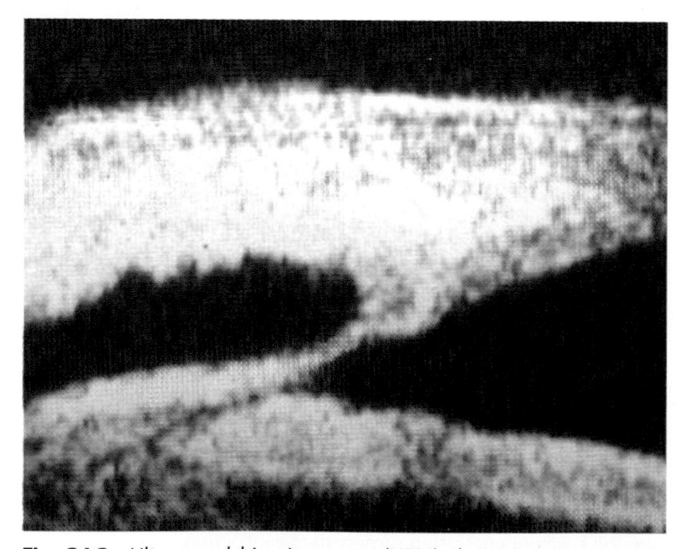

Fig. 24.2 Ultrasound biomicroscopy (UBM) showing a Descemet's window and deep scleral lake.

MIGS can be done as a standalone procedure or with cataract surgery, and have been defined by:

- Minimally invasive approach.
- Less conjunctival trauma.
- Modest efficacy.
- Early visual recovery.
- Less shallow anterior chambers/hypotony postoperatively.

The goal of MIGS is to reduce the need for medications in glaucoma, and they could be used in eyes with mild and occasionally moderate glaucoma, whereas traditional surgery is majorly targeted at cases where maximal medications have failed to achieve target IOP, or in advanced glaucomas. *MIGS provides IOP control to the mid-high teens with early visual rehabilitation and a reduction in the number of medications required.*

Indications for MIGS are as follows:

- Mild/moderate glaucoma.
- Primary open-angle glaucoma (POAG), pigmentary glaucoma, pseudoexfoliation glaucoma.
- Patients undergoing a cataract surgery.

Contraindications for the use of MIGS are angle closure and secondary glaucoma cases with trabecular scarring and prior glaucoma surgery. A very high baseline IOP is not ideal for MIGS. MIGS are also more expensive as compared to standard therapy.

Types of Implants

Three types of implants are being evaluated, namely:

- Trabecular—iStent, OMNI, Hydrus.

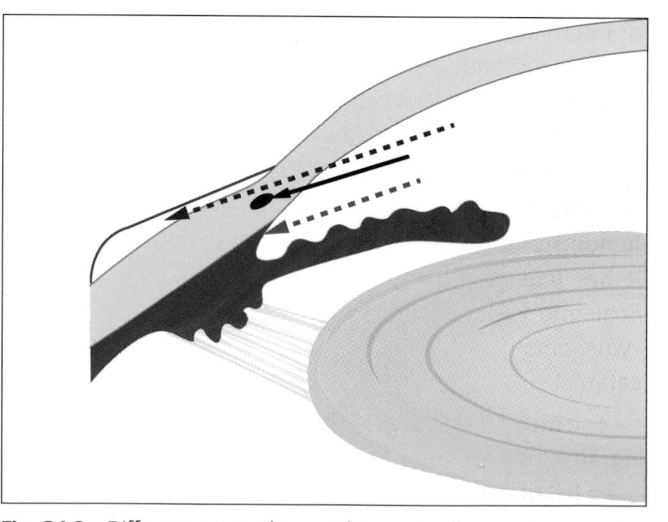

Fig. 24.3 Different approaches used in minimally invasive surgeries. *Blue arrow*, suprachoroidal; *black arrow*, trabecular approach to Schlemm's canal; and *brown arrow*, subconjunctival drainage.

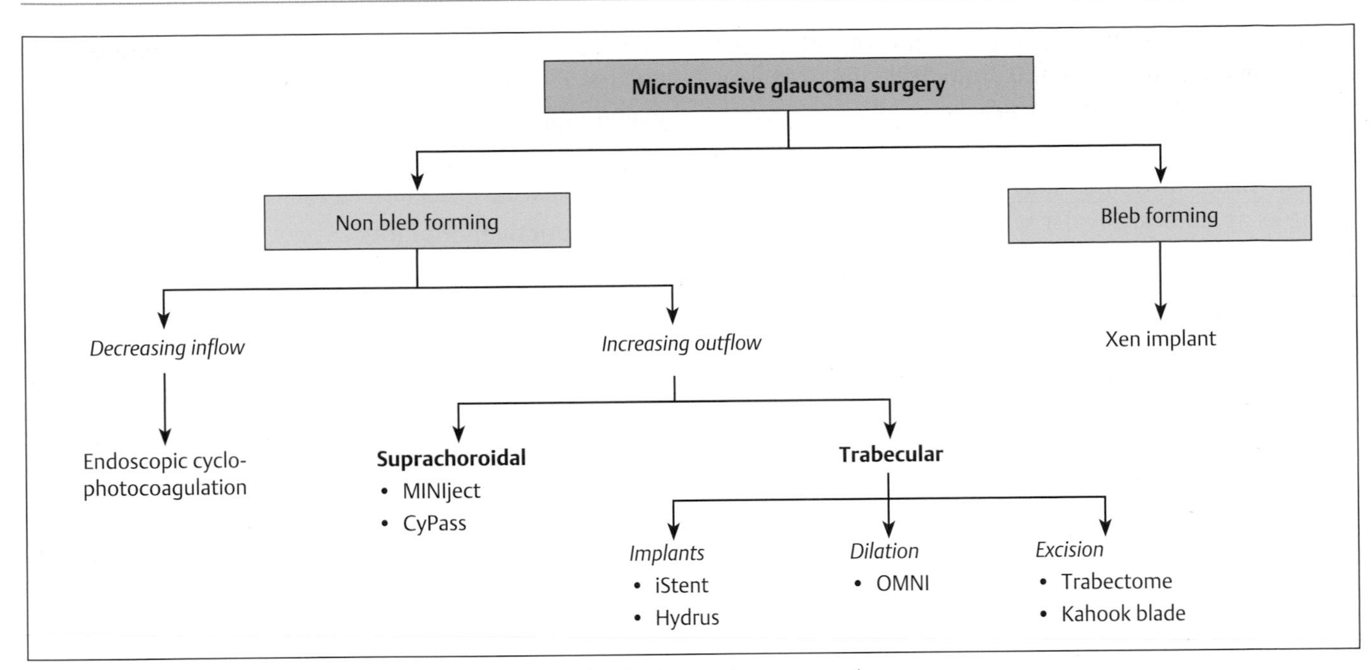

Flowchart 24.1 Types of microinvasive surgeries, their mode of action, and some examples.

- Suprachoroidal stents—iStent supra, MINIject, Solx gold shunt, CyPass.
- Subconjunctival implants—Xen, PRESERFLO/Innfocus, Express shunt (**Fig. 24.4**).

Trabecular implants increase trabecular outflow by bypassing the juxtacanalicular trabecular meshwork, which causes the most resistance to aqueous outflow. Suprachoroidal implants increase the uveoscleral outflow and the subconjunctival implants drain aqueous into the subconjunctival space. A few are discussed below.

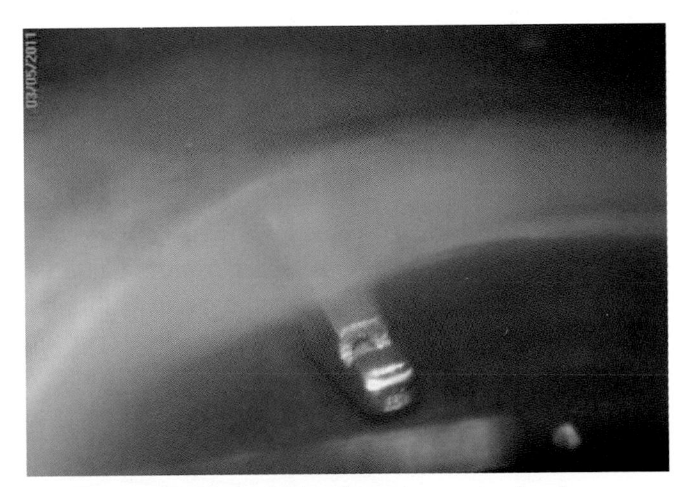

Fig. 24.4 Express shunt displaced into the anterior chamber.

Trabecular Stents

The *iStent inject* has been designed to connect the anterior chamber to Schlemm's canal. It is made of nonmagnetic titanium with heparin coating, a length of 360 µm and diameter of 230 µm. The iStent device has a sharp self-trephining tip at the leading edge with retention arches to fix the implant in place. It is preloaded on an injector system to inject the device at an angle. The leading edge is inserted into trabecular meshwork and the snorkel and lumen sit in the anterior chamber at the angle (**Fig. 24.5**). It has four holes in the part which is injected into the Schlemm's canal. An injector can simultaneously inject two stents into the angle. It is FDA approved for use with cataract surgery only.

The mean reduction in IOP was found to be 8.4 ± 3.6 mm Hg at 12 months and mean decrease in medications was 1.4 ± 0.8 in iStent with phacoemulsification.

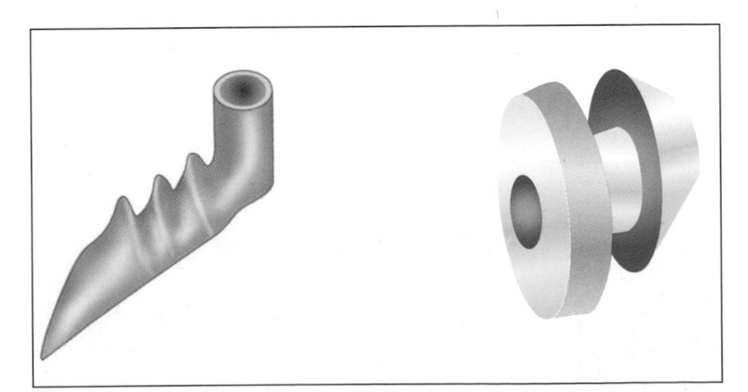

Fig. 24.5 iStent has a self-trephining tip and retaining arches to fix it in the Schlemm's canal, and a snorkel opening into the anterior chamber.

The most common complication reported with iStent is hyphema due to blood reflux from Schlemm's canal, or stent obstruction, seen in 4 to 30%.

Hydrus implant: This is a crescent-shaped, 8-mm-long implant made of nitinol alloy of nickel and aluminum, acting as an intracanalicular scaffold with multiple holes/collector channels in it to allow aqueous outflow through the trabecular meshwork. It is inserted into trabecular meshwork through a clear corneal incision (**Fig. 24.6**).

A randomized trial comparing the efficacy of cataract surgery alone versus Hydrus and cataract combined surgery showed that 80% of patients had >20% fall in IOP. Hydrus microstent and selective laser trabeculoplasty in POAG showed a similar decrease in IOP over 12 months. Complications seen are peripheral anterior synechiae and IOP spikes.

The *OMNI system* both viscodilates the canal of Schlemm and performs a trabeculotomy as it mechanically cuts through the trabecular meshwork.

Suprachoroidal Stents

MINIJect is a soft, microporous, flexible silicone implant placed in the supraciliary space. At 2 years all patients achieved a 20% IOP reduction with 48% of patients medication-free.

CyPass microstent is a 6.35-mm-long device made of polyamide with multiple holes in the shaft, which is inserted into the suprachoroidal space from the anterior chamber. It is guided into the suprachoroidal space through a guidewire with a tip, which disinserts the scleral spur and enters the suprachoroidal space. Reported adverse effects of CyPass were postoperative IOP elevation, transient hyphema, cataract progression, iritis, corneal edema, and malposition or dislocation of stent. Due to continuing loss of endothelial cells, 5 years following the implantation of CyPass, FDA has advised its withdrawal (**Fig. 24.7**).

Subconjunctival Implants

Xen Gel Implant—Ab Interno

The Xen Gel is a 6-mm-long porcine collagen and glutaraldehyde cross-linked implant, with a lumen diameter of 45 µm. The stent is manufactured in a dehydrated state when it is stiff; however, when injected into the eye, it swells up and becomes gel-like or soft after coming in contact with the aqueous. It is inserted from the anterior chamber into the subconjunctival space by a special injector (**Fig. 24.8**), creating a small fistula from the anterior chamber to the subconjunctival space with immediate formation of a bleb. It can also be combined with simultaneous injection of antimetabolites in the subconjunctival space to prevent fibrosis.

Xen Gel standalone implantation with MMC showed a 40% absolute success at 12 months with 89% qualified success for maintaining IOP at <18 mm Hg or a >20% reduction in IOP. A large multicenter study comparing Xen implant and trabeculectomy in POAG showed a mean pressure lowering of 46% at 12 months and a decrease in medications from 3 to 0 or one, with results similar to classic trabeculectomy.

The main complications of Xen Gel implant include the necessity for needling in up to 30% of patients, uveitic glaucoma, bleb leaks in up to 9%, dislocation/exposure

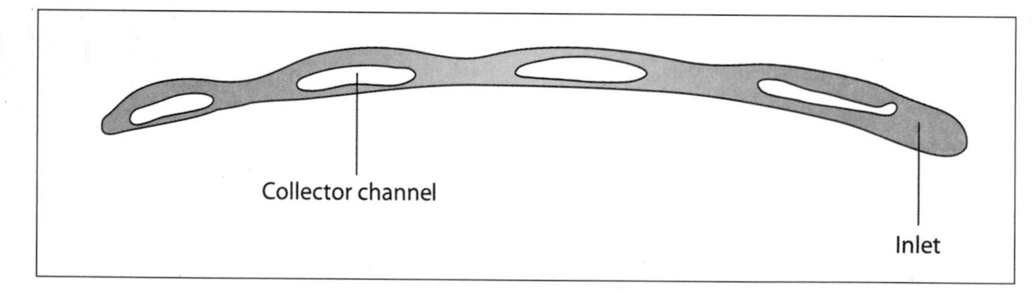

Fig. 24.6 Hydrus implant acts as an intracanalicular scaffold.

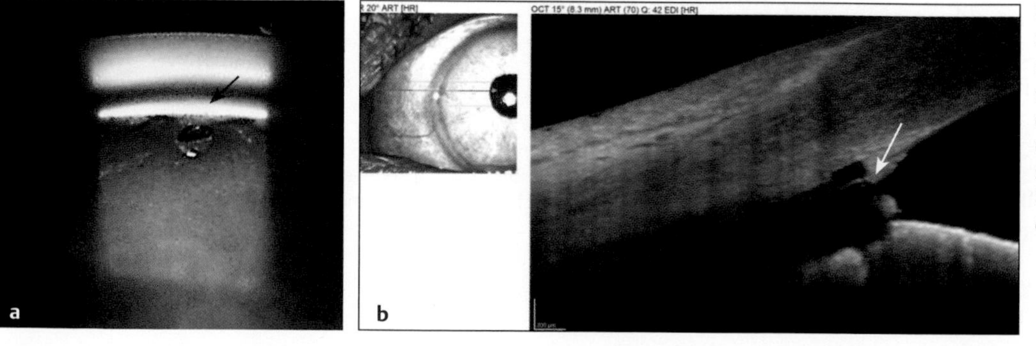

Fig. 24.7 (a) Opening of a CyPass implanted into the suprachoroidal space can be seen on gonioscopy (*black arrow*). **(b)** Anterior segment optical coherence tomography showing the placement of the implant between the sclera and choroid (*white arrow*).

of implant in 7%, and postoperative hyphema in 2%, with rare complications like malignant glaucoma and endophthalmitis. Trace amounts of residual polishing material in the needle sleeve have triggered a recall of batches of Xen around the world.

InnFocus/PRESERFLO Microshunt—Ab Externo

PRESERFLO, earlier called InnFocus microshunt, is an 8-mm-long tubular, ab externo device with a flange made of biostable material SIBS (polystyrene-isobutylene-styrene), a thermoplastic elastomer. It is inert, soft, and flexible (**Fig. 24.9**).

A small fornix-based conjunctival flap is raised, and MMC applied. A shallow scleral pocket is made 3 mm from the limbus, and a needle passed under it to reach the anterior chamber midway between the iris and cornea. The implant is threaded in with forceps, so that the fins are under the sclera. A 3-year follow-up of a single-site prospective, nonrandomized study on InnFocus alone or combined with cataract surgery showed 80% success rate keeping IOP at <14 mm Hg at 3 years. The qualified success rate was 95% and medication number reduced from 2.6 to 1.2. Transient hypotony and choroidal effusion may occur after placement of this shunt.

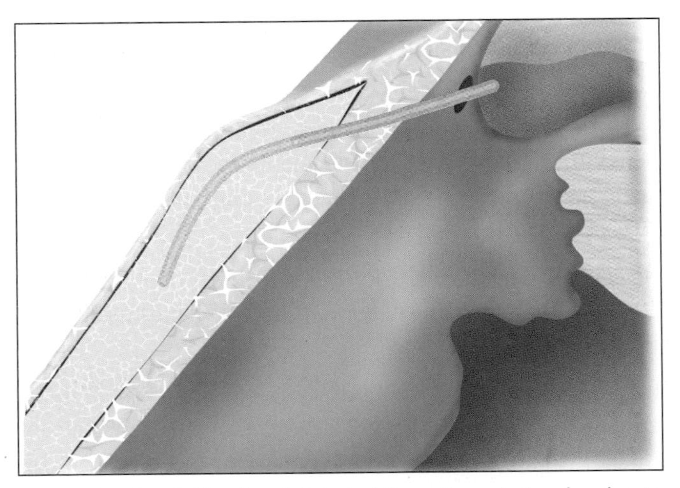

Fig. 24.8 Xen Gel implant is injected from the anterior chamber to the subconjunctival space.

Trabecular Surgeries

These target the dysfunctional trabecular meshwork in glaucoma, and a few examples are listed below:

- Ab interno trabeculectomy—trabectome.
- Excisional goniotomy—Kahook Dual Blade.
- Gonioscopy-assisted transluminal trabeculectomy (GATT)—illuminated cannula/6/0 polypropylene suture passed through a goniotomy incision.

Conclusion

MIGS target different aqueous outflow pathways with moderate efficacy to lower IOP in POAG without/with conjunctival scarring. They have potential advantages in primary glaucoma cases with mild-to-moderate glaucomas that don't tolerate glaucoma medications. Procedures targeting the subconjunctival space seem more efficacious, especially when done as a standalone procedure rather than combined with cataract surgery.

MIGS can lead to an IOP of mid-teens with few complications, which may be adequate in early glaucomatous damage. Long-term data on efficacy and safety is awaited, and as mentioned, out of the many being proposed, only a few see clinical evaluation. *The lack of long-term and comparative data makes choices difficult, and safety may not always outweigh efficacy.*

Cases

Case 1

A 60-year-old male was diagnosed to have an immature senile cataract and POAG, with moderate glaucomatous optic neuropathy, a superior arcuate scotoma in the right

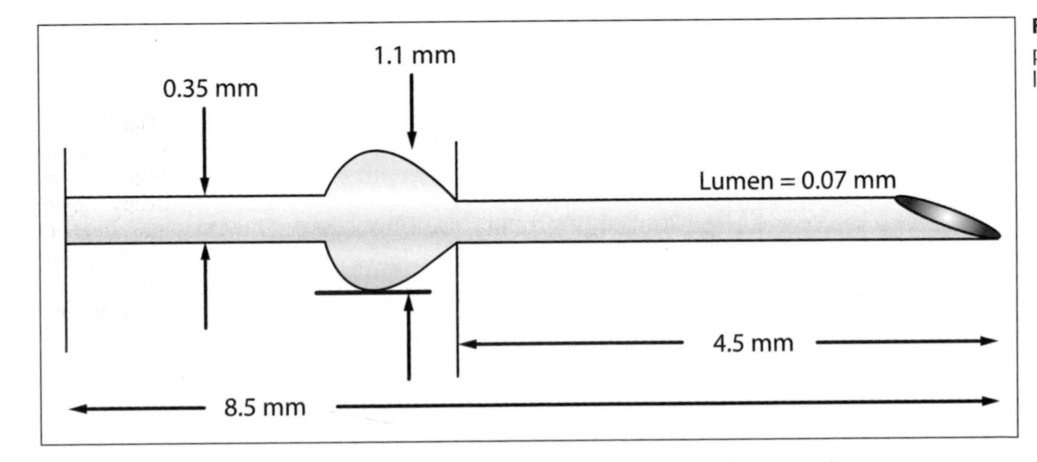

Fig. 24.9 InnFocus microshunt implant is inserted ab externo from the limbus to the anterior chamber.

eye, and a baseline IOP of 24 to 26 mm Hg in both eyes. He was started on a prostaglandin analog and after 4 weeks, although his IOP dropped to 18 to 20 mm Hg, he complained of redness of the eyes especially in the morning. He was switched to a combination of dorzolamide and timolol with which he had constant discomfort.

Points to consider

- Trabeculectomy would relieve the need for medications, but could exacerbate the cataract.
- As the baseline IOP was not high, a cataract surgery could reduce IOP by a few mm Hg and MIGS can lower it further.

As there was a visually significant cataract in the eye with the visual field defect, he was offered the possibility of having an iStent at the same time. After 6 months of cataract surgery with iStent, his IOP in the operated eye was 20 mm Hg, and he was advised to use timolol drops twice a day in both eyes to achieve an IOP of <15 mm Hg.

Case 2

A 60-year-old female underwent a cataract surgery and CyPass implantation in her left eye, and presented 1 year later with an IOP of 32 mm Hg on latanoprost and a combination of brimonidine–timolol (**Case 2-1**). Her specular count was 1800. Her perimetry showed a biarcuate scotoma in that eye with a documented progression over the last 2 years (**Case 2-1**).

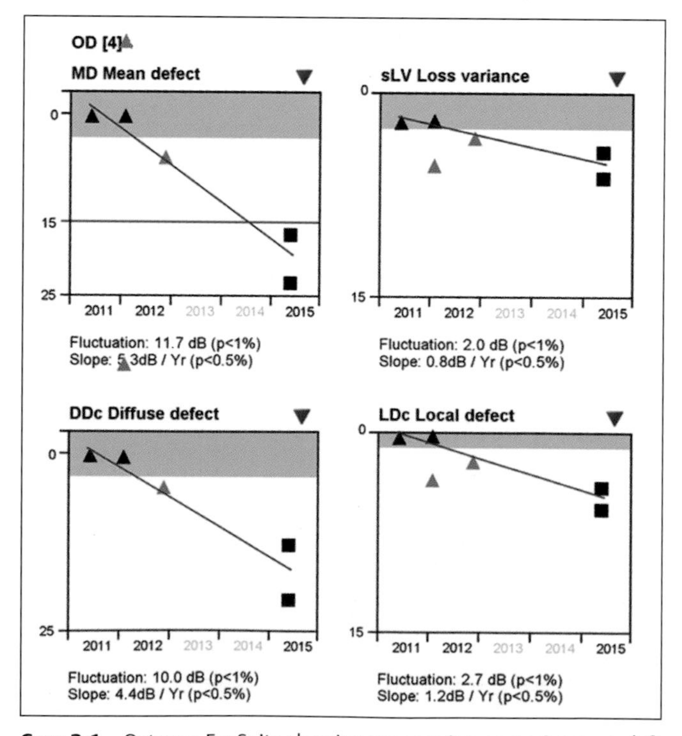

Case 2-1 Octopus EyeSuite showing progression on perimetry in left eye.

Points to consider

- CyPass suprachoroidal implant failed to control IOP.
- Corneal endothelial cell loss is significant.
- Occurrence of progression suggests the need for long-term low IOP.

In view of the medically uncontrolled, advanced glaucoma, a trabeculectomy was performed using MMC 0.2 mg/mL for 1 minute subconjunctivally. A year later her IOP was 10 to 12 mm Hg. She is under periodic review for corneal status, IOP, vision, and perimetry. The implant would be removed if endothelial loss continues.

Suggested Readings

Agrawal P, Bradshaw SE. Systematic literature review of clinical and economic outcomes of micro-invasive glaucoma surgery (MIGS) in primary open-angle glaucoma. Ophthalmol Ther 2018;7(1):49–73

Eldaly MA, Bunce C, ElSheikha OZ, Wormald R. Non-penetrating filtration surgery versus trabeculectomy for open-angle glaucoma. Cochrane Database Syst Rev [Internet]2014;(2). https://www.cochranelibrary.com/cdsr/doi/10.1002/14651858.CD007059.pub2/full?highlightAbstract=glaucom%7Cglaucoma

Fea AM, Ahmed IIK, Lavia C, et al. Hydrus microstent compared to selective laser trabeculoplasty in primary open angle glaucoma: one year results. Clin Exp Ophthalmol 2017;45(2):120–127

Healey PR, Clement, CI, Kerr NM, Tilden D, AghajanianL. Standalone iStent Trabecular Micro-bypass Glaucoma Surgery. J Glaucoma. 2021 Feb 15

King AJ, Shah A, Nikita E, et al. Subconjunctival draining minimally-invasive glaucoma devices for medically uncontrolled glaucoma. Cochrane Database Syst Rev 2018; 12:CD012742

Konopińska J, Lewczuk K, Jabłońska J, Mariak Z, Rękas M. Microinvasive Glaucoma Surgery: A Review of Schlemm's Canal-Based Procedures. Clin Ophthalmol. 2021;15: 1109–1118

Le JT, Bicket AK, Wang L, Li T. Ab interno trabecular bypass surgery with iStent for open-angle glaucoma. Cochrane Database Syst Rev 2019;3:CD012743

Rosdahl JA, Gupta D. Prospective studies of minimally invasive glaucoma surgeries: systematic review and quality assessment. Clin Ophthalmol 2020;14:231–243

Schlenker MB, Gulamhusein H, Conrad-Hengerer I, et al. Efficacy, safety, and risk factors for failure of standalone ab interno gelatin microstent implantation versus standalone trabeculectomy. Ophthalmology 2017;124(11):1579–1588

CHAPTER 25

Glaucoma Related to the Lens and Its Surgery

Overview

- Lens-Induced Glaucomas
  - Phacomorphic Glaucoma
  - Phacolytic Glaucoma
  - Lens Particle Glaucoma
  - Phacoanaphylactic Glaucoma
  - Phacotopic Glaucoma
- Intraocular Pressure Rise/Fall with Cataract Surgery in a Normal or Glaucomatous Eye
- Guidelines for Cataract/Filtering Surgery in POAG/PACG
- Clear Lens Extraction
- Cataract Surgery Together with Minimally Invasive Procedures
- Effect of Cataract Surgery on Imaging and Perimetry
- Cases
- Suggested Readings

Introduction

There is a close relationship between lens morphology and the trabecular meshwork, both in development and in acquired disorders. Various kinds of glaucoma and cataracts occur together, with some shared causative factors. The shared pathology starts from birth, with congenital anomalies occurring simultaneously, and this commonality continues through secondary insults such as trauma and uveitis, and on to senile cataracts and primary adult glaucomas.

Lens-Induced Glaucomas

The rise in intraocular pressure (IOP) secondary to lens changes can be attributed to either angle closure or trabecular outflow dysfunction in an open angle (**Table 25.1** and **Flowchart 25.1**).

Table 25.1 Pathophysiology of lens-induced glaucoma

Secondary angle closure	Secondary open angle
Phacomorphic glaucoma	Phacolytic glaucoma
Phacotopic glaucoma	Lens particle glaucoma
	Phacoanaphylactic glaucoma

Phacomorphic Glaucoma

This is the commonest form of lens-induced glaucoma seen in India, due to anteroposterior thickening of the lens, in an intumescent senile cataract and sudden hydration of the lens after trauma (**Fig. 25.1**). There is increased contact between the pupil and lens leading to an accumulation of aqueous behind the iris, and secondary angle closure. Expansion of the lens itself also leads to a peripheral push of the iris onto the trabecular meshwork, obstructing aqueous outflow and raising IOP.

There is a history of gradual diminution of vision due to cataractogenesis followed by acute pain associated with a further, sudden visual loss. On examination, a high IOP, corneal edema, and a shallow anterior chamber can be seen in a cataractous eye.

Management requires an initial medical control of IOP with systemic and topical glaucoma medications. Pilocarpine should be avoided as it may exacerbate the pupillary block. Lens extraction should be done after IOP control, and glaucoma medications need to be continued post surgery, with a taper over time, to maintain a target IOP based on the glaucomatous optic neuropathy present. If the attack has lasted many days, a combined cataract and filtering surgery may be required to achieve target IOP.

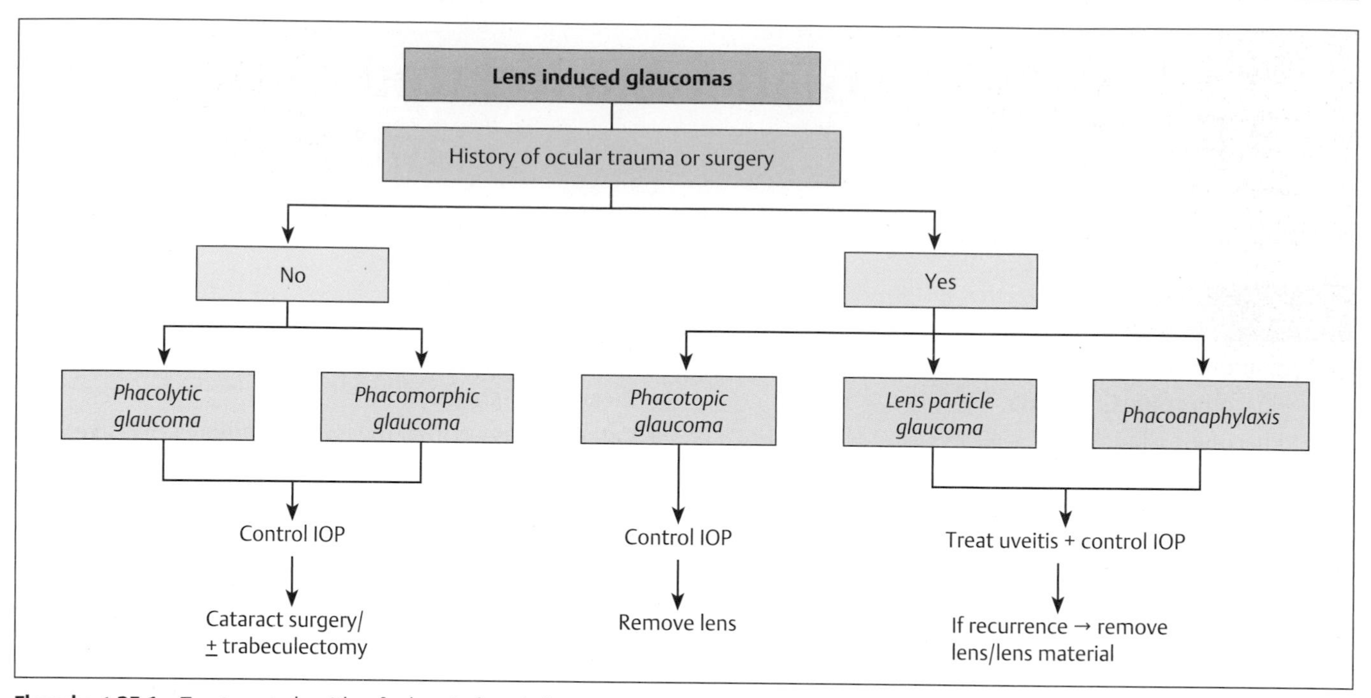

Flowchart 25.1 Treatment algorithm for lens-induced glaucomas. IOP, intraocular pressure.

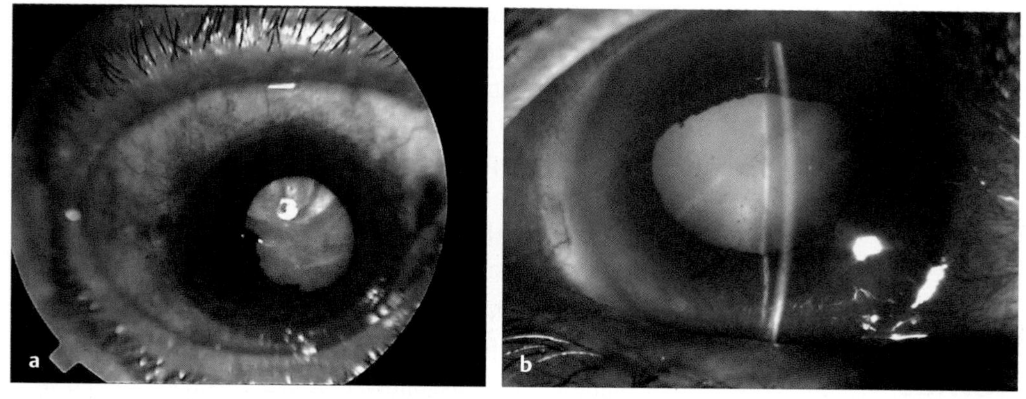

Fig. 25.1 **(a)** An intumescent immature senile cataract. **(b)** A mature senile cataract causing a very shallow anterior chamber and angle closure glaucoma.

Visual prognosis and IOP control depend upon the duration of the attack, with best results if IOP is controlled within 24 to 48 hours, and poor vision if duration is longer, especially if the attack lasts for weeks.

Phacomorphic glaucoma tends to occur in eyes predisposed to primary angle closure, and the fellow eye must be examined for an occludable angle, and an iridotomy done.

Phacolytic Glaucoma

In *hypermature or mature cataracts microscopic capsular breaks* may occur, which allow the normally sequestered lens proteins to leak out, and produce a severe inflammatory reaction.

There is a history of pain, photophobia, diminution of vision, and redness. On examination, the anterior chamber appears milky, with associated corneal edema and very high IOPs (**Fig. 25.2**). In early cases, flare may be observed, with lens particles forming a pseudohypopyon in the presence of a hypermature cataract.

Management consists of lowering the IOP with topical and systemic glaucoma medications, and the inflammation with topical steroids and cycloplegics. Once the eye quietens down, cataract surgery should be done, keeping in mind the possibility of weak zonules and a fragile capsule in hypermature cataracts. Trabeculectomy is generally not required.

Lens Particle Glaucoma

This is caused by inflammation and obstruction to trabecular outflow by *retained lens matter following trauma or surgery*. Signs of uveitis such as flare, cells, and synechiae may be seen, even weeks and months later.

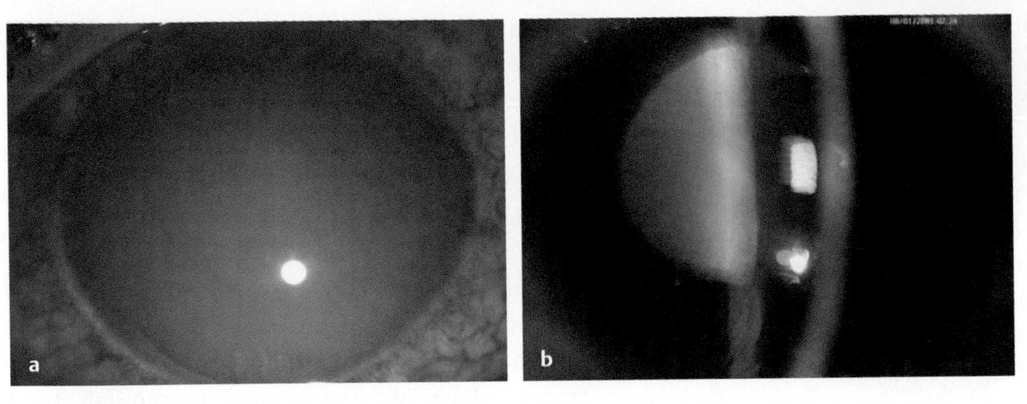

Fig. 25.2 **(a)** Ciliary and conjunctival congestion, corneal edema, and a milky appearance of the anterior chamber. **(b)** After resolution of the inflammatory response and control of intraocular pressure (IOP), a hypermature Morgagnian cataract can be seen.

Conservative management with glaucoma medications, topical steroids, and cycloplegics often suffices. In case recurrences occur or the IOP cannot be controlled, removal of the lens material has to be undertaken.

Phacoanaphylactic Glaucoma

This is seen as an *immune response triggered within 1 to 2 weeks of an ocular trauma or surgery*. It is a local type III hypersensitivity reaction.

Phacoanaphylaxis presents as granulomatous uveitis, with glaucoma only occurring occasionally, and the treatment is directed toward controlling inflammation and lowering IOP, if required.

Phacotopic Glaucoma

A subluxated or dislocated lens may lead to greater iridolenticular contact and a secondary angle closure glaucoma if prolonged, or direct pressure of the displaced lens on angle structures can hamper aqueous outflow. *Lens displacement can be a part of developmental abnormalities such as ectopia lentis or in hypermature cataracts or after trauma.*

Intraocular Pressure Rise/Fall with Cataract Surgery in a Normal or Glaucomatous Eye

An IOP rise after cataract surgery has been known to occur within 8 to 12 hours. This rise has been shown to be much higher in eyes with prior glaucoma as compared to those without glaucoma—reported to be as high as 44 mm Hg as compared to 32 mm Hg by Shingleton et al. The reasons for this rise are many—pre-existing trabecular dysfunction, use of viscoelastics, surgical inflammation, tight wound closure, pigment release, and lens particles.

A fall in IOP has been reported in some series after cataract surgery in primary open-angle glaucoma (POAG) and primary angle-closure glaucoma (PACG) eyes. The proposed mechanisms by which IOP lowering may occur after cataract surgery are:

- Iris/zonule movement backwards, stretching trabecular tissues.
- Reduction in glycosaminoglycans in the trabecular meshwork by fluidics during phacoemulsification.
- Inflammation inducing trabecular meshwork changes as in trabeculoplasty.
- Remodeling of trabecular meshwork due to ultrasound.

There is an ongoing debate on the effect of cataract surgery on IOP in POAG and PACG eyes. *In POAG eyes, a Cochrane review reported a decrease in IOP of 2 to 4 mm Hg.* Patients with an IOP of >21 mm Hg could have a fall of up to 5 mm Hg. For PACG eyes, a Cochrane review found that there was *no evidence from good quality randomized trials or nonrandomized studies of the effectiveness of lens extraction for control of IOP in chronic PACG.*

Most studies have looked to see if phacoemulsification lowered the IOP to <21 mm Hg, whereas suggested target IOPs today for even mild glaucoma are lower than that. The aim of glaucoma therapy is to achieve a "target" IOP appropriate for the severity of optic nerve damage, and lowering the IOP by a few mm Hg may not be sufficient to reach the necessary levels of IOP. However, *patients and surgeons may be lulled into a false sense of security, and patients may not return for regular reviews or therapy of their glaucoma unless they are forewarned that glaucoma medications may need to be continued even after cataract surgery if there is prior visual field loss.*

Guidelines for Cataract/Filtering Surgery in POAG/PACG

Cataract and glaucoma frequently coexist with a spectrum of presentations—advanced and medically uncontrolled glaucoma with cataract or mild glaucoma with cataract.

There is therefore a possibility of doing surgery for either one alone first followed by the second, or performing a combined surgery for the two together. In adults, it would make socioeconomic sense to do both surgeries together; however, the chance of complications increases, and the final reduction of IOP is not as good as after trabeculectomy alone. The choice of management also depends on the severity of glaucomatous neuropathy, with severe damage requiring low IOPs; and an IOP rise with phacoemulsification in such eyes could cause irreversible loss of vision. *In eyes with severe glaucoma, a trabeculectomy first is a better option.*

Cataract surgery prior to glaucoma surgery may do away with the possibility of failure of a prior trabeculectomy bleb with later cataract surgery. In PACG eyes with very shallow anterior chambers, phacoemulsification leads to a deeper anterior chamber, and glaucoma surgeries may have less intraoperative or postoperative complications. Unfortunately, this is offset by the fact that trabeculectomy in pseudophakic eyes may be less successful than in phakic eyes. *Lai et al found that 9.5% of PACG eyes have a significant fall in vision after phacoemulsification.*

It is also reported that a large number of eyes have progression of cataracts after trabeculectomy, and therefore a phacoemulsification done prior to or together with the glaucoma surgery may avoid a second surgery soon after glaucoma filtering surgery. *Progression of cataract is now infrequently seen, if releasable sutures are used and anterior chamber manipulations during the glaucoma surgery are minimized.* Glaucoma medications must be given pre- and postoperatively to control any rise in IOP that may occur. A careful and thorough removal of viscoelastics is essential.

Cataract surgery after trabeculectomy may compromise the function of a bleb due to postsurgical inflammation and a breakdown of the blood–aqueous barrier, and may even lead to bleb failure if effective steroids are not given for a longer duration of time. Cataract surgery performed soon after trabeculectomy leads to bleb failure more often, and *the ideal gap between surgeries is at least 3 months.* Following drainage device surgery, cataract surgery has not been seen to significantly alter IOP control.

Combined surgeries are inherently a compromise; the relatively watertight closure of a cataract now has an opening to allow flow of aqueous into the subconjunctival space, with possible shallowing of the anterior chamber and its attendant problems. Combined phacoemulsification with trabeculectomy is thought to have *more success in lowering IOP if done from two sites*, so that the surgical trauma and subsequent healing induced by the phacoemulsification incision and manipulations are kept away from the site of subconjunctival drainage of aqueous. *The IOP reduction in combined surgeries is reported to be less than a filtering surgery alone, while the eye is prone to complications of both surgeries.*

There are some **guidelines for cataract/trabeculectomy surgeries in POAG/PACG eyes with a visually significant cataract:**

- Visually significant cataracts with mild or moderate glaucomatous neuropathy, well controlled on one to two glaucoma medications, could have cataract surgery alone, and would need to continue with glaucoma medications as required after the surgery.
- In eyes with moderate glaucomatous neuropathy reaching target IOP on up to three to four medications, phacoemulsification alone or combined with a trabeculectomy can be done, with the patients counseled about the need for continued glaucoma medications.
- In eyes with severe glaucoma, it is thought best to do a trabeculectomy to control the IOP first followed 3 months later by cataract surgery. This avoids any damage to an already very compromised optic nerve that may occur due to the known rise in IOP after cataract surgery alone.

Clear Lens Extraction

Clear lens extraction is being suggested as a better way to widen the iridocorneal angle and prevent iridotrabecular contact compared to a laser iridotomy. The rationale put forward is that the lens is a major factor in causing anterior segment crowding in primary angle closure disease (PACD), and removal would deepen the anterior chamber. However, many studies have reported that the lens as a primary cause of PACD, that is, *exaggerated lens vault, occurs in less than 20 to 25% of eyes with PACD.* Also, the trabecular damage seen in eyes with PACG cannot be significantly altered by lens removal, even though there are many suggested hypotheses, as described above. *The EAGLE study randomized PAC or PACG eyes to clear lens extraction or laser iridotomy, and showed a difference in fall of IOP of only 1.18 mm Hg with cataract surgery as compared to iridotomy.* In acute PACG a comparison of iridotomy alone to a cataract surgery showed a greater chance of lower IOP in the long term with cataract surgery. Tham et al studied medically uncontrolled PACG eyes in which a clear lens extraction or trabeculectomy was done, and reported that phacoemulsification leads to the use of more glaucoma medications and had a higher IOP than after trabeculectomy (**Flowchart 25.2**).

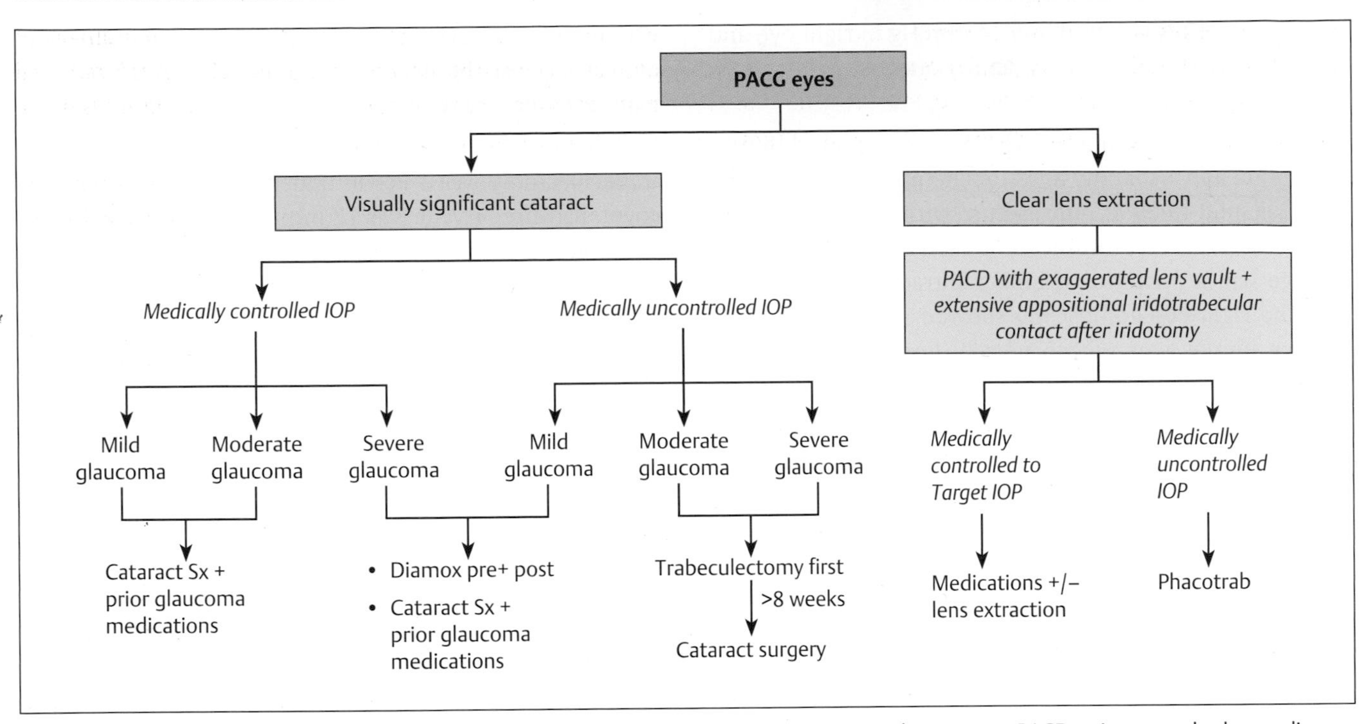

Flowchart 25.2 Role of cataract surgery in primary angle-closure glaucoma eyes. IOP, intraocular pressure; PACD, primary angle closure disease; PACG, primary angle-closure glaucoma.

As clear lens extraction is being proposed against the current standard of laser iridotomy in PACD eyes, it would be germane to study the complications and long-term problems of each. *Cataract surgery in the small eyes of PACD has to be done within a small anterior chamber volume of less than 1 mL, a corneal endothelium that is few millimeters away from a phaco probe, with an atonic and atrophic iris*, making a good capsulorrhexis and other maneuvers difficult. Even in eyes without glaucoma, intraoperative problems with PC rupture or vitreous loss have been reported in 1.95%, and long-term studies have shown that at 5 years cystoid macular edema was present in 3.5%, and corneal edema in 1% of eyes after phacoemulsification. There is a 42 times risk of retinal detachment surgery within 3 months of cataract surgery noted. Complications after a laser iridotomy are less dire, and include a postlaser spike of IOP, iritis, and hyphema.

Cataract Surgery Together with Minimally Invasive Procedures

Cataract surgery with minimally invasive devices is being evaluated in patients with early glaucoma on a single medication. The long-term efficacy and safety are still being reviewed, with some studies using multiple implants to improve success and some implants withdrawn by the FDA for corneal decompensation and other issues.

Effect of Cataract Surgery on Imaging and Perimetry

It is important to know that cataract surgery leads to changes in optical coherence tomography as well as perimetry parameters. *The retinal nerve fiber layer thickness on spectral domain optical coherence tomography shows increased values, and the global parameters on perimetry show an improvement. It is therefore best to reset a baseline after cataract surgery*. As the visual field index (VFI) is relatively unaffected by cataractogenesis, this has been found to remain unchanged.

To summarize, visual loss due to lenticular opacification is an indication for cataract surgery, but cataract surgery alone cannot be expected to reduce IOP to target levels in most glaucomatous eyes with visual field loss and high IOPs.

Cases

Case 1

An 83-year-old female presented with complaints of sudden painful diminution of vision in right eye for 1 week. On examination, best corrected visual acuity was perception of light with accurate projection of rays in only superior quadrant in the right eye and 6/12 in left eye, respectively. IOPs were 36 and 14 mm Hg in right eye and left eye, respectively, on maximal glaucoma medications in the right eye.

On slit-lamp examination, the right eye showed diffuse congestion and a shallow anterior chamber. The pupil was irregular, mid-dilated, nonreacting with patchy pupillary ruff atrophy, and an intumescent cataract (**Case 1-1**). The left eye had a posterior chamber intraocular lens in the bag. The right eye gonioscopy showed closed angles. The left eye fundus was within normal limits. The right eye posterior segment ultrasound was anechoic.

Points to consider

- High baseline IOP of 36 mm Hg.
- Duration of symptoms was 1 week.
- Inaccurate projection of light was present.

Diagnosis and Management

A diagnosis of right eye phacomorphic glaucoma, left eye Posterior chamber intraocular lens (PCIOL) was made. High IOPs with 1 week of symptoms and an inaccurate projection of rays suggest the necessity of a combined cataract and glaucoma surgery with a poor visual prognosis.

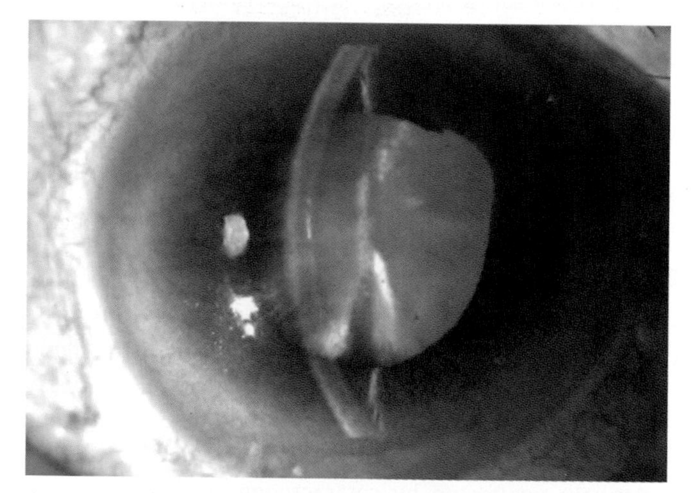

Case 1-1 Clinical picture of the right eye showing peripheral iridocorneal touch and an intumescent cataract.

The patient underwent a right eye two-site phaco with trabeculectomy, with PCIOL under intravenous mannitol cover. IOP after 1 year was 12 mm Hg, and there was total optic nerve head cupping seen. Vision improved only to 1/60 with inaccurate projection of light as was seen preoperatively.

Case 2

A 72-year-old male presented with complaints of sudden pain and redness along with diminution of vision in the right eye for 4 weeks. On examination, best corrected visual acuity was perception of light with accurate projection of rays in all quadrants in the right eye and 6/9 in the left eye, respectively. IOPs were 28 and 12 mm Hg in the right eye and left eye, respectively.

On slit-lamp examination, the right eye had anterior chamber flare and a few endothelial deposits with a deep anterior chamber and normal iris pattern. A hypermature cataract with anterior capsular calcific areas was seen. A relative afferent pupillary defect was present (**Case 2-1**). The left eye had an immature senile cataract. On gonioscopy, angles were open in both eyes with the right eye showing haziness over the trabecular meshwork. Fundus examination of the right eye was not possible, and the left eye was within normal limits. The right eye posterior segment ultrasound was anechoic.

Points to consider

- History of 4 weeks of redness and pain in the right eye.
- Relative afferent pupillary defect in the right eye.
- Signs of anterior segment inflammation.

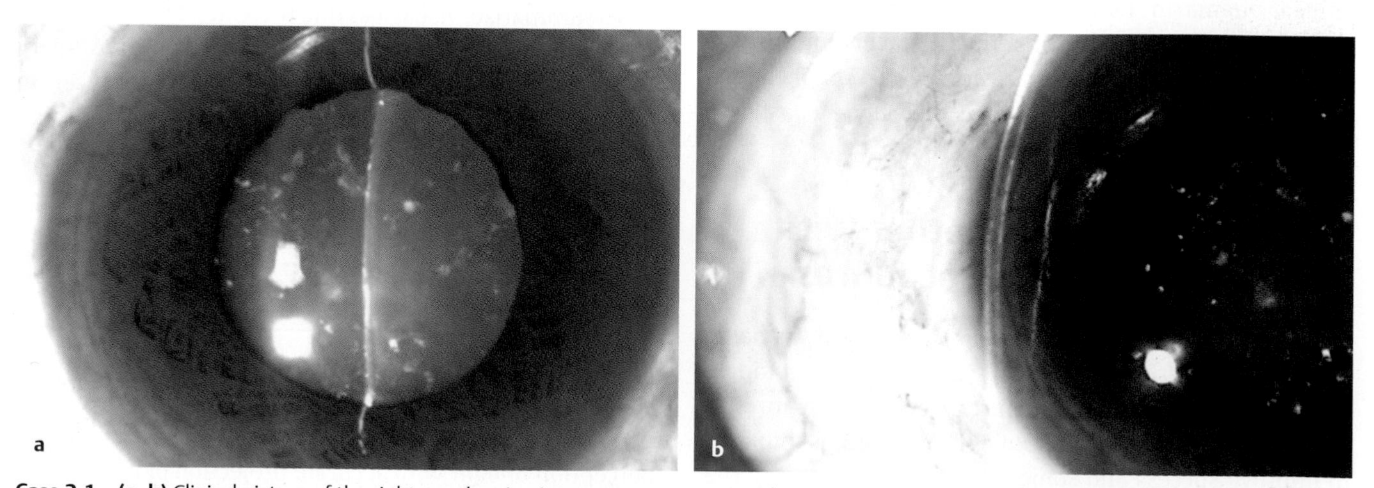

Case 2-1 **(a, b)** Clinical picture of the right eye showing intumescent cataract with anterior capsular calcification in a hypermature cataract, and a deep anterior chamber.

Diagnosis and Management

A diagnosis of resolving phacolytic glaucoma in the right eye, immature senile catract with nuclear sclerosis in the left eye was made and a guarded visual prognosis was explained. He was started on topical β-blocker/alpha agonist (fixed dose combination) and oral carbonic anhydrase inhibitors. Right eye phacoemulsification with PCIOL under intravenous mannitol cover was performed. Glaucoma medications were continued. Cup:disc ratio was found to be 0.8, with a vision of 6/36 in the right eye 2 months after surgery.

Case 3

A 65-year-old patient had a high IOP of 34 mm Hg on first postoperative day after cataract surgery, with blurring of vision and pain.

Points to consider

- High IOP in the first 2 to 7 days post cataract surgery is often due to retained viscoelastics in anterior chamber.
- If there is chronically raised IOP over 2 to 3 months, look for retained lens matter, a pre-existing glaucoma, or a steroid response.

Diagnosis and Management

A diagnosis of retained viscoelastic was made. Medical therapy was given to control IOP—timolol, brimonidine, and Diamox. He was reviewed regularly to taper medications gradually by asking to stop Diamox 3 days before review, then other drops one at a time, a week before a review till normal IOP was restored.

The IOP reduced to 18 mm Hg after 1 week on timolol and brimonidine, and all glaucoma medications were stopped after 3 weeks.

Case 4

A 65-year-old female complained of gradual diminution of vision in both eyes, with the right having a visual acuity of 6/36. She was a known diabetic and hypertensive. On examination, there was an immature senile cataract in both eyes with an IOP of 16 and 18 mm Hg and a cup:disc ratio of 0.8 in the right eye with significant thinning and pallor of the neuroretinal rim. The left eye had a cup:disc ratio of 0.6. Gonioscopy showed an open angle (**Case 4-1**). On perimetry there was extensive visual field loss on total deviation probability plot, but pattern deviation was not available as mean deviation threshold was exceeded in the right eye.

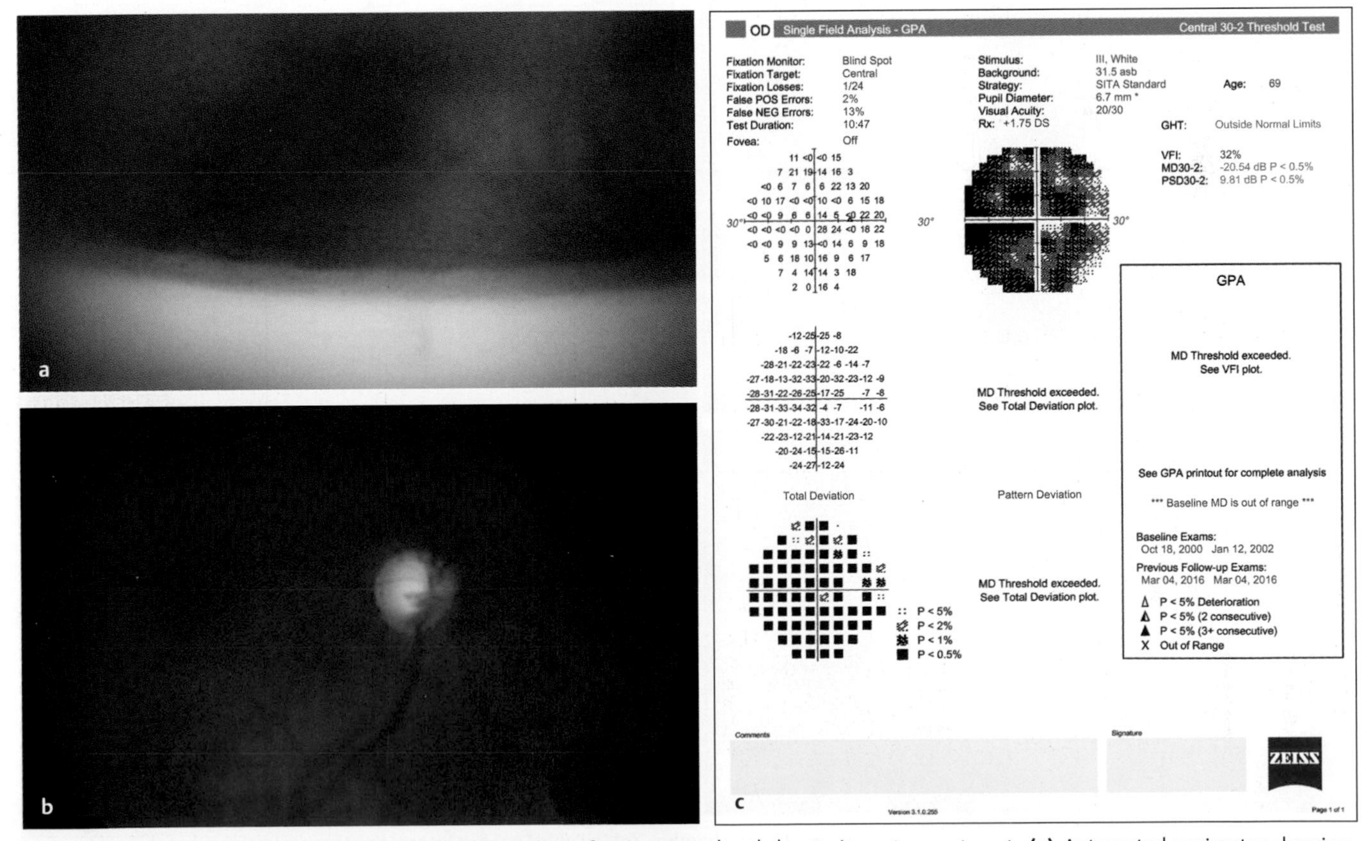

Case 4-1 **(a)** Open angle on gonioscopy. **(b)** Hazy view of optic nerve head due to immature cataract. **(c)** Automated perimetry showing extensive loss of retinal sensitivity, with a mean deviation of −20 dB.

Points to consider

- Possible moderate glaucomatous neuropathy.
- Visual acuity of 6/36.
- Immature senile cataract.

Diagnosis and Management

A diagnosis of POAG with immature senile cataract was made. IOP was controlled prior to phacoemulsification with a combination of dorzolamide and timolol, and additional oral acetazolamide was given before and after cataract surgery for 2 days. Her vision improved to 6/12 and she was advised repeat perimetry after 2 to 3 months.

Case 5

A 50-year-old lady with PACG had a baseline IOP of 36 mm Hg, and an IOP of 22 mm Hg on all topical glaucoma medications. On examination, there was a very shallow anterior chamber, a patent iridotomy, relatively clear lens, and a cup:disc ratio of 0.8 in both eyes having a thinned and pale neuroretinal rim. Gonioscopy showed an occludable angle and peripheral anterior synechiae over 200 degrees. On perimetry there was a superior arcuate scotoma breaking through to the periphery in the right eye (**Case 5-1**).

Points to consider

- Moderate severity of glaucoma requires a target IOP of <15 mm Hg.
- Very shallow anterior chamber.
- Life expectancy of 30+ years.

Diagnosis and Management

A diagnosis of PACG with moderate glaucomatous neuropathy in the right eye was made. The IOP fall after cataract surgery is likely to be small in the presence of extensive trabecular dysfunction.

A lens extraction was done as the surgeon feared a further shallowing of the anterior chamber after trabeculectomy. After 3 months her IOP continued to be 20 to 22 mm Hg on all tolerable topical glaucoma medications. A trabeculectomy was then performed and the IOP was 12 to 14 mm Hg off all medications after that.

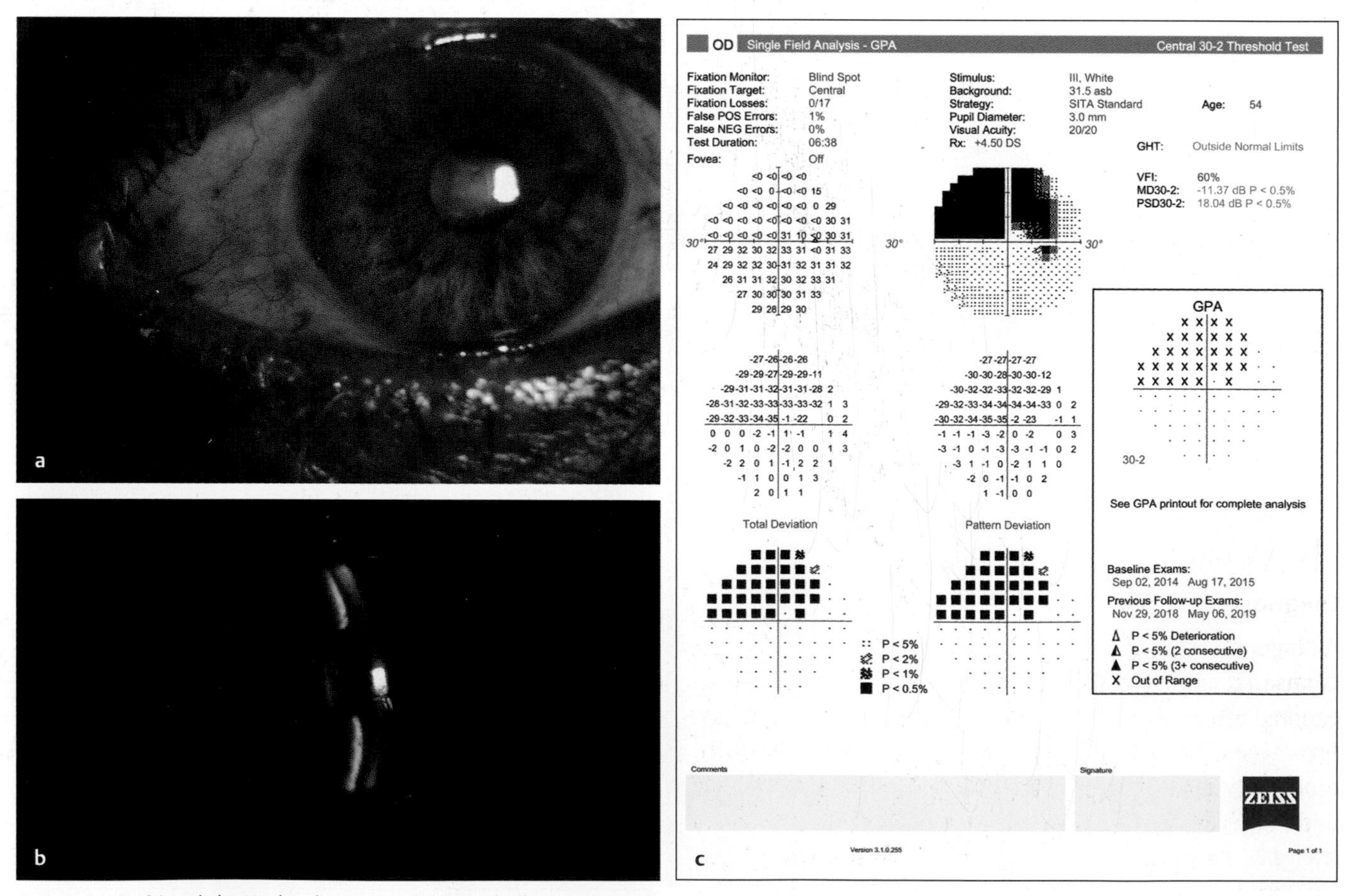

Case 5-1 (a, b) Early lenticular changes with a very shallow anterior chamber. **(c)** Reliable Swedish interactive threshold algorithm (SITA) standard field having a mean deviation of −11 dB, *visual field index* of 60%, and a superior arcuate scotoma that has broken into the periphery.

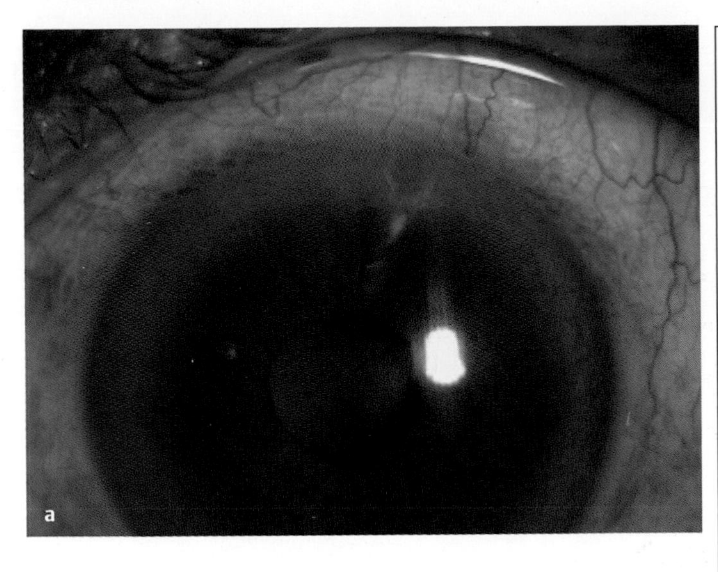

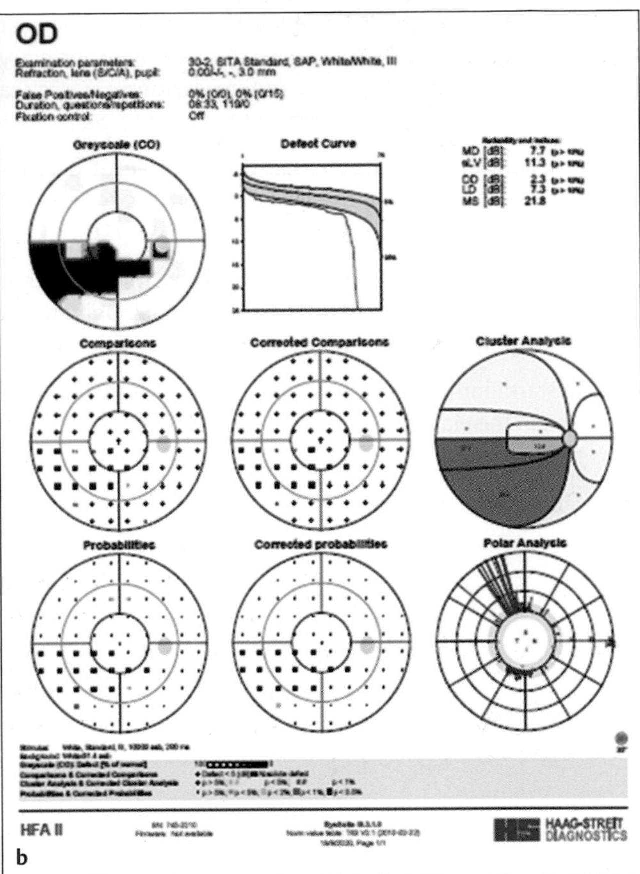

Case 6-1 **(a)** Anterior segment photograph showing a relatively featureless iris, pupillary ruff atrophy, and a patent iridotomy. **(b)** On reliable Octopus perimetry an inferior arcuate scotoma is present, with a corresponding polar analysis suggesting a loss of neuroretinal rim in the superotemporal area.

Case 6

A 56-year-old lady having PACG developed a cataract, reducing acuity to 6/18. On examination, there was a very shallow anterior chamber, and a patent iridotomy. Her last field showed an inferior arcuate scotoma. The IOP on timolol, brimonidine, and travoprost was 14 mm Hg, within target range for the moderate glaucomatous neuropathy (**Case 6-1**).

Points to consider

- IOP is well controlled on medication.
- Visually significant cataract.

Diagnosis and Management

A diagnosis of PACG with IMSC was made. The patient was counseled about the need for continued glaucoma medications after cataract surgery. Travoprost was stopped for a week. During phacoemulsification the iris prolapsed repeatedly and postoperatively there was corneal edema with severe inflammation. After 6 hours of surgery an IOP of 30 mm Hg was recorded and the patient was given oral acetazolamide with timolol and brimonidine drops. Oral glaucoma medications were stopped in a week and brinzolamide drops added. Steroid and antibiotic drops were continued for 6 weeks, when there was a best corrected vision of 6/9. Travoprost was restarted after 4 weeks.

Suggested Readings

Ahmad SS. Acute lens-induced glaucomas: a review. J Acute Dis 2017;6:47–52

Azuara-Blanco A, Burr J, Ramsay C, et al; EAGLE study group. Effectiveness of early lens extraction for the treatment of primary angle-closure glaucoma (EAGLE): a randomised controlled trial. Lancet 2016;388(10052):1389–1397

Ellant JP, Obstbaum SA. Lens-induced glaucoma. Doc Ophthalmol 1992;81(3):317–338

Friedman DS, Jampel HD, Lubomski LH, et al. Surgical strategies for coexisting glaucoma and cataract: an evidence-based update. Ophthalmology 2002;109(10):1902–1913

Jiang N, Zhao GQ, Lin J, et al. Meta-analysis of the efficacy and safety of combined surgery in the management of eyes with coexisting cataract and open angle glaucoma. Int J Ophthalmol 2018;11(2):279–286

Lai JS, Tham CC, Chan JC. The clinical outcomes of cataract extraction by phacoemulsification in eyes with primary angle-closure glaucoma (PACG) and co-existing cataract: a prospective case series. J Glaucoma 2006;15(1):47–52

Masis M, Mineault PJ, Phan E, Lin SC. The role of phacoemulsification in glaucoma therapy: a systematic review and meta-analysis. Surv Ophthalmol 2018;63(5):700–710

Murchison JF Jr, Shields MB. An evaluation of three surgical approaches for coexisting cataract and glaucoma. Ophthalmic Surg 1989;20(6):393–398

Papaconstantinou D, Georgalas I, Kourtis N, et al. Lens-induced glaucoma in the elderly. Clin Interv Aging 2009;4:331–336

Rhiu S, Hong S, Seong GJ, Kim CY. Phacoemulsification alone versus phacoemulsification combined with trabeculectomy for primary angle-closure glaucoma. Yonsei Med J 2010; 51(5):781–783

Shingleton BJ, Pasternack JJ, Hung JW, O'Donoghue MW. Three and five year changes in intraocular pressures after clear corneal phacoemulsification in open angle glaucoma patients, glaucoma suspects, and normal patients. J Glaucoma 2006;15(6):494–498

Tham CCY, Kwong YYY, Leung DYL, et al. Phacoemulsification versus combined phacotrabeculectomy in medically uncontrolled chronic angle closure glaucoma with cataracts. Ophthalmology 2009;116(4):725–731, 731.e1–731.e3

Vizzeri G, Weinreb RN. Cataract surgery and glaucoma. Curr Opin Ophthalmol 2010;21(1):20–24

CHAPTER 26 Low-Vision Aids for Glaucoma Patients

Overview

- Visual Impairment in Glaucoma
- Low-Vision Aids
  - Newer Technologies
  - General Measures
- Suggested Readings

Introduction

Glaucoma is one of the commonest causes of irreversible blindness around the world today, and *the ophthalmologist has to be prepared to help patients use their residual vision to the greatest extent possible.* Currently in India around 20% of individuals reaching an eye care facility have already lost vision in one eye, and about 10% have low vision/blindness in both eyes. The actual magnitude of the problem is unknown, as there are no nationwide surveys that have all the tools to identify glaucoma. Many cases go undocumented. *In developed countries about 11% of glaucoma patients are visually handicapped and 1 to 2% blind.*

Visual Impairment in Glaucoma

Glaucoma initially affects the two eyes asymmetrically and binocular vision largely reflects visual function in the better eye, with an overlap of the two visual fields compensating for scotomatous defects in either eye to varying extents. As scotomas enlarge in moderate and severe glaucomatous neuropathy, the peripheral field loss leads to patients bumping into objects, stumbling on uneven ground, difficulty using stairs, tripping over wires, etc., and an inability to see objects coming from the periphery, for example, while driving. Glare makes recognition of faces a problem, especially in outdoors. In the late stages patients commonly complain that they can see finer objects in the center, but lose the bigger picture.

Visual function is seen to be impaired in glaucoma in many ways listed below:

- Early glaucoma:
  - Decrease in contrast sensitivity.
- Moderate/severe glaucoma:
  - Loss of visual field—midperipheral at first and then peripheral and central.
  - Increased sensitivity to light: glare.
  - Diminution of contrast.
  - Delayed dark/light adaptation.
  - Abnormalities in color perception.
  - Difficulty reading.
  - Diminution of visual acuity.

A good evaluation of the patient's lifestyle, visual requirements, and current visual aids is very important to best improve visual function. Basic ophthalmic examination and glaucoma investigations should be performed to ascertain visual acuity, refractive status, contrast sensitivity, field loss, and medications being taken.

Low-Vision Aids

Low-vision aids enable patients to use their residual vision in the best possible manner, and reduce disability while performing activities of normal life. Minification makes images smaller, allowing them to fall within the constricted field of glaucoma patients, and is very useful.

Low-vision aids for glaucoma can be classified as:

- *Optical:*
  - Reverse telescopes: Handheld or spectacle mounted to minimize objects and thereby increase field (**Fig. 26.1**).
  - Sectoral prisms to increase field of vision.
  - High minus lenses to minify.
  - Magnifiers to help with central vision (**Fig. 26.2**).

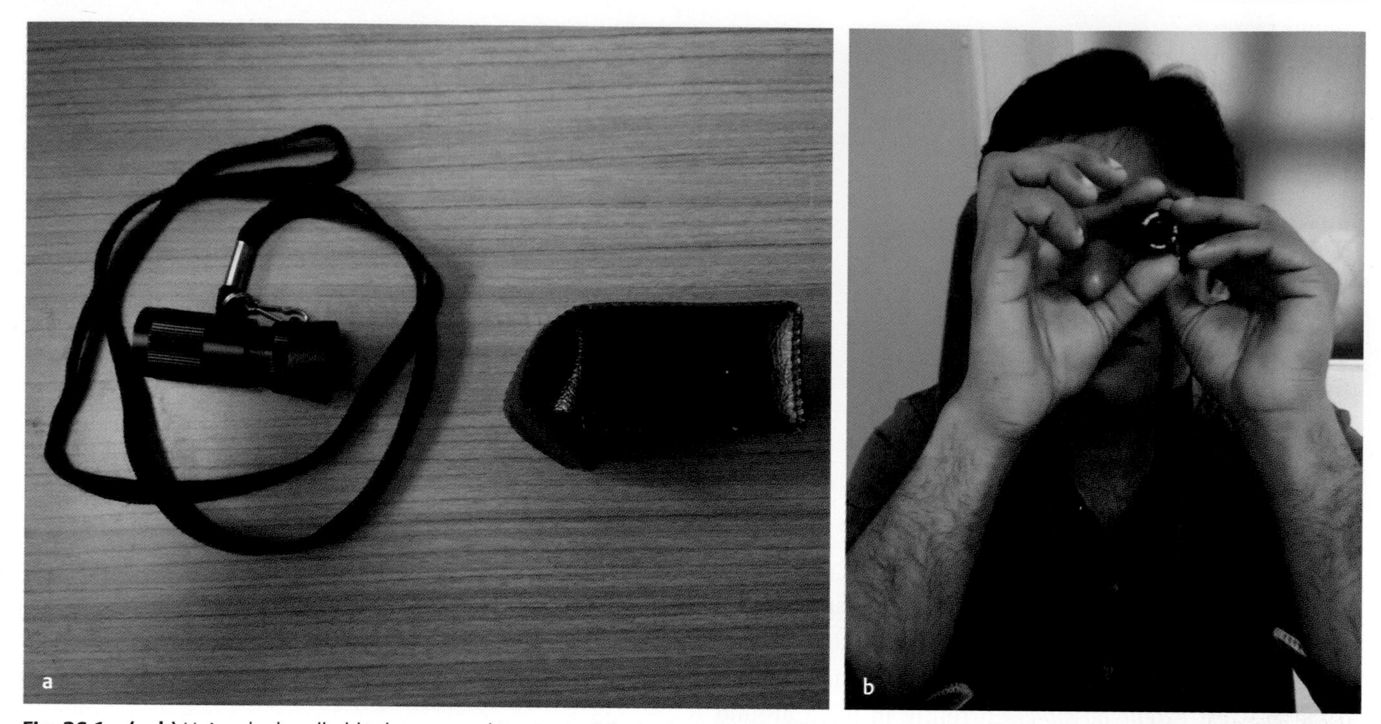

Fig. 26.1 **(a, b)** Uniocular handheld telescope and its usage. (The images are provided courtesy of Sneha Agarwal, New Delhi, India.)

- *Nonoptical:*
  - Rulers: To overcome tracking difficulties while reading, due to scotomas.
  - Filters: Yellow/orange filters to decrease glare (**Fig. 26.3**).
  - Lamps: LED lamps to improve illumination.
  - Visors: To decrease glare when out of the house.
  - Typoscopes: Dark plastic bands with a window to highlight area of interest.

Newer Technologies

- *HD CCTV desktop video magnifiers* capture images of interest and transfer them to a screen. They have multiple degrees of magnification, contrast, and color settings to adjust for best vision in a given individual. High-definition monitors allow even the smallest objects to be seen clearly and also do not have peripheral distortion of images.
- *Text to speech systems*: For example, JAWS (job access with speech), Window-Eyes 9, etc., provide speech outputs for common computer applications such as text, images, etc.
- *Smartphone/tablet*: Photographs taken by a camera can be used to see and magnify objects, and there are text-to-speech Apps that can be downloaded and used.
- *Computer settings* can be adjusted to increase contrast, while screens and filters can reduce glare.
- *Handheld video magnifiers* are small, light, and portable, and have LED lighting to improve visibility. They capture images of interest and transfer them to a 5- to 6-inch screen and can be used for reading books, newspapers, etc.

General Measures

Glare is caused by bright light—sunlight or fluorescent light—and can be decreased by *wearing a cap or visor when outside*, and the use of tinted spectacles or contrast-enhancing filters. Sunglasses that wrap around, block light from the periphery, also decrease glare. *Filters that are amber or yellow appear to reduce glare best.*

At home ambient light should be good to facilitate movement, with task lighting such as LED table lamps over the left shoulder for reading and other close work.

To prevent falls, *improving contrast at stairs by fluorescent or colored tape* is important as the peripheral visual field is

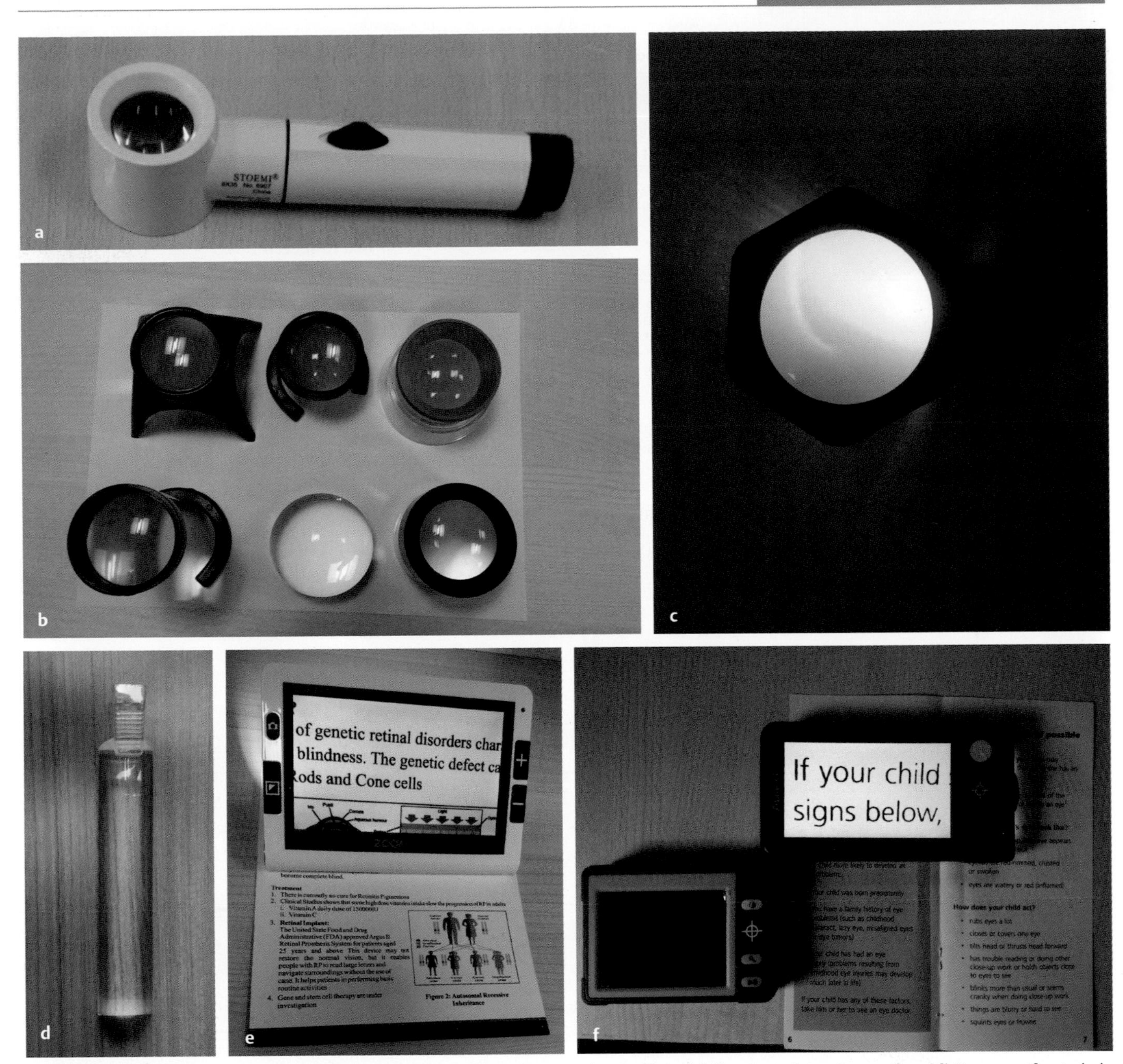

Fig. 26.2 **(a)** Handheld self-illuminated stand magnifier. **(b)** Various stand magnifiers. **(c)** Illuminated stand magnifier. **(d)** Bar magnifier to help read lines. **(e)** Portable video magnifier. **(f)** Video magnifier. (The images are provided courtesy of Sneha Agarwal, New Delhi, India.)

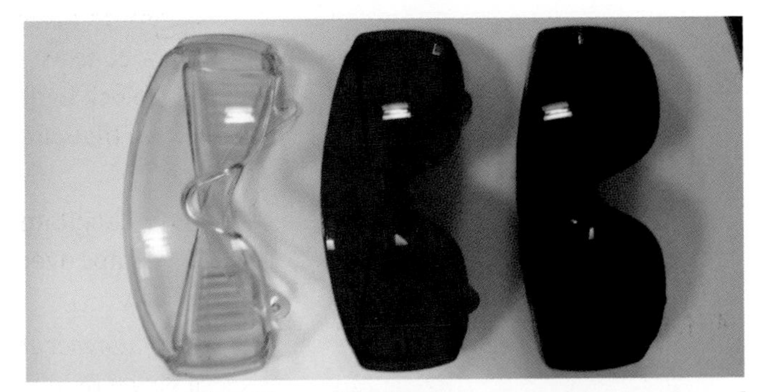

Fig. 26.3 Antiglare filters. (The images are provided courtesy of Sneha Agarwal, New Delhi, India.)

lost in glaucoma. Similarly, it must be ensured that there are no loose wires or objects that may pose as obstacles to walking. Installing hand rails along the wall helps to direct patients and afford some stability (**Table 26.1**).

The Government of India also provides assistance in many forms, and this can be ascertained at the Ministry of Social Justice & Empowerment.

Glaucoma should not be allowed to hinder a patient in his/her daily activities or work. The use of appropriate low-vision aids can improve the quality of life of almost all glaucoma patients, and should be tried and provided to all.

Table 26.1 Common activities affected by glaucoma can be improved to the extent possible by specific low-visual aids

		Possible solution
Activities—Distance	Television viewing Recognizing faces Blackboard work Watching movies	HD CCTV Amber/yellow filter Reverse telescope Reverse telescope
Activities—Intermediate	Cooking Computers Housework	Ambient lighting Text to speech Ambient lighting care with wires/stairs, etc.
Activities—Near	Reading Writing/signature	Handheld video magnifier Typoscope

Suggested Readings

Khanna A, Ichhpujani P. Low vision aids in glaucoma. J Curr Glaucoma Pract 2012;6(1):20–24

Rossetti L, Digiuni M, Montesano G, et al. Correction: blindness and glaucoma: a multicentre data review from 7 academic eye clinics. PLoS One 2016;11(3):e0151010

Sabel BA, Cárdenas-Morales L, Gao Y. Vision restoration in glaucoma by activating residual vision with a holistic, clinical approach: a review. J Curr Glaucoma Pract 2018;12(1):1–9

CHAPTER 27

Lifestyle Modifications for Glaucoma

Overview

- Associated Systemic Disease Control
- Preventing Intraocular Pressure Rise
- Lowering Intraocular Pressure
- Decrease Oxidative Stress
- Food and Supplements
- Suggested Readings

Introduction

Glaucoma is a multifactorial, chronic, progressive disease, which has been correlated with aging and stress. The major treatable factor is, of course, the intraocular pressure (IOP) with medications, laser, or surgery. However, lifestyle modifications may also help to lower IOP, decrease IOP fluctuations, as well as decrease the effects of oxidative stress on ocular tissues. As only a few glaucoma patients have a known gene responsible for the disease, environmental and lifestyle factors also influence it. This chapter discusses some of the lifestyle modifications which reduce the progression of glaucoma.

Associated Systemic Disease Control

A good control of associated systemic diseases such as hypertension, diabetes, and thyroid abnormalities is essential. Avoiding a night dose of hypertensive medications and checking blood pressure (BP) at night may help identify patients who are nocturnal dippers, that is, have a significantly low BP at night. Sleep apnea, identified by a history of snoring, may also be linked to glaucoma progression, especially in normal tension glaucoma. The role of diabetes in glaucoma pathology is still unclear, but well-controlled diabetes would reduce microangiopathies.

Physicians prescribing other medications should be informed that the patient has glaucoma, to help prevent any drug interactions, and exacerbation of the systemic problem or glaucoma. Steroids in any form such as inhalers, skin creams, etc., should be avoided as much as possible and a steroid-induced IOP rise looked for in case steroids are imperative.

Oxidative stress plays an important role in the pathogenesis of different types of glaucoma, both at the level of retinal ganglion cells and the trabecular meshwork. The diagnosis of glaucoma leads to additional stress, depression, and anxiety, adding to the ongoing pathology.

There are some suggested lifestyle changes that are thought to help, only as adjuncts to lowering IOP by all other means—medications, laser, and surgery.

Preventing Intraocular Pressure Rise

Some activities are known to raise IOP, and this may be seen more often and to a greater degree in patients having glaucoma, for example:

- Drink only a glass of liquid at a time, not a liter in the morning.
- Avoid any activity involving a Valsalva maneuver—chronic constipation, cough, etc.
- Avoid head down position, especially *shish asana* (headstand in yoga).
- Avoid blocking both nostrils at a time or breath holding.
- Avoid weight lifting.
- Avoid tight clothing around the neck, such as neck ties.

Lowering Intraocular Pressure

Some activities can lower IOP, even if only for the duration or a short while, for example:

- Aerobic exercise.
- Yoga.
- Meditation.

Yoga emphasizes postures and movements that relax the body, together with breathing exercises that provide increased oxygen to the body and brain. However, a glaucoma patient should avoid the following postures:

- Head stand.
- Downward facing dog.
- Standing forward bend.
- Plow.
- Legs up the wall.

Decrease Oxidative Stress

Oxidative stress-induced changes have been seen to occur in glaucomatous eyes at the ganglion cells and in the trabecular meshwork. This is also an integral part of aging, and glaucoma is an age-related disease. Oxidative stress could be decreased by:

- Dietary antioxidants.
- Omega 3 intake.
- Cessation of smoking.
- Meditation.

Food and Supplements

Glaucoma is a multifactorial disease that can currently only be treated by IOP reduction. However, certain foods and supplements help stabilize the disease.

Vitamin B3 has been shown in mice to reduce mitochondrial dysfunction and retinal ganglion cell damage. In these animals it has been shown to be neuroprotective, given orally or by intravitreal injection. Vitamins A and C are antioxidative, and would be expected to help in maintaining the health of the eye as well. The protective effect of such supplements on photoreceptors, in macular degeneration, was shown in Age-Related Eye Disease Study (AREDS), and could be extrapolated to glaucomatous neuropathy. Vitamin B12 has been shown to be neuroprotective, and its deficiency causes optic neuropathy.

Mitochondrial dysfunction increases ganglion cell susceptibility to injury in glaucoma. Co-enzyme Q10 and resveratrol support mitochondrial function and are powerful antioxidants, which may have a neuroprotective influence. Omega 3 fatty acids have been found to be beneficial in stabilizing glaucoma in some studies, by increasing ocular blood flow and lowering IOP with a neuroprotective action.

Fruits and vegetables rich in vitamins C and A and carotene are antioxidative, especially nitrate-rich dark leafy vegetables and fruits such as oranges. In certain cohort studies they have been shown to be associated with a reduced incidence and progression of primary open-angle glaucoma (POAG).

Flavonoids in tea reduce oxidative stress and improve blood flow. Dark chocolate also works through the presence of flavonoids. A couple of cups of coffee, caffeine, do not produce a significant IOP rise, but four to six cups a day may raise IOP in POAG patients.

Lifestyle modifications cannot treat glaucoma, but with increasing scientific research, these should be adjunctive measures to help reduce glaucoma-related morbidity.

Suggested Readings

Age-Related Eye Disease Study Research Group. A randomized, placebo-controlled, clinical trial of high-dose supplementation with vitamins C and E, beta carotene, and zinc for age-related macular degeneration and vision loss: AREDS report no. 8. Arch Ophthalmol 2001;119(10):1417–1436

Azumi I, Kosaki H, Nakatani H. Effects of metcobolamin (Methycobal) on the visual field of chronic glaucoma: a multicenter open study. Nippon Ganka Kiyo 1983;34:873–878

Sasaki T, Murata M, Amemiya T. Effect of long-term treatment of glaucoma with vitamin B-12. Glaucoma 1992;14:167–170

Williams PA, Harder JM, Foxworth NE, et al. Vitamin B3 modulates mitochondrial vulnerability and prevents glaucoma in aged mice. Science 2017;355(6326):756–760

Index

A
Adenosine receptor agonists, 252
Ahmed glaucoma valve (AGV), 320
Allergic conjunctivitis, 251
Alpha 2 agonists, 248
Angle recession, 216
Aniridia, 179–180
Anterior chamber angle structures, 25–27
ciliary body band, 26
iris, 26–27
Schwalbe's line, 25
scleral spur, 25
techniques to visualize, 28–30
trabecular meshwork, 25
Anterior chamber depth, 3–4
Anterior segment, 2–3, 161, 219
Anterior segment dysgenesis disorders, 176
Axenfeld-Rieger syndrome, 177–178
Peters anomaly, 178–179
Antiglare filters, 345
Aphakic glaucoma. *See* Pseudophakic glaucoma
Aqueous misdirection syndrome, 308–309
Aqueous misdirection/malignant glaucoma, 204
algorithm for management of, 206
clinical features, 205
pathophysiology, 205
ultrasound biomicroscopy of, 206
Arcuate scotoma, nonglaucomatous causes of, 50–57
Axenfeld-Rieger syndrome, 34, 177–178

B
b blockers (BBs), 248
Baerveldt implants, 319
Baseline intraocular pressure, 92
Bilateral eyelid edema and pigmentation, 255
Bleb-related endophthalmitis, 312
Blebitis, 312
Brimonidine, 248, 253

C
Cannabinoids, 252
Carbonic anhydrase inhibitors (CAIs), 250
Cataract surgery
case studies, 337–341
effect on imaging and perimetry, 337
in POAG/PACG, 335–336
IOP rise/fall with, 335
with minimally invasive procedures, 337
Cataractous or subluxated lens, 219
Cerebral spinal fluid hydrodynamics, 124
Childhood glaucomas
aniridia, 179–180
anterior segment dysgenesis disorders, 176
Axenfeld-Rieger syndrome, 177–178
Peters anomaly, 178–179
case studies, 186–189
causes of, 173
classification of, 173
examination, 182
genetic counseling for, 186
lifelong review, 185–186
management, 182
combined trabeculotomy with trabeculectomy, 184
glaucoma drainage devices, 185
goniotomy, 183
medications, 183
trabeculectomy with MMC, 184
trabeculotomy, 183
pathogenesis of, 173–174
primary congenital glaucoma (PCG), 174–177
prognosis, 186
secondary, 182
Sturge-Weber syndrome, 180–182
Cholinergic agonists, 250
Choroidal effusions, 307
Chronic hypotony, 313
Chronic uveitis, 202
Ciliary congestion, 2
Ciliary neurotrophic factor (CNTF), 253
Cirrus optical coherence tomography printout, 82
Clear lens extraction, 336–337
Closed globe injury
biomarkers for, 218
causing equatorial expansion, 216
clinical features of, 215–219
consequences of, 216
fundus photograph after, 218
ghost cell glaucoma, 220
management, 219–220
Combined trabeculotomy with trabeculectomy, 184
Congenital cataract surgery, 203
Cornea, 2–3
Cup:disc ratio, 14–15
Cyclodialysis, 217

D
Diagnosis of glaucoma
clinical evaluation, 271
diagnosis of change, 269
extraocular examination, 2
family history, 2
ocular examination
anterior chamber, 3–4
anterior segment, 2–3
iris, 4–5
lens, 5
visual status, 2
optic nerve head photography, 271–272
optical coherence tomography. *See* Optical coherence tomography
optical coherence tomography parameters for, 76
macular ganglion cell complex, 79
optic nerve head analysis, 79
retinal nerve fiber layer thickness, 77–79
perimetry. *See* Perimetry
retina, 5–6
systematic examination, 1–2
tonometry, 7–10
applanation, 7–9
digital palpation, 7
dynamic contour/Pascal tonometer, 10
noncontact tonometers, 9
ocular response analyzer (ORA), 10
rebound tonometer, 9
Schiotz indentation tonometers for, 9
tonopen, 9
Differential light sensitivity, 39
Digital palpation, 7
Direct gonioscopes, 24
Disc damage likelihood scale (DDLS), 16
Disc hemorrhages, 15–16
Dynamic contour/Pascal tonometer (DCT), 10

E
Eales' disease, 241
Early postoperative complications
aqueous misdirection syndrome, 308–309
choroidal effusions, 307
pupillary block, 308
shallow anterior chamber, 304–307
suprachoroidal hemorrhages, 308
Event-based analysis, 270

Exaggerated lens vault, 118
Extensive iridocorneal touch, 209
Extensive midperipheral anterior synechiae after uveitis, 208
Extraocular examination, 2
Extremely shallow anterior chamber post trabeculectomy, 205

F
Fixed drug combinations, 251
Floor effect, 86
Functional glaucomatous deficits, 269

G
Ganglion cell analysis, printout report of, 84
Glaucoma, 65
  ghost cell, 220
  management, long-term, 289
  staging system based on Humphrey visual fields, 69
Glaucoma drainage devices (GDDs), 185
  case studies, 325–326
  complications of, 323–324
  contraindications for using, 320
  indications for using, 320
  nonvalved implants, 319
  postoperative course, 323
  principle of, 319
  randomized control trials of
    Ahmed Baerveldt comparison study, 324
    primary tube *vs.* trabeculectomy study, 324–325
    tube *vs.* trabeculectomy study, 324
  surgical steps for
    nonvalved glaucoma drainage device, 322–323
    valved glaucoma drainage device, 321–322
  valved implants, 320
Glaucoma hemifield test (GHT), 46, 65
Glaucoma medical therapy
  algorithm for, 247, 251
  case studies, 254–257
  clinical baseline for starting, 247–248
  drug administration, 248
  failure of, 253
  glaucoma medications
    adenosine receptor agonists, 252
    cannabinoids, 252
    choice of, 251–252
    decreasing aqueous production, 248–250
    fixed drug combinations, 251
    hand out/instructions on use of, 253
    increasing trabecular outflow, 250
    increasing uveoscleral outflow, 250–251
    latanoprostene bunod, 0.024%, 252
    newer drug delivery systems, 252
    nonresponders, 253
  goal of, 269
  neuroprotection, 253
  permutations and combinations available in quest for, 247
  stem cell therapy, 253–254
Glaucoma progression
  algorithm depicting criteria for, 270
  case studies, 290–293
  detection difficulty, 269
  identifying, 270–271, 274
  management, 288–289
  Octopus EyeSuite for, 278–279
  printout, guided, 275
  quantification of, 270
  risk factors for, 288
  test for detecting
    frequency of testing and review of, 270
    ideal, 269–270
  therapeutic intervention effects on, 289
Glaucoma surgeries. *See also* Minimally invasive glaucoma surgeries
  advantages of, 295
  ideal features of, 295
  nonpenetrating, 327–328
  outcomes and postoperative interventions, 296
  pathways utilized in, 295
  trabeculectomy, 295
    case studies, 314–318
    concept, 296
    early postoperative complications, 304–309
    indications for, 296–297
    late complications, 309–314
    modifications, 300–303
    postoperative care, 303–304
    preoperative measures for, 297
    surgical procedure, 297–300
Glaucoma suspect management
  case studies, 107–110, 119–122
  primary angle-closure disease
    exaggerated lens vault, 118
    plateau iris syndrome, 118
    primary angle closure (PAC), 116–118
    primary angle-closure suspect, 116
    secondary angle closure, 118
  shallow anterior chamber
    anterior segment imaging, 115
    clinical features, 112–114
    diagnosing, 111–112
    evaluation, 114
    gonioscopy, 114–116
    management of eyes with, 115–116
    prevalence of, 111
  suspicion on basis of optic nerve head abnormalities, 107
  suspicion on basis of raised IOP, 105–106
Glaucomatous damage, clinical staging of, 92–96
  optic nerve head examination, 92–93
  perimetric staging, 93–96
Glaucomatous optic neuropathy
  hard and soft signs of, 6
  mild, moderate, and severe, 19–20
  pathophysiology of
    cerebral spinal fluid hydrodynamics, 12
    genetics, 12
    neurodegeneration, 11
    pressure dependent or mechanical factors, 11
    vascular perfusion factors, 11
  risk factor for, 23
  staging of, 18–21
Glaucomatous scotoma
  Anderson's criteria for diagnosing, 65–66
  classification of
    Aulhorn and Karmeyer, 66–67
    based on Humphrey visual fields, 69
    based on mean deviation, 67, 69
    based on optic nerve head, 67
    based on visual loss extent, 67
    case studies of, 72–74
    using staging, 69–70
  diagnosis on standard automated perimetry, 47–49
  illustration of staging, 70–71
Goldmann applanation tonometry, 8–9
Gonioscopes
  Goldmann and four-mirror, 24
  importance of, 24–25
  types of, 24
Gonioscopic patterns
  narrow angle, 30–33
  open angle, 30
Gonioscopy, 23
  case studies, 35–37
  grading systems for, 27–28
  in iridocyclitis, 32
  in neovascular glaucoma., 241
  indentation, 29–30
  manipulative, 28–29
  of eye with chronic anterior uveitis, 208
  primary open-angle glaucoma (POAG), 127
  recording, 33–35
Goniotomy, 183
Guided progression analysis (GPA), 273, 291

on optical coherence tomography, 280–282
printout, 274, 275
rate of progression, 290, 293

H

Handheld self-illuminated stand magnifier, 345
Humphrey field analysis (HFA), 45, 51
printouts, 277
single-field printout, 45
testing strategies on, 42

I

Indentation gonioscopy, 29–30
Indirect gonioscopes, 24
InnFocus microshunt, 331
Intractable secondary glaucoma, 233
Intraocular pressure
raised, 124
Intraocular pressure (IOP). *See also* Target intraocular pressure
baseline, 92
definition of, 91
extensive iridocorneal touch with, 209
measurement, 7
response to topical corticosteroid administration, 227
Intravitreal triamcinolone, 234
Iridocyclitis, gonioscopy in, 32
Iridodialysis, 216, 219
Iridotrabecular contact extent, 142
Iris, 4–5
Iris melanoma, 34
Iris neovascularization
ciliary congestion and mild corneal edema, 240
clinical presentation and management of, 240
management, 242–243
prevention and prognosis, 243–244
stages of, 240–241
Ischemic CRVO, 240–241

J

Juvenile open-angle glaucoma (JOAG)
anterior segment in, 161
case studies, 164–170
clinical features of, 161–162
definition of, 161
differential diagnoses of, 163
inheritance and genetics of, 161
management, 162–163
algorithm for, 164
prostaglandin (PG) analogs, 162
target IOP, 162
optic nerve head in patient with, 163
optic nerve heads (ONHs), 162–163
pathophysiology of, 161
prognosis, 164

K

Kinetic perimetry
history of, 39
procedure, 39–41

L

Large temporal iridodialysis, 217
Laser iridotomy, 256
Laser procedures in glaucoma
argon laser trabeculoplasty (ALT)
complications, 263
for primary open-angle glaucoma, 132
history of, 261
indications for, 262
postlaser therapy, 262–263
procedure, 262
prognostic factors for, 263
SLT, 261–262
case studies, 265–268
cyclophotocoagulation, 264
diode laser cyclophotocoagulation (DLCP), 264–265
laser iridoplasty, 263–264
laser peripheral iridotomy (LPI)
indications for, 259–260
postlaser therapy, 261
procedure, 260
with argon laser, 259
Latanoprostene bunod, 0.024%, 252
Late bleb dysfunction, 309–313
Lens, 5
Lens-induce glaucoma, 201
case studies, 337–341
lens particle glaucoma, 334–335
pathophysiology of, 333
phacoanaphylactic glaucoma, 335
phacolytic glaucoma, 334
phacomorphic glaucoma, 333–334
phacotopic glaucoma, 335
Limbal nodules, 233
Low vision aids, 343–346
classification of, 343–344
general measures, 344–345
newer technologies, 344

M

Macula report, 81
Malignant glaucoma. *See* Aqueous misdirection/malignant glaucoma
Manipulative gonioscopy, 28–29
Mean deviation, 46
Mid-dilated pupil with sphincter tears, 217
Minimally invasive glaucoma surgeries (MIGSs), 328–331
approaches used in, 328
case studies, 331–332
goals of, 328
implants types, 329
subconjunctival implants, 330–331
suprachoroidal stents, 330
trabecular stents, 329–330
indications and contraindications for, 328
types of, 328, 329
Molteno implants, 319

N

Neovascular glaucoma (NVG)
case studies, 244–246
clinical features, 239–242
definition of, 239
gonioscopy in, 241
management, 242–243
pathogenesis, 239
prevention and prognosis, 243–244
Nerve fibre layers, in optic nerve and retina, 40
Neurodegeneration, 123–124
Neuroprotection, 253
Neuroretinal rim, 14, 81
Nicotinamide, 253
Noncontact tonometers, 9
Nonglaucomatous optic atrophy *vs.* glaucomatous, 20
Nonpenetrating glaucoma surgeries (NPGSs), 327–328
Nonvalved implants, 319
Normal tension glaucoma (NTG)
algorithm for evaluation of, 130
PG analogs for, 132
Normative data, for optical coherence tomography, 76

O

Octopus EyeSuite for progression analysis, 278–279
Octopus perimetry, 292
Octopus type perimeter printouts, 47
Ocular examination
anterior chamber, 3–4
anterior segment, 2–3
iris, 4–5
lens, 5
visual status, 2
Ocular hypertension, 105–106
primary angle closure (PAC) with, 117–118
Ocular ischemic syndrome, 241
Ocular response analyzer (ORA), 10
Ocular trauma, 215
Open globe injuries, 220–221
Optic cup, 13–14
Optic disc, 5–6
Optic nerve and retina, nerve fibre layers in, 40
Optic nerve head, 254
abnormalities, suspicion on basis of, 107

analysis, 81, 85
Optic nerve head examination, 5–6, 92
clinical role of, 12
cup:disc ratio, 14–15
disc hemorrhages, 15–16
in glaucomatous neuropathy, 13
neuroretinal rim, 14
normal optic nerve head, 12–13
optic cup, 13–14
optic nerve head size and shape, 13
peripapillary atrophy, 16–17
physiological cupping, 18
retinal nerve fiber layer defects, 17–18
vascular signs, 16
Optic nerve heads (ONHs), 162–163
Optical coherence tomography, 256. *See also* Retinal nerve fiber layer optical coherence tomography report
case studies, 86–90
combined structural and functional assessment with, 288
event analysis, 280, 281
factors leading to misinterpretation in, 86
fallacies of, 75
guided progression analysis on, 280–282
importance in glaucoma, 75
inter-eye asymmetry measure, 278
macula report, 81
normative data for, 76
optic nerve head analysis, 81, 85
parameters for glaucoma diagnosis, 76, 278, 291
macular ganglion cell complex, 79, 280
optic nerve head analysis, 79, 280
retinal nerve fiber layer thickness, 77–79, 279
principle of, 75–76
printout reading, 77
progression diagnosis, 280
rate of progression, 293
spectral domain, 76
Spectralis tracking laser tomography analysis, 283
swept source, 76
trend analysis, 280, 281
Oral carbonic anhydrase inhibitors, 250

P

Pachymetry, 129
Palpebral large papillae, 233
Patient-related artifacts, 86
Pattern deviation, 46
Pattern standard deviation (PSD), 46
Perimeter printouts, 47
Perimetric artifacts, 50
Perimetry, 269, 272–278
case studies, 58–62
definition of, 39
event-based analysis, 272–273, 276
frequency for diagnosing progression, 274
kinetic, 39–41
history of, 39
procedure, 39–41
pointwise linear regression, 273
primary open-angle glaucoma (POAG), 127
static, 41–50
algorithms, 41, 42
arcuate scotoma, nonglaucomatous causes of, 50–57
glaucoma hemifield test (GHT), 46
glaucomatous scotoma diagnosis, 47–49
mean deviation, 46
patient parameters, 41–42
pattern deviation, 46
pattern standard deviation (PSD), 46
perimeter printouts, 47
perimetric artifacts, 50
reliability parameters, 46
strategies, 41, 42
test parameters, 42–45
total deviation, 46
visual field index (VFI), 46–47
visual field loss patterns, 49
trend-based analysis, 273
Peripapillary atrophy, 16–17
Peters anomaly, 178–179
Phacoanaphylactic glaucoma, 335
Phacolytic glaucoma, 334
Phacomorphic glaucoma, 333–334
Phacotopic glaucoma, 335
Physiological cupping, 18
Pigment dispersion syndrome, 31
Pigment dispersion syndrome and pigmentary glaucoma, 194–195
Pilocarpine, 250
Plateau iris, 33
Plateau iris syndrome, 118
Postkeratoplasty therapy, 230
Primary angle closure (PAC), 32, 116–118
Primary angle-closure disease
exaggerated lens vault, 118
plateau iris syndrome, 118
primary angle closure (PAC), 116–117
with ocular hypertension, 117–118
primary angle-closure suspect, 116
secondary angle closure, 118
Primary angle-closure disease (PACD)
case studies, 154–159
classification of, 141–142
clinical features of
primary acute angle-closure glaucoma, 150–151
primary angle closure, 145–149
primary angle closure with hypertension, 149–150
primary angle-closure glaucoma, 151–153
clinical staging, 141
pathophysiology of
anatomic predisposition, 142–143
genetics, 143
iridotrabecular contact extent, 142
physiological factors, 143
relative pupillary block hypothesis, 143
prevalence of, 141
provocative tests for, 143, 145
Primary angle-closure suspect, 116
Primary congenital glaucoma (PCG), 33, 174–177
Primary glaucomas, 173
Primary open-angle glaucoma (POAG), 271
case studies, 134–139
cataract/filtering surgery in, 335–336
clinical features, 125–127
follow-up, 133
investigations
gonioscopy, 127
pachymetry, 129
perimetry and imaging, 127
management, 129
laser trabeculoplasty, 132
medical, 131–132
pattern deviation plots, 131
surgery, 132–133
target IOP range setting, 130–131
normal tension glaucoma in, 129
pathophysiology of
cerebral spinal fluid hydrodynamics, 124
genetics, 124
neurodegeneration, 123–124
pressure dependent or mechanical factors, 123
raised intraocular pressure, 124
vascular perfusion factors, 123
predisposing and risk factors for developing, 125
prognosis for, 134
randomized control trials in, 133
rates of change in, 269
risk factors for progression reported in, 131
Prostaglandin (PG) analogs, 250
Pseudoexfoliation syndrome, 31
clinical features, 192
management, 193
ocular examination, 192–193
pathogenesis, 192
Pseudophakic glaucoma
after anterior chamber intraocular lens, 202

after congenital cataract surgery, 204
clinical features of, 202–203
complications, 204
definition of, 201
etiology of, 201–202
factors contributing to, 202
intraocular lens in sulcus, 203
management, 203–204
prevalence of, 201
prognosis, 204
vitreous in wound, 203
with chronic uveitis after posterior capsular rupture, 203
Pupillary block, 308
Pupillary reaction, 4

R

Rebound tonometer, 9
Red green disease, 86
Relative pupillary block hypothesis, 143
Reliability parameters, 46
Retina examination, 5–6
Retinal dialysis, 217
Retinal nerve fiber layer, 254
analysis, 82
defects, 17–18, 290
Retinal nerve fiber layer optical coherence tomography report
key parameters table, 81
neuroretinal rim thickness plots, 81
patient information/details, 79–80
quality scores/signal strength, 80
retinal nerve fiber layer circular tomogram, 81
retinal nerve fiber layer deviation map, 81
retinal nerve fiber layer quadrant and clock-hour maps, 81
retinal nerve fiber layer thickness map, 80–81
retinal nerve fiber layer thickness plots, 81
vertical and horizontal tomograms, 81
Retinal sensitivity to recorded values, relationship of, 40
Rho-associated protein kinase inhibitors, 250

S

Schiotz indentation tonometers, 9
Sclera, 2
Secondary angle closure, 118, 191–192
Secondary glaucomas, 173, 182
aqueous misdirection/malignant glaucoma, 204
clinical features, 205
management of
algorithm for, 206
pathophysiology, 205
ultrasound biomicroscopy of, 206
case studies, 195–198, 209–213
closed-angle, 191
definition of, 191, 201
open-angle, 191
pigment dispersion syndrome and pigmentary glaucoma, 194–195
pseudoexfoliation syndrome with glaucoma
clinical features, 192
management, 193
ocular examination, 192–193
pathogenesis, 192
pseudophakic or aphakic glaucoma
clinical features of, 202–203
complications, 204
definition of, 201
etiology of, 201–202
factors contributing to, 202
management, 203–204
prevalence of, 201
prognosis, 204
uveitic glaucoma
clinical features of, 207–208
management, 208–209
pathophysiology of, 207
prognosis, 209
Secondary open and angle closure, 34
Segmentation errors, 86
Selective laser trabeculoplasty (SLT), 261
Shallow anterior chamber, 304–307
Single field reading
algorithm, 42
glaucoma hemifield test (GHT), 46
illustrating, 50, 52–57
mean deviation, 46
patient parameters, 41–42
pattern deviation, 46
pattern standard deviation (PSD), 46
reliability parameters, 46
test parameters, 42–45
total deviation, 46
visual field index (VFI), 46–47
Spectralis macula thickness map change report, 286
Spectralis optical coherence tomography printout, 83
Spectralis tracking laser tomography analysis, 283
Static perimetry, 41–50
algorithms, 41, 42
arcuate scotoma, nonglaucomatous causes of, 50–57
glaucomatous scotoma diagnosis, 47–49
perimeter printouts, 47
perimetric artifacts, 50
single field reading
glaucoma hemifield test (GHT), 46
mean deviation, 46
patient parameters, 41–42
pattern deviation, 46
pattern standard deviation (PSD), 46
reliability parameters, 46
test parameters, 42–45
total deviation, 46
visual field index (VFI), 46–47
strategies, 41, 42
visual field loss patterns, 49
Steroid-induced glaucoma
case studies, 233–238
clinical features, 229–231
definition of, 227
management, 231
discontinuation of steroid, 231
guidelines, 232
nonsteroidal anti-inflammatory drops, 231
treatment algorithm for, 232
pathophysiology, 229
prognosis, 233
risk factors for, 227–228
route, duration, and doses related to, 228–229
steroid potency, 228
Steroid-induced ocular hypertension, 227
Steroids
anti-inflammatory effect of, 228
effect on trabecular outflow channel, 230
Sturge-Weber syndrome, 180–182
Subconjunctival implants, 330–331
Suprachoroidal hemorrhages, 308
Suprachoroidal stents, 330
Swedish interactive threshold algorithm (SITA), 41
Systematic examination, 1–2

T

Target intraocular pressure
absolute or threshold, clinical recommendations of, 97–99
case studies, 101–104
definition of, 91
factors determining
baseline IOP, 92
clinical staging of glaucomatous damage, 92–96
limitations of setting, 99
methods of determining
formula-based values, 97
percentage reduction in IOP, 96–97
threshold/absolute cutoff value, 96
over time, reassessing, 99–101
range setting for primary open-angle glaucoma, 130–131
range, setting and achieving, 97
Tendency oriented perimetry (TOP), 41
Test parameters, 42–45
Text to speech systems, 344

Tonometers, comparison of, 7
Tonometry, 7–10
applanation, 7–9
digital palpation, 7
dynamic contour/Pascal tonometer, 10
noncontact tonometers, 9
ocular response analyzer (ORA), 10
rebound tonometer, 9
Schiotz indentation tonometers for, 9
tonopen, 9
Tonopen, 9
Topical carbonic anhydrase inhibitors, 250
Total deviation, 46
Trabecular meshwork
in late traumatic glaucoma, 220
recession and moderate pigmentation of, 256
tears in, 217
Trabecular stents, 329–330
Trabeculectomy, 295, 336
bleb, 204
case studies, 314–318
concept, 296
early postoperative complications, 304–309
aqueous misdirection syndrome, 308–309
choroidal effusions, 307
pupillary block, 308
shallow anterior chamber, 304–307
suprachoroidal hemorrhages, 308
in eye with uveitic glaucoma, 209
indications for, 296–297
late complications, 309–314
blebitis, 312
chronic hypotony, 313
failure of surgery, 309
late bleb dysfunction, 309–313
modifications, 300–303
postoperative care, 303–304
preoperative measures for, 297
surgical procedure, 297–300
with MMC, 184
Trabeculotomy, 183
Traumatic glaucoma
case studies, 222–225
chemical injuries, 221
closed globe injury
biomarkers for, 218
causing equatorial expansion, 216
clinical features of, 215–219
consequences of, 216
ghost cell glaucoma, 220
management, 219–220
definition of, 215
etiology of, 215
open globe injuries, 220–221
Traumatic layered hyphema, 217
Trend-based analysis, 270

U

Ultrasound biomicroscopy (UBM), 219
Uniocular handheld telescope, 344
Uveitic glaucoma
clinical features of, 207–208
management, 208–209
pathophysiology of, 207
prognosis, 209
Uveitis, extensive midperipheral anterior synechiae after, 208
Uveitis-glaucoma-hyphema (UGH) syndrome, 203

V

Valved implants, 320
Vascular perfusion factors, 123
Vascular signs, 16
Vernal keratoconjunctivitis, 230
Viscosurgical device, 202
Visual field
definition of, 39
perimetry for measuring. *See* Perimetry
Visual field (VF) loss, 91
Anderson's criteria for diagnosing, 65–66
importance of classifying, 65
patterns, 49
Visual field index (VFI), 46–47
Visual impairment in glaucoma, 343
Visual status, 2

X

Xen gel implant, 330–331

Z

Zonular dialysis, 217